This book is due for return not later than the last
date stamped below, unless recalled sooner.

THE ANTIMICROBIAL AGENTS
ANNUAL/3

THE ANTIMICROBIAL AGENTS ANNUAL

EDITORIAL BOARD

THE ANTIMICROBIAL AGENTS ANNUAL/3

Editors

PHILLIP K. PETERSON
Department of Medicine, Hennepin County Medical Center,
Minneapolis, MN, U.S.A.

JAN VERHOEF
Department of Clinical Microbiology, University Hospital,
Utrecht, The Netherlands

ELSEVIER
Amsterdam – New York – Oxford

ISBN 0 444 90494 8

ISSN 0168-938 X

Published by
Elsevier Science Publishers B.V. (Biomedical Division)
P.O. Box 211
1000 AE Amsterdam
The Netherlands

Sole distributor for the USA and Canada
Elsevier Science Publishing Co. Inc.
52 Vanderbilt Avenue
New York, NY 10017
USA

Printed in the Netherlands

CONTRIBUTORS

A.M. ANGELES
Section of Infectious Diseases, Boston University Medical Center, The Evans Memorial Department of Clinical Research, The University Hospital of the Boston University Medical Center, 88 East Newton Street, Boston, MA 02118, U.S.A.

R.W. AUCKENTHALER
Division des Maladies Infectieuses, Hôpital Cantonal Universitaire, 1211 Genève 4, Switzerland

J.S. BAKKEN
Department of Medical Microbiology, Creighton University, 2500 California Street, Omaha, NE 68178, U.S.A.

H.H. BALFOUR Jr
Clinical Microbiology Laboratory, University of Minnesota Hospitals, Box 437, Mayo Memorial Building, 420 Delaware Street, S.E., Minneapolis, MN 55455, U.S.A.

J.G. BARTLETT
Division of Infectious Diseases, Department of Medicine, Johns Hopkins Hospital, Blalock 111, 600 North Wolfe Street, Baltimore, MD 21205, U.S.A.

T. BERGAN
Department of Microbiology, Institute of Pharmacy, University of Oslo, P.O. Box 1108, Blindern, 0317 Oslo 3, Norway

J.R.A. BRANDT
Institute of Tropical Medicine, 155 Nationalestraat, 2000 Antwerp, Belgium

C.C. CAMPBELL
Malaria Branch, Division of Parasitic Diseases, Center for Infectious Diseases, Centers for Disease Control, Public Health Service, US Department of Health and Human Services, Atlanta, GA 30333, U.S.A.

C. CARBON
Hôpitaux de Paris, C.H.U. Bichat, 46 Rue Henri Ruchard, 75877 Paris Cédex, France

Contributors

E. COLLATZ
Laboratoire de Microbiologie Médicale, Université Pierre et Marie Curie, Rue de l'Ecole de Médecine, 75270 Paris Cédex 06, France

K.B. CROSSLEY
Infectious Diseases Section, Department of Internal Medicine, St. Paul-Ramsey Medical Center, St. Paul, MN 55101, U.S.A.

P. DEMEDTS
Institute of Tropical Medicine, 155 Nationalestraat, 2000 Antwerp, Belgium

R. DOLIN
Infectious Disease Unit, University of Rochester School of Medicine and Dentistry, 601 Elmwood Avenue, Rochester, NY 14642, U.S.A.

H.L. DUPONT
The University of Texas, Health Sciences Center, 1728 Freeman Building, 6431 Fannin, Houston, TX 77030, U.S.A.

G.M. ELIOPOULOS
Department of Medicine, New England Deaconess Hospital, 185 Pilgrim Road, Boston, MA 02215, U.S.A.

C.D. ERICSSON
Program in Infectious Diseases and Clinical Microbiology, University of Texas Medical School at Houston, P.O. Box 20708, JFB 1.722, Houston, TX 77225, U.S.A.

L. EYCKMANS
Institute of Tropical Medicine, 155 Nationalestraat, 2000 Antwerp, Belgium

G.J. GALASSO
Department of Health & Human Services, National Institutes of Health, Public Health Service, Shannon Building, Room 111, Bethesda, MD 20892, U.S.A.

J.N. GALGIANI
Section of Infectious Diseases (III), Veterans Administration Medical Center, The University of Arizona, Health Sciences Center, Tucson, AZ 85724, U.S.A.

P.R.J. GANGADHARAM
Division of Mycobacterial Diseases, Department of Medicine, National Jewish Center for Immunology and Respiratory Medicine, 1400 Jackson Street, Denver, CO 80206, U.S.A.

S. GEERTS
Institute of Tropical Medicine, 155 Nationalestraat, 2000 Antwerp, Belgium

N.H. GEORGOPAPADAKOU
Department of Chemotherapy, Hoffmann-La Roche Inc., Nutley, NJ 07110, U.S.A.

D.N. GERDING
Department of Medicine, Infectious Diseases Section, Veterans Administration Medical Center, 54th Street and 48th Avenue, Minneapolis, MN 55417, U.S.A.

P.L. GIGASE
Institute of Tropical Medicine, 155 Nationalestraat, 2000 Antwerp, Belgium

I.M. GOULD
Regional Microbiology Laboratory, City Hospital, Grampian Health Board, Aberdeen AB9 8AU, Scotland, U.K.

B.M. GREENE
Division of Geographic Medicine, Department of Medicine, Case Western Reserve University, University Hospitals of Cleveland, Cleveland, OH 44106, U.S.A.

D. GREENWOOD
Department of Microbiology, University Hospital, Queen's Medical Centre, Nottingham NG7 2UH, U.K.

C.B. HALL
Department of Pediatrics, University of Rochester Medical Center, 601 Elmwood Avenue, Rochester, NY 14642, U.S.A.

K.L. HARTSHORN
Department of Medicine, Infectious Disease Unit, Massachusetts General Hospital and Harvard Medical School, Fruit Street, Boston, MA 02114, U.S.A.

P.E. HERMANS
Division of Infectious Diseases, Mayo Clinic and Mayo Medical School, Rochester, MN 55905, U.S.A.

M.S. HIRSCH
Department of Medicine, Infectious Disease Unit, Massachusetts General Hospital and Harvard Medical School, Fruit Street, Boston, MA 02114, U.S.A.

I.M. HOEPELMAN
Department of Internal Medicine, Clinical Microbiology & Laboratory of Infectious Diseases, and U-Gene Research, University Hospital, Catharijnesingel 101, 3511 GV Utrecht, The Netherlands

W.T. HUGHES
Division of Infectious Diseases, St. Jude Children's Research Hospital, 332 North Lauderdale, Memphis, TN 38101, U.S.A.

G. HUMBERT
Infectious Diseases Department, Hôpital Charles Nicolle, 1 Rue de Gérmont, 76038 Rouen Cédex, France

R.R. JACOBSON
Clinical Branch, Public Health Service, Gillis W. Long Hansen's Disease Center, Carville, LA 70721, U.S.A.

J.E. KAPUSNIK
Division of Clinical Pharmacy, School of Pharmacy, Room C-152, University of California, San Francisco, CA 94143-0622, U.S.A.

D.A. KATZENSTEIN
Division of Virology, Office of Biologics Research and Review, Center of Drugs and Biologics, 8800 Rockville Pike, Bethesda, MD 20892, U.S.A.

C.A. KAUFFMAN
Division of Infectious Diseases, University of Michigan, Veterans Administration Center, 2215 Fuller Road, Ann Arbor, MI 48105, U.S.A.

V. KUMAR
Institute of Tropical Medicine, 155 Nationalestraat, 2000 Antwerp, Belgium

B. LEV
Unit of Infectious Diseases, Chaim Sheba Medical Center, Affiliated to the Tel-Aviv University, Sackler School of Medicine, Tel-Hashomer 52621, Israel

J.M. LOOS
Microbiology-Immunology, Baylor College of Medicine, Infectious Diseases Hospital, The Methodist Hospital, 6565 Fannin, M.S. 910, Houston, TX 77030, U.S.A.

B.J. LUFT
  Division of Infectious Diseases, Department of Medicine, Health Sciences
  Center, T-15, 080, State University of New York at Stony Brook, Stony Brook,
  NY 11794-8153, U.S.A.

J. MILLS
  Division of Infectious Diseases, Department of Medicine, The Medical Service,
  Room 5H22, San Francisco General Hospital, 1001 Potrero Avenue, San
  Francisco, CA 94110, U.S.A.

P. NGUYEN-DINH
  Malaria Branch, Division of Parasitic Diseases, Center for Infectious Diseases,
  Centers for Disease Control, Public Health Service, US Department of Health
  and Human Services, Atlanta, GA 30333, U.S.A.

R.L. NICHOLS
  Tulane University School of Medicine, Department of Surgery, 1430 Tulane
  Avenue, New Orleans, LA 70112, U.S.A.

S.R. NORRBY
  Department of Infectious Diseases, Umeå University Hospital, 901 85 Umeå,
  Sweden

G.B.A. OKELO
  Department of Medicine, University of Nairobi, P.O. Box 30588, Nairobi,
  Kenya

P. PIOT
  Department of Microbiology, Institute of Tropical Medicine, 155 Nationalestraat, 2000 Antwerp, Belgium

P.A. PIZZO
  Pediatric Branch, Clinical Oncology Program, Division of Cancer Treatment,
  National Cancer Institute, National Institutes of Health, Bethesda, MD 20892,
  U.S.A.

S.L. REED
  Division of Infectious Diseases, H-811F, UCSD Medical Center, University of
  California, 225 Dickinson Street, San Diego, CA 92103-9981, U.S.A.

J.S. REMINGTON
  Department of Immunology and Infectious Diseases, Research Institute, Palo
  Alto Medical Foundation, 860 Bryant Street, Palo Alto, CA 94301, U.S.A.

Contributors

M. RUBIN
Pediatric Branch, Clinical Oncology Program, Division of Cancer Treatment, National Cancer Institute, National Institutes of Health, Bethesda, MD 20892, U.S.A.

E. RUBINSTEIN
Unit of Infectious Diseases, Chaim Sheba Medical Center, Affiliated to the Tel-Aviv University, Sackler School of Medicine, Tel-Hashomer, 52621, Israel

M.A. SANDE
Department of Medicine, The Medical Service, Room 5H22, San Francisco General Hospital, 1001 Potrero Avenue, San Francisco, CA 94110, U.S.A.

C.C. SANDERS
Department of Medical Microbiology, Creighton University, 2500 California Street, Omaha, NE 68178, U.S.A.

W.E. SANDERS Jr
Department of Medical Microbiology, Creighton University, 2500 California Street, Omaha, NE 68178, U.S.A.

A.M. SUGAR
Section of Infectious Diseases, Boston University Medical Center, The Evans Memorial Department of Clinical Research, The University Hospital of the Boston University Medical Center, 88 East Newton Street, Boston, MA 02118, U.S.A.

H. TAELMAN
Clinical Department, Institute of Tropical Medicine, 155 Nationalestraat, 2000 Antwerp, Belgium

R.W. TOFTE
Section of Infectious Diseases, Park Nicollet Medical Center, Minneapolis, MN 55416, U.S.A.

G. VAN DER GROEN
Department of Microbiology, Institute of Tropical Medicine, 155 Nationale-straat, 2000 Antwerp, Belgium

K.L. VOSTI
Department of Medicine, Division of Infectious Diseases, Stanford University School of Medicine, Stanford, CA 94305, U.S.A.

E.E. WACK
   Section of Infectious Diseases (III), Veterans Administration Medical Center, The University of Arizona, Health Sciences Center, Tucson, AZ 85724, U.S.A.

F.A. WALDVOGEL
   Clinique Médicale Thérapeutique, Hôpital Cantonal Universitaire, 1211 Geneva 4, Switzerland

M. WÉRY
   Institute of Tropical Medicine, 155 Nationalestraat, 2000 Antwerp, Belgium

J.D. WILLIAMS
   Department of Medical Microbiology, The London Hospital Medical College, Turner Street, London, E1 2AD, U.K.

D.N. WILLIAMS
   Internal Medicine Department, Section of Infectious Diseases, Park Nicolett Medical Center, 5000 West 39th Street, Minneapolis, MN 55416, U.S.A.

T.W. WILLIAMS Jr
   Microbiology-Immunology, Baylor College of Medicine, Infectious Diseases Hospital, The Methodist Hospital, 6565 Fannin, M.S. 910, Houston, TX 77030, U.S.A.

R. WISE
   Department of Medical Microbiology, Dudley Road Hospital, Dudley Road, Birmingham, B18 7QH, U.K.

A. ZWAHLEN
   Hôpital de Zone à St-Loup, 1349 Pompaples, Switzerland

INTRODUCTION

Within a year after the publication of the *Antimicrobial Agents Annual 1, Annual 2* was published. Many physicians, pharmacologists, pharmacists and microbiologists have expressed great interest in this annual series and have found the first two volumes both stimulating and useful. The enthusiasm with which *Annuals 1 and 2* were received illustrates the great need for concise summaries and critical commentaries of the most recent literature in the field of antimicrobial treatment. We have therefore adhered in *Annual 3* to the same objectives and overall structure as those of the previous volumes. Again, we are very fortunate that so many outstanding contributors have been willing to continue their contribution to this series. They were requested to gather and synthesize the most recent information on antibiotics or antimicrobial treatment which is often diffusely spread over numerous journals. The authors have evaluated new reports and incorporated the most recent information in this book.

It stands to reason that developments in some groups of antimicrobial agents are more dynamic than others (e.g. cephalosporins and quinolones remain classes of agents about which knowledge is rapidly expanding). Data on these agents have therefore received major attention and are discussed in detail.

For some agents scarcely any new information had appeared since the publication of *Annual 2* (e.g. chloramphenicol, fusidanes, lincosamides, macrolides, nitrofurantoins). For the sake of completeness, however, we have included the relevant chapters more or less unchanged. The chapter on interferons has also been reprinted without major change.

We believe that the current topics chosen for *Annual 3* are both timely and of great potential interest to a wide audience. We are indeed grateful to the authors, all well-known authorities, who undertook such a difficult task.

We do hope that this Annual will also find its way to the infectious disease specialist, clinical microbiologist, pharmacist etc.

We again want to express our thanks to all the contributors to *Annual 3,* who have responded to the special demands of this type of publication, and to our colleagues of Elsevier Science Publishers, who have made timely publication a reality.

As Editors, we remain open to suggestions from our colleagues.

PHILLIP K. PETERSON
JAN VERHOEF

CONTENTS

Contents

ANTIFUNGAL AGENTS

ANTIPARASITIC AGENTS

xvi

Contents

CHAPTER 1

Aminoglycosides (aminocyclitols)

GUY HUMBERT, CLAUDE CARBON and EKKEHARD COLLATZ

Despite the development of many new antimicrobial compounds from other classes of antibiotics, the time-tested aminoglycosides will continue to play an important, although changing, role in the therapy of bacterial infections for some time to come.

The mechanisms by which resistance to these drugs occurs, the molecular bases of their toxicity, and the kinetics of their antibacterial effects are now better understood. It appears virtually impossible to develop a totally non-toxic yet microbiologically active new compound. Hence, efforts to reduce nephro- or ototoxicity, mainly by shortening treatment and reducing the number of daily injections, would appear to be clinically relevant.

ACTIVITY

Habekacin (1-N-HABA-dibekacin), one of the two aminoglycosides currently under clinical study (1), has been further evaluated with respect to its antimicrobial spectrum and its susceptibility to aminoglycoside-modifying enzymes (2–5). A feature which tends to distinguish this drug from most of the aminoglycosides currently in clinical use is its relatively low susceptibility to enzymic modification. Habekacin was found to be stable against aminoglycoside-modifying enzymes, except for AAC(2′) and AAC(6′)-IV (2). No cross-resistance to this drug was observed in gram-negative bacteria, such as Serratia marcescens and Pseudomonas aeruginosa, which were resistant to multiple aminoglycosides, including amikacin. However, it was not clear whether these strains were producers of an AAC(6′), the enzyme most frequently responsible for amikacin resistance in these species (6). In an extensive survey of the susceptibility of P. aeruginosa to aminoglycosides, habekacin was found to be slightly more active than amikacin, while there was no difference in the incidence of resistance to the two drugs (5). Habekacin was reported to have potent antibacterial activity against strains of Staphylococcus aureus and S. epidermidis, even against those highly resistant to gentamicin and amikacin (4).

Antimicrobial Agents Annual 3
P.K. Peterson and J. Verhoef, editors
© Elsevier Science Publishers BV, 1988

Mechanism of action

The molecular events underlying the bactericidal action of the aminoglycosides are still being unravelled. One model that has been proposed claims to accommodate what is known about aminoglycoside-ribosome interactions, aminoglycoside-induced membrane damage, and transmembrane accumulation of these drugs (7). Upon the demonstration of an altered distribution of newly synthesized periplasmic proteins in *Escherichia coli* cells treated with streptomycin, Davis and colleagues argued that misreading plays an indirect but essential role in the bactericidal action of aminoglycosides, in that misread proteins would create 'channels' across the inner membrane. These channels, of unknown nature, would permit increasing influx of drug (with ensuing increased misreading) until the intracellular concentration was sufficient to block initiating ribosomes, and consequently protein synthesis, irreversibly (7). Misreading, or rather altered misreading, was implicated in the change of susceptibility of *Haemophilus influenzae* to aminoglycosides. Studying clinical isolates resistant to 10–20 μg of 2-deoxystreptamine compounds per ml, but susceptible to streptomycin, Levy et al (8) ascribed resistance to a ribosomal alteration resulting in reduced misreading and associated reduced drug accumulation across the inner membrane.

The effect of astromicin (fortimicin A) on the cytoplasmic membrane of *S. marcescens* was studied by Umeda et al (9). From analysis of micrographs of thin-sectioned and freeze-fractured cells they concluded that astromicin caused the loss of membrane components, i.e. proteins and probably also phospholipids. It also caused the formation of fragile spheroplasts. The inhibition by several 2-deoxy-streptamine aminoglycosides of the initiation of DNA replication was described by Matsunaga et al (10) in a temperature-sensitive mutant of *E. coli*. This inhibition was considered to be a consequence of cytoplasmic membrane damage and subsequent interruption of DNA-membrane attachment which was assumed to be required for the initiation of chromosome replication. While the antibiotics used (habekacin, dibekacin, gentamicin) did not interfere with DNA elongation, such an effect of a kanamycin derivative, 1-*N*-eicosanoyl-3″-*N*-(trifluoroacetyl)kanamycin, was observed when SV40 DNA replication was studied in vitro, but the inhibition effect was ascribed to the substituents rather than the kanamycin moiety (11).

The mechanisms of synergism between aminoglycosides and β-lactam antibiotics has been reviewed, particularly with enterococci (12). Alteration of the enterococcal cell envelope through β-lactam action, entailing enhanced intracellular uptake of aminoglycosides, was presented as the key event leading to synergism. The possibility of a concomitant effect of aminoglycosides on penicillin-binding proteins (13) was not considered. Streptococci of the viridans group were recently found to respond differently to aminoglycoside + β-lactam combinations and no stimulation of streptomycin uptake by penicillin was observed (14).

Predictions of the absence of synergism or the presence of antagonism cannot be made with precision (15–17). There is also no strict correlation between synthesis of aminoglycoside-modifying enzymes and absence of synergy in gram-negative bacilli. Synergy between amikacin and cefotaxime was observed in several species of Enterobacteriaceae synthesizing an AAC(6')-4 (18).

Resistance mechanisms

Molecular cloning of aminoglycoside resistance genes and the preparation of DNA probes representative of these genes (19) have made it possible to study the distribution of these genes within bacterial populations and, in one instance, the movement of a resistance gene from gram-positive to gram-negative bacteria (20). On the other hand, efforts are still being made to develop assays for the identification of aminoglycoside-modifying enzymes (21). These may be helpful as long as probes for particular genes are not available.

Genes for which DNA probes (which were not strictly intragenic in all cases) have been prepared include those coding for APH(3')-I and APH(3')-II (22), APH(3')-III (23–25), AAD(2″) (26, 27), AAD(4') (25), AAC(3')-IV (28), and AAC(6')-APH(2″) (24, 25). Next to allowing the identification of the genes in question, some of the probes have also been useful in providing indications as to whether these genes were chromosome- or plasmid-borne (24, 25). The apparently chromosomal APH(3')-III and AAC(6')-APH(2″) genes from several clinical isolates of *S. aureus* were found to be transferable, to *S. aureus* and *S. epidermidis*, by a conjugative process (29) somewhat reminiscent of a mode of a transposon-mediated aminoglycoside resistance transfer which has been investigated in depth in streptococci (30–33). First identified in a high-level kanamycin-resistant strain of *Streptococcus pneumoniae*, the transposable element Tn*1545* carries, in addition to an APH(3')-III gene, the determinants of resistance to macrolides and tetracycline. It was found to transfer into several enterococcal species, as well as into *S. aureus* and *Listeria monocytogenes*, and to transpose into their chromosomes (30). The element also transposed to the chromosome of *E. coli* and *Bacillus subtilis* and was able to transform the latter (31). The authors speculate that the properties of this conjugative transposon could explain the sudden emergence and dissemination of multiple resistance to antibiotics within pneumococci. The further observation that an APH(3')-III gene, found in *Campylobacter coli* (23), was identical to that carried by Tn*1545* (33) led the authors to extend their speculation and suggest that resistance gene transfer to extremely distantly related organisms may occur via transformation and subsequent transposition involving Tn*1545*-like elements (or else recombination); they implicated an ancillary role of selective pressure in the occurrence of such a rare event of resistance gene transfer (20). Incidentally, an APH(3')-III gene was also detected in a strain of *C. coli* isolated from an animal (34) and it was found to be structurally related to the APH of Tn*1545* (B. Papadopoulos, unpublished observation). (The APH(3') nomenclature used here, at variance with that used in Refs 25 and 34, is as described in Ref. 20.)

The effect of antibiotic usage, or selective pressure, on the incidence and dissemination of bacterial resistance has been the subject of several studies and reviews, especially with respect to the use of amikacin (18, 35–40).

In the 10 years of amikacin use, resistance to this drug has not increased markedly and there seems to be fair agreement among most authors that the exclusive, or almost exclusive, use of amikacin within a given institution does not markedly favor the selection of amikacin-resistant bacteria. Some authors maintain that even in instances where an increase in amikacin consumption appeared to be paralleled by an increase in the isolation of resistant organisms, antibiotics other than amikacin may have been the effective selectors (35, 36). Also, a tendency was observed towards a decrease in resistance to gentamicin and tobramycin, but to various degrees in different species (37–39).

While fluctuations in the incidence of amikacin resistance during (quasi)exclusive amikacin usage are slight, they can go in either direction. For example, under such a policy, resistance to amikacin by *Pseudomonas aeruginosa* may increase moderately (38) or decrease marginally (39) or markedly (40).

However rare, amikacin resistance may increase to a remarkable extent in certain niches, be it through spread of a resistant strain or through dissemination of a resistance plasmid among different bacterial genera. Over 50% of the *P. aeruginosa* strains isolated in a Greek hospital were resistant to multiple antibiotics, including amikacin, and at least 60% of these produced an AAC(6′) enzyme (41). Approximately 25% of the coagulase-negative staphylococci, but no *S. aureus*, isolated in several units of two Canadian hospitals became amikacin-resistant, with no concomitant decrease in resistance to tobramycin and gentamicin. Probably two stably linked aminoglycoside resistance determinants had been selected (41).

The rapid dissemination of closely related aminoglycoside resistance plasmids among several genera belonging to the family Enterobacteriaceae has been observed in a hospital in Chile (42). The resistance gene, coding for AAC(6′)-4, was found to be expressed under the control of the regulatory elements of a TEM-I-type β-lactamase gene, carried by the ubiquitous transposable element Tn3, to which it was fused. The acetyltransferase gene was located, in a polycistronic arrangement, next to an AAD(3″)(9) gene (43). A gene organization of this kind could explain how efficient co-selection of related and unrelated resistance determinants may occur. It would also make it very likely that combination therapy with a TEM-I-susceptible β-lactam would have enhanced the selection of amikacin resistance, while combination with cefotaxime, for example, might not (18).

CLINICAL PHARMACOLOGY

In a cross-over study in human volunteers receiving a single dose of gentamicin, no significant effect of circadian cycle on antibiotic pharmacokinetics was observed after two periods of fasting (45). In contrast, dietary protein loading resulted in a significant decrease in the elimination half-life and in an increase in total body clearance compared with fasting subjects. These results suggest that a controlled diet is required when pharmacokinetic studies are performed in volunteers. Thus, variations in protein intake could partly explain interindividual variations in aminoglycoside kinetics observed in patients. Bergeron and Marois (46) showed that short-term (3 days) therapy with gentamicin combined with an antibiotic which accumulates in different parts of the kidney results in synergy. However, it should be stressed that these results could also be explained by the kinetics of antimicrobial action (time-dependent killing and lack of post-antibiotic effect of β-lactam antibiotics and conversely dose-dependent effect and pronounced post-antibiotic effect of aminoglycoside) rather than by the action of the drug in different parts of the renal parenchyma.

Moore et al (47) have examined the relationship between plasma aminoglycoside levels, minimum inhibitory concentration (MIC) for the infecting organism and therapeutic outcome in 236 patients who participated in 4 clinical trials of 3 different aminoglycosides. They found a strong association between clinical response and maximal or mean peak antibiotic levels/MIC ratios.

Hendeles and Neims (48) demonstrated that routine peak and trough measurements of aminoglycosides in serum are unnecessary in patients between 3 months and 18 years of age unless duration of therapy extends beyond 10 days, renal function is impaired or there is a clinical need for higher doses or shorter intervals, or a potential nephrotoxin has been administered in the previous 3 months.

ADVERSE EFFECTS

Nephrotoxicity

Experimental studies   Nephrotoxicity of aminoglycosides is in part related to the renal accumulation of the antibiotics. The method most often used to estimate accumulation of these drugs is homogenization of renal tissue with subsequent centrifugation and assay of the supernatant. However, this method could fail to detect tissue-bound aminoglycoside. Based upon the findings that aminoglycosides are stable in solutions with a pH ranging from 2 to 10 and are not destroyed by high temperatures, Gilbert and Kohlhepp (49) proposed a new sodium hydroxide digestion method for measurement of tobramycin concentrations in the rat kidney. Digestion with 1.0 N sodium hydroxide at 70°C for 15 minutes significantly increased the amount of assayable tobramycin. This method has now to be used to study the relationship between aminoglycoside accumulation in the kidney and the degree of renal failure. It would also seem interesting to use new models for the study of aminoglycoside nephrotoxicity, e.g. cells in culture. Schwertz et al (50) used a pig kidney epithelial cell line (LLC-PK$_1$) which has properties similar to those of renal proximal tubule cells. They demonstrated that manifestations of gentamicin toxicity parallel those reported in the whole animal, thus making the LLC-PK$_1$ cell in culture a valid system for elucidating the mechanism of aminoglycoside alterations in renal epithelium.

Bergeron and Bergeron investigated the influence of endotoxin on the intrarenal distribution of aminoglycosides. The endotoxin-injected rats accumulated significantly more aminoglycosides in their kidneys than normal animals (51). This finding was demonstrated using two different techniques: autoradiography of tobramycin uptake by the proximal and distal tubules (52) and microbiological assays in different parts of the kidney (53). The authors concluded that by increasing the total amount of drug within the kidney, endotoxin might increase the nephrotoxic potential of aminoglycosides.

It has been recently suggested that vancomycin when given concomitantly with aminoglycosides may increase the frequency of aminoglycoside nephrotoxicity. Wood et al (54) studied the influence of vancomycin on tobramycin nephrotoxicity in male Fischer rats. When compared with controls, animals receiving vancomycin alone exhibited no detectable renal toxicity when, at the dose used, tobramycin alone was toxic. When compared with tobramycin alone, the combination of vancomycin and tobramycin caused earlier and more severe toxicity. These experimental data confirm the clinical results of Farber and Moellering in 1983: in their retrospective study, the rate of nephrotoxicity for vancomycin alone was calculated to amount to less than 5%, rising to 35% when vancomycin was given together with aminoglycosides (55). However, the mechanism by which vancomycin enhances aminoglycoside nephrotoxicity is still not clear at present.

Clinical studies   Williams et al (56) analyzed data from 60 patients treated with amikacin. The variables most highly associated with nephrotoxicity were days of therapy and number of doses. Only 1 patient developed nephrotoxicity before the 6th day of amikacin therapy and the risk of nephrotoxicity increased after 9 or 10 days of treatment. In contrast with the findings of others, these authors did not find any correlation between peak or trough aminoglycoside serum concentrations and nephrotoxicity. Among numerous risk factors for nephrotoxicity analyzed in 338 patients, Sawyers et al (57) also found that duration of therapy was the factor most strongly associated with nephrotoxicity, followed in order by serum levels of aminoglycoside 1 hour after administration, total dose of aminoglycoside, and liver disease. The interaction of liver disease and aminoglycosides was recently reviewed by Moore et al (58). In 179 hospitalized patients who had been enrolled in a prospective randomized trial of nafcillin/tobramycin versus cefotaxime treatment, a clear interaction was demonstrated between tobramycin use and liver disease. The specific mechanism by which liver disease could increase the risk of renal dysfunction is unknown. One hypothesis was suggested: liver disease enhances renin release and stimulation of the renin-angiotensin system resulting in renal vasoconstriction. Usually, the kidney can compensate for this action with an increased production of prostaglandin E_2. Aminoglycosides inhibit prostaglandin production and thus favor renal vasoconstriction and a reduced renal cortical blood flow.

Ototoxicity

Some recent studies provide interesting information on the pathophysiology of the ototoxic potential of aminoglycosides. Study of the kinetics of entry of different drugs into inner ear tissues and fluids showed no correlation between the drug concentrations and their degree of toxicity. These results demonstrate that selective aminoglycoside ototoxicity cannot be explained by a preferential uptake of drugs in the afflicted tissue or in the perilymph (59). Data obtained from experiments with isolated crista ampullaris of the inner ear of the guinea-pig suggest that aminoglycosides and polyamines share common pathways of active transport and that the transport of gentamicin can be reduced in the presence of other aminoglycosides (60). A multistep model of aminoglycoside toxicity has been proposed by Schacht (61). The initial step is an electrostatic interaction between aminoglycosides and the plasma membrane. The resulting displacement of calcium accounts for acute effects, but the action is reversible and antagonized by divalent cations. An energy-dependent uptake process is required for the expression of toxicity. Subsequently the drug binds to phosphatidylinositol biphosphate inhibiting its hydrolysis and preventing its physiologic functions. This hydrolysis results in a signal cascade to mobilize intracellular calcium stores. Other functions regulated by polyphosphoinositides, such as synthesis of prostaglandins, are also potentially affected, as well as intracellular reactions which are controlled by calcium polyamines.

Lerner et al (62) reported a prospective comparative blinded trial of ototoxicity of amikacin and gentamicin. From this small study (70 patients evaluable for ototoxicity) it was concluded that the auditory and vestibular toxicity of both drugs was similar. In an univariate analysis a weak association was observed between ototoxicity and nephrotoxicity and also between ototoxicity and mean trough aminoglycoside serum levels. With regard to evaluation of toxicity through randomized trials of aminoglycosides, Evans et al (63) draw attention to the fact that, among 42 trials, the proportion of patients eligible for analysis was 19% regarding auditory toxicity. Twenty-nine per cent of the trials reported that evaluators were blinded to treatment group assignments. Auditory toxicity was an end-point in 23 trials. Only 1 study reported a significant difference in favor of netilmicin over tobramycin. Generally the trials are considerably smaller in sample size than is required for the detection of small to moderate differences in risk. Both qualitative overviews and pooled analyses of a quantitative overview may be useful in deciding whether to devote the effort and resources necessary to conduct large-sample trials.

CLINICAL USES

Despite the development of new or improved compounds from other classes of antibiotics (carbapenems, monobactams, 5-fluoroquinolones etc.), aminoglycosides continue to have a valuable role in the treatment of various infectious diseases, in particular those acquired in hospital. In January 1986, during a symposium held in Mexico, aminoglycoside uses were discussed. The conclusions of this meeting were published in a special issue of *American Journal of Medicine (Suppl. 6B)*. The main indications for aminoglycoside therapy and the principal infections treated were reviewed and discussed by Siegenthaler et al (64). Except for some urinary tract infections, aminoglycosides are mainly used in combinations and essentially with a β-lactam antibiotic because of their frequent synergistic interaction. This combination appears to be particularly beneficial and is widely accepted for the treatment of severe bacterial infections in immunocompromised patients. The recent development of newer more active and less toxic β-lactams has led some authors to advocate the use of β-lactam combinations in the empiric treatment of febrile neutropenic cancer patients. Nevertheless, the analysis of randomized controlled trials showed that the response rates obtained with a two β-lactam combination are similar and not superior to those obtained with a β-lactam + aminoglycoside combination (65). The former combination implies a non-negligible risk of antagonism or of β-lactamase induction. Thus, in this clinical setting, the combination of an aminoglycoside with a β-lactam active against *Pseudomonas* is probably still the best empiric therapy available (66). In 118 oncology patients, netilmicin or tobramycin in conjunction with piperacillin was equally effective, but ototoxicity was less severe and more often reversible with netilmicin (67). In fact, in immunocompromised hosts, amikacin is still the drug of choice: it is the most synergistic aminoglycoside and in large multicenter surveillance programs which were carried out over 5 years, its unrestricted use did not result in a significant increase in amikacin resistance rate (68, 69).

Ps. aeruginosa endocarditis is a life-threatening infection, antimicrobial therapy consisting of 6-weeks treatment with a semisynthetic penicillin, such as ticarcillin, combined with an aminoglycoside. The unusually high doses of aminoglycosides used in the treatment of this infection led to an assessment of the toxicity of tobramycin in 13 cases of pseudomonal endocarditis where patients underwent high-dose therapy (8 mg/kg/d) and in 13 cases of gram-negative infections where patients underwent conventional therapy (3 mg/kg/d). Although the sample studied was relatively small, the results suggest that patients receiving high-dose tobramycin do not appear to be at greater risk for developing nephrotoxicity than patients receiving conventional therapy. The risk of ototoxicity, especially in the high-frequency range, can be minimized by monitoring tobramycin serum concentrations to adjust to appropriate doses and serial audiograms (70).

Meier et al (71) also reported the successful treatment of a pancreatic abscess due to *Nocardia asteroides* with amikacin. This study and the previous results obtained in the treatment of disseminated nocardiosis confirm the therapeutic interest of this drug.

DOSING

Several experimental studies have been devoted recently to the efficacy of once-daily dosing of aminoglycosides. In a guinea-pig model of *Pseudomonas pneumoniae*, it was demonstrated that high peak concentrations with prolonged dosing intervals were more efficacious than lower levels maintained with intermittent therapy in normal animals. Conversely in neutropenic animals, once-daily dosing of aminoglycoside was not so effective because of significant regrowth occurring at the end of each 24-hour dosing interval. However, when intermittent mezlocillin therapy was added to the tobramycin regimens in this neutropenic model, single high daily doses of the aminoglycoside were as effective as the conventional intermittent tobramycin + mezlocillin combination therapy (72).

Aminoglycoside activity in vivo appeared to be affected by the interval between doses but not by the bacterial inoculum size of *Ps. aeruginosa* in a thigh infection model of the mouse. An inverse pattern was observed with ceftazidime and ticarcillin (73). In the same model, Vogelman et al (74) have shown that the post-antibiotic effects of tobramycin, as well as of imipenem and ciprofloxacin, allowed maximal cidal activity to be achieved without constantly maintaining drug levels above the MIC. These in vivo experiments argue for the use of large spaced doses of aminoglycosides.

Two studies performed in human volunteers described the lack of major side-effects of relatively high single daily doses of either 4.5 mg/kg netilmicin (75) or 5.1 mg/kg tobramycin (76) on renal or auditory functions. However, these studies cannot allow prediction of events which could occur in patients treated for more than 1 week with such high single daily doses of an aminoglycoside. Comparative clinical studies are warranted to establish the true benefits and the cost-effectiveness of such a therapeutic method.

An implantable drug pump has been developed for delivering aminoglycosides in human subjects. Various antibiotics including amikacin have been shown to maintain their stability in the pump. The use of this new delivery system has proved to be effective in eradicating experimentally induced osteomyelitis in animals. Preliminary results in man seem to confirm these experimental data (77). This technique offers the advantage of high local and low systemic levels of antibiotic, a low incidence of side-effects, and a decreased length of hospitalization. However, further clinical studies including a larger number of patients and with a long follow-up are warranted.

FUTURE DIRECTIONS

In 1986, no newer aminoglycoside derivative has been synthesized or identified. Only two studies referred to *O*-demethyl-fortimicin-A-sulfate (3-ODMF), a semisynthetic derivative of fortimicin A under investigation since 1980.

Sennello et al (78) investigated the pharmacokinetics of 3-ODMF in 16 healthy adult volunteers. Intramuscular or intravenous doses of 3-ODMF ranging from 0.25 to 16 mg/kg were administered. The half-life of the drug in plasma averaged 2.0 hours after intramuscular injection and 2.7 hours after intravenous infusion. Plasma drug clearance was dose- and route-independent. The mean 0-48 hour urinary recovery after intramuscular injection and intravenous infusion was 90 and 102%, respectively. The results indicated that, like other aminoglycosides, the drug is almost entirely cleared by renal mechanisms. Serieys et al (79) evaluated the efficacy of 3-ODMF given to 28 hospitalized patients with acute urinary tract infections at a dose of 2–5 mg/kg for 7-14 days. The treatment was successful in 53.5% of the patients; 35.5% relapsed due to severe underlying disease. In 10.7% of the patients, 3-ODMF was discontinued or given in reduced doses because of an increase in serum creatinine during therapy. The clinical and bacteriologic results were satisfactory but did not differ from those usually obtained with aminoglycosides in the treatment of gram-negative urinary tract infections.

Because of the failure to identify less toxic, yet active agents during the past 10 years, little can be expected in terms of new developments in aminoglycoside research. As concluded by Price, 'it seems safe to assume that the current armamentarium of aminoglycosides is all that will be available for use in the foreseeable future' (1).

REFERENCES

1. Price KD (1986) The potential for discovery and development of improved aminoglycosides. *Am. J. Med., 80(6B)*, 182.
2. Okamoto R, Iobe S (1986) Antibacterial activity of HBK. *Chemotherapy (Tokyo), 34, Suppl. 1*, 1.
3. Goto S, Ogawa M, Tsuji A et al (1986) Antibacterial activity of HBK, a new derivative of dibekacin. *Chemotherapy (Tokyo), 34, Suppl 1*, 11.
4. Oguri T, Hayashi Y (1986) Antibacterial activity of HBK against various clinical isolates. *Chemotherapy (Tokyo), 34, Suppl 1*, 41.
5. Thabaut A, Meyran M (1986) Etat actuel de la sensibilité de *Pseudomonas aeruginosa* aux aminosides en France. *Pathol. Biol., 34*, 621.
6. Shimizu K, Kumoda T, Hsieh WC et al (1985) Comparison of aminoglycoside resistance patterns in Japan, Formosa and Korea, Chile and the United States. *Antimicrob. Agents Chemother., 28*, 282.
7. Davis BD, Chen L, Tai PC (1986) Misread protein creates membrane channels: an essential step in the bactericidal action of aminoglycosides. *Proc. Natl Acad. Sci. USA, 83*, 6164.
8. Levy J, Burns JL, Mendelman PM et al (1986) Effect of tobramycin on protein synthesis in 2-deoxystreptamine aminoglycoside-resistant clinical isolates of *Haemophilus influenzae. Antimicrob. Agents Chemother. 29*, 474.
9. Umeda A, Murata K, Amako K (1986) Astromicin-induced membrane damage in *Serratia marcescens. Antimicrob. Agents Chemother., 30*, 398.
10. Matsunaga K, Yamaki H, Nishimura T, Tanaka N (1986) Inhibition of DNA replication initiation by aminoglycoside antibiotics. *Antimicrob. Agents Chemother., 30*, 468.

11. Yamaki H, Ariga H, Tanaka N (1986) Inhibition of SV40 DNA replication *in vitro* by 1-*N*-acyl-3″-*N*-(trifluoroacetyl) kanamycin. *Biochem. Biophys. Res. Commun., 136*, 322.

12. Moellering R, Eliopoulos GM, Allan JD (1986) Beta-lactam/aminoglycoside combinations: interactions and their mechanisms. *Am. J. Med., 80(5C)*, 30.

13. Gutmann L, Tomasz A (1981) Degradation of the penicillin binding proteins in aminoglycoside-treated group A streptococci. *FEMS Microbiol. Lett., 10*, 323.

14. Miller MH, El-Sokkary MA, Feinstein SA, Lowy FD (1986) Penicillin-induced effects on streptomycin uptake and early bactericidal activity differ in viridans group and enterococcal streptococci. *Antimicrob. Agents Chemother., 30*, 763.

15. Courvalin P, Carlier C, Collatz E (1980) Plasmid-mediated resistance to aminocyclitol antibiotics in group D streptococci. *J. Bacteriol., 143*, 541.

16. Thauvin C, Eliopoulos GM, Wernnersten C et al (1985) Antagonistic effect of penicillin-amikacin combinations against enterococci. *Antimicrob. Agents Chemother., 28*, 78.

17. Courvalin P, Carlier C (1981) Resistance to aminoglycoside-aminocyclitol antibiotics in bacteria. *J. Antimicrob. Chemother., 8, Suppl A*, 57.

18. Acar JF, Goldstein FW, Ménard R, Blériot JP (1986) Strategies in aminoglycoside use and impact on resistance. *Am. J. Med., 80(6B)*, 82.

19. Tenover F (1986) Studies of antimicrobial resistance genes using DNA probes. *Antimicrob. Agents Chemother., 29*, 721.

20. Trieu-Cuot P, Courvalin P (1986) Evolution and transfer of aminoglycoside resistance genes under natural conditions. *J. Antimicrob. Chemother., 18, Suppl C*, 93.

21. Lovering AM, White OL, Reeves DS (1986) Identification of individual aminoglycoside-inactivating enzymes in a mixture by HPLC determination of reaction products. *J. Antimicrob. Chemother., 18*, 139.

22. Young SA, Tenover FC, Gootz TD et al (1985) Development of two DNA probes for differentiating the structural genes of subclasses I and II of the aminoglycoside-modifying enzyme 3′-aminoglycoside phosphotransferase. *Antimicrob. Agents Chemother., 27*, 739.

23. Lambert T, Gerbaud G, Trieu-Cuot P, Courvalin P (1985) Structural relationship between the genes encoding 3′-aminoglycoside phosphotransferases in *Campylobacter* and Gram-positive cocci. *Ann. Inst. Pasteur (Paris), 136B*, 135.

24. El Solh N, Moreau N, Ehrlich SD (1986) Molecular cloning of *Staphylococcus aureus* chromosomal aminoglycoside resistance genes. *Plasmid, 15*, 104.

25. Dickgiesser N, Kreiswirth BN (1986) Determination of aminoglycoside resistance in *Staphylococcus aureus* by DNA hybridization. *Antimicrob. Agents Chemother., 29*, 930.

26. Tenover FC, Gootz TD, Gordon KP et al (1984) Development of a DNA probe for the structural gene of the 2″-*O*-adenyltransferase aminoglycoside-modifying enzyme. *J. Infect. Dis., 150*, 678.

27. Groot Obbink DJ, Ritchie LJ, Cameron FH et al (1985) Construction of a gentamicin resistance gene probe for epidemiological studies. *Antimicrob. Agents Chemother., 28*, 96.

28. Chaslus-Dancla E, Gerbaud G, Lafont JP et al (1986) Nucleic acid hybridization with a probe specific for 3-aminoglycoside acetyltransferase type IV: a survey of resistance to apramycin and gentamicin in animal strains of *Escherichia coli*. *FEMS Microbiol. Lett., 34*, 265.

29. El Solh N, Allignet J, Bismuth R et al (1986) Conjugative transfer of staphylococcal antibiotic resistance markers in the absence of detectable plasmid DNA. *Antimicrob. Agents Chemother.*, *30*, 161.

30. Courvalin P, Carlier C (1986) Transposable multiple antibiotic resistance in *Streptococcus pneumoniae*. *Mol. Gen. Genet.*, *205*, 291.

31. Courvalin P, Carlier C (1987) Tn*1545*: a conjugative shuttle transposon. *Mol. Gen. Genet.*, *206*, 259.

32. Caillaud F, Carlier C, Courvalin C (1987) Physical analysis of the conjugative shuttle transposon Tn*1545*. *Plasmid*, *17*, 58.

33. Caillaud F, Trieu-Cuot P, Carlier C, Courvalin P (1987) Nucleotide sequence of the kanamycin resistance determinant of the pneumococcal transposon Tn*1545*: evolutionary relationships and transcriptional analysis of *aphA-3* genes. *Mol. Gen. Genet.*, *207*, 509.

34. Rivera MJ, Castillo J, Martin C et al (1986) Aminoglycoside phosphotransferases APH(3')-IV and APH(3'') synthesized by a strain of *Campylobacter coli*. *J. Antimicrob. Chemother.*, *18*, 153.

35. Young LS, Hindler J (1986) Aminoglycoside resistance: a worldwide perspective. *Am. J. Med.*, *80(6B)*, 15.

36. Gerding DN, Larson TA (1986) Resistance surveillance programs and the incidence of gram-negative bacillary resistance to amikacin from 1967 to 1985. *Am. J. Med.*, *80(6B)*, 22.

37. Phillips I, King A, Shannon K (1986) Prevalence and mechanisms of aminoglycoside resistance: a ten year study. *Am. J. Med.*, *80(6B)*, 48.

38. Saavedra S, Vera D, Ramirez-Ronda CH (1986) Susceptibility of aerobic gram-negative bacilli to aminoglycosides: effects of 45 months of amikacin as first-line aminoglycoside therapy. *Am. J. Med.*, *80(6C)*, 65.

39. Ruiz-Palacios GM, Ponce de Leon S, Sifuentes J et al (1986) Control of emergence of multiresistant gram-negative bacilli by exclusive use of amikacin. *Am. J. Med.*, *80(6C)*, 71.

40. Giamerellou H, Van Landuyt HW, Bolaert J, Gilbert B et al (1986) Surveillance of aminoglycoside resistance: European data. *Am. J. Med.*, *80(6C)*, 76.

41. Touliatou K, Korotzanis G et al (1986) Nosocomial consequences of antibiotic usage. *Scand. J. Infect. Dis.*, *18*, *Suppl 49*, 182.

42. Hammerberg O, Elder D, Richardson H, Landis S (1986) Staphylococcal resistance to aminoglycosides before and after introduction of amikacin in two teaching hospitals. *J. Clin. Microbiol.*, *24*, 629.

43. Tran Van Nhieu G, Goldstein FW, Pinto ME et al (1986) Transfer of amikacin resistance by closely related plasmids in members of the family Enterobacteriaceae isolated in Chile. *Antimicrob. Agents Chemother.*, *29*, 833.

44. Tran Van Nhieu G, Collatz E (1987) Primary structure of an aminoglycoside 6'-*N*-acetyltransferase, AAC(6')-4, fused in vivo with the signal peptide of the Tn*3*-encoded β-lactamase. *J. Bacteriol.*, *169*, in press.

45. Dickson CJ, Schwartzman MS, Bertino JS (1986) Factors affecting aminoglycoside disposition: effects of circadian rhythm and dietary protein intake on gentamicin pharmacokinetics. *Clin. Pharmacol. Ther.*, *39*, 325.

46. Bergeron MG, Marois Y (1986) Benefit from high intrarenal levels of gentamicin in the treatment of *E. coli* pyelonephritis. *Kidney Int.*, *30*, 481.

47. Moore RD, Lietman PS, Smith CR (1987) Clinical response to aminoglycoside thera-

py: importance of the ratio of peak concentration to minimal inhibitory concentration. *J. Infect. Dis.*, *155*, 93.

48. Hendeles L, Neims A (1986) Identification of children for whom routine monitoring of aminoglycoside serum concentrations is not cost effective. *J. Pediatr.*, *109*, 897.

49. Gilbert DN, Kohlhepp SJ (1986) New sodium hydroxide digestion method for measurement of renal tobramycin concentrations. *Antimicrob. Agents Chemother.*, *30*, 361.

50. Schwertz DW, Kreisberg JI, Venkatachalam MA (1986) Gentamicin-induced alterations in pig kidney epithelial (LLC-PK1) cells in culture. *J. Pharmacol. Exp. Ther.*, *236*, 254.

51. Bergeron MG, Bergeron Y (1986) Influence of endotoxin on the intrarenal distribution of gentamicin, netilmicin, tobramycin, amikacin and cephalothin. *Antimicrob. Agents Chemother.*, *29*, 7.

52. Bergeron MG, Bergeron Y, Marois Y (1986) Autoradiography of tobramycin uptake by the proximal and distal tubules of normal and endotoxin-treated rats. *Antimicrob. Agents Chemother.*, *29*, 1005.

53. Bergeron MG, Lessard C, Turcotte A (1986) In vitro uptake of gentamicin and tobramycin by rat renal tubules in the presence or absence of *Escherichia coli* endotoxin. *J. Antimicrob. Chemother.*, *18*, 375.

54. Wood CA, Kohlhepp SJ, Kohnen PW, Houghton DC, Gilbert DN (1986) Vancomycin enhancement of experimental tobramycin nephrotoxicity. *Antimicrob. Agents Chemother.*, *30*, 20.

55. Farber BF, Moellering Jr RC (1983) Retrospective study of the toxicity of preparations of vancomycin from 1974 to 1981. *Antimicrob. Agents Chemother.*, *23*, 138.

56. Williams PJ, Hull JH, Sarubbi FA, Rogers JF, Wargin WA (1986) Factors associated with nephrotoxicity and clinical outcome in patients receiving amikacin. *J. Clin. Pharmacol.*, *26*, 79.

57. Sawyers CL, Moore RD, Lerner SA, Smith CR (1986) A model for predicting nephrotoxicity in patients treated with aminoglycosides. *J. Infect. Dis.*, *153*, 1062.

58. Moore RD, Smith CR, Lietman PS (1986) Increased risk of renal dysfunction due to interaction of liver disease and aminoglycosides. *Am. J. Med.*, *80*, 1093.

59. Dulon D, Aran JM, Zajic G, Schacht J (1986) Comparative uptake of gentamicin, netilmicin and amikacin in the guinea pig cochlea and vestibule. *Antimicrob. Agents Chemother.*, *30*, 96.

60. Williams SE, Smith DE, Schacht J (1987) Characteristics of gentamicin uptake in the isolated crista ampullaris of the innear ear of the guinea pig. *Biochem. Pharmacol.*, *36*, 89.

61. Schacht J (1986) Molecular mechanisms of drug induced hearing loss. *Hearing Res.*, *22*, 297.

62. Lerner SA, Schmitt BA, Seligsohn R, Matz GJ (1986) Comparative study of ototoxicity and nephrotoxicity in patients randomly assigned to treatment with amikacin or gentamicin. *Am. J. Med.*, *80*, Suppl 6B, 98.

63. Evans D, Buring J, Mayrent S, Rosner B, Colton T, Hennekens C (1986) Qualitative overview of randomized trials of aminoglycosides. *Am. J. Med.*, *80*, 39.

64. Siegenthaler WE, Bonetti A, Luthy R (1986) Aminoglycoside antibiotics in infectious diseases. An overview. *Am. J. Med.*, *80*, Suppl 6B, 2.

65. Dejace P, Klastersky J (1986) Comparative review of combination therapy: two betalactams versus betalactam plus aminoglycosides. *Am. J. Med.*, *80*, Suppl 6B, 29.

66. Gaya H (1986) Combination therapy and monotherapy in the treatment of severe infection in the immunocompromised host. *Am. J. Med.*, *80*, Suppl 6B, 149.

67. Bernstein JM, Gorse GJ, Linzmayer MI, Pegram PS, Levin RD, Brummett RE, Markowitz N, Saravolatz LD, Lorber RR (1986) Relative efficacy and toxicity of netilmicin and tobramycin in oncology patients. *Arch. Intern. Med., 146,* 2329.

68. Gerding DN, Larson TA (1986) Resistance surveillance programs of the incidence of Gram negative bacillary resistance to amikacin from 1967 to 1985. *Am. J. Med., 80, Suppl 6B,* 22.

69. Berk SL, Alvarez S, Ortega G, Verghese A, Holtsclaw-Berk SA (1986) Clinical and microbiologic consequences of amikacin use during a 42-month period. *Arch. Intern. Med., 146,* 538.

70. Rybak MJ, Boike SC, Levine DP, Erickson SR (1986) Clinical use and toxicity of high-dose tobramycin in patients with pseudomonal endocarditis. *J. Antimicrob. Chemother., 17,* 115.

71. Meier B, Metzger U, Muller F, Siegenthaler W, Luthy R (1986) Successful treatment of a pancreatic *Nocardia asteroides* abscess with amikacin and surgical drainage. *Antimicrob. Agents Chemother., 29,* 150.

72. Kapusnik JE, Sande MA (1986) Challenging conventional aminoglycoside dosing regimens: the value of experimental models. *Am. J. Med., 80, Suppl 6B,* 179.

73. Gerber AU, Bangerter T, Creter U, Feller C (1986) Impact of bacterial inoculum size and initial treatment free interval on antimicrobial efficacy in vivo: In: *Abstracts, 26th Interscience Conference on Antimicrobial Agents and Chemotherapy, New Orleans, LA, 1986,* No. 573.

74. Vogelman B, Leggett J, Gudmundsson S, Totsuka K, Ebert S, Craig WA (1986) Pharmacokinetic parameters and comparative cidal activity of eight antibiotics in vivo against. *P. aeruginosa.* In: *Abstracts, 26th Interscience Conference on Antimicrobial Agents and Chemotherapy, New Orleans, LA, 1986,* No. 576.

75. Pierre C, Blanchet F, Seta N, Chaigne P, Faurisson F, Labrarre C, Sterkers O, Amiel C, Carbon C (1986) Renal and auditory tolerance of once daily dosing of netilmicin in healthy volunteers. In: *Abstracts, 26th Interscience Conference on Antimicrobial Agents and Chemotherapy, New Orleans, LA, 1986,* No. 29.

76. Petty BG, Baumgardner JV, Lietman PS (1986) Comparison of the renal effects of single *vs* thrice daily dosing of tobramycin in healthy volunteers. In: *Abstracts, 26th Interscience Conference on Antimicrobial Agents and Chemotherapy, New Orleans, LA, 1986,* No. 30.

77. Perry CR, Ritterbusch JK, Rice SH, Davenport K, Burdge RE (1986) Antibiotics delivered by an implantable drug pump. *Am. J. Med., 80, Suppl 6B,* 222.

78. Senello LT, Wilson DS, Afarian J, Holtam LS, Norman G, Rollins DE, Tolman KG (1986) Single-dose pharmacokinetics of 3-O-demethyl-fortimicin A in humans after intravenous or intramuscular administration. *Antimicrob. Agents Chemother., 29,* 400.

79. Serieys C, Bergogne-Berezin E, Prokocimer Ph, Declercq D (1986) Etude clinique et bactériologique de l'O-déméthyl-fortimicine-A-sulfate dans l'infection urinaire. *Pathol. Biol., 34,* 490.

CHAPTER 2

Antimycobacterial drugs

PATTISAPU R.J. GANGADHARAM

Basic and clinical studies with antimycobacterial drugs continue in several parts of the world. This is because of the recognition of the grim fact that the major mycobacterial diseases, tuberculosis and leprosy, have not shown a significant decline in their incidence, particularly in the developing and underdeveloped countries. Worldwide there is an increasing problem of some serious mycobacterial diseases, e.g. the *Mycobacterium avium* complex (MAC) disease, among acquired immunodeficiency syndrome (AIDS) patients. There is concern that even in developed countries, the rapid decline in morbidity as a result of chemotherapy has now more or less stabilized, with a risk of increased morbidity and mortality mostly due to immigrant populations.

In spite of such awareness amongst clinicians and epidemiologists, there does not seem to be equal response on the part of pharmaceutical manufacturers to launch vigorous programs to discover new antimycobacterial drugs. Many of the drugs which have been developed mainly for other bacterial, viral and parasitic diseases are also tested for their possible antimycobacterial activity. Unfortunately, most of these studies have not gone beyond in-vitro screening. One reason for such limited approaches may be due to the thinking that control of tuberculosis and mycobacterial diseases cannot be achieved by chemotherapy alone, but by some innovative immunobiologic manipulations. As such, many pharmaceutical industries are diverting their attention from conventional drug discovery to immunobiologic modulations in the hope that eradication of tuberculosis, leprosy and other mycobacterial diseases, if at all possible, can be realized through this approach. With this attitude, even the few scientists who were involved in chemotherapy of mycobacterial diseases are now channelling their efforts towards immunobiologic approaches against these diseases.

On the positive side, scientific investigations of antimycobacterial drugs are continuing. Studies are being conducted in several parts of the world for better

Research work included in this review was supported by research grants (AI 15049, AI 21897 and AI 42544) from the National Institutes of Health, the Upjohn Company and the American Cyanamid Company.

Antimicrobial Agents Annual 3
P.K. Peterson and J. Verhoef, editors
© Elsevier Science Publishers BV, 1988

and more appropriate application of the available antimycobacterial drugs individually, and in combined chemotherapy programs, both in controlled clinical trials and under field conditions. The prototypes of the controlled clinical trials which were established on a world-wide basis in the past 30 years, thanks to the pioneering efforts of the British Medical Research Council and its collaborating organizations, are still used to assess the efficacy of drug combinations. Likewise, new mechanisms of toxicity of the existing antimycobacterial drugs are being delineated and development of close analogs of the existing drugs, e.g. rifampin, are being reported. Also, the usefulness of several antimycobacterial drugs has been evaluated in diseases other than those for which they were originally intended.

Another welcome feature is the application of molecular biology and molecular pharmacology to antimycobacterial chemotherapy. In the past year, studies have appeared on sustained release of antimycobacterial drugs using direct implantations inside the body, or osmotic pumps. Similarly, encapsulation of some drugs into liposomes (phospholipid vesicles) has been investigated by us and others to effect targeted delivery to appropriate sites of bacterial proliferation.

This Chapter summarizes knowledge of antimycobacterial drugs accumulated mostly during the past year and which has appeared subsequent to earlier versions of this Chapter (1, 2). In most cases, what was discussed previously is not repeated, and therefore the present Chapter is to be used as a companion to those appearing in *Annuals 1* and *2*. For convenience the same order of discussion of the drugs is maintained; however, in view of recent developments, some drugs have been pooled together for a more coherent understanding. For instance, several analogs of rifampin, e.g. cyclopentyl rifampin, rifabutin, CGP7040 etc., are included in the section on rifampin instead of individual sections as was done earlier.

Rifampin

Rifampin by virtue of its unique properties continues to be the most important drug for tuberculosis, leprosy and non-tuberculosis mycobacterial diseases, as well as for many non-mycobacterial diseases. As the key member in regimens for short-course chemotherapy, rifampin will continue to be very important in the treatment of tuberculosis. While its use in leprosy and other non-tuberculosis mycobacterial diseases is a logical extension of its role in tuberculosis chemotherapy, its use in non-mycobacterial diseases has been debated as discussed earlier (1, 2). The use of rifampin in combination with other drugs has disclosed several toxic manifestations which are directly or indirectly due to its use. Earlier literature has shown that intermittent administration of rifampin frequently results in the so-called 'flu' syndrome (3) and, during the past year, several other toxicities due to such usage have been recognized. Finally several analogs of rifampin have been investigated; some, e.g. rifabutin and cyclopentyl rifampin, were introduced earlier and previously discussed (1, 2). Several excellent reviews of rifampin have appeared in recent years (4, 5).

Discussion in this section is grouped as follows: (a) Treatment of tuberculosis, (b) treatment of non-tuberculosis mycobacterial diseases, (c) influence on the metabolism and toxicity of other drugs, (d) toxic manifestations, and (e) rifampin analogs.

Role of rifampin in the treatment of tuberculosis

Short-course chemotherapy of tuberculosis has been acknowledged worldwide as the most effective form of chemotherapy of tuberculosis (6). Several studies have been reported from many countries with variations in duration of treatment, number and nature of drugs used in the intensive and continuation phases, and different doses of the drugs. Some other studies have dealt with more specialized conditions such as lymph node tuberculosis (7), gastrointestinal tuberculosis (8), tuberculosis of the penis (9) and tuberculous disease of the female reproductive organs (10). In all these studies, the positive results obtained have been attributed primarily to rifampin, making it the drug of choice. On the other hand, it has been mentioned that short-course chemotherapy will not be adequate for tuberculosis in AIDS patients (11), and longer courses of treatment with triple or quadruple therapy followed by maintenance isoniazid are generally necessary. Sensitive methods like high-performance liquid chromatography (HPLC) techniques were standardized not only for estimation of free rifampin, but also its principal metabolite, 2,5-desacetyl rifampin in serum (12). Some of these studies tried to correlate the serum concentrations of the free drug and its metabolites with clinical response.

Role of rifampin in treatment of non-tuberculosis mycobacterial diseases

One of the cardinal properties of rifampin, besides its specific action against *M. tuberculosis*, is its specific role in the treatment of *M. kansasii* disease (13). As mentioned earlier, just as isoniazid is recognized as the mandatory drug of choice in the treatment of pulmonary tuberculosis, rifampin happens to be the most valuable drug in the treatment of *M. kansasii* disease, unless contraindicated for other reasons. In fact, several authors (14, 15) including our group (16) have suggested the use of rifampin for short-course chemotherapy of *M. kansasii* disease. However, it was realized that *M. kansasii* may develop resistance to rifampin. Indeed, acquired drug resistance to rifampin by *M. kansasii* was reported by Davidson and Waggoner (17) over 10 years ago, soon after its introduction in the United States. Recent studies, by Ahn et al dealt with similar experience using controlled clinical trials, and these investigators have suggested the use of sulfamethoxazole derivatives as an alternative form of chemotherapy for patients with rifampin-resistant isolates (18).

The role of rifampin in the treatment of regular and dapsone-resistant leprosy has been extensively investigated using combined treatment with rifampin and dapsone (19). Since rifampin alters the metabolism of dapsone, adjustment of the dose of dapsone is necessary. Use of rifampin in the treatment of cutaneous infections due to *M. chelonei* and the disease caused by *M. malmoense* has been established (20, 21). *M. malmoense* isolates are generally resistant to isoniazid, but susceptible to rifampin and ethionamide. Several studies have confirmed the penetration of rifampin into mouse (22) and human monocyte-derived macrophages (23) as well as its activity against persistent bacilli of *M. tuberculosis*, *M. leprae* and several of the non-tuberculosis mycobacteria (24).

Toxic reactions due to rifampin

Extensive clinical experience with rifampin has uncovered several toxic manifestations. Most important among these is the so-called 'flu' syndrome, which manifests more frequently when rifampin is given intermittently than daily (3).

Recent studies have mentioned renal failure and hemolysis, often encountered on intermittent administration of rifampin and associated with the 'flu' syndrome. Mattson and Janne (25) indicated that the 'flu' syndrome was caused by mild intravascular hemolysis which was quantitatively different from serious reactions, such as massive hemolysis and renal failure. Fortunately, renal failure was reversible, and quite frequently the symptoms disappeared when the drug was discontinued (25). In rare cases, rifampin had to be abandoned indefinitely. Prednisolone did not seem to prevent hemolysis and renal failure due to rifampin. Leukopenia has been ascribed to intermittent rifampin therapy (26). Myalgia caused by myoglobinemia and myoglobinuria may be associated with the 'flu' syndrome (27). Acute transplant rejection episodes were observed when rifampin was prescribed in poorly tolerant renal transplant recipients (28). Rejection occurred despite giving double the daily doses of steroids. The detrimental effect of rifampin was due both to its capacity as an enzymatic inducer of steroid metabolism and to its interference with active mechanisms involved in specific transplantation tolerance as discussed earlier (2). Discoloration of soft contact lenses by rifampin has been reported (29). In contrast to the evidence arising from clinical situations, animal studies have not confirmed the immunobiologic toxicity of rifampin and dapsone (30).

Influence of rifampin on the metabolism of other drugs

As discussed previously (1, 2), rifampin induces its own metabolism as well as the metabolism of several other drugs. Concomitant administration of rifampin with other drugs often necessitates alteration of the dose of these drugs and guidelines for assessing the imputability of hepatic drug interactions caused by rifampin have been published (31). For instance, the dose of theophylline for asthmatic patients has to be increased when rifampin is given. Adrenal crisis was reported when rifampin was given along with steroids to patients with adrenal insufficiency. Studies continue to come out dealing with the influence of rifampin on the metabolism of ketoconazole (32), cyclosporin (33), verapamil (34), antipyrine (35), digoxin

(36), phenobarbital (37), and phenytoin (38), besides extensive work on its influence on the metabolism and bioavailability of isoniazid (39).

Rifampin analogs

Rifabutin

Laboratory and clinical studies with rifabutin (previously called ansamycin or LM 427) have continued. Tsukamura et al (40) showed that the in-vitro activity of rifabutin against *M. tuberculosis* was 2–4 times greater than that of rifampin. Rifampin-resistant mutants isolated from H_{37} Rv strain were 160 times more resistant to rifampin, and 128 times more resistant to rifabutin than the parent strain. The responses to rifabutin of rifampin-resistant strains isolated from patients under rifampin therapy differed from strain to strain: 4 of the 8 strains tested were resistant to 40 μg/ml rifabutin, but the other 4 strains were less resistant, and one of the 4 was susceptible to 1.25 μg/ml of rifabutin.

The response of naturally rifampin-resistant MAC strains was different from that of *M. tuberculosis* strains. Of 40 strains tested, 32 showed natural resistance to rifampin (40 μg/ml or more) and 19 were susceptible to 1.25 μg/ml of rifabutin. Thus, the natural resistance to rifampin did not always accompany resistance to rifabutin. These authors confirmed the earlier findings that MAC strains, which are frequently (>80%) resistant to rifampin, are commonly (70%) susceptible to 1.25 μg/ml of rifabutin. Although a relationship between the serotype and susceptibility to rifabutin has not clearly been demonstrated, MAC strains with serotypes 4, 8 and 16 are often susceptible to rifabutin. Rifabutin is more active than rifampin against *M. tuberculosis*, *M. bovis*, *M. kansasii*, *M. marinum*, *M. xenopei*, *M. haemophilum*, *M. scrofulaceum*, *M. nonchromogenicum* and *M. terrae*. Among these, the greatest differences have been noted with *M. marinum*, *M. xenopei* and *M. haemophilum*.

The division of tuberculosis control at the Centers for Disease Control (CDC) in Atlanta reported the results of a large-scale trial of rifabutin used in the treatment of 821 patients with life-threatening mycobacterial disease (41). In this study 604 patients had AIDS and disseminated MAC disease, 36 were immunosuppressed and had disseminated MAC disease, 138 were patients with disabling progressive MAC pulmonary disease or other forms of localized MAC disease, and 43 patients had rifampin-resistant *M. tuberculosis* infections. Patients with normal hepatic and hematopoietic function were randomly assigned to either a high (300 mg) or a low (150 mg) dose of rifabutin, while choice of companion drugs was left to the patient's physician.

Death was the most common cause for stopping treatment and by the end of 2 years, only 25% of the patients remained on rifabutin. About 6% of the patients stopped treatment because of suspected adverse drug reactions, although the adverse reactions were not related to the rifabutin dosage, and were lower in patients with localized disease than in those with disseminated disease. Although one-third of the patients with disseminated disease showed clinical improvement during therapy, documented eradication of MAC disease in these patients was uncommon. Sputum culture conversion occurred in 15% of the patients with pulmonary MAC disease and 29% with drug-resistant tuberculosis. No relationship was seen between rifabutin dosage and sputum conversion. However, among all categories of patients, those randomized to the higher dose of rifabutin had a greater 1 year survival (46%) than those randomized to the lower dose (29%), and those not eligible for randomization (18%). While these preliminary data suggest that rifabutin is safe and well tolerated, conclusions regarding its efficacy in the treatment of mycobacterial disease, particularly infections caused by MAC organisms in patients with AIDS, await results of large-scale studies. Controlled clinical trials along these lines are being contemplated for the near future.

A long-acting derivative of rifabutin, 3-azinomethylrifamycin (FEC-22250) was investigated by Della Bruna et al (42). This drug has been shown to have a long half-life in animals and good oral absorption as well as a broad antibacterial spectrum including activity against mycobacteria. In experimental tuberculosis using $H_{37}Rv$ strain, FEC-22250 showed an efficacy 14 times greater than that of rifampin and is therapeutically active when administered once every 3 weeks. Further investigations of this drug are clearly warranted.

Rifapentine

Investigations are continuing on rifapentine (previously called cyclopentyl rifampin or DL-473). Tsukamura et al (43) carried out detailed in-vitro studies on comparative antimycobacterial activities of rifapentine with rifampin. Their results indicated that:

a. The in-vitro growth-inhibitory activity of rifapentine against *M. tuberculosis* strains was approximately twice that of rifampin. All rifampin-susceptible strains were susceptible to rifapentine and all rifampin-resistant strains were resistant to rifapentine.

b. About 80% of MAC strains isolated from patients who did not receive rifampin earlier were resistant to rifampin, at a concentration of 40 μg/ml or more. Of these 'naturally rifampin-resistant' strains, approximately 75% were resistant to rifapentine at the same concentration. However, the remaining 25% of the strains were more or less susceptible to rifapentine.

c. MAC strains (serotypes 1 and 2) were often resistant to rifapentine, whereas those having serotype 16 were often susceptible to rifapentine.

d. Antimycobacterial spectra of rifapentine and rifampin were almost identical. However, the growth-inhibitory activity of rifapentine against *M. tuberculosis*, *M. kansasii* and *M. szulgai* was twice that of rifampin.

Wylie et al (44) studied the relative uptake and distribution of radiolabelled rifapentine and rifampin into the subcellular organelles of mouse peritoneal macrophages using analytic fractionation on sucrose density gradients. In serum-free solution, uptake of rifapentine was thrice that of rifampin; in the presence of serum, uptake of both drugs was less and equal. Almost all of the cell-associated drug was found in the cytosol and no difference in distribution was detected between the two rifampins. It was concluded that the prolonged action of rifapentine compared to rifampin in chemotherapy of tuberculosis cannot be attributed to better penetration of the macrophages (44). In contrast to its activity in vitro rifapentine did not show any activity in vivo against MAC infections in beige mice. (Gangadharam and Perumal, unpublished observations).

Newer analogs (the CGP series)

Recently, 3 new rifampin derivatives, CGP-7040, CGP-27557 and CGP-29861, were compared with rifampin in several pharmacokinetic and experimental chemotherapy investigations (45–47). The biologic half-lives of these drugs were considerably longer than that of rifampin (45). The half-life, in hours, for CGP-7040 was 47 in mice, over 120 in rabbits and 80 in dogs; the corresponding figures were 20, 70 and 15 for CGP-27557; 45, 100 and 15 for CGP-29861; and only 6 hours in the mouse and 4 hours in the rabbit, for rifampin. The drug concentrations in these animal species increased approximately proportionally to the dose administered. The serum binding capacity of these compounds was similar to rifampin, and the drugs accumulated in the liver to a lesser extent than rifampin.

Studies carried out in human volunteers have given similar data: the half-life of CGP-7040, CGP-27557 and CGP-29861 were 30, 8 and 40 hours, respectively, as compared to 4 hours for rifampin. Unlike rifampin, food had no influence on the absorption of CGP-7040 and CGP-27557, whereas the absorption of CGP-29861 was twice as high when taken after breakfast. All 3 drugs showed slower absorption and lower peak concentrations in the blood than pure rifampin.

Antimycobacterial activities in vitro and in vivo of these compounds also showed interesting properties, warranting further investigations (46). In vitro, these 3 compounds showed similar activities against gram-positive and gram-negative bacteria as well as tubercle bacilli; all were similar to rifampin. CGP-7040 was superior to rifampin against non-tuberculosis mycobacteria. In vivo, the 3 compounds were less active against experimental staphylococcal infections than rifampin. In murine tuberculosis, with short duration of treatment, the ED_{50} of CGP-7040 was comparable to that of rifampin, whereas CGP-27557 and CGP-29861 were 5 times more active than rifampin. With longer treatment periods and different dosage intervals, CGP-27557 and CGP-29861 proved to be several times more active than rifampin, as evidenced by enumeration of tubercle bacilli in the lungs; they also proved to be tuberculocidal at lower dosages. LeCoeur et al (47) assessed the role of CGP-29861, given either in the initial or in the continuation phase of experimental short-course chemotherapy of tuberculosis.

FUTURE DIRECTIONS

Rifampin will continue to be the most important antimycobacterial drug in the foreseeable future. Approaches will be made not only to substantiate its activity in short-course chemotherapy programs but also its interactions with other drugs and its immunobiologically related toxicities. In addition, new derivatives with prolonged half-lives and reduced toxicity will be sought. It is not unrealistic to anticipate that some of these drugs will be introduced as possible competitors to rifampin. Recent investigations have focused on the mode of administration of rifampin, at least in experimental animal models. Two or 3 such approaches are being investigated in several centers including ours (48). (Gangadharam and Düzgünes, unpublished observations). One is to study the liposome-encapsulated form of rifampin with a targeted type of delivery inside the host. Other approaches include implantation procedures (48) and osmotic pumps. Another important development, about which considerable research has accumulated in recent years, is the use of combination forms of chemotherapy using rifampin, isoniazid and pyrazinamide (49). Some preparations (e.g. Rifater) have been investigated in several parts of the world (50). It is hoped that combination forms will not only eliminate the errors in the drug dosage systems (49), but also will ensure better compliance in drug intake, especially in self-administered protocols (51).

Isoniazid

Isoniazid is considered to be the most powerful, most bactericidal, best tolerated and cheapest drug available today. As mentioned earlier (1, 2) its use is considered mandatory in all forms of treatment of tuberculosis. Its use as a chemoprophylactic agent is still being pursued (52) in spite of fear of hepatotoxicity, which is due mostly to the influence of rifampin (53) as discussed earlier (2). In most features of antimycobacterial action it is similar, and in many other considerations (e.g. cost, toxicity, etc.) superior to rifampin. As indicated previously (1, 2), most of the killing of tubercle bacilli in combination chemotherapy is due to isoniazid, and the companion drug, be it a powerful drug like rifampin, or a weak drug like thioacetazone or para-aminosalicylic acid, will be useful only in killing drug-resistant mutants of isoniazid. Its importance in short-course chemotherapy and chemoprophylaxis programs continues and several large-scale clinical experiences have been reported (54, 55). Many of these deal not necessarily with the treatment of tuberculosis *per se*, but with the occurrence of toxic manifestations, some of which were not considered important previously (1, 2). Some of these deal not only with hepatotoxicity, which was highlighted in *Annual 2* (2), but with neurotoxicity, another important toxic manifestation of isoniazid (53, 56). Similarly, some of the biologic properties of isoniazid, especially its mutagenic potential, are being re-explored.

The current review deals with: the role of isoniazid in the treatment of tuberculosis and other mycobacterial diseases especially in short-course chemotherapy; chemoprophylaxis; the onset of toxicity, metabolism and inactivation in relation to the occurrence of toxic manifestations; modern procedures of estimation in biologic systems; and finally its role in mutagenesis and DNA repair.

Several reports dealt with successful application of short-course chemotherapy regimens containing isoniazid, both in controlled clinical trials as well as under program conditions (54, 55). Some of these studies dealt with supervised intermittent chemotherapy in rural areas (57). Similarly, long-term assessment of its role in combination with streptomycin in the treatment of tuberculosis of the spine in children, and with rifampin in the treatment of tuberculosis meningitis have been reported (58, 59).

Several studies on chemoprophylaxis using isoniazid have been reported (55, 60) despite fears of hepatotoxicity (61). An interesting outcome is the follow-up of one large-scale trial conducted in Eastern European countries by the International Union Against Tuberculosis (IUAT) (62). This study assessed the efficacy of toxicity of isoniazid preventive therapy regimens of 12, 24 and 52 weeks' duration. The data obtained from this study was reanalyzed by Snider et al (63) to obtain the cost-effectiveness of the 3 alternative regimens. Over a wide range of assumptions, a regimen of 24 weeks' duration was found to be more cost-effective than either the 12- or 52-week regimens. Using these base estimations, the cost per case prevented with the 24-week regimen was $7,112.00 compared with $16,024 for the 52-week regimen. Among a cohort of 100% treated, each additional case prevented with the 52-week regimen would cost $80,807; thus, a shorter course of isoniazid preventive chemotherapy is relatively cost-effective compared to the current policy. It should be recognized that even the lowest cost within the chemoprophylaxis program is several times greater than any immunization procedure.

Studies on inactivation or metabolism of isoniazid still continue and have been extended to children (64). Likewise, the inactivation status has been correlated with the occurrence of toxicity, particularly hepatotoxicity (65, 66). The rate of inactivation of isoniazid did not seem to influence the clearance of phenytoin; rifampin, which is shown to be a strong inducer of elimination of phenytoin, was not influenced by isoniazid in either the slow or rapid acetylators (38). Interest in the measurement of isoniazid and rifampin particularly to assess the rate of inactivation etc. continued using modern techniques like HPLC (12).

Several studies dealt with the effect of isoniazid on brain function and other neurologic manifestations, and occurrences of pellagra encephalopathy in tuberculosis patients on isoniazid therapy have been reported (66, 67). Similarly the changes in brain amino acid levels, particularly gamma-aminobutyric acid (GABA) in Huntington disease patients on isoniazid therapy have been reported (68). Increase in GABA following isoniazid treatment in animals was discussed earlier (1, 2) and another study reported similar findings with man (69).

Another interesting toxic manifestation of isoniazid is shown to occur when it is administered along with cheese and wine (70). Administration of isoniazid in patients who have taken old cheese and wine resulted in a hypersensitive crisis due to the interaction between monoamine oxidase inhibitors. Histamine accumulates in old cheese on prolonged keeping, and if the quantity of the cheese taken by patients is high, consumption of isoniazid results in high levels of histaminase, acting on histamine, which in turn precipitates symptoms of headache, palpitation, severe general flushing, conjunctival effusion, and dyspnea with dangerous consequences. Contrary to these negative reports, a possible therapeutic role for isoniazid has been reported in the treatment of postural cerebellar tremors in multiple sclerosis (117).

The mutagenic role of isoniazid was investigated with a DNA repair assay using isolated human or rat hepatocytes as metabolic systems (118) as well as DNA excision repair and mutagenicity studies using *Salmonella typhimurium*. With rat hepatocytes, isoniazid appeared to be weakly mutagenic and did not induce significant increases in hepatocellular DNA-excision repair. With isolated hepatocytes of two human subjects, isoniazid appeared also weakly mutagenic. However, with hepatocytes of two other human subjects, the drug was found to be highly mutagenic. Comparable results were obtained for the induction of hepatocellular DNA-excision repair. Thus, the concern of the possible mutagenicity of isoniazid continues, although to a limited extent.

FUTURE DIRECTIONS

Isoniazid will continue to be an important drug in the treatment of tuberculosis and other mycobacterial diseases for several years to come. Research on isoniazid will continue along several lines. It will continue to be used in short-course chemotherapy regimens of tuberculosis. The chemoprophylaxis program will continue in spite of the arguments against it. This is all the more important because of the failure of BCG vaccination (71) and the absence of a potent immunization procedure against tuberculosis. The toxicity of isoniazid will continue to be investigated especially that related to liver and brain functions. However, these findings will probably not deter its widespread use. Concerns regarding its mutagenicity may not be as serious as discussed earlier (1, 2) and hopefully will end as academic investigations.

Pyrazinamide

Among the 4 important drugs in short-course chemotherapy regimens, pyrazinamide occupies an important place, especially due to its sterilizing activity on persisting bacilli. Essentially the same types of investigations with this drug have been performed in the last year as in previous years. Some of the more important contributions which may alter our attitude towards pyrazinamide are discussed here.

Mitchison and Nunn (72) analyzed the role of individual drugs and the influence of initial drug resistance in short-course chemotherapy regimens. Their analysis indicated that pyrazinamide is a bactericidal drug and the rifampin + pyrazin-amide combination has a sterilizing activity that prevents emergence of resistance; the activity of this combination is greater than that of isoniazid and streptomycin. Failure rate in patients with initial resistance to isoniazid, streptomycin or both was high (30%) in the streptomycin + isoniazid + pyrazinamide regimens, and moderate (17%) in the isoniazid + rifampin regimens. It decreased as the number of drugs was increased and as the duration of treatment with rifampin was prolonged. A comparison of the 2-month culture findings and relapse rates after the end of chemotherapy, in patients with initially susceptible and resistant organisms, suggested that almost all the sterilizing activity in short-course chemotherapy regimens was due to rifampin and/or pyrazinamide. In experimental models of short-course chemotherapy, Grosset et al (73) showed that pyrazinamide enables the prevention of emergence of resistance to rifampin.

Acocella et al (22) studied the penetration of rifampin, pyrazinamide and pyrazinoic acid, the principal metabolite of pyrazinamide, into dead, resident and stimulated mouse peritoneal macrophages. The degree of penetration was studied using ^{14}C-labelled compounds at concentrations corresponding to the peak, trough and intermediate serum concentrations observed in human subjects after administration of therapeutic doses. Their results indicated that the 3 compounds penetrated inside macrophages rapidly, and at lower concentrations the uptake of the 3 drugs was practically complete. With increasing concentrations, the absolute amounts of drugs inside the intracellular compartment increased. Comparison of the degree of penetration of the 3 drugs into the 3 types of macrophages suggested that the process of transfer through the macrophage wall is of a passive nature, and not related to the metabolic state of the cells. Analysis of the binding of the 3 drugs to intracellular proteins indicated that more binding sites are probably available for rifampin than for pyrazinamide or its metabolite.

Using the same conditions, Acocella et al (22) studied the killing effect of rifampin, pyrazinamide and pyrazinoic acid on macrophage-ingested live *M. tuberculosis*. The same concentrations as in earlier studies were used and numbers of viable bacilli were observed at 3, 18, 24, 48 and 72 hours after ingestion. Greater killing was observed between 48 and 72 hours and there was no difference between rifampin, pyrazinamide and its metabolite in this regard.

In contrast to these reports, Ikeda and Lee (74) found a negligible effect of pyrazinamide on intracellularly multiplying mycobacteria. Using a silicone-coated slide culture method and mycobacterium-infected mouse peritoneal macrophages, these authors showed that pyrazinamide, either alone or combined with other drugs, under several experimental conditions, had little effect on the intracellular multiplication of tubercle bacilli. According to these authors (74), the unique capacity of pyrazinamide to inhibit intracellular mycobacteria, which was quoted as evidence for excellent clinical results of short-course chemotherapy with regimens containing this drug, was not borne out by their studies.

Recent studies have also shown that pyrazinamide could antagonize the action of some drugs. Tsukamura and Ichiyama (75) found an antagonistic effect of pyrazinamide to ofloxacin, which shows less activity in the lungs and more in the liver because of its rapid excretion via the lungs (76). Ofloxacin treatment markedly reduced the colony-forming unit (CFU) counts from the liver, while pyrazinamide treatment did not have any effect. On the other hand, in mice treated with both ofloxacin and pyrazinamide, the numbers of viable bacteria in the liver increased by 3–4 weeks, thus demonstrating antagonism of the activity of ofloxacin by pyrazinamide. In contrast to the studies in vivo, no antagonism was seen between the two drugs in vitro (75).

An interesting observation was made by Heifets et al (77) who showed that pyrazinamide, even at high concentrations, is not active in vitro against MAC, whether or not the organisms are pyrazinamidase-positive. These authors also suggested that the pyrazinamidase test, which is used by many workers as an indirect method for testing susceptibility of pyrazinamide (78), is not useful for such purposes when dealing with MAC. On the other hand, several studies dealt with the usefulness of the pyrazinamidase test in susceptibility testing of pyrazinamide for *M. tuberculosis* (79). Similarly, other studies (80) have appeared on rapid indirect pyrazinamide susceptibility testing using radiometric methods, similar to those reported by Heifets and Iseman (81).

FUTURE DIRECTIONS

Pyrazinamide will continue to be an important drug in the chemotherapy of mycobacterial diseases, particularly in short-course chemotherapy of tuberculosis. Studies may also continue on its use in the treatment of other non-tuberculosis mycobacterial diseases, and perhaps in leprosy, though it is questionable whether its use in the treatment of MAC disease will be pursued. Similarly, the role of other rifampin analogs on altering pyrazinamide toxicity and metabolism will be investigated.

Ethambutol

Ethambutol continues to be used in the 3-drug regimens of conventional chemotherapy of tuberculosis, and in the 4-drug regimens in the initial phase of short-course chemotherapy. Recent studies have dealt with its role in short-course chemotherapy of tuberculosis of lymph nodes and other areas (7). Some attempts have been made to prepare new derivatives (82), though progress has been slight in this area.

Besides MAC disease discussed earlier (2), recent studies have indicated its usefulness in the treatment of disease caused by *M. chelonei* and other non-tuberculosis mycobacterial organisms. The optic neuritis induced by ethambutol is still being carefully studied (83). More recently, blue-yellow color vision changes were found as early symptoms of ocular toxicity of ethambutol (84). Retino-neuritis due to ethambutol was documented only with high doses (> 20 mg/kg/d), an observation confirming earlier findings. Pau (85) who reviewed this literature indicated various guidelines which may help decide on the nature and frequency of the onset of toxicity. He occasionally observed a clinical picture of reddish optic disc, retinal hemorrhages, a fine granular pigment alteration of the macular region, and loss of vision for more than 1 year with an optic disc pallor – all of which suggest toxic retinitis or retino-neuritis, rather than neuritis. These observations were confirmed by electrophysiologic findings.

During the past year, a few other observations were made concerning the mycobactericidal activity of ethambutol. Using an in-vitro model of monocyte-derived macrophages, which has direct relevance to the in-vivo effects in human subjects, Crowle et al (86) showed that ethambutol inhibited and killed tubercle bacilli within the cells at the same concentrations as in bacteriologic culture medium. When the drug was added 2 days after infection, ethambutol killed intra-macrophage bacilli at lower concentrations than in the bacteriologic culture medium. The concentrations of ethambutol that proved mycobactericidal in human macrophages are easily achieved clinically. It was speculated that this enhanced killing is due to the defective cell walls created by ethambutol. The effect of ethambutol on the cell walls of mycobacteria and inhibition of mycolic acid synthesis was reviewed earlier (1, 2).

Another important contribution to our understanding of ethambutol activity was by Heifets et al (87) who determined its minimal inhibitory (MIC) and bactericidal (MBC) concentrations against MAC and *M. tuberculosis* organisms using radiometric (Bactec) methods. These authors found the MICs to be lower in liquid than in solid medium. The broth determined MICs for susceptible *M. tuberculosis* and most of the MAC strains were comparable to serum levels. Ethambutol produced bactericidal effects against both *M. tuberculosis* and MAC and the MIC/MBC ratios were in the same range for both species. It was proposed that MICs, MBCs and MIC/MBC ratios should be considered as important criteria for susceptibility testing of MAC and *M. tuberculosis* in future clinical trials.

Finally, Cheema et al reported several studies (88–90) on the action of ethambutol on the phospholipid composition and metabolism of *M. smegmatis*. Ethambutol inhibited phospholipid biosynthesis in the organism, and induced leakage of major components into the growth medium. The levels of phosphatidyl ethanolamine decreased significantly, while other phospholipids were not affected. It was postulated that alterations in phospholipids may be responsible for maintenance of drug permeability barriers.

FUTURE DIRECTIONS

Ethambutol may continue to be an important drug for mycobacterial diseases, particularly those caused by MAC and rapid growers. Its use in the treatment of tuberculosis may remain about the same, unless another powerful drug replaces it. Its use in the treatment of leprosy may be extended. It is unlikely that derivatives of ethambutol will be pursued with vigor to uncover better substitutes.

Streptomycin

As in the previous year, many studies have dealt with the effect of streptomycin on non-mycobacterial organisms and in the treatment of non-infectious diseases; the latter arose because of its effects on the vestibular function of animals and man. The few studies on mycobacterial diseases dealt with its use in short-course chemotherapy, in combination chemotherapy for tuberculosis and non-tuberculosis mycobacterial diseases, in drug susceptibility testing, or assays in various biologic fluids. For convenience, various studies dealing with this drug are discussed below as: (a) its role in treatment of tuberculosis and other mycobacterial diseases; (b) methods of estimation; and (c) biosynthesis and other molecular biologic aspects.

Treatment of tuberculosis and other mycobacterial diseases

Streptomycin continues to be an important drug in short-course chemotherapy of tuberculosis. Of particular relevance is its usefulness in the treatment of tuberculosis meningitis in children (91). Drug susceptibility studies are done on tubercle bacilli and non-tuberculosis mycobacteria obtained from patients under various treatment programs, as well as from AIDS patients. In many of these studies, recent methods (e.g. radiometric (Bactec)), were used.

Methods of estimation

Methods of determining streptomycin using the established microbiologic procedures as well as recent techniques involving HPLC have been adopted (92). An interesting review of the physicochemical methods for determining streptomycin and other antibiotics in tissues and fluids including milk, particularly of food-producing animals, has appeared (93). The pharmacokinetics of this drug along with other drugs in tuberculosis patients with and without complications have been reported (94).

Biosynthesis and other molecular biologic aspects

Studies of various molecular biologic aspects of streptomycin have continued in the past year. The biosynthetic pathways of streptomycin from *Streptomyces griseus*, the source from which this antibiotic was originally obtained, have been studied (95). Similarly, the characterization and cloning of a gene from *S. griseus*, coding for streptomycin phosphorylating activity and characterization of streptomycin phosphotransferase were established (96). The effect of streptomycin on respiration and growth characteristics, on mutation frequencies, nucleotide sequences, cross-linking to 30S subunits, and on the stoichiometry of GTP hydrolysis in a poly(U)-dependent cell-free system were studied (97).

FUTURE DIRECTIONS

Streptomycin may continue to be an important drug in short-course chemotherapy regimens for tuberculosis. However, its use for this purpose may diminish should a more powerful, orally administered, drug be developed. If liposome-entrapped streptomycin proves to be efficacious, its use may replace the conventional method of administration. On the other hand, its use in the treatment of the wide variety of non-tuberculosis diseases may not continue because of the availability of several other drugs. It will still be used by molecular biologists, mostly for academic purposes, and it may find a place in immunobiology, mainly as a probe to study the transport and activity of drugs inside macrophages and other cells.

Capreomycin

Capreomycin is used to a limited extent as a second-line drug for the treatment of drug-resistant tuberculosis. Even here, it has not found much use, except for rare situations where all other available drugs have failed. It has limited usefulness in the treatment of non-tuberculosis mycobacterial diseases. During the last year, no significant contributions dealing with this drug have appeared.

Kanamycin

As in previous years, most of the research work on this drug have dealt with non-mycobacterial systems. A few studies, however, dealt with its toxic manifestations and mechanisms of their development. The contributions regarding this drug in the past year will be discussed as follows: (a) molecular biology and mechanisms of resistance development; (b) methods of estimation; (c) effect on body functions; and (d) ototoxicity.

Molecular biology and mechanisms of resistance development

The activity of kanamycin against several non-acid-fast organisms has been exploited for study of the mechanism of resistance development, plasmid-mediated functions, and the role of aminoglycoside transferase enzymes in the development of resistance (98). In fact, kanamycin aminotransferase has been used as a probe to study the development of resistance among gram-positive and gram-negative organisms, to other aminoglycoside antibiotics like tobramycin, gentamicin etc. The use of sponges incorporating kanamycin in outpatient dental surgery practice has been advocated (99). Likewise, attempts have been made to synthesize kanamycin derivatives with possible antiviral activity. In contrast to these various studies, very few dealt with mycobacteria.

Methods of estimation

Many approaches to determine kanamycin concentrations in biologic fluids have been made using modern technology. Thus, the use of gas chromatography, HPLC, fluorescence polarization immunoassay, and radioenzymatic assay using kanamycin 6'-acetyltransferase and microcrystallography were reported (100–103).

The effect of kanamycin on the central nervous system using the rabbit knee joint model (104), and the contractile response of guinea-pig urinary bladder (105) have been investigated. Of particular importance were studies on the ototoxicity of kanamycin in several animal species. Detailed studies were performed using morphologic, electrophysiologic and scanning electronmicroscopic procedures, in albino and pigmented guinea-pigs given different doses of this drug under varying conditions of administration. These studies were primarily aimed at investigating the relation of aminoglycoside ototoxicity to melanin pigment. A significantly lower incidence of hearing loss and of hair cell degeneration were seen in albino animals than in pigmented animals, supporting the hypothesis that the affinity of kanamycin for inner ear melanin may be responsible for the difference in ototoxicity between albino and pigmented animals (106). Other studies have investigated the dissociation of the concentration of kanamycin in plasma and perilymph from an ototoxic effect (107). The magnitude of ototoxicity due to kanamycin was related to the total daily dose alone, and not the dosing schedule. This lack of a relationship between the dosing schedule and the magnitude of ototoxicity is the opposite of that reported for the nephrotoxicity resulting from gentamicin, tobramycin and netilmicin. Another interesting study dealt with the age dependence of ototoxicity due to kanamycin (108); a greater susceptibility of younger mice to hearing sensitivity was seen than in older mice which did not demonstrate any loss of hearing sensitivity. The role of methyluracil in preventing the ototoxic action of kanamycin has been investigated (109).

FUTURE DIRECTIONS

The role of kanamycin in the chemotherapy of mycobacterial diseases is slowly decreasing. It will soon be replaced by amikacin, which is less toxic, more acceptable and more efficacious.

Amikacin

Interest continues in the chemotherapeutic activity of amikacin, an aminoglycoside antibiotic closely related to kanamycin. We have completed several studies dealing with this drug (110; Gangadharam et al, in preparation). These include its activity under in-vitro dynamic conditions simulating those existing in vivo, in experimental MAC infections of beige mice, and on the phagocytosis and intracellular multiplication of MAC inside macrophages from beige, C57B1/6 and S/W mice. Constant exposure and in-vitro human model studies demonstrated a rapid bactericidal action of amikacin against MAC. Pulsed exposure studies revealed a minimum of 48 hours exposure to be necessary for complete bactericidal action. Amikacin showed rapid killing of the organisms inside the beige mouse, and administration of the drug in 1, 2 or 3 doses a day did not make any difference. In contrast to its high activity in vitro and in vivo, its activity inside macrophages was not apparent. At 2.5, 5 and 10 $\mu g/ml$, amikacin did not show any demonstrable activity on either phagocytosis or intracellular multiplication of MAC inside resident or activated peritoneal macrophages from any of the 3 strains of mice. The lack of activity of amikacin against intracellular MAC may be due to inefficient permeation of the drug inside the macrophages.

Wallace et al (111) investigated amikacin, along with several other drugs, in the treatment of non-pulmonary infections due to *M. fortuitum*. Among 123 patients with such infections, those with localized disease received a single drug, preferably sulfonamide, while patients with advanced disease received amikacin or amikacin + cefoxitin, followed by sulfonamide, based on susceptibilities in vitro. Response to therapy was excellent: 68 (90%) with *M. fortuitum* and 34 (72%) with *M. chelonei* infections were successfully treated. Cultures became negative within 6 weeks after stopping chemotherapy, except for sternal osteomyelitis for which a mean period of 12 months following therapy was needed in 80% of cases. Relapses were rare except in patients with disseminated disease, and drug resistance developed in only 1 patient. These studies thus demonstrated the value of amikacin-containing regimens, and benefit of chemotherapy based on susceptibility in vitro. In parallel, these authors (112) studied the nature of development of resistance in these organisms to amikacin and other aminoglycosides and antibacterial agents. Aminoglycoside-susceptible strains of *M. fortuitum* and *M. chelonei* contained an aminoglycoside acetyltransferase (3)-III or IV. No additional enzymes were seen with laboratory or clinically acquired aminoglycoside resistance. Plasmids of several sizes were present in some susceptible isolates of both species, but acquired resistance was not associated with a change in the apparent size or number of these plasmids. Isolates with acquired resistance to amikacin were resistant to the other 2-deoxystreptamine aminoglycosides, but showed little or no change in MIC to streptomycin, suggesting either a difference in cellular uptake between the two groups of drugs or, more likely, different binding sites on the ribosome. Based on these studies, these authors (112) concluded that mutational resistance is the probable mechanism of acquired resistance in *M. fortuitum* and *M. chelonei* to antibacterial agents including amikacin.

An interesting study compared nephrotoxicity of two amikacin sulfate formulations in rats (113). The nephrotoxicity of Amikin and Pierene were compared using a nephrotoxicity protocol in rats. The two formulations were administered subcutaneously twice a day for 9 days at doses of amikacin ranging from 50 to 350 mg/kg/d. As expected, microscopic examination of the kidneys revealed dose-dependent renal damage in Amikin/Pierene-treated rats. The dose-response curves of the two formulations were not parallel, suggesting that the mechanisms of nephrotoxicity due to Pierene and Amikin may differ. An analysis of variance revealed that Pierene was significantly more nephrotoxic than Amikin over the common dosage levels (125, 200, 275 mg/kg/d). A possible explanation for this difference may be due to the content of 3-*N*-aminohydroxybutyric acid kanamycin A (BB-K29) in the two formulations. The Pierene product was found to contain 9–14% by weight of this relatively inactive, but acutely toxic, impurity while Amikin contained less than 1%. BB-K29, though essentially inactive microbiologically, was found to be nephrotoxic in rats.

FUTURE DIRECTIONS

Amikacin will soon replace kanamycin in the treatment of both mycobacterial and non-mycobacterial diseases. Its role in the treatment of disease caused by MAC, especially in AIDS patients, and by rapid growers like *M. fortuitum* and *M. chelonei* is promising. Its high activity in vitro and in vivo, but poor activity inside macrophages, again raises doubts about its usefulness in established infections, at which stage most of the mycobacteria will reside inside the macrophages. Since permeability factors are likely to influence its action, preparations using liposomes or other carriers with a targeted delivery objective, may be useful. Such studies are underway in our laboratories. The variations in the toxic potential of different formulations should be a warning on the possible dangers of highly toxic formulations available in several parts of the world. Likewise, the possibility should be considered that the increase in resistance to amikacin among gram-negative organisms may be followed by resistance of mycobacterial isolates.

Clofazimine

Clofazimine continues to be an important drug in the treatment of leprosy. As such, almost all studies reported in the last year concerning its clinical use, pharmacokinetics, discovery of other analogs, and the assessment of a newly identified toxic manifestation in the gastrointestinal tract, had relevance to the management of leprosy.

FUTURE DIRECTIONS

Clofazimine will continue to be an important drug, at least in the treatment of leprosy, and perhaps in the treatment of disease caused by MAC. However, its toxicity, mainly to the gastrointestinal tract following prolonged usage, should be an important consideration. If this is established, it will act as a deterrent to continuous and increased use of this drug. Several clofazimine analogs will be investigated, mainly to achieve higher serum levels and greater activity than the parent drug. Investigations on the immunopharmacologic aspects of clofazimine and its analogs will continue.

Ethionamide and prothionamide

Little work has been reported on these two drugs in the past year. A regimen containing prothionamide was investigated in South Africa in a group of 150 tuberculosis patients (114). The patients received a combination of rifampin, pyrazinamide and a preparation known as Isoprodian, which contains isoniazid and prothionamide and diphenylsulfone. All the drugs were given daily for 5 months and early analysis showed disappointing results. There were 5 treatment failures, 27 relapses and 17 patients who did not complete the prescribed regimen. Drug susceptibility in vitro of MAC strains obtained from AIDS patients showed universal resistance to ethionamide, along with other drugs (115). On the other hand, most of the *M. malmoense* strains showed susceptibility in vitro to ethionamide, and regimens containing rifampin and ethionamide were useful in treating this disease (21).

FUTURE DIRECTIONS

It is likely that ethionamide will continue to be used in the retreatment of drug-resistant tuberculosis, MAC or other non-tuberculosis mycobacterial diseases. Even though earlier studies indicated some value of prothionamide in leprosy, recent studies have not confirmed this. Prothionamide has been shown to be equal in toxicity to ethionamide, and is unlikely to replace ethionamide.

Para-aminosalicylic acid (PAS)

The few papers on PAS that have appeared during the past year dealt with its role in conventional forms of treatment of tuberculosis. As short-course chemotherapy of tuberculosis is gaining importance, necessitating discontinuation of conventional methods, PAS is becoming obsolete. Nevertheless, PAS is considered in rare cases of multiple-drug-resistant patients as the only available drug.

Even in these cases its use is limited because it is a weak bacteriostatic drug with all its added disadvantages.

As discussed in the last review (2), its use in the treatment of ulcerative colitis was investigated. Another study dealt with reduction of toxicity of PAS by charcoal and the effect of the charcoal/drug ratio on antidotal efficacy (116). At a charcoal/drug ratio of 50:1, less than 5% of the dose was absorbed, but when the ratio was increased to 2.5:1, 37% of the drug was absorbed. Even though the actual dose ratio in acute intoxication by the drug is not known, large doses (50–100 g) of activated charcoal should be used. Besides these studies, no important literature has accumulated on this drug in the past year.

Thiacetazone

In many developing countries, thiacetazone continues to be included in the standard conventional regimen comprising isoniazid and thiacetazone, with or without streptomycin or ethambutol. Wherever financially and operationally feasible, this regimen is replaced by short-course chemotherapy regimens. In rare circumstances, the use of thiacetazone as the only available drug is contemplated in the treatment of multiple-drug-resistant tuberculosis cases. Besides general reports of chemotherapy programs, no new information has been published on this drug.

Cycloserine

The few studies reported on cycloserine dealt with the susceptibility of tuberculosis and non-tuberculosis mycobacterial strains, especially from AIDS patients, and the possible use of this drug in combination with other drugs in retreatment regimens.

Summary

Mycobacterial diseases continue to be important ailments in the world. In developing and underdeveloped countries, tuberculosis and leprosy are still rampant, and extensive use of chemotherapy and immunization procedures have not made a significant dent in the epidemiologic picture. Similarly, in developed countries, mycobacterial diseases are important opportunistic infections in AIDS patients. In these countries, tuberculosis has increased slightly recently, perhaps due to increased migration of populations from developing and underdeveloped countries. These problems add to an increase in drug resistance, which makes control programs difficult. While the available drugs are being thoroughly investigated, there is a necessity to discover new drugs which are highly active, because soon many of the existing drugs will become either ineffective or unavailable in several parts of the world.

Ironically, as indicated in the introduction and earlier versions of this Chapter (1, 2), interest in the development of antimycobacterial drugs is not as active as it should be. Appeals from international agencies such as the World Health Organization and the International Union Against Tuberculosis are making little headway in the discovery of additional drugs for these purposes. On the other hand, many scientists are applying modern technology to modification of delivery of existing drugs. Attempts to modify delivery systems using liposome-encapsulated targeted systems, or by sustained release preparations, are being evaluated in experimental animals. Should these results be successful, they can probably be extended to man. Finally, a marriage between the different approaches to chemotherapy of tuberculosis and leprosy, which were divergent until recently, is a welcome and healthy development. Hopefully such unified and synergistic approaches will soon yield profitable results to achieve global control of these important diseases.

ACKNOWLEDGMENTS

I am grateful to Ms Kishori Parikh, Drs V.K. Perumal, R. Taylor, N.R. Podapati and L. Kesavalu for assistance in literature sorting and to Ms Corine Eckman for excellent secretarial assistance.

REFERENCES

1. Gangadharam PRJ, Iseman MD (1986) Antimycobacterial drugs. In: Peterson PK, Verhoef J (Eds), *The Antimicrobial Agents Annual 1*, p 17. Elsevier, Amsterdam.
2. Gangadharam PRJ, Iseman MD (1987) Antimycobacterial drugs. In: Peterson PK, Verhoef J (Eds), *The Antimicrobial Agents Annual 2*, p 14. Elsevier, Amsterdam.
3. Aquinos M (1973) Adverse reactions to daily and intermittent rifampicin and their management. In: Burley DM (Eds), *Rifampicin and Current Policies in Antituberculosis Chemotherapy*. Ciba Laboratories, Horsham, Sussex, U.K.
4. Ramakrishnan CV (1987) Rifampicin – a look back. *Lung India, 5*, 19.
5. Bagga SS, D'Costa L (1985) Present therapeutic status of rifampin. *Clinician, 49*, 375.
6. Gomi J, Aoyagi T, Fukuhara Y et al (1985) The short course therapies by Ryoken's method. *Kekkaku, 60*, 435.
7. McGavin CR (1985) Short course chemotherapy for tuberculosis of lymph nodes: a controlled trial. *Br. Med. J., 290*, 1106.
8. Skutil V, Varsa J, Obsitnik M (1985) Six month chemotherapy for urogenital tuberculosis. *Eur. Urol., 11*, 170.
9. Tanikawa K, Matsushita K, Ohkoshi M (1985) Tuberculosis of the penis: report of the case and review of the literature. *Acta Urol. Jpn., 31*, 1065.
10. Sutherland AM (1985) Drug treatment of tuberculosis of the female genital tract. *J. Obstet. Gynecol., 6*, 51.
11. Doble N, Hykin P, Shaw R, Keal EE (1985) Pulmonary *Mycobacterium tuberculosis* in acquired immune deficiency syndrome. *Br. Med. J., 291*, 849.
12. Ramana Rao G, Murthy SSN (1984) High pressure liquid chromatographic assay of rifampicin and isoniazid in dosage forms. *Indian J. Pharm. Sci., 46*, 181.
13. Gruneberg RN, Emmerson AM, Cremer AWF (1985) Rifampicin for nontuberculous infections. *Chemotherapy (Basel), 31*, 324.

14. Schraufnagel DE, Leech JA, Schraufnagel MM et al (1984) Short course chemotherapy for mycobacteriosis kansasii? *Can. Med. Assoc. J.*, *130*, 34.
15. Ahn CH, Lowell JR, Ahn SS, Ahn SI, Hurst GA (1983) Short-course chemotherapy for pulmonary disease caused by *Mycobacterium kansasii*. *Am. Rev. Respir. Dis.*, *128*, 1048.
16. Gangadharam PRJ, Pratt PF (1982) Experimental short course chemotherapy of *Mycobacterium kansasii* disease (Abstract). *Bull. Int. Un. Tuberc.*, *57*, 64.
17. Davidson PT, Waggoner R (1976) Acquired resistance to rifampicin by *Mycobacterium kansasii*. *Tubercle*, *57*, 271.
18. Ahn CH, Wallace RJ, Steele LC, Murphy DT (1987) Sulfonamide-containing regimens for disease carried by rifampin-resistant *Mycobacterium kansasii*. *Am. Rev. Respir. Dis.*, *135*, 10.
19. Warndorff Van Diepen T, Mengistu G (1985) Relapse rate and incidence of dapsone resistance in lepromatous leprosy patients in Addis Ababa: risk factors and effect of short-term supplementary treatment. *Int. J. Lepr.*, *53*, 189.
20. Bendelac A, Cambazard F, Fougerat J et al (1985) Cutaneous infections due to *Mycobacterium chelonei*: report of one case and review of the literature. *Ann. Dermatol. Venereol.*, *112*, 319.
21. Connolly MJ, Magee JG, Hendrick DJ, Jenkins PA (1985) *Mycobacterium malmoense* in the North-East of England. *Tubercle*, *66*, 211.
22. Acocella G, Carlone NA, Cuffini AM, Cavallo G (1985) The penetration of rifampicin pyrazinamide and pyrazinoic acid into mouse macrophages. *Am. Rev. Respir. Dis.*, *132*, 1268.
23. Crowle AJ, May M (1981) Preliminary demonstration of tuberculo-immunity in vitro. *Infect. Immun.*, *31*, 453.
24. Nesthus I, Haneberg B, Glette J, Solberg CO (1985) The influence of antimicrobial agents on macrophage-associated Staphylococcus aureus. *Acta Pathol. Microbiol. Immunol. Scand. Sect. B*, *93*, 189.
25. Mattson K, Janne J (1982) Mild intranasal hemolysis associated with flu-syndrome during intermittent rifampin treatment. *Eur. J. Respir. Dis.*, *63*, 68.
26. Van Assendelft AHW (1985) Leucopenia in rifampicin chemotherapy. *J. Antimicrob. Chemother.*, *16*, 407.
27. Qunibi WY, Godwin J, Eknoyan G (1980) Toxic nephropathy during continuous rifampin therapy. *South. Med. J.*, *73*, 791.
28. Farge D, Charpentier B, Simonneau G et al (1985) Rifampin and acute cellular rejection in renal transplantation. *Nephrologie*, *6*, 53.
29. Harris J, Jenkins P (1985) Discoloration of soft contact lenses by rifampicin. *Lancet*, *2*, 1133.
30. Nagata Y, Kohsaka K, Ito T (1985) Negative observations on immunologic side effects of rifampin and dapsone in mice. *Int. J. Lepr.*, *53*, 421.
31. Danon G, Lagier G, Begaud B, Couzigou P (1985) Guidelines for assessment of infectability of hepatic drug reaction. *Thérapie*, *40*, 247.
32. Craven PC, Engelhard D, Stutman HR et al (1985) Interaction of ketoconazole with rifampin and isoniazid. *N. Engl. J. Med.*, *312*, 1061.
33. Howard P, Bixler TJ, Gill B (1985) Cyclosporin-rifampin drug interaction. *Drug Intell. Clin. Pharm.*, *19*, 763.
34. Rahn KH, Mooy J, Bohm R, Van der Vet A (1985) Reduction of bioavailability of verapamil by rifampin. *N. Engl. J. Med.*, *312*, 920.
35. Abrahamson FP, Lutz MP (1986) The kinetics of induction by rifampin of alpha$_1$ acid

glycoprotein and antipyrine clearance in the dog. *Drug Metab. Dispos., 14*, 46.

36. Marcus FI (1985) Pharmacokinetic interactions between digoxin and other drugs. *J. Am. Coll. Cardiol., 5, Suppl A*, 82A.

37. Noda A, Sendo T, Ohno K et al (1985) Effect of rifampin and phenobarbital on the fate of isoniazid and hydrazine in vivo in rats. *Toxicol. Lett., 25*, 313.

38. Kay L, Kampmann JP, Svendsen TL et al (1985) Influence of rifampicin and isoniazid on the kinetics of phenytoin. *Br. J. Clin. Pharmacol., 20*, 323.

39. Timbell JA, Park BK, Harland SJ (1985) A study of the effects of rifampicin on isoniazid metabolism in human volunteer subjects. *Hum. Toxicol., 4*, 279.

40. Tsukamura M, Mizuno S, Toyana H, Ichiyama S (1986) Comparison of in vitro antimycobacterial activities of ansamycin and rifampicin. *Kekkaku, 61*, 497.

41. O'Brien RJ, Lyle MA, Johnson MW, Geiter LJ, Snider DE (1986) Preliminary experience with rifabutine (ansamycin LM-427) in the treatment of life-threatening mycobacterial disease. *Bull. Int. Un. Ag. Tuberc., 61*, 11 (Abstract No. A008).

42. Della Bruna C, Ungheri D, Sebben G, Sanfilippo A (1985) Laboratory evaluation of a new long-acting 3-azinomethylrifamycin FCE 22250. *J. Antibiot., 38*, 779.

43. Tsukamura M, Mizuno S, Toyana H (1986) In vitro antimycobacterial activity of rifapentine (comparison with rifampicin) *Kekkaku, 61*, 633.

44. Wylie GL, Scoging A, Lowrie DB (1986) Uptake and intracellular distribution of rifamycin DL-473 and rifampicin in mouse macrophages. *Bull. Int. Un. Ag. Tuberc., 61*, 11 (Abstract No. A007).

45. Tosch W, Batt E (1986) Pharmacokinetics of new long-acting rifamycin derivatives in animals. *Bull. Int. Un. Ag. Tuberc., 61*, 9 (Abstract No. A003).

46. Vischer WA, Gowrishankar R, Ashtekar DR, Costa-Pereira R, Subramanyam D, Kump W, Traxler P (1986) Antitubercular activity in vitro and in vivo of new long-acting rifamycin derivatives. *Bull. Int. Un. Ag. Tuberc., 61*, 8 (Abstract No. A002).

47. LeCoeur H, Truffob-Penot C, Grosset J (1986) Activity of CGP-29861, a new long lasting rifamycin derivative against *Mycobacterium tuberculosis* in the mouse. *Bull. Int. Un. Ag. Tuberc., 61*, 10 (Abstract No. A005).

48. Mathur IS, Gupta HP, Srivastava SK et al (1985) Evaluation of subdermal biodegradable implants incorporating rifampicin as a method of drug delivery in experimental tuberculosis of guinea pigs. *J. Med. Microbiol., 20*, 387.

49. Acocella G, Angel JH (1986) Short course chemotherapy of pulmonary tuberculosis: a new approach to drug dosage in the initial intensive phase. *Am. Rev. Respir. Dis., 134*, 1283.

50. Hong Kong Chest Service/British Medical Research Council (1986) Clinical study of a combined preparation of isoniazid, rifampicin and pyrazinamide (Rifater 3) in 3-times weekly regimens for pulmonary tuberculosis. *Bull. Int. Un. Ag. Tuberc., 61*, 19 (Abstract No. A026).

51. Sbarbaro JA (1986) Reality versus the academic milieu. *Am. Rev. Respir. Dis., 134*, 1109.

52. Grzybowsi S (1986) Isoniazid prophylaxis. *J. Am. Med. Assoc., 255*, 1615.

53. Gangadharam PRJ (1986) Isoniazid, rifampin and hepatotoxicity. *Am. Rev. Respir. Dis., 133*, 963.

54. Fox W (1985) Modern short-course regimens in the treatment of tuberculosis. *Pneumoftiziologie, 34*, 122.

55. Dutt AK, Moers D, Stead WW (1986) Short-course chemotherapy for extrapulmonary tuberculosis: nine years' experience. *Ann. Intern. Med., 104*, 7.

56. Devadatta S, Gangadharam PRJ, Andrews RH et al (1960) Peripheral neuritis due to isoniazid. *Bull. WHO, 23*, 587.

37

57. Kan GQ, Zhang LX, Wu JC, Mal ZL (1985) Supervised intermittent chemotherapy for pulmonary tuberculosis in a rural area of China. *Tubercle*, *66*, 1.
58. Griffiths DLI, Seddon H, Ball J et al (1985) A 10 year assessment of controlled trials of inpatient and outpatient treatment and of plaster-of-Paris jackets for tuberculosis of the spine in children on standard chemotherapy: studies in Masan and Pausan, Korea. *J. Bone Jt Surg.*, *67*, 103.
59. Hermida-Escobedo C, Peredo-Velarde MA (1985) Evaluation of rifampicin-isoniazid treatment in tuberculous meningitis. *Rev. Lat. Am. Microbiol.*, *27*, 277.
60. Perst RE (1985) Family tuberculosis contacts: resource contingent management. *Fam. Pract.*, *2*, 30.
61. Israel HL (1974) Stop isoniazid prophylaxis. *Ann. Intern. Med.*, *80*, 672.
62. Thompson NJ (1982) Efficacy of various durations of isoniazid preventive therapy for tuberculosis: five years of follow-up in the IUAT trial. *Bull. WHO*, *60*, 555.
63. Snider DE, Caras GJ, Kaplan JP (1986) Preventive therapy with isoniazid: cost effectiveness of different durations of therapy. *J. Am. Med. Assoc.*, *255*, 1579.
64. Paire M, LaVarenne J, Rodet MF (1984) Isoniazid inactivation in children. *Thérapie*, *39*, 625.
65. Pereira Filho RA, Seva-Pereira A, De Magalhaes AFN, Ramalho AS (1985) Isoniazid acetylation in hepatic cirrhosis. *Rev. Paul. Med.*, *103*, 276.
66. Ohnishi A, Chua CL, Kuroiwa Y (1985) Axonal degeneration distal to the site of accumulation of vesicular profiles in the myelinated fiber axon in experimental isoniazid neuropathy. *Acta Neuropathol.*, *67*, 195.
67. Ishii N, Nishihara Y (1985) Pellagra encephalopathy among tuberculous patients: its relation to isoniazid therapy. *J. Neurol. Neurosurg. Psychiatry*, *48*, 628.
68. Perry IL, Wall RA, Hansen S (1985) Brain amino compounds in a Huntington's patient on isoniazid therapy. *Neurology*, *35*, 755.
69. Bernasconi R, Klein M, Martin P et al (1985) The specific protective effect of diazepam and valproate against isoniazid-induced seizures is not correlated with increased GABA levels. *J. Neural. Transm.*, *63*, 169.
70. Kottegoda SR (1985) Cheese, wine and isoniazid. *Lancet*, *2*, 1074.
71. Tuberculosis Prevention Trial, Madras (1979) Trial of BCG vaccines in South India for tuberculosis prevention. *Indian J. Med. Res.*, *70*, 349.
72. Mitchison DA, Nunn AJ (1986) Influence of initial drug resistance on the response to short-course chemotherapy of pulmonary tuberculosis. *Am. Rev. Respir. Dis.*, *133*, 423.
73. Grosset J, Truffot-Pernot C, Poggi S et al (1985) The prevention of rifampicin resistance with pyrazinamide. *Rev. Mal. Respir.*, *2*, 205.
74. Ikeda N, Lee K (1986) Symposium on the latest topics concerning pyrazinamide (Nagasawa S, Shinoda A, Chairmen). *Kekkaku*, *60*, 25.
75. Tsukamura M, Ichiyama S (1986) Antagonistic effect of pyrazinamide against antituberculosis activity of ofloxacin in mice. *Kekkaku*, *62*, 67.
76. Tsukamura M (1985) Antituberculosis activity of ofloxacin (DL-8280) in experimental tuberculosis in mice. *Am. Rev. Respir. Dis.*, *132*, 915.
77. Heifets LB, Iseman MD, Crowle AJ, Lindholm-Levy PJ (1986) Pyrazinamide is not active against *Mycobacterium avium* complex. *Am. Rev. Respir. Dis.*, *134*, 1287.
78. McClatchy JK, Tsang AY, Cernich MS (1981) Use of pyrazinamide activity in *Mycobacterium tuberculosis* as a rapid method for determination of pyrazinamide susceptibility. *Antimicrob. Agents Chemother.*, *20*, 565.
79. Jakschik M (1985) Pyrazinamidase activity and sensitivity to pyrazinamide of tuberculosis bacteria. *Prax. Klin. Pneumol.*, *39*, 136.

80. Ashtekar DR, Fernandez F, Kale RN et al (1985) Rapid indirect pyrazinamide susceptibility testing of *Mycobacterium tuberculosis*. *IRCS Med. Sci.*, *13*, 736.

81. Heifets LB, Iseman MD (1985) Radiometric method for testing susceptibility of mycobacteria to pyrazinamide. *J. Clin. Microbiol.*, *21*, 200.

82. Mazumdar VK, Dey DC (1985) Preparation and evaluation of ethambutol derivatives. *Indian J. Pharm. Sci.*, *47*, 179.

83. Gupta PR, Purohit SD, Sharma RG, Agarwal KC (1984) Ethambutol induced optic neuritis in two brothers. *Indian J. Tuberc.*, *31*, 128.

84. Polak BCP, Leys M, Van Lith GHM (1985) Blue-yellow colour vision changes as early symptoms of ethambutol oculotoxicity. *Ophthalmologica*, *191*, 223.

85. Pau H (1985) Retinoneuritis due to myambutol (ethambutol). *Klin. Monatsbl. Augenheilkd.*, *187*, 25.

86. Crowle AJ, Sbarbaro JA, Judson FN, May MH (1985) The effect of ethambutol on tubercle bacilli within cultured human macrophages. *Am. Rev. Respir. Dis.*, *132*, 742.

87. Heifets LB, Iseman MD, Lindholm-Levy P (1986) Ethambutol MIC's and MBC's for *Mycobacterium avium* complex and *Mycobacterium tuberculosis*. *Antimicrob. Agents Chemother.*, *30*, 927.

88. Cheema S, Khuller GK (1985) Metabolism of phospholipids in *Mycobacterium smegmatis* ATCC 607 in the presence of ethambutol. *Indian J. Med. Res.*, *82*, 207.

89. Cheema S, Khuller GK (1985) Phospholipid composition and ethambutol sensitivity of *Mycobacterium smegmatis* ATCC 607. *Indian J. Exp. Biol.*, *23*, 511.

90. Cheema S, Asotra S, Khuller GK (1985) Ethambutol induced leakage of phospholipids in *Mycobacterium smegmatis*. *IRCS Med. Sci.*, *13*, 843.

91. Ramachandran P, Durai Pandian M, Nagarajan M et al (1986) Three chemotherapy studies of tuberculous meningitis in children. *Tubercle*, *67*, 17.

92. Kurosawa N, Kuribayashi S, Owada E, Ito K (1985) Determination of streptomycin in serum by high-performance liquid-chromatography. *J. Chromatogr. Biomed. Appl.*, *34*, 379.

93. Okigbo ON, Richardson GH (1985) Detection of penicillin and streptomycin in milk by impedance microbiology. *J. Food Protect.*, *48*, 979.

94. Petrenko VI (1985) Pharmacokinetics of isoniazid, rifampicin and streptomycin in tuberculous patients with chronic pulmonary heart. *Probl. Tuberkl.*, *63*, 34.

95. Distler J, Klier K, Piendl W et al (1985) Streptomycin biosynthesis in *Streptomyces griseus*. I. Characterization of streptomycin idiotrophic mutants. *FEMS Microbiol. Lett.*, *30*, 145.

96. Distler J, Mansouri K, Plepersberg W (1985) Streptomycin biosynthesis in *Streptomyces griseus*. II. Adjacent genomic location of biosynthetic genes and one of two streptomycins resistance genes. *FEMS Microbiol. Lett.*, *30*, 151.

97. Smailou SK, Gavrilova LP (1985) Effect of streptomycin on the stoichiometry of GTP hydrolysis in a poly(U)-dependent cell free translation system. *FEBS Lett.*, *192*, 165.

98. Townsend DE, Bolton S, Ashdown N, Grubb WB (1985) Transfer of plasmid-borne aminoglycoside resistance determinants in staphylococci. *J. Med. Microbiol.*, *20*, 169.

99. Livshits YaG, Timofeeva GA, Sadkov SA et al (1986) The use of antiseptic sponge with kanamycin in outpatient dental surgery. *Stomatologiya (Moscow)*, *65*, 50.

100. Kubo H, Kobayashi Y, Nishikawa T (1985) Rapid method for determination of kanamycin and dibekacin in serum by use of high-pressure liquid chromatography. *Antimicrob. Agents Chemother.*, *28*, 521.

101. Nakaya KI, Sugitani A, Yamada F (1985) A new ECD gas chromatographic determination of kanamycin in beef. *J. Food Hyg. Soc. Jpn*, *26*, 443.

102. Yalcindag ON (1985) Identification of some aminoglycoside antibiotics with micro-cristallography. *J. Pharm. Belg.*, *40*, 249.

103. Weber A, Smith AL, Opheim KE (1985) Radioenzymatic assays for aminoglycosides with kanamycin 6′-acetyltransferase. *J. Clin. Microbiol.*, *21*, 419.

104. Schurman DJ, Kajiyama G (1985) Antibiotic absorption from infected and normal joints using a rabbit knee joint model. *J. Orthop. Res.*, *3*, 185.

105. Yoshida M, Koeda T (1985) Effects of aminoglycoside antibiotics on the contractile response of guinea-pig urinary bladder. *Chemotherapy (Tokyo)*, *33*, 447.

106. Wasterstrom SA, Bredberg G, Lindquist NG et al (1986) Ototoxicity of kanamycin in albino and pigmented guinea pigs. I. Amorphologic and electrophysiologic study. *Am. J. Otol.*, *7*, 11.

107. Davis RR, Brummett RE, Bendrick TW, Himes DL (1984) Dissociation of maximum concentration of kanamycin in plasma and perilymph from ototoxic effect. *J. Antimicrob. Chemother.*, *14*, 291.

108. Prieva BA, Yanz JL (1984) Age dependent changes in susceptibility to ototoxic hearing loss. *Acta Otolaryngol.*, *98*, 428.

109. Neschetnaya LB (1986) Experimental morphologic data on the preventive effect of 4-methyluracil upon ototoxic action of monomycin and kanamycin. *Zh. Ushn. Nos. Gorl. Bolezn.*, *46*, 13.

110. Kesavalu L, Gangadharam PRJ, Perumal VK, Podapati NR, Iseman MD (1987) Chemotherapeutic activity of amikacin against *Mycobacterium avium intracellulare*. In: *Abstracts, 87th Annual Meeting of American Society for Microbiology, Atlanta, GA*, Abstract No. U67.

111. Wallace Jr RJ, Swenson JM, Silcox VA, Bullen MG (1985) Treatment of nonpulmonary infections due to *Mycobacterium fortuitum* and *Mycobacterium chelonei* on the basis of in vitro susceptibilities. *J. Infect. Dis.*, *152*, 500.

112. Wallace Jr RJ, Hall SI, Bobey DG et al (1985) Mutational resistance as the mechanism of acquired drug resistance to aminoglycosides and antibacterial agents in *Mycobacterium fortuitum* and *Mycobacterium chelonei*. *Am. Rev. Respir. Dis.*, *132*, 409.

113. Williams PD, Reilly CM, Hottendorf GH (1985) Comparative nephrotoxicity of 2 amikacin sulfate formulations in rats. *Curr. Ther. Res. Clin. Exp.*, *37*, 1030.

114. Largton ME, Cowie RL (1985) Failure of a prothionamide containing oral antituberculosis regimen. *S. Afr. Med. J.*, *68*, 881.

115. Kiehn TE, Edwards FF, Brannon P et al (1985) Infections caused by *Mycobacterium avium* complex in immunocompromised patients: diagnosis by blood culture and fecal examination, antimicrobial susceptibility tests and morphological and seroagglutination characteristics. *J. Clin. Microbiol.*, *21*, 168.

116. Olkkola KT (1985) Effect of charcoal-drug ratio on antidotal efficacy of oral activated charcoal in man. *Br. J. Clin. Pharmacol.*, *19*, 767.

117. Hallett M, Lindsey JW, Adelstein LD, Riley PO (1985) Controlled trial of isoniazid therapy for severe postural cerebellar tremor in multiple sclerosis. *Neurology*, *35*, 1374.

118. Neis JM, Harp SW, Roelofs HMJ et al (1986) Mutagenicity and DNA-excision repair induced by isoniazid after metabolic activation by isolated human and rat hepatocytes. *Cancer Lett.*, *30*, 103.

CHAPTER 3

Antibiotic therapy for leprosy

ROBERT R. JACOBSON

Progress in leprosy, as with most diseases, continues to be measured in inches and feet rather than miles. Monotherapy with dapsone or clofazimine is still widely employed to treat leprosy and is usually effective if taken regularly. Compliance continues to be a problem because of the 3–7 years required to treat paucibacillary (indeterminate, tuberculoid and borderline-tuberculoid) cases and the necessity for lifetime therapy in multibacillary (mid-borderline, borderline-lepromatous and lepromatous) patients. Relapse is common and a serious problem with primary and secondary dapsone resistance has arisen so that monotherapy can no longer be recommended. Also it is hoped that multidrug therapy utilizing rifampin will allow a shortened treatment interval. Current recommendations in the United States and those of the World Health Organization (WHO) are shown in Table 1. The U.S. approach is to continue dapsone (or clofazimine) several years for paucibacillary cases and indefinitely in multibacillary cases after an initial course of combination drug therapy. Trials currently underway will determine whether 6 months therapy for paucibacillary cases and 2 years for multibacillary patients as recommended by WHO are sufficient. These will require at least a decade of follow-up to measure adequately the relapse rate; thus, it may be 5–10 more years before the issue is resolved to everyone's satisfaction.

This year saw publication of a landmark article (1) describing the results of 20 years of supervised sulfone monotherapy followed by discontinuance in multibacillary cases in Malaysia. They found a relapse rate of about 1% per year. This undoubtedly represents the best one could do with monotherapy and underscores the need to use multidrug therapy. A study (2) in India suggests that reinfection as well as relapse may occur in endemic areas, but this is not documented. Monotherapy works much better for paucibacillary disease which is more common than multibacillary with a long-term relapse rate of only 2.4% noted in a recent study (3) of cases who defaulted before completing therapy. Few control programs do this well, however, and the shortened treatment period that multidrug therapy may allow could be an important advance. The success possible with multidrug therapy for paucibacillary patients is illustrated in an Ethiopian trial (4) where

Antimicrobial Agents Annual 3
P.K. Peterson and J. Verhoef, editors
© Elsevier Science Publishers BV, 1988

Table 1   *Current leprosy treatment recommendations*

Type of disease	GWL Hansen's Disease Center		WHO regimens
	Patients infected with dapsone-sensitive *M. leprae*	Patients infected with dapsone-resistant *M. leprae*	All patients
Paucibacillary	Dapsone 100 mg/d for 4–7 years depending on classification + Rifampin 600 mg/d for first 6 months*	Clofazimine 50–100 mg/d for 4–7 years depending on classification † + Rifampin 600 mg/d for first 6 months*	Dapsone 100 mg/d for 6 months, unsupervised + Rifampin 600 mg once monthly for 6 months, supervised
Multibacillary	Dapsone 100 mg/d for life + Rifampin 600 mg/d for first 3 years*,**	Clofazimine 50–100 mg/d for life + Rifampin 600 mg/d for first 3 years*	Dapsone 100 mg/d with clofazimine 50 mg/d, both unsupervised + Rifampin 600 mg with clofazimine 300 mg both given once monthly, supervised ††

*Rifampin is occasionally given in a dose of 600 mg once monthly.
**Clofazimine is occasionally added as a third drug, particularly if the sensitivity of the patient's bacilli to dapsone is unknown.
† If the patient will not take clofazimine, rifampin + ethionamide (250 mg/d) is substituted and the combination continued for the same time intervals as clofazimine.
†† Treatment with all 3 drugs is continued at least 2 years and preferably to bacterial negativity.

nearly 90% completed the standard WHO 6-month regimen.

The search for a method simpler than the mouse footpad technique to perform drug sensitivity testing and to measure bacterial viability continues. A recent report (5) details simple fluorescent staining techniques yielding a more accurate measure of viability than the morphologic index, but confirmation is needed. Several investigators (6) utilize measurement of decay of adenosine triphosphate levels in *Mycobacterium leprae* exposed to various drugs for sensitivity testing, but it must be considered investigational until controlled trials of this and other methods are done. The neonatally thymectomized Lewis rat (NTLR) has been demonstrated (7) to be superior to the mouse footpad technique for detecting persistent viable bacilli in clinical drug trials, but the large number of bacilli required necessitates large biopsies and limit its usefulness. Reports of primary (8) and secondary (9) dapsone resistance continue to appear. Primary resistance fortunately continues to be mostly low-level, so dapsone generally remains an effective component of multidrug therapy. Although mostly low-level, primary resistance seems to be a relatively new occurrence since strains of *M. leprae* isolated by several groups prior to 1977 showed (10) no evidence of resistance to even low dapsone levels.

Dapsone

Dapsone has been used for the treatment of leprosy since the 1940s, and remains the most commonly prescribed drug today in spite of a significant problem with dapsone-resistant *M. leprae* infecting many patients. The drug is weakly bactericidal for *M. leprae* and its mechanism of action involves competitive inhibition with para-aminobenzoic acid for the enzyme, dihydropteroate synthetase, thereby blocking the synthesis of dihydrofolic acid. When dapsone resistance develops, the change is not reversed by multiple passages in the mouse footpad, suggesting that it is genotypic (11). Dapsone also has anti-inflammatory activity and a recent study (12) suggests that this is due to an antioxidant action of the drug exerted by quenching oxygen intermediates from polymorphonuclear leukocytes without affecting phospholipid transmethylation of the cell membranes. Others (13) have noted a mild suppression of the immune response in borderline leprosy patients with reactive lesions.

Monitoring dapsone intake is considered vital if short-term multidrug therapy is to be a success and a number of methods are being evaluated. Most investigators continue to use the spot test for urinary dapsone which utilizes filter papers impregnated with a modified Ehrlich's reagent. A hemagglutination inhibition test is reportedly (14) much more sensitive, but the older spot test is simpler and considered sufficient by most investigators (15, 16).

ADVERSE EFFECTS

Hemolytic anemia is the most common adverse effect and it may be more severe in those with a glucose-6-phosphate dehydrogenase (G-6-PD) deficiency. Agranulocytosis is the most serious complication, but in the last few years an apparent small increase in the incidence of the dapsone syndrome has generated some interest. This was first reported in the early days of sulfone therapy; in the most severe cases exfoliative dermatitis, a generalized lymphadenopathy, hepatosplenomegaly, fever and a hepatitis may develop, and deaths have occurred. Most reported cases have less than the full symptom complex (17). Patients usually recover with therapy which consists of discontinuing the dapsone and giving corticosteroids. Sharma et al (18) reported 3 cases occurring in 1200 patients given dapsone and another report (19) details its occurrence in 2 brothers being treated for multibacillary leprosy. Whether the prevalence of this problem has increased because higher average doses of dapsone are used today or it is simply being recognized and reported with greater regularity is unknown. Toxicity problems from the sulfonamides have been noted more frequently in patients who are slow acetylators (20), but whether the same is true of the sulfones is not known. Another report (21) notes that dapsone is apparently safe during pregnancy.

FUTURE DIRECTIONS

There seems to be little interest in the development of new sulfones, but a long-acting preparation given intra-adiposely once monthly is under investigation in clinical trials (22).

Rifampin and other rifamycins

Rifampin (rifampicin) is discussed in detail in Chapters 2 and 16. It is markedly bactericidal for *M. leprae* with a single dose of 600 mg or more rapidly killing the bacilli as measured in the mouse footpad. Studies with the NTLR (7) suggest that a higher dose (1500 mg) is more rapidly bactericidal, but the results did not attain statistical significance. Persistent viable bacilli remain (23) even after high doses, but their significance in terms of attempts to shorten therapy remain uncertain. Groenen et al (24) suggest that the marked bactericidal activity of higher or more frequent doses of rifampin may result in more frequent reactive episodes in both paucibacillary and multibacillary leprosy cases, but this has yet to be confirmed by others.

Rifampin's relatively high cost among anti-leprosy drugs has been a stimulus to find ways of maximizing its effectiveness. Thus probenecid reportedly (25) increased serum levels produced by a 300 mg dose, but it is difficult to see any advantage to this since just 600 mg once monthly is apparently very effective in the WHO regimens. Mehta et al (26) studied the effects of dapsone and clofazimine on rifampin's pharmacokinetics in leprosy cases. Dapsone had no effect, but clofazimine reduced rifampin's absorption and the combination of dapsone and clofazimine also reduced rifampin's serum levels. Though statistically significant, the changes observed are unlikely to be significant clinically.

ADVERSE EFFECTS

Although hepatotoxicity is rifampin's major side effect, particularly when it is given with a thioamide, other serious side effects may occasionally occur. Two groups report (27, 28) single cases of acute renal failure in patients receiving 1500 and 600 mg of rifampin once monthly, both of whom eventually recovered. Although too much weight should not be given to a single case-report, its occurrence in a patient receiving only 600 mg once monthly (28) is of some concern since that is the keystone of the WHO regimens and it had been thought that this was unlikely at that dose level. A fixed drug eruption has also been reported (29) in a leprosy patient on intermittent rifampin, but the problem had no serious sequelae.

FUTURE DIRECTIONS

Although at least one clinical trial is underway using ansamycin to treat multibacillary leprosy cases, it, rifapentine, and other rifamycins are unlikely to improve on the results attained to date with rifampin. Thus, future efforts are likely to concentrate more on maximizing the effectiveness of rifampin than on new drug development.

Clofazimine

Clofazimine is also reviewed in Chapter 2 because of its activity against other mycobacteria, but its major application is in the treatment of leprosy. It was approved in December 1986, by the Food and Drug Administration for the treatment of leprosy in the United States, so it is no longer considered investigational.

Clofazimine has been used to treat leprosy since the 1960s and although it was originally given only to those with sulfone-resistant disease, it is now widely prescribed as part of multidrug therapy in the standard WHO multibacillary regimen. It is also used extensively for the management of both reversal (Type 1) and erythema nodosum leprosum (ENL, Type 2) reactions occurring in leprosy cases during chemotherapy. It is weakly bactericidal for *M. leprae*, but its mechanisms of action for this and its apparent anti-inflammatory effects in reactive episodes are unknown. About 63% of a 100 mg dose is absorbed from the gastrointestinal tract. It accumulates at multiple tissue sites and clears very slowly after being discontinued. Its half-life has been estimated at 70 days.

During the year under review a second case infected with clofazimine-resistant *M. leprae* has been reported (30). Interestingly the patient had never received clofazimine, so the meaning of this result, if it can be confirmed by others, is uncertain. The previously reported case (31) was not confirmed on subsequent mouse footpad studies (32).

ADVERSE EFFECTS

Many patients find the skin pigmentation produced by clofazimine cosmetically unacceptable. This diminishes gradually as the disease clears even though the patient may remain on clofazimine. Its accumulation in the bowel wall can lead to edema of the wall with effacement of the mucosa producing obstructive symptoms. This is uncommon in patients who are taking 100 mg/d or less, but mild abdominal pain may occur. The gastrointestinal effects of clofazimine were recently studied (33) in 15 patients receiving 100 or 300 mg daily over a 3-month interval. Mild diarrhea occurred in 4 and fecal fat excretion increased in 1 patient, but no changes were produced in the jejunal mucosa except for clofazimine crystals in the lamina propria of 1 case. A study (34) in rats fed clofazimine demonstrated increased deposition of the drug in Peyer's patches. Crystal-containing epithelioid cell granulomas were noted within the patches and the draining mesenteric lymph nodes. These changes occurred after only a few doses and whether they have any relation to the enteropathy observed in man is unknown.

FUTURE DIRECTIONS

Attempts to develop derivatives of clofazimine that are non-pigmenting and/or demonstrate increased bactericidal activity continue. Though unsuccessful to date, this work will continue because of its importance to leprosy control efforts.

Ethionamide and prothionamide

These two preparations may be considered identical from the point of view of activity and toxicity. Both are bactericidal for *M. leprae*, intermediate between dapsone/clofazimine and rifampin in this regard. Ethionamide is readily absorbed from the gastrointestinal tract and is rapidly distributed throughout the body with a half-life of about 3 hours. The effect of prothionamide on the metabolic distribution of dapsone and rifampin was recently studied (35) and no significant changes were observed.

ADVERSE EFFECTS

Hepatitis and various gastrointestinal complaints are the major side effects. A recent study (36) of 100 patients, e.g. found hepatitis twice as common in a regimen containing prothionamide, dapsone and rifampin as in one with clofazimine substituted for the prothionamide. Another (37) found ethionamide and prothionamide as acceptable as dapsone to patients, but the doses employed were low (125–250 mg).

FUTURE DIRECTIONS

Attempts have been made to find derivatives with greater activity and less toxicity, so far without success. Ultimately, alternative drugs now under study are likely to replace them in most control programs.

Other drugs

Thiacetazone is still used to treat leprosy in many Third World countries mainly because of its low cost. Since it is only bacteriostatic against *M. leprae*, most control programs are gradually abandoning its use in favor of the standard WHO multidrug therapy regimens. The aminoglycosides streptomycin, amikacin and kanamycin are bactericidal against *M. leprae* when given in high doses in mouse footpad studies (38) and streptomycin was occasionally used to treat leprosy in the past. Because of their high cost and the need to give them by injection for prolonged periods, they are of relatively little value for the management of leprosy cases.

Desoxyfructoserotonin is bacteriostatic for *M. leprae* and although it may also have some immunostimulatory activity (39), it has attracted little interest as an anti-leprosy drug thus far.

The quinoline ciprofloxacin showed (40) no activity against *M. leprae* in the mouse footpad system. However, the authors note that the pharmacokinetics of the drug may be quite different in the mouse, so that the findings are not necessarily applicable to human leprosy. This and other quinolines are undergoing further study and there is considerable hope that at least one important new anti-leprosy drug will emerge from this group.

There is extensive research activity (41) directed toward elucidating the structure and genetics of *M. leprae* which it is hoped will lead to new drug development. Unfortunately it will obviously be many years before new drugs could evolve from such basic research.

Immunotherapy

It is believed that leprosy develops only in those patients with a specific defect in their cell-mediated immune response to *M. leprae*. Thus, when exposed to the bacillus, these individuals will allow it to grow to varying degrees depending upon the extent of the defect. Current antimicrobial therapy obviously has proven very successful in destroying nearly all viable *M. leprae*. A tiny number of persistent viables remain, however, and relapse is always possible. There is therefore a considerable interest in immunotherapy which might reverse the immune defect and at the same time assist, or even circumvent, conventional antimicrobial therapy for this disease. Vaccination with a mixture of heat-killed *M. leprae* and BCG is reportedly (42) effective in this regard, but this work needs confirmation by others. At least one trial of transfer factor (43) and more recently interferon-γ (44) also demonstrated some activity. Other reports (45) also suggest that the defect is potentially correctable. Thus, we are likely to see a continued high level of interest and research in this approach to treatment.

Summary

Although there were no major developments in the year under review, important progress continues to be made in the therapy of leprosy. Most important is the continued success of short-term multidrug therapy with relatively few relapses to date. It will be several years before we can adequately gauge the success of this approach, but thus far the results are surprisingly good. The promise the quinolines hold for yielding an important new anti-leprosy drug is encouraging and more data should be available within the next year. Work on the structure and genetics of *M. leprae* is making important progress and though clinical application of these findings may be several years away, it bodes well for the future of leprosy control and treatment. Our knowledge of the immune defect in leprosy patients also continues to increase rapidly and with our better understanding of the problem the chances of a successful immunotherapeutic approach increase.

REFERENCES

1. Waters MFR, Rees RJW, Laing ABG, Fah KK, Meade TW, Parikshak N, North WRS (1986) The rate of relapse in lepromatous leprosy following completion of 20 years of supervised sulfone therapy. *Lepr. Rev., 57*, 101.
2. Almeida JG, Jesudasan K, Christian M, Chacko CJG (1986) Relapse rates in lepromatous leprosy according to treatment regularity. *Int. J. Lepr., 54*, 16.
3. Jesudasan K, Bradley D, Christian M (1985) Are defaulters with paucibacillary leprosy a problem? *Indian J. Lepr., 57*, 354.
4. Becx-Bleumink M (1986) Implementation of multidrug therapy in the ALERT leprosy programme in the Shoa Region of Ethiopia: first results with paucibacillary patients. *Lepr. Rev., 57*, 111.
5. Odinsen O, Nilson T, Humber DP (1986) Viability of *Mycobacterium leprae*: a comparison of morphologic index and fluorescent staining techniques in slit-skin smears and *M. leprae* suspensions. *Int. J. Lepr., 54*, 403.
6. Kvach JT, Neubert TA, Palomino JC, Heine HS (1986) Adenosine triphosphate content of *Mycobacterium leprae* isolated from armadillo tissue by percoll buoyant density centrifugation. *Int. J. Lepr., 54*, 1.
7. Gelber RH, Humphres RC, Fieldsteel AH (1986) Superiority of the neonatally thymectomized Lewis rat (NTLR) to monitor a clinical trial in lepromatous leprosy of the two regimens of rifampin and dapsone. *Int. J. Lepr., 54*, 273.
8. Gonzalez AB, Hernandez O, Suarez O, Gonzalez-Abreu E, Rodriguez JE (1986) Survey for primary dapsone resistance in Cuba. *Lepr. Rev., 57*, 341.
9. Dos Santos Damasco MH, Talhari S, Viana SM, Signorelli M, Saad MHF, Andrade LMC (1986) Secondary dapsone-resistant leprosy in Brazil: a preliminary report. *Lepr. Rev., 57*, 5.

10. Shepard CC, Rees RJW, Levy L, Pattyn SR, Ji Baohong, Dela Cruz EC (1986) Susceptibility of strains of *Mycobacterium leprae* isolated prior to 1977 from patients with previously untreated lepromatous leprosy. *Int. J. Lepr.*, *54*, 11.

11. Prabhakaran K, Harris EB, Hastings RC (1986) Dapsone-resistance in *Mycobacterium leprae*: a genotypic change. *IRCS Med. Sci.*, *14*, 829.

12. Miyachi Y, Niwa Y (1985) Anti-inflammatory action mechanisms of dapsone. *Acta Dermatol.*, *80*, 213.

13. Rao SSL, Stanley JNA, Kiran KU, Rao TD, Rao PR, Pearson JMH (1986) The effect of dapsone in high and normal dosage on the clinical and cell-mediated immune status of patients with borderline (BT-BL) leprosy. *Lepr. Rev.*, *57*, 19.

14. DeWit M, Balakrishnan S, Kumar A (1985) Application of HI test for dapsone in urine under field conditions. *Indian J. Lepr.*, *57*, 318.

15. Van Asbeck-Raat AM, Becx-Bleumink M (1986) Monitoring dapsone self-administration in a multidrug therapy programme. *Lepr. Rev.*, *57*, 121.

16. Huikeshoven H, Madarang MG (1986) Spot test for detection of dapsone in urine: an assessment of its validity and interpretation in monitoring dapsone self-administration. *Int. J. Lepr.*, *54*, 21.

17. Johnson DA, Cattau Jr EL, Kuritsky JN, Zimmerman HJ (1986) Liver involvement in the sulfone syndrome. *Arch. Intern. Med.*, *146*, 875.

18. Sharma VK, Kaur S, Kumar B, Singh M (1985) Dapsone syndrome in India. *Indian J. Lepr.*, *57*, 807.

19. Jamrozik K (1986) Dapsone syndrome occurring in two brothers. *Lepr. Rev.*, *57*, 57.

20. Neil H, Spielberg SP, Grant DM, Tang BK, Kalow W (1986) Differences in metabolism of sulfonamides predisposing to idiosyncratic toxicity. *Ann. Intern. Med.*, *105*, 179.

21. Kahn G (1985) Dapsone is safe during pregnancy. *J. Am. Acad. Dermatol.*, *13*, 838.

22. Pieters FAJM, Zuidema J, Merkus FWHM (1986) Sustained release properties of an intra-adiposely administered dapsone depot injection. *Int. J. Lepr.*, *54*, 383.

23. Walters MFR, Rees RJW, Pearson JMH, Laing ABG, Hemly HS, Gelber RH (1978) Rifampicin in lepromatous leprosy: nine years experience. *Br. Med. J.*, *1*, 133.

24. Groenen G, Janssens L, Kayembe T, Nollet E, Coussens L, Pattyn SR (1986) Prospective study on the relationship between intensive bactericidal therapy and leprosy reactions. *Int. J. Lepr.*, *54*, 236.

25. Panka R, Lal S, Rao RS (1985) Effect of probenecid on serum rifampicin levels. *Indian J. Lepr.*, *57*, 329.

26. Mehta J, Gandhi IS, Sane SB, Wamburkar MN (1985) Effect of clofazimine and dapsone on rifampicin pharmacokinetics in multibacillary and paucibacillary leprosy cases. *Indian J. Lepr.*, *57*, 297.

27. Dedhia NM, Almeida AF, Khanna UB, Mittal BV, Acharya VM (1986) Acute renal failure – a complication of new multidrug regimen for treatment of leprosy. *Int. J. Lepr.*, *54*, 380.

28. Chen HS, Yeh JC, Yang CS, Lin JF, Lin ML (1984) Acute interstitial nephritis associated with renal failure induced by rifampin – a case report. *J. Formosan Med. Assoc.*, *83*, 1053.

29. Naik RPC, Balachandran C, Ramnarayan K (1985) Fixed eruption due to rifampicin. *Indian J. Lepr.*, *57*, 648.

30. Kar HK, Bhatia VN, Harikrishnan S (1986) Combined clofazimine and dapsone resistant leprosy: a case report. *Int. J. Lepr.*, *54*, 389.

31. Warndorff-Van Diepen T (1982) Clofazimine resistant leprosy: a case report. *Int. J. Lepr.*, *51*, 39.
32. Levy L (1986) Clofazimine resistant *M. leprae*. *Int. J. Lepr.*, *54*, 137.
33. Bhasin DK, Kumar B, Broor SL, Kaur S, Malik AM, Mehra SK (1985) Effect of clofazimine: detailed studies of small intestine functions. *Indian J. Lepr.*, *57*, 364.
34. Levine S, Saltzaman A (1986) Clofazimine enteropathy: possible relation to Peyer's patches. *Int. J. Lepr.*, *54*, 392.
35. Mathur A, Venkatesan A, Girdhar BK, Bharadwaj VP, Girdhar A, Bagga AK (1986) A study of drug interactions in leprosy. I. Effect of simultaneous administration of prothionamide on metabolic disposition of rifampicin and dapsone. *Lepr. Rev.*, *57*, 33.
36. Kar HK, Balakrishnan S, Kumar GV, Sirumban P, Roy RG (1985) Hepatitis and multidrug therapy in leprosy with special reference to prothionamide. *Indian J. Lepr.*, *57*, 78.
37. Stanley JNA, Pearson JMH, Ellard GA (1986) Ethionamide, prothionamide, and thiacetazone self-administration: studies of patient compliance using isoniazid-marked formulations. *Lepr. Rev.*, *57*, 9.
38. Gelber RH, Henika PR, Gibson JB (1984) The bactericidal activity of various aminoglycoside antibiotics against *Mycobacterium leprae* in mice. *Lepr. Rev.*, *55*, 341.
39. Ambrose EJ, Antia NH, Birdi TJ, Mahadevan PR, Mester L, Mistry NF, Mukherjee F, Shetty V (1985) The action of deoxyfructose serotonin on intracellular bacilli and on host response in leprosy. *Lepr. Rev.*, *56*, 199.
40. Banerjee DK (1986) Ciprofloxacin (4-quinolone) and *Mycobacterium leprae*. *Lepr. Rev.*, *57*, 159.
41. Jacobs WR, Docherty MA, Curtiss III R, Clark-Curtiss JE (1986) Expressions of *Mycobacterium leprae* genes from a *Streptococcus mutans* promoter in *Escherichia coli* K-12. *Proc. Natl Acad. Sci. USA*, *83*, 1926.
42. Convit J, Aranzazu N, Ulrich M, Pinardi ME, Reyes O, Alvarado J (1982) Immunotherapy with a mixture of *Mycobacterium leprae* and BCG in different forms of leprosy and in Mitsuda-negative contacts. *Int. J. Lepr.*, *50*, 415.
43. Hastings RC (1977) Transfer factor as a probe of the immune deficit in lepromatous leprosy. *Int. J. Lepr.*, *45*, 281.
44. Nathan CF, Kaplan G, Levis WR, Nusrat A, Witmer MD, Sherwin SA, Job CK, Horowitz CR, Steinman RM, Cohn ZA (1986) Local and systemic effects of intradermal recombinant interferon-γ in patients with lepromatous leprosy. *N. Engl. J. Med.*, *315*, 6.
45. Mohogheghpour N, Gelber RR, Engleman EG (1987) T cell defect in lepromatous leprosy is reversible in vitro in the absence of exogenous growth factors. *J. Immunol.*, *138*, 570.

CHAPTER 4

Aztreonam

J.D. WILLIAMS

Since the publication of *Annual 2* relatively few new data on aztreonam have appeared in the literature and the discussion which follows continues to represent a current perspective regarding this agent.

Aztreonam is the first member of a new class of β-lactams to be available for treatment of patients. The monocyclic β-lactams differ from the heterocyclic structures of other β-lactams in that activation of the β-lactam ring is by way of a sulfonic acid substituent in the 1-position (Fig. 1) (1).

Monocyclic compounds might be expected to differ in many respects from classical β-lactams and this is in fact the case. This review will focus upon the differences which are seen between monocyclic and heterocyclic β-lactams.

ACTIVITY

The activity of aztreonam is specifically directed against aerobic gram-negative bacteria. The mode of action is similar to that of other β-lactams active against gram-negative bacteria, namely by inactivation of he penicillin-binding proteins (PBP), aztreonam having particular affinity for PBP-3 (2, 3), producing filament formation.

The in-vitro activity against aerobic gram-negative bacteria is shown in Table 1.

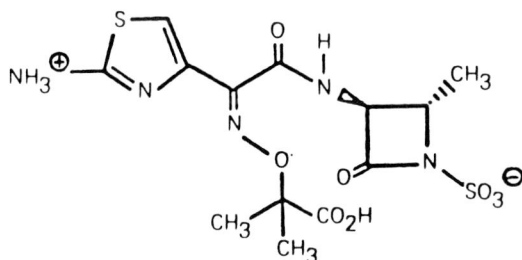

Fig. 1   Structure of aztreonam.

Antimicrobial Agents Annual 3
P.K. Peterson and J. Verhoef, editors
©Elsevier Science Publishers BV, 1988

Table 1   *Activity of aztreonam against aerobic gram-negative bacteria*

Organism	Minimum inhibitory concentration (mg/l)		
	Mode	MIC_{90}	95% range
Escherichia coli	0.25	0.5	0.12–1
Citrobacter	0.25	0.5	0.12–1
Klebsiella pneumonia	0.5	0.5	0.25–1
Proteus mirabilis	0.12	0.25	0.06–4
Proteus vulgaris	0.12	0.25	0.06–4
Providencia	0.1	0.25	<0.1–0.5
Enterobacter spp.	0.5	4	0.12–50
Serratia	0.5	1	0.12–2
Pseudomonas spp.	2	8	1–64
Acinetobacter	2	8	1–64
Neisseria gonorrhoeae	0.03	0.12	0.03–0.25
Haemophilus influenzae	0.03	0.06	0.03–0.12
Fusobacterium	1		64

Many studies have shown that the activity against Enterobacteriaceae is fairly uniform with a 95% range of susceptibility of 0.03–1 mg/l (4–6). Very few strains overall fall outside this range, although occasional reports of higher inhibitory levels have been reported when specially selected collections of multiresistant isolates have been tested (7, 8). *Pseudomonas, Alcaligenes, Enterobacter* and *Acinetobacter* are less susceptible than enterobacteria with minimal inhibitory concentrations (MICs) within a range of 0.5–4 mg/l (9) and hemophilic organisms such as *Neisseria gonorrhoeae* and *Haemophilus influenzae* are more susceptible than Enterobacteriaceae with MICs within the 0.01–0.12 mg/l range (10, 11). Occasional strains fall outside these ranges, but one feature of the numerous in-vitro studies is the uniformity of results. Different values have been reported for shigellae where strains from the United Kingdom (11, 12) appear more sensitive than strains from the United States (5); this may represent either strain or methodological differences.

The organisms against which aztreonam has no useful activity are listed in Table 2. The number of species is large and includes many organisms which are part of the normal flora as well as common pathogens. Again, uniform results have been reported from a large number of in-vitro studies (5, 9, 11). Infections with these organisms are not likely to respond to aztreonam therapy nor (as will be shown later) are these organisms likely to be eradicated from the skin or mucous membranes.

Other microbiological features of importance are the stability to gram-negative β-lactamases, the ability to induce chromosomally mediated β-lactamases, the

Table 2   *Bacteria against which aztreonam has little or no activity*

Organism	Minimum inhibitory concentration (mg/ml)	
	Range	Mode
Streptococci Groups A, C, G	8–64	32
Streptococci Group D	>128	>128
Streptococcus pneumoniae	64	64
Staphylococcus aureus	1024	1024
Coagulase-negative staphylococci	>100	>100
Bacteroides fragilis	0.5–128	64
Bacteroides asaccharolyticus	0.1–128	16
Anaerobic cocci	1–128	128
Clostridium	>128	>128

ability to elicit resistance in infecting organisms during treatment, and the extent of cross-resistance to aztreonam, if resistance is present to other β-lactam antibiotics. Table 3 lists some of these general properties of aztreonam in comparison with selected representative β-lactams. This problem cannot be presented too simplistically, however, because there are always exceptions to general rules and the relative importance of different mechanisms of resistance varies considerably among bacterial species. Aztreonam is stable to most of the wide range of transferable and some chromosomal β-lactamases against which this antibiotic has been examined (9, 10). Reports have been published on slow hydrolysis by PSE-2 enzyme detectable by bioassay (9) and more rapid hydrolysis by the chromosomal enzyme of *Klebsiella oxytoca* (13). Aztreonam is a poor inducer of chromosomally mediated β-lactamases (13) which are reported to be of increasing clinical significance (14, 15). Aztreonam is also able to inhibit chromosomal β-lactamases (16). When β-lactam resistance in gram-negative bacteria is due to intrinsic problems of passage through the outer membrane, the resistance appears to apply to all β-lactam antibiotics. Organisms in which this is likely to be of common occurrence include *Pseudomonas aeruginosa* (17) and *N. gonorrhoeae*. When enzymic mechanisms are present, the cross-resistance will depend on the type of enzyme present as to whether or not the antibiotic is a candidate substrate for that particular enzyme. The selection of resistant mutants during treatment is not a prominent feature of any β-lactam antibiotic. Resistant strains may emerge due to selection of a proportion of a heterogeneous population or by inducing enzymic mechanisms (18). At the present time, this has not been reported to be a significant feature of aztreonam. Aztreonam is a poor inducer (19) and a poor substrate (20) for β-lactamases.

Table 3   *Microbiological features of aztreonam compared to selected β-lactam antibiotics*

	Ampicillin	Mezlocillin	Carboxy-penicillin	Cefal-otin	Cefoxitin	Ceftazidime	Thienamycin	Aztreonam
Spectrum								
Gram-positive	+	+	±	++	±	±	+	–
Gram-negative aerobic	+	+	+	+	+	++	++	++
Gram-negative anaerobic	±	±	±	–	++	–	++	–
Stability to β-lactamase								
Staphylococcal	–	–	–	+	+	+	+	+
Transferable Gram-negative	–	–	–	–	+	+	+	++
Chromosomal Gram-negative	±	±	+	–	+	±	±	+
β-Lactamase-inducing ability	+	±	±	+	++	±	++	–
Cross-resistance								
Intrinsic mechanism	+	+	+	+	+	+	–	+
β-Lactamase mechanism	+	+	+	+	–	–	–	–
Selection of resistance mutants on therapy	–	±	–	–	–	–	±	–

Effect on gastrointestinal flora

Most forms of antibiotic therapy result in some eradication of the normal bacterial flora and the replacement of this flora by other organisms resistant to the antibiotics being exhibited. For example, tetracycline may lead to the overgrowth of *Proteus* or *Candida* species in a patient, whereas ampicillin therapy may be complicated by the emergence of *Klebsiella* species and cephalosporin therapy by the appearance of *P. aeruginosa*. Broad-spectrum activity against a wide range of organisms can be a disadvantage if large amounts of the normal flora have been ablated. Several studies have been made of aztreonam in both animals and man. It was expected that the narrow antimicrobial spectrum might remove only gram-negative aerobes and leave most other organisms intact.

The effect of aztreonam on the gastrointestinal flora in man has been extensively studied by Van der Waaij (21). Doses of aztreonam of 60–1500 grams were given orally each day to 10 volunteers and the fecal flora was monitored. There was usually a dramatic reduction in Enterobacteriaceae even on the lowest dosage to 10 or fewer organisms per gram of feces. The fall in anaerobic flora was 'limited' and 'insignificant'. *Candida* species were not affected and only one subject showed an increase in enterococci. A dose of 300 grams a day in most subjects produced feces from which Enterobacteriaceae could not be isolated. Two volunteers were unaffected and the reason for this requires further investigation.

Extensive studies of the effect of aztreonam on the gastrointestinal flora of animals have recently been reported (22). Aztreonam does not change the indigenous intestinal microflora in the hamster model (23). A study of hemorrhagic cecitis in a hamster model showed that latamoxef and cefoperazone were both as capable of inducing fatal infections as clindamycin. Aztreonam and ceftazidime did not suppress the anaerobic flora nor did they produce hemorrhagic cystitis (24). In cancer patients treated prophylactically with intravenous aztreonam, gram-negative bacteria in the stools were greatly reduced (25).

CLINICAL PHARMACOLOGY

Aztreonam displays no exceptionally different pharmacological properties from those of other parenterally administered β-lactam antibiotics that are not absorbed orally (26, 27). The properties are summarized in Table 4. Modification of dosage is advised in patients with renal failure, cirrhosis of the liver and in patients undergoing dialysis. These modifications can be directly related to the creatinine clearance and other measurements. The modifications can be summarized as follows: In patients with renal failure the usual initial dose is given and subsequent doses are reduced to one-quarter of the normal dose (28). An additional one-eighth dose can be given after a period of hemodialysis or peritoneal dialysis. In severe alcoholic cirrhosis the dosage needs to be reduced by 20–25%, but reduced dosages are not required in other forms of liver disease (29).

Table 4   *Pharmacological properties of aztreonam in healthy volunteers after dose of 500 g intravenously and intramuscularly*

	i.v.	i.m.
Mean peak level	58 mg/l	22 mg/l
Time to peak	5 min	1 h
Serum half-life	1.7 h	
Urine excretion		
Active	66%	
Inactive	7%	
Volume of distribution	12.6 l	
Urine concentrations 0-2 h	1400 mg/l	
Serum protein binding	60%	

ADVERSE EFFECTS

Hypersensitive reactions are an important limitation to the use of β-lactam antibiotics. In the case of cephalosporins there is the possibility of cross-allergenicity with penicillins (30). Thus, it is important to know whether monobactams also produce allergic responses, and, in particular, whether there is cross-allergenicity with penicillins or cephalosporins.

Detailed studies have been undertaken by Saxon et al (31, 32). Studies in rabbits indicated that anti-penicillin and anti-cephalosporin antibodies did not react with aztreonam. Antibodies against aztreonam raised in rabbits reacted with the side-chains rather than the β-lactam nucleus. A series of experiments in 36 human volunteers indicated that IgE did not develop in any subject; one developed an IgG antibody against the side-chains (not cross-reacting with penicillins or cephalosporins). Studies in 41 patients with IgE-reactive skin tests to penicillin showed no reaction to aztreonam or its products. These investigations suggest that there is very little cross-reactivity between aztreonam and other β-lactam antibiotics. Jensen et al (33) treated 15 hypersensitive patients with aztreonam. All patients had *Pseudomonas* infection complicating cystic fibrosis; allergic reactions to the β-lactams included 7 with anaphylactic reactions to penicillins (5) or cephalosporins (2), generalized urticaria and 7 with generalized reactions to cephalosporins (6) and/or penicillins (4). The only side effect noted with aztreonam was phlebitis in one patient. This is fairly convincing evidence of lack of cross-allogenicity.

The experimental data therefore suggest that aztreonam should have a reduced potential for immunological reactions compared with other β-lactams. No doubt, as increasing numbers of patients are treated with this compound, it will be possible to determine the incidence of allergic phenomena. In early studies the incidence of 'rash' was 1.5% of 1771 patients treated (34). To date, 134 patients with a history of penicillin and/or cephalosporin therapy have been treated with aztreonam and only one had a hypersensitivity reaction or urticarial rash (34).

The most frequently reported side-effects have been local reaction (1.7%), skin rash (1.8%), nausea (0.6%) and diarrhea (0.8%). The overall incidence of side-effects and abnormal laboratory results necessitating discontinuation of aztreonam was 2.1% (35).

CLINICAL USES

In determining the possible clinical role of aztreonam one should consider those infections where aerobic gram-negative rods are frequent pathogens. In particular, aztreonam might be used where an aerobic gram-negative was the only likely pathogen; if there is a likelihood of mixed infections with other organisms, additional antibodies would be needed.

The types of infection for which aztreonam could be considered are shown in Table 5. Many studies are now available showing the efficacy of aztreonam in many of these conditions. It is not possible in this short review to assess these reports critically, many of which are preliminary, but Table 6 summarizes some of the results and cure rates reported in different categories of infection. At this stage most investigators have treated small numbers of patients and reported their results in conference proceedings. The 5 studies summarized in Table 6 are those in which sufficient data have been presented to allow preliminary assessment of the clinical efficacy of aztreonam. Most investigators agree that aztreonam is effective in severe gram-negative bacterial infections and should take its place alongside aminoglycosides, the expanded-spectrum cephalosporins and quinolones as an appropriate agent for treatment of these infections.

Interactions with other antibiotics

Although one of the advantages of aztreonam is the limited spectrum which enables known aerobic gram-negative infection to be treated with a single agent, it

Table 5   *Infections where aztreonam might be a therapeutic possibility*

Used alone	*Used in combination*
Urinary tract infection	Abdominal sepsis
(including bacteremia from this source)	(with anti-anaerobe therapy)
Biliary tract infection	Respiratory tract
Gonorrhea	(with antipneumococcal therapy)
Gram-negative osteomyelitis	Septicemia in leukemics
	(with anti-gram-positive therapy)
	Neonatal meningitis
	(with antistreptococcal therapy)

Table 6   *Results of therapy with aztreonam in various infections*

Infection	No. of patients and type	Results	Ref.
Gram-negative pneumonia	19 patients including some hospital-acquired *Pseudomonas* and enterobacteria, some also given gram-positive drugs	13 cured, 6 improved, 2 resistant *Pseudomonas* emerged on treatment	36
Gram-negative pneumonia	47 patients; 2/3 treated with aztreonam, 1/3 with tobramycin; almost all hospital-acquired; some given gram-positive drugs	Of 26 aztreonam, 8 cured and 93% showed oral improvement compared to 50% for tobramycin; organism eradication 92% for aztreonam. 57% for tobramycin; superinfection rate high	37
Urinary tract infection	159 hospital-acquired: I. Aztreonam 3 daily doses II. Aztreonam 2 daily doses III. Cefamandole 3 daily doses	I. Cure rate 92% II. Cure rate 83% III. Cure rate 70% Superinfection with enterococci in aztreonam and *Pseudomonas* in cefamandole group.	38
	35 aztreonam-treated patients compared with 17 gentamicin-treated; difficult group of patients with underlying abnormalities	Aztreonam 35/35 cures but 6 with relapse, 6 re-infection; gentamicin 14/17 cures but 1 relapse, 4 re-infection, high rate of colonization with Group D streptococci, aztreonam group	39
Gram-negative osteomyelitis, with purulent arthritis	20 patients, 17 with osteomyelitis and 3 with purulent arthritis	All responded, culture negative in 14 days. 1 recurrence and 2 relapses with gram-positive organisms	40
Serious gram-negative infection	Bacteremia 12, respiratory 7, cystic fibrosis 16, bone and joints 12, UTI 24, abdominal 4 occasionally combined with complementary drugs when needed, e.g. anti-anaerobe	Clinical cure or improvement 88%; eradication of organisms; no details of superinfection	41
Uncomplicated gonorrheal infection	Comparison of 209 patients treated with aztreonam 1 g single dose with 201 treated with spectinomycin 2 g single dose	97% of each group cured	42
Gram-negative septicemia	112 patients including 41 ex-urinary-infection	Microbiological cure in 97; clinical cure in 75; partial cure in 16	43
Gonorrhea	1 g single dose in 32 patients	All cured	44
Peritonitis in CAPD	27 episodes combined with gram-positive therapy	22 clinical success; 21 microbiological success	45

CAPD = continuous ambulatory peritoneal dialysis.

is inevitable that aztreonam will be used in combination with other antibiotics. The rationale for these combinations will be to complement its activity with antibiotics acting against other organisms in mixed infections and to exploit any synergistic opportunities which may emerge. Preliminary studies indicate that aztreonam does not impair the activity of penicillins, erythromycin or vancomycin against staphylococci; nor do these agents interfere with aztreonam activity against gram-negative bacilli (46). An extensive study by Nakatomi and Neu shows an antagonism between erythromycin and aztreonam (47). Some synergy with aminoglycosides has been reported in about 60% of *Pseudomonas* and Enterobacteriaceae strains.

DOSING

The recommended dosage for urinary tract infection is 0.5 or 1 gram 8- or 12-hourly and for systemic infections of differing severity the dose is from 3 to 8 grams a day at intervals of 6–12 hours. The intravenous route is needed when a single dose exceeds 1 gram, but doses of 1 gram or less can be given by intramuscular injection (48). In children with cystic fibrosis and *Pseudomonas aeruginosa* infections a dose of 200 mg/kg/d divided into 4 doses has been recommended (49).

FUTURE DIRECTIONS

Although extensive studies have been carried out on structure-activity relationships of monocyclic β-lactams (1), aztreonam is the only compound currently available for use in patients. Other compounds are being developed and it seems likely that further derivatives of aminobactamic acid will emerge (50, 51).

REFERENCES

1. Cimarusti CM, Sykes RB (1984) Monocyclic beta-lactam antibiotics. *Med Res. Rev., 4*, 1.
2. Imada A, Kitano K, Kintaka K et al (1981) Sulfazecin and isosulfazecin: novel beta-lactam antibiotics of bacterial origin. *Nature (London), 289*, 590.
3. Sykes RB, Bonner DP, Bush K et al (1981) Monobactams – monocyclic beta-lactam antibiotics produced by bacteria. *J. Antimicrob. Chemother., 8, Suppl E*, 1.
4. Wise R, Andrews JM, Hancox J (1981) SQ 26776, a novel beta-lactam: an in-vitro comparison with other antimicrobial agents. *J. Antimicrob. Chemother., 8, Suppl E*, 39.
5. Neu HC, Labthavikal P (1981) Antibacterial activity of a monocyclic beta-lactam, SQ 26776. *J. Antimicrob. Chemother., 8, Suppl E*, 111.
6. Jacobus NV, Ferreira MC, Barza M (1982) In vitro activity of aztreonam, a monobactam antibiotic. *Antimicrob. Agents Chemother., 22*, 832.

7.   Acar JF, Kitzis MD, Goldstein FW (1981) In vitro activity of SQ 26,776 against multi-
     ple resistant enterobacteria – preliminary results. *J. Antimicrob. Chemother., 8, Suppl
     E*, 97.

8.   Brogden RN, Heel RC (1986) Aztreonam: a review of its antibacterial activity, phar-
     macokinetic properties and therapeutic use. *Drugs, 31*, 96.

9.   Livermore DM, Williams JD (1981) In-vitro activity of SQ 26776 against Gram-nega-
     tive bacteria and its stability to their beta-lactamases. *J. Antimicrob. Chemother., 8,
     Suppl E*, 29.

10. Phillips I, King A, Shannon K, Warren C (1981) SQ 26776 in vitro antibacterial activi-
     ty and susceptibility to beta-lactamases. *J. Antimicrob. Chemother., 8, Suppl E*, 103.

11. Percival A, Thomas E, Hart CA, Karayiannis P (1981) In vitro activity of monobac-
     tam SQ 26,277 against Gram-negative bacteria. *J. Antimicrob. Chemother., 8, Suppl
     E*, 49.

12. Reeves DS, Bywater MJ, Holt HA (1981) Antibacterial activity of SQ 26776 against
     antibiotic resistant enterobacteria including *Serratia* spp. *J. Antimicrob. Chemother.,
     8, Suppl E*, 57.

13. Then RL (1984) Interaction of Ro 17-2301 (AMA-1080) with beta-lactamases.
     Chemotherapy (Basel), 30, 394.

14. Livermore DM, Williams RJ, Lindridge MA et al (1982) *Pseudomonas aeruginosa* iso-
     lates with modified beta-lactamase inducibility effects on beta-lactam sensitivity. *Lan-
     cet, 2*, 1466.

15. Sanders CC, Sanders Jr WE (1985) Microbial resistance to newer generation beta-lac-
     tam antibiotics: clinical and laboratory implications. *J. Infect. Dis., 151*, 399.

16. Neu HC, Labthavikul P (1983) In vitro activity and beta-lactamase stability of a
     monobactam SQ 26,917 compared with those of aztreonam and other agents. *Anti-
     microb. Agents Chemother., 24*, 227.

17. Livermore DM, Williams RJ, Williams JD (1981) In vitro activity of MK 0787 (*N*-
     formimidoyl thienamycin) against *Pseudomonas aeruginosa* and other Gram-negative
     rods and its stability to their beta-lactamases. *J. Antimicrob. Chemother., 8*, 351.

18. Curtis NAC, Eisenstadt RL, Rudd C, White AJ (1986) Inducible Type 1 beta-lacta-
     mases of Gram-negative bacteria and resistance to beta-lactam antibiotics. *J. Antimi-
     crob. Chemother., 17*, 51.

19. Livermore DM (1983) *Resistance Mechanisms of Pseudomonas aeruginosa to Antibiot-
     ics.* Thesis, University of London.

20. Bush K, Freudenburger JS, Sykes RB (1982) Interaction of aztreonam and related
     monobactams with beta-lactamases from Gram-negative bacteria. *Antimicrob. Agents
     Chemother., 22*, 414.

21. Van der Waaij D, Hofstra W (1982) Effect of aztreonam on the colonisation resistance
     of the digestive tract: consequences for selective decontamination. In: *Abstracts, 22nd
     Interscience Conference on Antimicrobial Agents and Chemotherapy, Miami Beach, FL,
     1982.* Abstract No. 137. American Society for Microbiology, Washington, DC.

22. Van der Waaij D (1985) Selective decontamination of the digestive tract with oral az-
     treonam and temocillin. *Rev. Infect. Dis., 7, Suppl. 4*, S628.

23. Fernandes PB, Bonner DP, Sykes RB (1983) Aztreonam, a new concept in beta-lac-
     tam antibiotics. *Compr. Ther., 9(5)*, 21.

24. Weinberg DS, Fernandes PB, Kao C-C, Clark JM, Bonner DP, Sykes RB (1986) Eval-
     uation of aztreonam, cefoperazone, latamoxef and ceftazidime in the hamster model.
     J. Antimicrob. Chemother., 18, 729.

25. Bodey GP, Jadeja L, Swabb E et al (1983) Pharmacokinetic studies of aztreonam. In: *Program and Abstracts, 23rd Interscience Conference on Antimicrobial Agents and Chemotherapy, Las Vegas, 1983*, Abstract No. 41. American Society for Microbiology, Washington, DC.

26. Swabb EA, Sugerman AA, Platt TB et al (1982) Single dose pharmacokinetics of the monobactam aztreonam in healthy subjects. *Antimicrob. Agents Chemother., 21*, 944.

27. Swabb EA, Singhvi SM, Leitz MA, Frantz M, Sugerman AA (1983) Metabolism and pharmacokinetics of aztreonam in healthy subjects. *Antimicrob. Agents Chemother., 24*, 394.

28. Mihingu JCL, Scheld WM, Bolton ND et al (1983) Pharmacokinetics of aztreonam in patients with varying degrees of renal dysfunction. *Antimicrob. Agents Chemother., 24*, 252.

29. MacLeod CM, Bartley EA, Payne JA, Devlin RG (1983) Aztreonam handling in cirrhosis. In: Spitky KH, Karrer K (Eds), *Proceedings, 13th International Congress of Chemotherapy, Vienna, 1983, PS 4.2*, p. 7. Egermann, Vienna.

30. Batchelor FR, Dewdney JM, Weston RD et al (1966) The immunogenicity of cephalosporin derivatives and their cross reaction with penicillin. *Immunology, 10*, 21.

31. Saxon A, Hassner A, Swabb EA et al (1984) Lack of cross reactivity between the monobactam aztreonam and penicillin in penicillin allergic subjects. *J. Infect. Dis., 149*, 16.

32. Saxon A, Swabb EA, Adkinson NF (1985) Investigation into the immunologic cross reactivity of aztreonam with other beta-lactam antibiotics. *Am. J. Med., 78, Suppl 2A*, 19.

33. Jensen T, Koch C, Pedersen SS, Hobby N (1987) Aztreonam for cystic fibrosis patients who are hypersensitive to other beta-lactams. *Lancet, 1*, 1319.

34. Henry SA, Bendash CB (1985) Aztreonam: worldwide overview of the treatment of patients with Gram-negative infection. *Am. J. Med., 78, Suppl 2A*, 57.

35. Newman TJ, Dreslinski GR, Tadros SS (1985) Safety profile of aztreonam in clinical trials. *Rev. Infect. Dis., 7, Suppl 4*, 648.

36. Greenberg RN, Reilley PM, Luppen KL et al (1985) Aztreonam therapy for Gram-negative pneumococci. *Am. J. Med., 78, Suppl 2A*, 31.

37. Schentag JJ, Vari AJ, Winslade NE et al (1985) Treatment with aztreonam or tobramycin in critical care patients with Gram-negative pneumonia. *Am. J. Med., 78, Suppl 2A*, 34.

38. Childs SJ (1985) Aztreonam in the treatment of urinary tract infection. *Am. J. Med., 78, Suppl 2A*, 44.

39. Settler FR, Moyer JE, Schram M et al (1984) Aztreonam compared with gentamicin for treatment of serious urinary tract infection. *Lancet, 2*, 1315.

40. Pribyl C, Salzer R, Beskin RJ et al (1985) Aztreonam in the treatment of serious orthopaedic infections. *Am. J. Med., 78, Suppl 2A*, 51.

41. Scully B, Neu HC (1983) Aztreonam therapy of critically ill patients. In: Spitky KH, Karrer K (Eds), *Proceedings, 13th International Congress of Chemotherapy, Vienna, 1983, ST*, p 61. Egermann, Vienna.

42. Miller LK, Sanchez PL, Berg SW et al (1983) Effectiveness of aztreonam, a new beta-lactam antibiotic against penicillin-resistant gonococci. *J. Infect. Dis., 148*, 612.

43. Pierard D, Boelaert J, Van Landuyt HW et al (1986) Aztreonam treatment of Gram-negative septicemia, *Antimicrob. Agents Chemother., 29*, 359.

44. Gottlieb A, Mills J (1985) Effectiveness of aztreonam for the treatment of gonorrhea. *Antimicrob. Agents Chemother., 27*, 270.

45. Dratwa M, Glupczynski Y, Lameire N, Verschraegen G, Boelaert J, Van Landhuyt H, Verbeeven D, Lauwers S (1987) Treatment of gram-negative peritonitis in CAPD patients with aztreonam. In: *Abstracts, 3rd European Congress of Clinical Microbiology, The Hague, 1987*, No. 294.
46. Tanaka SK, Bonner DP, Sykes RB (1983) In vitro activity of aztreonam in combination with aminoglycosides and other beta-lactam against Gram-positive and Gram-negative bacteria. In: Spitky KH, Karrer K (Eds), *Proceedings, 13th International Congress of Chemotherapy, Vienna, 1983, SS 4. 1/3, 27/1*. Egermann, Vienna.
47. Nakatomi M, Neu HC (1986) The effect of the combination of erythromycin with new beta-lactam antibiotics against gram-negative aerobic respiratory pathogens. *Chemioterapia, 5*, 379.
48. Product monograph (1984) *Azactam® (Aztreonam): Clinical and Laboratory Studies*. Squibb.
49. Reed MD, Aronoff SC, Stern RC, Yamashita TS, Myers CM, Friedhoff LT, Blumer JL (1986) Single dose pharmacokinetics of aztreonam in children with cystic fibrosis. *Pediatr. Pulmonol., 2*, 282.
50. Matsuda K, Nagashima M, Nakagawa S et al (1986) In vitro antibacterial activity of BO 1165, a new monobactam antibiotic. *J. Antimicrob. Chemother., 17*, 747.
51. Nakoo M, Kondo M, Imada A (1986) Bactericidal and bacteriolytic activities of caramanam and its effect on bacterial morphology. *J. Antimicrob. Chemother., 17*, 433.

CHAPTER 5

β-Lactamase inhibitors

I.M. GOULD and R. WISE

There are several mechanisms of resistance to β-lactam antibiotics and the most important is probably enzymatic destruction by β-lactamases. These enzymes are ubiquitous and many different types exist. It has proved difficult to develop antibiotics (in particular orally absorbed compounds) with stability to a wide range of these enzymes and this has encouraged the development of enzyme inhibitors to enhance the activity of labile compounds against resistant strains.

All inhibitors that have been developed as far as clinical use are β-lactams. Many β-lactam antibiotics inhibit β-lactamases, particularly the newer more enzyme-stable agents. Our brief will be those agents that do not have useful antibiotic activity in their own right but whose proven or potential use is as β-lactamase inhibitors.

For the structure of clavulanic acid, penicillanic acids and other microbial metabolites which are β-lactamase inhibitors, the reader is referred to *Annual 1*.

The last year has not seen any major advances in the field. Clavulanic acid combinations with amoxicillin and ticarcillin are now marketed more widely and oral and intravenous combinations of sulbactam with ampicillin and cefoperazone are also available in some countries. No clinical trials of new agents are reported, although in vitro studies on new penicillanic acid derivatives have been (1, 2).

The clinical relevance of β-lactam degradation in the patient and the therapeutic importance of the protection of labile penicillins by β-lactamase inhibitors or the use of β-lactamase-stable agents has been accepted in many infections, but there is still much debate regarding upper and lower respiratory tract infections (3). Evidence is slowly accumulating of the clinical benefits of using β-lactamase stable agents (4) in this setting.

ACTIVITY

Mechanism of action

Details of the mechanism of action of β-lactamase inhibitors are discussed in *Annual 1*. In summary, all the clinically useful β-lactamase inhibitors to date are suic-

Antimicrobial Agents Annual 3
P.K. Peterson and J. Verhoef, editors
©Elsevier Science Publishers BV, 1988

63

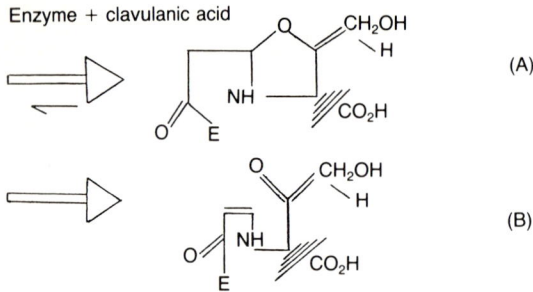

Fig. 1 Mechanism of action of β-lactamase inhibitors. Formation of enzyme-inhibitor complex (A) followed by conversion to an irreversibly inactivated complex (B). After Neu (5).

ide inhibitors with a mechanism of action similar to that of clavulanic acid. An enzyme-inhibitor complex is formed by competitive inhibition (Fig. 1) (5) and is followed by conversion to an irreversibly inactivated complex (6–8).

It is common for modest synergy to occur with β-lactam antibiotics against susceptible bacteria. This could be due to a low level of membrane-bound β-lactamase or a direct inhibitory activity on cell-wall-synthesizing enzymes: clavulanate and YTR-830 show strongest affinity for penicillin-binding protein-2 (PBP-2) of some organisms (9). The importance of the former has recently been discussed in the context of *Staphylococcus aureus* of intermediate methicillin resistance (10). Regarding the latter, it is possible that at sub-minimum inhibitory concentrations (MIC), binding to PBP-2 could counteract the filament-forming tendency of some penicillins (Greenwood called this a 'complementation effect') (11).

Spectrum of activity *(see also Annual 1 and Refs 12, 13)*

Clavulanate

Clavulanate has only weak antibacterial activity of its own except for its activity against penicillin-sensitive *Neisseria gonorrhoeae* (MIC 1.25 μg/ml) and *Legionella pneumophila* (0.2–0.4 μg/ml). It gives very good inhibition of the majority of plasmid-mediated penicillinases such as staphylococcal, TEM-1 and 2, SHV-1, PSE-1, 2, 3 and 4, PIT-2 and, to a lesser extent, OXA-1, 2 and 3, all known chromosomally mediated penicillinases and also a few cephalosporinases such as those produced by *Proteus vulgaris, Bacteroides* species and *Pseudomonas cepacia*. Essentially, it has good activity against Richmond and Sykes Class II-V enzymes but little affinity for Class I (e.g. chromosomal cephalosporinase JT-414 *E. coli, Enterobacter cloacae* NCTC-10005, *P. aeruginosa* A). Penetration into the periplasmic space of gram-negative bacteria is not usually a problem.

King et al (14) and Crump and Cansdale (15) have noticed induction of Type

1 chromosomal β-lactamase by clavulanate and consequent antagonism of the combined penicillin in *Providencia rettgeri, E. cloacae, Morganella morganii* and *Providencia stuartii*. Recent data suggest that this induction is variable between strains (16). Further studies on this point are needed.

Levels of clavulanate needed for apparent maximal inhibition of β-lactamase depend upon the enzymes, organisms and possibly methodology employed, but in general, by plate MIC, 0.5 μg/ml of clavulanate, when combined with amoxicillin, has a marked effect, often maximal in gram-positive organisms, *N. gonorrhoeae* and *Haemophilus influenzae*. However, Enterobacteriaceae and *Pseudomonas* species, possibly due to permeability problems, often need 5 or even 10 μg/ml by plate MIC for maximal effect, although in vivo it does not seem, from available evidence, that these levels need to be attained. Kill curve studies in our own laboratories (17) and animal studies (18) highlight possible fallacies in MIC data. Lapointe and Lavallee have recently shown much better synergy between amoxicillin/clavulanate than trimethoprim/sulfamethoxazole, particularly when cidal activity was studied (19).

Hunter et al (20) noticed, surprisingly, that clavulanate often reduces MICs in methicillin-resistant *Staphylococcus aureus* and *S. epidermidis*. Other authors have found this with sulbactam. This is probably due to inhibition of coincidental β-lactamase production (rather than, say, an effect on the target-site PBPs). The *Bacteroides fragilis* group are also susceptible to the effects of clavulanate which particularly reduces MICs for organisms resistant to penicillin, ampicillin and ticarcillin, but less so for the acylureido-penicillins. This is probably because other mechanisms may often be involved as well, e.g. permeability and affinity to PBPs.

Mycobacterium tuberculosis and *Nocardia* species have been reported as being susceptible to combinations of clavulanate and amoxicillin, possibly an observation of great significance that requires further study. Many penicillins and cephalosporins have been reported to be potentiated in vitro, including ampicillin, amoxicillin, carbenicillin, ticarcillin, piperacillin, penicillin G, mezlocillin, azlocillin, mecillinam, cefalotin, cefaloridine, cefotetan, cefoperazone, cefotiam, cefotaxime and cefsulodin.

Sulbactam and other penicillanic acid derivatives (See also Annual 1 and Refs 21, 22)

With the exception of *N. gonorrhoeae, N. meningitidis, Acinetobacter calcoaceticus* and *Pseudomonas acidovorans*, sulbactam does not have useful antibacterial activity. It tends to be active against the same groups of β-lactamases as clavulanate but it is 2–5 times less potent, although its protective effect extends beyond clavulanate to include *Proteus, Providencia, Citrobacter* and *Enterobacter* species and also *Serratia marcescens* (23, 24). However, it is not such a strong inducer of Type 1 β-lactamases.

The 6β-bromo and 6β-iodo compounds have been compared with clavulanate and sulbactam for their ability to potentiate ampicillin activity against a wide range of ampicillin-resistant organisms in vitro (25, 26). We have found clavulanate to be the most potent followed by 6β-bromo- and then 6β-iodo-penicillanic acids, all being more active than sulbactam. The halo-penicillanic acids were more effective than clavulanate in TEM and *H. influenzae* (25). Penicillanic acid derivatives (in combination with ampicillin) were active against many different enzymes and bacteria, from levels of 0.5 μg/ml rising to 32 μg/ml (25).

Retsema et al (27) have described enzymes inhibited by sulbactam: 90% of ampicillin-resistant *S. aureus*, *B. fragilis* and *H. influenzae* were killed by 3.12 μg of sulbactam and 3.12 μg of ampicillin. Interestingly, all 14 strains of methicillin-resistant staphylococci were inhibited by 12.5 μg/ml of each (similar findings to those previously mentioned for clavulanate). For cephalosporinase-producing strains of *E. aerogenes*, *E. cloacae*, *S. marcescens*, *Prov. stuartii* and *P. mirabilis*, the sulfone is more active than clavulanate, although neither is very impressive. Clavulanate is more active than sulbactam against penicillinase-producing *N. gonorrhoeae* (28). However, Jones et al (29) found sulbactam most inhibitory against 8 strains of *Legionella*. One important factor in limiting the activity of penicillanic acid sulfones against gram-negative bacteria may be the penetration into the periplasmic space (5).

The combination of sulbactam with cefoperazone enhances the already marked activity of the latter against Enterobacteriaceae and broadens the spectrum to include all *Haemophilus* species, *Bacteroides* species, most *Acinetobacter* species and many *Pseudomonas* species, although there is little beneficial effect on gram-positive bacteria (22, 30, 31).

YTR-830 has less inherent antibacterial activity (32, 33) than clavulanate, but its β-lactamase-inhibiting properties are greater than sulbactam, indeed similar to clavulanate (9, 34) with a similar spectrum to those of sulbactam. It is more stable in solution than clavulanic acid (34) and does not appear to induce β-lactamase (35). Of the newer β-lactamase inhibitors it is the one with the most potential (36). Recently Chin and Neu have reported in vitro studies on 6-acetylmethylene penicillanic acid (AMPA) (1). It showed excellent broad-spectrum β-lactamase inhibition with extracted enzymes but was inferior to clavulanate and sulbactam with intact bacteria. Other penicillanic acid derivatives (BL-P2013 and BL-P2090) were inferior to clavulanic acid against *M. tuberculosis* (2).

Resistance mechanisms

Bacteria isolated from 3 patients treated by File et al (37) with Timentin (clavulanate + ticarcillin) had significant increases in MICs during therapy. None was the cause of clinical treatment failure, but one organism (*P. aeruginosa*) developed in vitro resistance, the mechanism of which is unknown.

The only method of resistance described as developing on treatment with β-lactamase inhibitors is enzyme induction by clavulanate in a previously susceptible organism.

Differences in permeability or amounts of β-lactamase produced may account for differences in effect with different organisms, but class of enzyme is probably most important. An example of permeability problems can be seen with some *P. aeruginosa* highly resistant to ticarcillin due to plasmid β-lactamase production. Clavulanate will only synergise with ticarcillin in strains where it can penetrate.

As clavulanate inhibits most plasmid-mediated enzymes, it is anticipated that amoxicillin + clavulanate will exert a lower selective pressure than amoxicillin does on its own. The low frequency of emergence of plasmid mutants while on treatment with Augmentin was noted in a study of fecal flora in 104 patients with urinary tract infections treated for 10 days: 22.3% of the *E. coli* were resistant to amoxicillin at the end of the therapy, but only 2.6% were resistant to Augmentin (38). However, increases in total Enterobacteriaceae fecal counts of 2 or 3 logs occur after oral therapy and clavulanate in feces is undetectable (39). Brumfitt et al (40) recently reported the elimination of fecal staphylococci after a 7-day course of oral Augmentin in healthy volunteers.

CLINICAL PHARMACOLOGY (*Table 1*)

Clavulanate

Clavulanate is well adsorbed and the pharmacokinetics at least in terms of serum elimination half-life are well matched to those of amoxicillin and ticarcillin; both are now available in combination with clavulanate. Tissue penetration is generally very good including inflammatory blister fluid, peritoneal fluid, pleural fluid, bile, bone (41), gallbladder, pus, tonsils (42), and subcutaneous fat. Two recent studies have suggested that sputum penetration, although not as good as previously quoted

Table 1 *Clinical pharmacology of clavulanate and sulbactam*

	Clavulanate	Sulbactam
Absorption	good	poor (good in prodrug form)
Peak serum level	4 μg/ml after 125 mg p.o.	1.4 μg/ml after 500 p.o.
		4.9 μg/ml after 250 p.o.
		as prodrug
Peak serum level	8 μg/ml after 200 mg i.v.	43 μg/ml after 1 g.i.v.
Half-life	1 h	1 h
Elimination	renal	renal
Protein binding	22%	20%
Half-life hemodialysis	70 min	140 min
Tissue penetration	good	good
Effect of probenecid	none	$t_{\frac{1}{2}}$ increased to 1.5 h

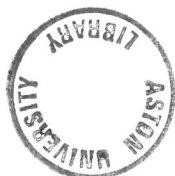

(see *Annual 2*, p. 62), is still satisfactory for therapy of chest infection due to β-lactamase-producing *H. influenzae* and *B. catarrhalis*. Mean maximum sputum concentrations were about 0.4 and 0.2 μg/ml after 200 mg i.v. and 250 mg p.o. respectively (43, 72). A recent publication has confirmed satisfactory penetration of clavulanate into cerebrospinal fluid (CSF) in inflamed meninges (44). A mean peak of 0.25 μg/ml of clavulanate was reached in the CSF 2 hours after 0.2 g given intravenously, a penetration of 8.4%. This level should be satisfactory for therapy of β-lactamase-producing *H. influenzae*, but ideally larger doses of clavulanate could be given.

In patients with renal failure or in neonates, the parallel excretion rates of clavulanate and amoxicillin or ticarcillin no longer hold and excretion of the penicillin is impaired more: e.g. the $t_{\frac{1}{2}\beta}$ for clavulanate is around 164 min and for amoxicillin 232 min in patients with a creatinine clearance of 20 ml/min. In patients on hemodialysis the $t_{\frac{1}{2}\beta}$ is around 120 min for amoxicillin and 70 min for clavulanate. Recovery in dialysate is around 40% of the administered dose. Details of pharmacokinetic studies in renal impairment have recently been published (45, 46).

Sulbactam

Sulbactam is well adsorbed when combined with ampicillin as a mutual prodrug. We have studied sultamicillin, the mutual prodrug of sulbactam and ampicillin, and showed doubling of the expected serum levels of ampicillin and sulbactam, had both been given separately (47). The pharmacokinetics and tissue penetration are very similar to those of ampicillin. Tissue penetration is good with 96% of the serum level present in peritoneal fluid. Penetration is also high into blister fluid, sputum, middle ear (48), appendix, bile, gallbladder, myometrium (49), abscess pus and umbilical cord blood (50). CSF penetration is low in uninflamed meninges but can be up to 30% of serum levels in meningitis. Elimination is primarily renal with the half-life increased to 21 hours in terminal renal failure, but the pharmacokinetics of ampicillin or cefoperazone and sulbactam remain well matched. However, with hepatic dysfunction, cefoperazone elimination is disproportionately decreased (51). Breast milk contains 1-2% of the dose in common with some other β-lactams (50).

ADVERSE EFFECTS AND DRUG INTERACTIONS

Both clavulanate and the penicillinate derivatives are well tolerated and trials to date have not revealed any major toxicity problems. With both, gastrointestinal effects are observed quite frequently after oral administration but are rarely severe enough to interfere with patient compliance. Augmentin appears to induce more nausea and sultamicillin more diarrhea (52). Occasionally, patients on high-dose clavulanate (250 mg) vomit, but nausea is less prevalent with lower doses or when the drug is taken with meals.

Clavulanate combined with amoxicillin or ticarcillin and sulbactam with ampicillin have had extensive clinical evaluation for toxicity and all combinations seem to retain the safety of the original *β*-lactam component (see *Annual 1*, for details).

Recently reported, however, are 23 patients treated with ticarcillin, clavulanic acid and tobramycin: 43.5% developed a positive direct antiglobulin ('Coombs') test but no hemolysis (53). This is probably related to non-immunologic protein adsorption to the membrane of erythrocytes similar to that reported for cefalotin.

Marked changes in intestinal flora have been noted with cefoperazone + sulbactam (54) and problems of diarrhea are anticipated with this combination. Pain after intramuscular injection of sulbactam is a common complaint, but this can be prevented by the use of lignocaine.

CLINICAL USES

The *β*-lactamase inhibitors have obvious therapeutic advantages where infection is due to *β*-lactamase-producing organisms or where such organisms may be coincidentally present, but not exerting a direct pathogenic effect as in the respiratory tract. Here failure of therapy with agents normally active against the infecting agent may be due to inactivation by commensal organisms which produce *β*-lactamases. With combination *β*-lactam therapy they may also protect other agents prescribed simultaneously from inactivation.

Currently, in the United Kingdom, amoxicillin is available for oral or intravenous administration in combination with clavulanate (Augmentin) and sulbactam may soon be available in combination with ampicillin for intravenous use. Also now available, the combination of clavulanate with ticarcillin (Timentin) for parenteral use gives a broader spectrum of action than Augmentin and should prove useful in seriously ill patients. Similarly, in certain countries, trials of sulbactam in combination with cefoperazone have been carried out and this combination is marketed in the Far East. Data are accumulating showing that sulbactam and clavulanate are efficacious and well tolerated in children (55, 56).

Evidence is accumulating of the clinical advantage of *β*-lactamase inhibitors in combination with ampicillin/amoxicillin for upper and lower respiratory infection. Two trials recently published (4, 57) are the best clinical evidence to date of the superiority of Augmentin over conventional therapy in this setting.

Clavulanate + amoxicillin (Augmentin)

Both oral and intravenous preparations are now available by prescription in many parts of the world and extended experience indicates that it is satisfactory therapy for a wide range of infections involving *β*-lactamase-positive and -negative organisms (see *Annual 1*, for details of therapeutic trials). We recommend its use as first-line therapy for upper and lower respiratory tract infections including otitis media, bronchitis and pneumonia, soft tissue infections, biliary tract sepsis, peritonitis and genitourinary infection, and in the prophylaxis of genitourinary and intra-abdominal sepsis. A recent trial in our unit demonstrated its efficacy as an alternative to metronidazole in the prophylaxis of appendicectomy (58). Extensive pharmacokinetic and therapeutic experience of oral Augmentin in children is reported in a recent publication (59).

As a first-line agent for serious sepsis, it is probably satisfactory on its own for community-acquired pneumonia (excluding *Legionella* and atypical organisms), intra-abdominal sepsis, pyelonephritis and septicemia, but there is no experience of its use in meningitis or endocarditis. For serious sepsis in immunosuppressed patients or as acquired in hospital it should be combined with an aminoglycoside or other agent active against organisms producing Type 1 chromosomal β-lactamases. The importance of induction of these enzymes by clavulanate in the clinical setting is uncertain. Of interest will be trials in otitis media and streptococcal pharyngitis comparing the success of Augmentin versus penicillin or ampicillin in eradicating the pathogens.

Clavulanate + ticarcillin (Timentin)

Theoretically the combination of clavulanate + ticarcillin is a promising one due to the broad spectrum of ticarcillin. Organisms such as *Ent. cloacae* and *P. aeruginosa* resistant to ampicillin and amoxicillin and which produce Type 1 chromosomal enzymes poorly inhibited by clavulanate may be susceptible to ticarcillin alone. However, in vitro results have been disappointing in some ticarcillin-resistant gram-negative bacteria, especially *P. aeruginosa, Serratia* spp., *Enterobacter* spp. and *Citrobacter* spp., probably due to production of large amounts of plasmid β-lactamases and/or induction of chromosomal β-lactamases by clavulanate (60–63). Discrepancies between disc diffusion testing and broth susceptibility studies are reported (17, 60) and need further studies.

Kosmidis et al (64) have reported extensive experience with Timentin 5.2 g 6-hourly in serious sepsis with ticarcillin-resistant organisms, with encouraging results. Even infection due to Timentin-resistant *P. aeruginosa* appear to respond, although many organisms were not eradicated. Their results are surprisingly good in view of the small doses of clavulanate given and are presumably due to irreversible inactivation of β-lactamase after only short periods of exposure to clavulanate.

Extensive clinical experience in serious sepsis is reported in two recent publications (65, 66). Results are as one would expect from data in vitro including satisfactory response when used as empiric therapy for febrile neutropenics. Persistent *S. aureus* infections required vancomycin therapy in 2 patients despite in vitro sensitivity to Timentin. Satisfactory results are also reported in pneumonia, cystic fibrosis, urinary tract infection, skin and soft tissue infections, gram-positive and gram-negative osteomyelitis (although associated with emergence of resistance in *P. aeruginosa*) prophylaxis and therapy of intra-abdominal sepsis, pelvic inflammatory disease, endomyometritis and septicemia. Comparison with standard therapies was satisfactory. Its place is yet to be defined, but it may well be a useful agent in combined therapy with an aminoglycoside, quinolone or cephalosporin for serious sepsis. It should be used with caution as sole therapy for serious infection.

Sulbactam + ampicillin

Sulbactam in combination with ampicillin either orally or parenterally has been used now to treat many hundreds of patients with serious infection in largely non-comparative therapeutic trials and to a lesser extent in comparative trials of therapy and prophylaxis. In therapeutic trials about 40% of organisms have been ampicillin-resistant. Results have been satisfactory, the agent performing as well as the standard regimes used for comparison, and eradication of ampicillin-resistant organisms being as frequent as ampicillin-sensitive ones (see *Annual 1*, for details of clinical trials).

Results of trials indicate that the combination is appropriate for soft tissue, upper and lower respiratory, genitourinary, intra-abdominal and septicemic infections (55), but there are no reports of trials as therapy for bacterial meningitis caused by β-lactamase-producing organisms. Oral therapy for gonorrhea as a single dose of 0.5 or 1 g sulbactam and 1 or 2 g ampicillin respectively in combination with probenecid is satisfactory but does not affect the incidence of postgonococcal

Table 2   *Dosing for β-lactamase inhibitors*

Drug	Dose	Indication
Augmentin p.o.*	375 mg clavulanate 125 mg + amoxicillin 250 mg q. 8 h	lower urinary tract infections
	750 mg clavulanate 250 mg + amoxicillin 500 mg q. 6–8 h	soft tissue, respiratory infections and upper urinary infections
Augmentin i.v.*	1.2 g clavulanate 0.2 g + amoxicillin 1.0 g q. 4-8 h	for serious infections
Timentin i.v.*, **	3 or 5 g ticarcillin + 0.1 or 0.2 g clavulanate q. 4–8 h	for serious infections
Sulbactam + ampicillin i.v.*	1–3 g (1:1 or 1:2 ratio) q. 6 h	for serious infections

* Increase dosage interval in renal failure for all drugs.
** Decrease dose of ticarcillin if creatinine clearance < 40 ml/min.

urethritis. Results in respiratory infections are perhaps most disappointing with poor bacteriologic responses sometimes accompanied by poor clinical response. Post-treatment colonization with *Branhamella* species or even failure to eradicate *Haemophilus* species or hemolytic streptococci was relatively common. This may be explained by inadequate and/or infrequent dosing, but further trials are required.

Because of its good antianaerobic activity, sulbactam + ampicillin is useful in prophylaxis of genitourinary and intra-abdominal infections; comparative trials indicate that it is satisfactory for prophylaxis in appendicectomy, biliary, upper gastrointestinal, gynecologic and urinary tract surgery (55, 67).

Sulbactam + cefoperazone

Limited clinical experience with sulbactam + cefoperazone confirms its efficacy as a therapeutic agent in a wide spectrum of infections (68–70) including pneumonia (71), urinary tract infection, biliary infections, septicemia (69), gynecologic infections, pelvic inflammatory disease and peritonitis, with the combination giving significantly higher cure rates than cefoperazone alone (70).

DOSING

For a summary of recommended doses and their indications, see Table 2.

FUTURE DIRECTIONS

β-Lactamase inhibitors are certainly here to stay and further development of new inhibitors is definitely indicated. Those presently available are not ideal in that they are not active against some clinically important β-lactamases nor are their pharmacokinetic properties ideally matched in some instances to the associated β-lactamase antibiotic. The availability of inhibitors on their own is also a potential area of use to be combined with the most appropriate β-lactam for a specific occasion and for increasing dosage relative to the combined penicillin for therapy in inaccessible sites, e.g. CSF in meningitis.

REFERENCES

1. Chin NX, Neu HC (1986) β-Lactamase inhibition by acetylmethylene penicillanic acid compared to clavulanate and other penicillanic acid derivatives. In: *Abstracts, Interscience Conference on Antimicrobial Agents and Chemotherapy, New Orleans, 1986*, p 1296. American Society For Microbiology, Washington, DC.

2. Sorg TB, Cynamon MH (1987) Comparison of four *β*-lactamase inhibitors in combination with ampicillin against *Mycobacterium tuberculosis. J. Antimicrob. Chemother., 19*, 59.
3. Roos K, Grahn E, Holm SE (1986) Evaluation of beta-lactamase activity and microbial interference in treatment failures of acute streptococcal tonsilitis. *Scand. J. Infect. Dis., 18*, 313.
4. McLeod DT, Ahmad F, Capewell S et al (1986) Increase in bronchopulmonary infection due to *Branhamella catarrhalis. Br. Med. J., 292*, 1103.
5. Neu HC (1985) Contribution of beta-lactamases to bacterial resistance and mechanisms to inhibit beta-lactamases. *Am. J. Med., 79, Suppl 5B*, 2.
6. Fisher J, Charnas RL, Bradley SM, Knowles JR (1981) Inactivation of RTEM *β*-lactamase from *E. coli*: interaction of peam sulfones with enzyme. *Biochemistry, 20*, 2726.
7. Labia R, Lelievre V, Peduzzi J (1980) Inhibition kinetics of three R-factor-mediated *β*-lactamases by a new *β*-lactam sulfone (CP 45899). *Biochim. Biophys. Acta, 611*, 351.
8. Fisher JF, Knowles JR (1980) The inactivation of beta-lactamases by mechanism-based reagents. In: Sandler M (Ed.), *Enzyme Inhibitors as Drugs*, p 209. MacMillan, London.
9. Moosdeen F, Williams JD, Yamabe S (1985) Inhibition of *β*-lactamase, binding to PBPs and morphological changes affected by YTR 830, a new penicillinate sulphone. In: Ishigami J (Ed), *Recent Advances in Chemotherapy*, p 1272. University of Tokyo Press, Tokyo.
10. McDougal LK, Thornsberry C (1986) The role of *β*-lactamase in staphylococcal resistance to penicillinase-resistant penicillins and cephalosporins. *J. Clin. Microbiol., 23*, 832.
11. Greenwood D, O'Grady F, Baker P (1979) An in vitro evaluation of clavulanic acid, a potent, broad-spectrum *β*-lactamase inhibitor. *J. Antimicrob. Chemother., 13*, 121.
12. Van Landuyt HW, Lambert A (1981) Comparative activity of BRL 25000 with amoxicillin against resistant clinical isolates. In: Nelson JD, Grassi C (Eds), *Current Chemotherapy and Infectious Diseases, Vol 1*, p 334. American Society for Microbiology, Washington, DC.
13. Sutherland R, Beale AS, Boon RJ et al (1985) Antibacterial activity of ticarcillin in the presence of clavulanate potassium. *Am. J. Med., Suppl. 5B*, 13.
14. King A, Gransden WR, Phillips I (1983) The effect of clavulanic acid on the susceptibility to ticarcillin of Enterobacteriaceae and *Pseudomonas aeruginosa* that produce chromosomally and plasmid-determined *β*-lactamases. In: Spitzky KM, Karrer K (Eds), *Proceedings, 13th International Conference on Chemotherapy, Vienna, 1983, Vol. 2*, 89/56. Egermann, Vienna.
15. Crump J, Cansdale S (1982) Enterobacter resistant to amoxycillin/clavulanate (Letter to Editor) *Lancet, 2*, 500.
16. Farmer TH, Reading C (1987) Induction of the *β*-lactamases of a strain of *Pseudomonas aeruginosa, Morganella morganii* and *Enterobacter cloacae. J. Antimicrob. Chemother., 19*, 401.
17. Gould IM, Dent J, Wise R (1987) In-vitro bacterial killing kinetics of ticarcillin/clavulanic acid. *J. Antimicrob. Chemother., 19*, 307.
18. Dijkmans BAC, Vaishnav J, Mattie H (1985) Efficacy of amoxycillin and benzylpenicillin combined with clavulanic acid against *Bacteroides fragilis* in vitro and in experimentally infected mice. *Scand. J. Infect. Dis., 17*, 311.
19. Lapointe JR, Lavallee C (1987) Antibiotic interaction of amoxycillin and clavulanic

acid against 132 β-lactamase positive *Haemophilus* isolates: a comparison with some other oral agents. *J. Antimicrob. Chemother., 19*, 49.

20. Hunter PA, Coleman K, Fisher J, Taylor D (1980) In vitro synergistic properties of clavulanic acid, with ampicillin, amoxycillin and ticarcillin. *J. Antimicrob. Chemother., 6, 455*.

21. Retsema JA, English AR, Girard AE et al (1983) Sulbactam and ampicillin: synergistic antibacterial activity against hospital isolates of Enterobacteriaceae, methicillin-resistant staphylococcus and anaerobes. In: *Proceedings, 13th International Conference on Chemotherapy, Vienna, Vol 1/23*, p 1. Egermann, Vienna.

22. Jones RN, Wilson HW, Thornsberry C, Barry AL (1985) In vitro antimicrobial activity of cefoperazone-sulbactam combinations against 554 clinical isolates including a review and β-lactamase studies. *Diagn. Microbiol. Infect. Dis., 3*, 489.

23. Greenwood D, Eley A (1982) In vitro evaluation of sulbactam, a penicillanic acid sulphone with β-lactamase inhibitory properties. *J. Antimicrob. Chemother., 10*, 117.

24. Yamaguchi A, Hirata T, Sawai T (1983) Kinetic studies on inactivation of *Citrobacter freundii* cephalosporinase by sulbactam. *Antimicrob. Agents Chemother., 24*, 23.

25. Wise R, Andrews JM, Patel N (1981) 6-β-Bromo and 6-β-iodo penicillanic acid, two novel β-lactamase inhibitors. *J. Antimicrob. Chemother., 7*, 531.

26. Neu HC (1983) β-Lactamase inhibitory activity of iodopenicillanate and bromopenicillanate. *Antimicrob. Agents Chemother., 17*, 615.

27. Retsema JA, English AR, Girard AE (1980) CP-45,899 in combination with penicillin or ampicillin against penicillin-resistant *Staphylococcus, Haemophilus influenzae* and *Bacteroides. Antimicrob. Agents Chemother., 17*, 615.

28. Wise R, Andrews JM, Bedford KA (1980) Clavulanic acid and CP-45899: a comparison of their in vitro activity in combination with penicillins. *J. Antimicrob. Chemother., 6*, 197.

29. Jones RN, Barry APC, Thornsberry C (1983) Collaborative in vitro investigations of sulbactam/ampicillin against clinically relevant bacterial pathogens in the United States. In: *Proceedings, 13th International Conference on Chemotherapy, Vienna, Vol 1/23*, p 6. Egermann, Vienna.

30. Yokota T (1985) Bacteriological studies of sulbactam/cefoperazone. In: Ishigami J (Ed.), *Recent Advances in Chemotherapy*, p 23. University of Tokyo Press, Tokyo.

31. Veno K (1985) Bacteriological studies against anaerobes. In: Ishigami J (Ed), *Recent Advances in Chemotherapy*, p 23. University of Tokyo Press, Tokyo.

32. Aronoff S, Lambrozzi P, Yamabe S (1985) In vivo and in vitro comparison of YTR 830 and clavulanate combined with amoxicillin against *Staphylococcus aureus*. In: Ishigami J (Ed.), *Recent Advances in Chemotherapy*, p 1268. University of Tokyo Press, Tokyo.

33. Aronoff S, Labrozzi P, Jacobs M, Yamabe S (1985) In vivo comparison of YTR 830 and clavulanate combined with amoxicillin against *Citrobacter freundii* and *Proteus mirabilis*. In: Ishigami J (Ed), *Recent Advances in Chemotherapy*, p 1270. University of Tokyo Press, Tokyo.

34. Ishida N, Hyodo A, Hanehara C et al (1985) YTR 830, a novel β-lactamase: comparative in vitro and in vivo studies with clavulanic acid and sulbactam. In: Ishigami J (Ed.), *Recent Advances in Chemotherapy*, p 1274. University of Tokyo Press, Tokyo.

35. Kitzis MD, Gutmann L, Yamabe S, Acar JF (1985) Evaluation of new β-lactamase inhibitor YTR 830. In: Ishigami J (Ed), *Recent Advances in Chemotherapy*, p 1276. University of Tokyo Press, Tokyo.

36. Jacobs MR, Aronoff SC, Johenning S et al (1986) Comparative activities of the *β*-lactamase inhibitors YTR 830, clavulanate, and sulbactam combined with ampicillin and broad-spectrum penicillins against defined *β*-lactamase-producing aerobic gram-negative bacilli. *Antimicrob. Agents Chemother., 29*, 980.

37. File Jr TM, Tan JS, Salstrom S et al (1984) Timentin versus piperacillin or moxalactam in the therapy of acute bacterial infections. *Antimicrob. Agents Chemother., 26*, 310.

38. Iravani A, Richard GA. Quoted by Leng B (1982) Augmentin in the treatment of urinary tract infections due to amoxycillin-resistant bacteria. In: Croyden EAP, Michel MF (Eds), *Proceedings, European Symposium on Augmentin, 1982*, p 153. Elsevier, Amsterdam.

39. Motohiro T, Tanaka K, Koga T et al (1985) Effect of BRL 25000 (clavulanic acid-amoxicillin) on bacterial flora in human faeces. *Jpn. J. Antibiot., 38*, 478.

40. Brumfitt W, Franklin I, Grady D, Hamilton-Miller JMT (1986) Effect of amoxicillin-clavulanate and cephradine on the fecal flora of healthy volunteers not exposed to a hospital environment. *Antimicrob. Agents Chemother., 30*, 335.

41. Grimer RJ, Karpinski MRK, Andrews JM, Wise R (1986) Penetration of amoxycillin and clavulanic acid into bone. *Chemotherapy, 32*, 185.

42. Federspil P, Koch A, Schatzle W, Tiesler E (1986) Timentin – clinical and pharmacokinetic evaluation in otorhinolaryngology. *J. Antimicrob. Chemother., 17*, 103.

43. Maesen FPV, Davies BI, Baur C (1987) Amoxycillin/clavulanate in acute purulent exacerbative bronchitis. *J. Antimicrob. Chemother., 19*, 373.

44. Bakken JS, Bruun JN, Gaustad P, Tasker TCG (1986) Penetration of amoxicillin and potassium clavulanate into the cerebrospinal fluid of patients with inflamed meninges. *Antimicrob. Agents Chemother., 30*, 481.

45. Dalet F, Amada E, Cabrera E (1986) Pharmacokinetics of the combination of ticarcillin with clavulanic acid in renal insufficiency. *J. Antimicrob. Chemother., 17*, 57.

46. Horber FF, Frey FJ, Descoeudres C et al (1986) Differential effect of impaired renal function on the kinetics of clavulanic acid and amoxicillin. *Antimicrob. Agents Chemother., 29*, 614.

47. Hartley S, Wise R (1982) A three-way crossover study to compare the pharmacokinetics and acceptibility of sultamicillin at two dose levels with that of ampicillin. *J. Antimicrob. Chemother., 10*, 49.

48. Voelker MS, Nightingale CH, Quintiliami R et al (1985) Sultamicillin use in otitis media: penetration of sulbactam, a beta-lactamase inhibitor, and ampicillin. *Curr. Ther. Res. Clin. Exp., 38*, 738.

49. Schwiersch U, Lang N, Wildfeuer DA (1986) Concentration of sulbactam and ampicillin in serum and the myometrium. *Drugs, 31, Suppl 2*, 26.

50. Foulds G (1986) Pharmacokinetics of sulbactam/ampicillin in humans: a review. *Rev. Infect. Dis., 8, Suppl 5*, S503.

51. Usada Y, Sekine O, Aoki N et al (1985) Pharmacokinetics of antibiotics combined with *β*-lactamase inhibitors in patients with renal and/or hepatic dysfunctions. In: Ishigami J (Ed), *Recent Advances in Chemotherapy*, p 1310. University of Tokyo Press, Tokyo.

52. Kaleida PH, Bluestone CD, Blatter MM (1986) Sultamicillin (ampicillin-sulbactam) in the treatment of acute otitis media in children. *Pediatr. Infect. Dis., 5*, 33.

53. Williams ME, Thomas D, Harman CP et al (1985) Positive direct antiglobulin tests due to clavulanic acid. *Antimicrob. Agents Chemother., 27*, 125.

54. Iwato S, Sato Y, Kusumoto Y et al (1985) The influence of new cephens on the intesti-

nal flora. In: Ishigami J (Ed), *Recent Advances in Chemotherapy*, p 2603. University of Tokyo Press, Tokyo.

55. Lode H, Kass EH (Eds) (1986) Enzyme-mediated Resistance to β-Lactam Antibiotics: A Symposium on Sulbactam/Ampicillin. *Rev. Infect. Dis., 8, Suppl 5.*

56. Schaad UB, Pfenninger J, Wedgwood-Krucko J (1987) Sequential intravenous-oral amoxycillin/clavulanate (Augmentin) therapy in paediatric hospital practice. *J. Antimicrob. Chemother., 19*, 385.

57. Boston PF, Gowers E, Rose AJ (1986) Augmentin compared with oxytetracycline for chest infections in general practice. *Br. J. Dis. Chest, 80,* 148.

58. Drumm J, Donovan IA, Wise R, Lowe P (1985) Metronidazole and Augmentin in the prevention of sepsis after appendicectomy. *Br. J. Surg., 72,* 571.

59. *The Japanese Journal of Antibiotics (February*, 1985).

60. Manian FA, Alford RH (1986) Discrepancies between disk diffusion and broth susceptibility studies of the activity of ticarcillin plus clavulanic acid against ticarcillin-resistant *Pseudomonas aeruginosa. Antimicrob. Agents Chemother., 30,* 35.

61. Tausk F, Stratton CW (1986) Effect of clavulanic acid on the activity of ticarcillin against *Pseudomonas aeruginosa. Antimicrob. Agents Chemother., 30,* 584.

62. Verbist L, Verhaegen J (1986) Susceptibility of ticarcillin-resistant gram-negative bacilli to different combinations of ticarcillin and clavulanic acid. *J. Antimicrob. Chemother., 17, Suppl C,* 7.

63. Pulverer G, Peters G, Kunstmann G (1986) In-vitro activity of ticarcillin with and without clavulanic acid against clinical isolates of gram-positive and gram-negative bacteria. *J. Antimicrob. Chemother., 17, Suppl C,* 1.

64. Kosmidis J, Stathakis C, Boletis J, Daikos GK (1983) Ticarcillin/clavulanic acid combination in serious infections: clinical pharmacokinetic and in vitro evaluation. In: *Proceedings, 13th International Conference on Chemotherapy, Vienna, 1983 Vol. 3/97,* p 56. Egermann, Vienna.

65. Neu HC (Ed.) (1985) Beta-lactamase inhibition: therapeutic advances. *Am. J. Med., 79, Suppl 5B.*

66. Leigh DA, Phillips I, Wise R (Eds) (1986) Timentin – ticarcillin plus clavulanic acid: a laboratory and clinical perspective. *J. Antimicrob. Chemother., 17, Suppl C.*

67. Dorflinger T, Madsen PO (1985) Antibiotic prophylaxis on transurethral surgery: a comparison of sulbactam-ampicillin and cefoxitin. *Infection, 13,* 66.

68. *The Japanese Journal of Antibiotics (October,* 1984).

69. Kunii O (1985) Clinical evaluation of sulbactam/cefoperazone in the field of internal medicine. In: Ishigami J (Ed), *Recent Advances in Chemotherapy*, p 23. University of Tokyo Press, Tokyo.

70. Nishiura T (1985) Clinical evaluation of sulbactam/cefoperazone in the surgical field. In: Ishigami J (Ed), *Recent Advances in Chemotherapy*, p 23. University of Tokyo Press, Tokyo.

71. Hara K, Saito A, Suzuyama Y (1985) Well controlled comparative clinical trial of sulbactam/cefoperazone and cefotaxime in the treatment of respiratory infections. *Chemotherapy (Tokyo), 33,* 159.

72. Gould IM, Legge JS, Reid TMS (1987) Amoxycillin/Clavulanic acid levels in respiratory secretions. *J. Antimicrob. Chemother.,* in press.

CHAPTER 6

The cephalosporins and cephamycins

CHRISTINE C. SANDERS, JOHAN S. BAKKEN
and W. EUGENE SANDERS Jr

The purpose of this Chapter is to review the literature concerning cephalosporin and cephamycin antibiotics published during 1986 and early 1987. The reader is referred to our Chapters in the previous two issues of this *Annual* (1, 2) for information published prior to this time.

The general characteristics of a number of currently used cephalosporins and cephamycins are listed in Table 1. Their characteristics have been updated since the table was published in the second issue of the *Annual* (2). A number of reviews and proceedings of symposia concerning the cephalosporins and cephamycins have been published in the last 12 months (3–15). They provide extensive details on the properties and uses of the agents listed in Table 1.

ACTIVITY/RESISTANCE

Inducible β-lactamases

The inducible, chromosomally-mediated β-lactamases of certain non-fastidious gram-negative bacilli that are responsible for broad-spectrum cephalosporin resistance continue to be the subject of intensive investigation. In the last 12 months, major advances have been made in delineating which β-lactams are powerful reversible inducers of the enzymes and which are efficient selectors of stably derepressed mutants that express greatly elevated levels of the enzymes (16–19). It is extremely important to separate these two properties since most drugs that are efficient inducers are poor selectors and vice versa (19–21). Thus, it would be misleading to discuss the 'inducer potential' of any compound without first identifying whether reversible induction or selection of stably derepressed mutants is being considered. From the numerous studies performed to date, it appears that the cephamycins and imipenem are extremely potent reversible inducers regardless of

Antimicrobial Agents Annual 3
P.K. Peterson and J. Verhoef, editors
©Elsevier Science Publishers BV, 1988

Table 1.   *Overview of the cephalosporins and cephamycins*

	Clinically important spectra[a]						Clinical indications[d]	
	Strepto-cocci[b]	Staphylo-cocci[c]	*Haemo-philus*	Enterics	*Pseudo-monas*	*B. fragilis* group	Gonorrhea	Meningitis
First-generation cephalosporins	±	+	±	+[R]	0	0		
Cefalotin							0	0
Cefazolin							0	0
Ceforanide							0	0
Cefaclor							0	0
Second-generation cephalosporins	±	+	±	++[R]	0	0		
Cefamandole							0	0
Cefuroxime			+				+	+
Cefonicid							(+)	0
Cephamycins	0	0	+	++[R]	0	+[R]		
Cefoxitin							+	0
Cefotetan							+	0
Third-generation cephalosporins	0	0	+	+++[R]	±	+[R]		
Cefotaxime	±	±					+	+
Moxalactam							0	+
Cefoperazone					+[R]	±	(+)	0
Ceftizoxime	±	±					+	+
Ceftriaxone	±	±					+	+
Ceftazidime					+[R]		*[e]	+
Cefmenoxime	±	±					*	(+)
Cefsulodin			0	0	+[R]	0	0	(+)

[a]Infections caused by these organisms may respond to therapy with the drug indicated. Spectrum for each major group is indicated. Only exceptions to the group profile are indicated for specific drugs. 0 = not indicated; +/− = indicated only under very special circumstances; + = indicated but may not be drug of choice (number of pluses indicates relative percent of strains susceptible); R = some strains resistant.

[b]Streptococci excluding enterococci. None of the drugs listed is active against enterococci.

[c]None of the drugs listed is active against methicillin-resistant staphylococci.

[d]Indications for single dose treatment of gonorrhea including that due to penicillin-resistant strains and for treatment of meningitis. 0 = not indicated; + = indicated and approved by FDA; (+) = data insufficient for approved indication but approval likely with additional data.

[e]* = insufficient data.

organism or inducer concentration examined (1, 2, 16–19). Certain compounds, like desacetylcefotaxime, first- and second-generation cephalosporins, and potassium clavulanate are variable inducers enhancing enzyme levels in some but not all strains examined. This variability appears to be dependent not only upon the

Side-chain Toxicity[f]	Excretion[g] urine (bile)	Adjust dose[i] R (L)	Removed by dialysis H(P)[i]	Serum T½[j] (h)	Dose interval[j] (h) M/S	Recent reviews, symposia	
							First-generation cephalosporins
						6, 10, 14	
0	60-80[h]	+(0)	+(+)	0.7	4/4		Cefalotin
0	90	+(0)	+(0)	1.4	8-12/6		Cefazolin
0	90	+	+	2.8	12/12		Ceforanide
0	60-85	±(0)	0	0.8	8/[k]		Cefaclor
							Second-generation cephalosporins
						6, 14	
+	65-85	+(0)	+(0)	0.6	4-8/4-6	11	Cefamandole
0	90	+(0)	+(+)	1.2	8/6		Cefuroxime
0	90	+(0)	0	4.5	24/24		Cefonicid
						3	*Cephamycins*
0	85	+(0)	+(0)	0.8	4-8/4-6	8, 9	Cefoxitin
+	60-75 (12)	+	+	3.5	12		Cefotetan
							Third-generation cephalosporins
						3,5,6,7,13-15	
0	55[h]	±(0)	+(+)	1.1	6-8/4-6		Cefotaxime
+	75-90	+(0)	+(0)	2.3	8-12/6		Moxalactam
+	25-30 (70)	0(+)	±	1.9	12/6-8	12	Cefoperazone
0	85	+(0)	+	1.9	8-12/8		Ceftizoxime
0	40-60 (11-65)	±(0)	0(0)	5.8-8.7	24/12[l]	4	Ceftriaxone
0	90	+(0)	+(+)	1.8	8-12/8		Ceftazidime
+	72 (11)	+	+(+)	1.5	6-8		Cefmenoxime
0	65	+	+	1.6	6-8		Cefsulodin

[f]Bleeding and disulfiram reactions associated with methylthiotetrazole side-chain. 0 = drug does not possess side-chain; + = drug possesses side-chain and toxicity has been demonstrated; (+) = drug possesses side-chain, data on toxicity limited.

[g]Percent of dose eliminated by route indicated. Bile listed only when significant percent eliminated by this route.

[h]Metabolized to desacetylated derivative.

[i]Dosage adjustment needed in presence of renal (R) or liver (L) disease. Removed by hemo- (H) or peritoneal (P) dialysis.

[j]Values shown are for adults. Dose interval shown for mild to moderate (M) and severe (S) infections. Values in parentheses are tentative.

[k]not applicable.

[l]12 h interval for meningitis.

drug and species examined, but also upon the particular strain examined (19). In general, the penicillins and third-generation cephalosporins are poor reversible inducers unless extremely high, superinhibitory concentrations are examined (16-19). Selection of stably derepressed mutants does not occur with imipenem, while most of the newer cephalosporins are highly efficient selectors (17-23).

The genetics responsible for inducible β-lactamases in Enterobacteriaceae have also been extensively studied over the last 12 months (24-27). A recent review by Lindberg and Normark (25) detailed the genetic system responsible for these enzymes as it is now understood. It appears that the structural gene, *amp*C is under both positive and negative control by an adjacent regulatory region *amp*R. This region must be present for induction to occur. However, mutations leading to stable derepression occur outside the *amp*R-*amp*C region in a non-adjacent area of the chromosome designated *amp*D. Thus, stable derepression may not be due to a mutation in a conventional repressor gene. Recent studies by Gates et al (28) suggest that the genetic region responsible for the inducible chromosomal β-lactamase in *Pseudomonas aeruginosa* may be more complex than that in the Enterobacteriaceae. This organism, unlike most Enterobacteriaceae, undergoes sequential derepression which involves at least 2 mutational events. The β-lactamase product of each stage of derepression is different, suggesting perhaps 2 structural genes under control of the same repressor. Clearly, much more investigation will be required before the expression of these chromosomal enzymes so important to cephalosporin resistance is fully understood.

The mechanism by which inducible, chromosomally-mediated β-lactamases produce resistance to the newer cephalosporins continues to be the subject of numerous investigations (16, 18, 19, 29, 30). Hydrolysis of ceftriaxone, cefotaxime, cefsulodin, cefpiramide, cefoperazone, cefmenoxime, and other β-lactam antibiotics by the chromosomal cephalosporinase produced by various Enterobacteriaceae and *P. aeruginosa* was demonstrated in several studies (16, 18, 19, 29). Studies by Phelps et al (30) emphasized the importance of enzyme affinity in the resistance mediated by chromosomal cephalosporinases. These investigators showed that in many instances both ceftazidime and BMY-28142 were equally resistant to hydrolysis but only the latter possessed appreciable activity against strains producing high levels of cephalosporinase. The major difference found between the 2 compounds was a lower affinity of the enzyme for BMY-28142. Thus, affinity of the enzyme for a β-lactam drug was a better indicator for resistance than susceptibility of the drug to hydrolysis. All factors involved in resistance to newer β-lactams mediated by chromosomal cephalosporinases were reviewed by Sanders and Sanders (19). Studies by these authors showed that affinity of the enzyme for a drug, susceptibility to hydrolysis, rate of drug permeation, and numbers of lethal targets in the cell all determine the effect of derepression of chromosomal cephalosporinases on the activity of β-lactam antibiotics. Anionic cephalosporins were most affected while zwitterionic penems, penams and carbapenems were least affected by derepression of these enzymes. The former penetrated less well, had multiple lethal targets, and were bound avidly by the chromosomal cephalosporinases. The latter penetrated rapidly, had few lethal targets and may or may not be bound by the cephalosporinase. Thus, multiple factors, not merely resistance to hydrolysis, must be taken into account before any accurate predictions of drug activity in the presence of β-lactamase can be made.

Other β-lactamases

Livermore and Jones recently described a novel-plasmid-mediated β-lactamase in *P. aeruginosa* that was responsible for resistance to cefoperazone and cefsulodin but not cefotaxime, ceftazidime, ceftriaxone or moxalactam (31). This enzyme, designated NPS-1, had a pI of 6.5, hydrolyzed cephalosporins less rapidly than benzylpenicillin and did hydrolyze oxacillin at a rate one-half of that of benzylpenicillin. Enzymes mediating resistance to moxalactam and cefoxitin have been demonstrated in various species of *Bacteroides* including *B. fragilis, B. thetaiotaomicron* and *B. bivius* (32–35). Disturbing features of these enzymes that have been recently delineated include the transmissibility of one *B. fragilis* β-lactamase of pI 8.1 (34) and the broad-spectrum, high-level resistance mediated by a second *B. fragilis* enzyme that requires a zinc cofactor (33). This latter enzyme is similar to those found in *P. maltophilia* and *Flavobacterium odoratum* and is insusceptible to inhibition by sulbactam or potassium clavulanate.

Other resistance mechanisms

Resistance to cephalosporins mediated by non-enzymatic mechanisms was reported in clinical isolates of *Neisseria gonorrhoeae* and *Escherichia coli*. Non-penicillinase-producing strains of *N. gonorrhoeae* that are resistant to penicillin have been described recently (36, 37). These chromosomally resistant strains possess altered penicillin-binding proteins and are 4- to 16-fold less susceptible to cefoxitin and 16- to 256-fold less susceptible to cefotaxime. A recent report by Bakken et al (38) emphasized the importance of outer-membrane permeability upon susceptibility to cephalosporins. A clinical isolate of *E. coli* recovered from a child after 8 weeks of ceftazidime therapy was found to be resistant to this third-generation drug only. This selective resistance to ceftazidime was found to be due to altered outer-membrane proteins (OMPs). Since ceftazidime is the poorest penetrating drug among the newer cephalosporins, such selective resistance via this mechanism was not surprising. However, the ability of potassium clavulanate to reverse this resistance via a direct effect upon the OMPs was unexpected. Thus, it appears that potassium clavulanate, in addition to functioning as a β-lactamase inhibitor, may potentiate the effects of certain β-lactam drugs via a permeabilizing effect.

CLINICAL PHARMACOLOGY

A number of papers, describing various aspects of the clinical pharmacology of the new cephalosporins, appeared in the literature in the last year. The salient features of the drugs in clinical use are summarized in Table 1. Specific pharmacokinetic details may be found in recent papers dealing with concentrations in vitreous humor (39) and cerebrospinal fluid (40-42), and the influence of hemodialysis and chronic ambulatory peritoneal dialysis (CAPD) on cephalosporin clearance (43–51).

ADVERSE EFFECTS AND DRUG INTERACTIONS

The cephalosporins and cephamycins continue to be among the safest antimicrobial agents. In a recent review, Midtvedt stressed that misuse constitutes the most serious side effect of the newer β-lactam antibiotics (52). From data presented in 2 large reviews (14, 15), it appears that the adverse effects relative to renal, hepatic and hematopoietic parameters usually are mild, reversible and of a similar low magnitude for all third-generation cephalosporins. However, the growing number of reports on superinfections and emergence of resistance during clinical use of expanded spectrum cephalosporins raises serious concern about the safety and efficacy of these agents. These topics are covered in detail in a separate section of this Chapter.

Coagulopathies

The literature cited in *Annual 2* (2) established that prolongation of the prothrombin time observed with certain new cephalosporins is caused by the NMTT group attached in the 3-position of the dihydrothiazine ring (Table 1). This has been reiterated in a recent review by Sattler et al (53). The release of free NMTT has been proposed to result from hepatic metabolism with excretion of the side chain into plasma or bile (with enterohepatic reabsorption) or by direct release into the small intestine. Aronoff et al (11) showed that the free NMTT moiety was rapidly cleared from plasma in volunteers with normal renal function. With diminished renal function cefamandole and NMTT plasma levels remained high. Furthermore, renal failure caused significant reduction in NMTT protein-binding, and this was attributed directly to metabolic alterations occurring in patients with uremia. Thus, prolonged and elevated NMTT plasma levels are more likely to occur in patients with reduced renal function or those who are malnourished or hypoproteinemic. This renders these patients at greater risk for developing hypoprothrombinemia and bleeding due to the interference of NMTT with γ-carboxylation of glutamic acid (1, 2). In a prospective, double-blind multicenter study Nichols et al (54) demonstrated a higher incidence of hypoprothrombinemia in patients with peritonitis than in those with pneumonia. They also observed that moxalactam induced the highest average increase in prothombin time when compared with either ceftizoxime or cefotaxime. A close correlation between the degree of ileus and development of coagulopathy in moxalactam-treated patients was also evident. Washida et al (55) evaluated prospectively coagulation profiles in 40 otherwise healthy patients treated with cefmenoxime for complicated urinary tract infections. Twenty of 40 patients received 10 mg of vitamin K_2 intravenously on the first day of therapy. Reversible changes in coagulation, unassociated with clinical bleeding, were observed in 3 of the patients that were not given supplemental vitamin K. Brown et al (56) confirmed an increased risk of bleeding with moxalactam by a multivariate analysis of 1493 patients treated with various antibiotics. The rate of bleeding with moxalactam therapy was 22.2%. However, 8.2% of patients given cefoxitin also developed clinically significant bleeding, and the authors speculated that other chemical moieties on the cephalosporin nucleus were possible responsible. To date, only cephalosporins with a *N*-methylthiotetrazole (NMTT) side chain (cefmetazole, moxalactam, cefoperazone, cefmenoxime, cefamandole, cefotetan) have been implicated in causing vitamin-K-reversible hypoprothrombinemia. However, Agnelli et al (57) recently questioned whether or not the NMTT side chain is the culprit in cephalosporin-induced hypoprothrombinemia. They found changes of equal magnitude in the prothrombin time following cefamandole and ceftriaxone treatment in their study of 30 patients with various serious infections. No changes were observed in the prothrombin time of patients treated with ceftazidime. Ceftriaxone contains a thriazine ring rather than the NMTT side chain, and both moieties are connected to the β-lactam ring by a sulfhydryl group in the 3-position. It has previously been shown that glutathione reduces the inhibitory effect of NMTT on prothrombin synthesis, which may indicate that the sulfhydryl group of NMTT plays an important role in causing coagulopathy (58). The support of this was the observation that ceftazidime, which does not contain a free sulfhydryl group, did not induce hypoprothrombinemia (57). Kerremans et al (59) have recently suggested that individual variations in *S*-methylation of heterocyclic thiol metabolites of cephalosporins may be responsible for individual differences in susceptibility to cephalosporin-induced hypoprothrombinemia.

Disulfiram-like reactions

It has been established that cephalosporins containing the NMTT side chain may cause a disulfiram-like reaction to alcohol (1, 2), but the details of the mechanisms responsible are still unsettled. Kitson postulated that the free NMTT-side chain is oxidized in vivo to form a dimer which has considerable structural similarity to disulfiram (60). Freundt, however, argues that the intact cefamandole molecule is responsible, contending that 'cefamandole is not metabolized in humans' (61). NMTT alone was found to inhibit the metabolic convertion of radiolabeled ethanol to $^{14}CO_2$ to the same extent as moxalactam in a study by Turcan et al (62). Aronoff et al (11) have recently shown that free NMTT does appear in plasma of patients treated with cefamandole. It therefore seems plausible that the NMTT-moiety, either alone or in the dimer form proposed by Kitson (60) is the responsible factor.

Hematologic suppression

Rashes, fever and/or eosinophilia with accompanying neutropenia may occur in 5-15% of patients treated with cephalosporins for more than 10 days (2, 14, 15). It is still unsettled whether neutropenia results from a direct toxic effect of β-lactam drugs on granulocytopoiesis, IgG immune-complex-mediated destruction of immature granulocytes, or both.

Hypersensitivity reaction

A syndrome consisting of generalized puritic rash and arthritis was observed by Murray et al (63) in children taking cefaclor. By 1985 more than 600 cases had been reported to Eli Lilly and Company prompting a warning in the package insert (64). Kammer and Short estimated that 1.5% of patients taking cefaclor will develop this reaction (65). Although children under 2 years of age are most commonly affected, the syndrome may develop in adults as well (64, 66). Approximately two-thirds of the cases occur upon second administration of cefaclor, and previous hypersensitivity reactions to other classes of antibiotics are frequently found in the medical history. The rash usually appears 1-2 weeks after initiation of therapy, develops centrally and/or peripherally, and may be purpuric, maculopapular or even erythema-multiform-like. There are few specific derangements in laboratory parameters, but most patients will manifest leukocytosis. Upon withdrawal of cefaclor the symptoms are usually readily reversible. No cross-allergy with other cephalosporins has been noted. It is presently unclear whether it is cefaclor itself or the specific base, to which cefaclor is added, that is the antigenic determinant (66). Although the risk for important sequelae from this adverse reaction appears low, it would appear prudent to use alternative agents for the therapy of bacterial upper respiratory infections in children.

CLINICAL USES

The cephalosporins continue to be the most widely prescribed antibiotic group in the United States (67). A number of reviews addressed the general use of cephalosporins (2, 3, 5-7, 68, 69) and specific drugs (4, 8, 9). Individual publications were largely confirmatory of findings described in *Annual 2*. Cefotetan, a cephamycin, was the only new drug approved for clinical use by the Food and Drug Administration in 1986. For the first time in its history, the *Medical Letter* (68) recommended cephalosporins as antimicrobial drugs of first choice for therapy of certain bacterial infections (5 species within Enterobacteriaceae, *Haemophilus ducreyi* and *N. gonorrhoeae*). This recommendation appeared to be based primarily upon an attempt to avoid the use of aminoglycosides and possible associated nephro- and/or ototoxicity. However, the *Medical Letter* remained undecided as to whether or not the third-generation cephalosporins will eventually replace the aminoglycosides for 'gram-negative coverage' in patients with suspected sepsis. It also did not explain why a cephalosporin was listed as a preferred agent for treatment of infections due to certain organisms with inducible β-lactamases when in the past, the *Medical Letter* has warned about the potential for such organisms to develop resistance rapidly. Neu has recently reviewed the areas of appropriate use of new antibiotic agents (70), and concludes that emergence of resistance to expanded-spectrum cephalosporins has complicated therapy of difficult infections. At the present time there are not sufficient data to resolve many of the controversies regarding the appropriate use of these new agents.

Neutropenia

The recent literature on empiric antibiotic therapy of febrile neutropenic cancer patients has focused on the question of whether β-lactam monotherapy is as efficacious as combination therapy (71-76). Although several investigators conclude that ceftazidime monotherapy is as efficacious as standard regimens (71-73, 75), others have found less satisfactory results with β-lactam monotherapy and advocate a β-lactam aminoglycoside combination (77-81). Valid comparisons of results from separate trials are difficult to make since many studies used different definitions of clinical response (81). It is noteworthy that among approximately 2000 patients with neutropenia and fever, microbiologically documented infections and/or bacteremia were only found in approximately 30% and 20%, respectively (71-73, 75, 77-80). Gram-positive organisms accounted for a substantial number of cases with bacteremia, and most investigators admit that additional antibiotic coverage with compounds like vancomycin, may be needed initially or added later for patients that do not show a favorable clinical response to β-lactam monotherapy (71, 72, 76-80). Young states that the most important deciding factor in the outcome in these patients appears to be the severity and duration of neutropenia and whether it resolves, since successful treatment of infection is usually related to a rise in the neutrophil count (81).

A disturbing observation was that resistance to third-generation cephalosporins among gram-negative bacilli isolated from hospitalized patients was significantly more common in patients previously treated with one of the newer cephalosporins (81, 82). While Verhagen et al (75) successfully used ceftazidime to treat neutropenic patients with *P. aeruginosa* bacteremia, Bragman et al (83) noted emergence of ceftazidime resistance and therepeutic failure in 33% of similar patients with systemic *P. aeruginosa* infections. It remains unresolved whether β-lactam monotherapy offers adequate protection as presumptive therapy for patients with granulocytopenia and fever. However, available evidence tends to support the superiority of combination therapy for gram-negative bacteremia in such patients (70, 84).

Specific infections

Meningitis The Board of the American Academy of Pediatrics has recently reviewed the diagnosis and management of meningitis in pediatric patients (85). Cephalosporins have not been recommended as agents for initial antimicrobial chemotherapy in meningitis in children or neonates. Second- or third-generation cephalosporins have been recommended only as alternate agents in patients that would not tolerate penicillins, chloramphenicol or aminoglycosides. However, Neu contends in a recent review that cefotaxime, ceftizoxime, ceftazidime or ceftriaxone should be the drugs of choice for adults with meningitis due to *E. coli* or *Klebsiella pneumoniae* (70).

In a multicenter randomized trial, 107 patients aged 3 months to 16 years with bacterial meningitis were initially given either cefuroxime or ampicillin plus chloramphenicol (86). Clinical cure rates were identical (95%) with 1 death in each group. Chloramphenicol and ampicillin sterilized the cerebrospinal fluid (CSF) earlier than cefuroxime, thus the authors felt that additional investigation would be necessary to demonstrate the equivalence of cefuroxime. They recommended standard therapy. Prado et al (57) evaluated ceftriaxone dosed twice daily for the treatment of meningitis in 24 pediatric patients. Two patients infected with *Enterobacter hafnia* and pneumococci failed, while the remaining 22 patients were cured. CSF ceftriaxone concentrations were consistently above the minimum inhibitory concentrations (MICs) of all the isolated pathogens including one *P. aeruginosa*. Thus, the results of these recent clinical trials of newer cephalosporins in bacterial meningitis continue to be encouraging, but less than definitive.

Sexually transmitted diseases Grimes et al (88) examined the patterns of antibiotic treatment between 1966 and 1983 for acute sexually transmitted pelvic inflammatory disease (PID) in women of reproductive age. Although cephalosporins emerged as the most frequently prescribed antibiotic for hospitalized patients, the authors suggested that this trend may be unwise due to the prevalent involvement of *Chlamydia trachomatis* in this syndrome. Cefoxitin + probenecid or ceftriaxone, either one followed by tetracycline, has recently been recommended by the *Medical Letter* for non-hospitalized patients with PID (69).

Mills et al recently reviewed the literature on trials of different β-lactam drugs (89) in single-dose therapy of uncomplicated gonococcal infections. Oral or parenteral second- and third-generation drugs were each more than 90% efficacious. Uncomplicated gonorrhea due to penicillin-sensitive and penicillinase-producing *N. gonorrhoeae* (PPNG) strains was successfully treated with cefoxitin and probenecid (90) or cefuroxime axetil with or without probenecid (91-93) in over 90% of patients. Anogenital and pharyngeal gonorrhea responded less well, but the addition of probenecid improved the cure rate observed with cefuroxime axetil (91). At present, ceftriaxone is the recommended drug of choice in the treatment of anorectal or pharyngeal gonorrhea (69). In a recent study by Laga et al (94), a single 125 mg i.m. dose of ceftriaxone cured all 62 neonates with gonococcal ophthalmia neonatorum (54% of strains PPNG), as well as 18 of 18 neonates with oropharyngeal gonococcal infection. Bowmer et al (95) found that a single intramuscular dose of 250 or 500 mg ceftriaxone cured 129 of 132 men with chancroid. A 27-year-old man with documented hypersensitivity to penicillin was treated intramuscularly with ceftriaxone at 1 g daily for 14 days for asymptomatic neurosyphilis (96). Following ceftriaxone therapy, serum and CSF IgG reactivity to all lues-associated antigens steadily decreased. The authors suggested that ceftriaxone may provide a useful alternative therapy for penicillin-allergic patients with neurosyphilis.

Obstetric and gynecologic infections   Cefotetan was compared to moxalactam or cefoxitin by Poindexter et al (97) in a study of young women with pelvic infections. One of 118 patients treated with cefotetan had an unsatisfactory clinical response while all of the patients treated with either moxalactam or cefoxitin were cured. Two prospective investigations compared cefoxitin with piperacillin for the treatment of pelvic infections (98, 99). Both studies demonstrated equal efficacy, with cure rates ranging from 86 to 93%.

Respiratory infections   A randomized study of patients with pneumonia, comparing the safety and efficacy of cefamandole with ceftriaxone, was recently described by Bittner et al (100). A total of 37 patients were evaluated, and all but one patient had underlying diseases. Although gram-negative bacilli comprised only 19% of pre-therapy isolates, they accounted for 6 of 7 cases (86%) with bacteriologic and 3 of 4 cases (75%) with clinical failure. In another randomized multicenter trial in hospitalized patients with pneumonia (101) satisfactory clinical responses were observed in 91% of ceftazidime-treated patients and 83% of cefamandole-treated patients. Clinical failures were caused by mixed infections with gram-positive and gram-negative bacteria. Two of 23 patients with pneumococcal pneumonia failed ceftazidime therapy, which correlates with the poor in vitro activity of this agent against many gram-positive pathogens.

Antibiotic therapy of respiratory tract infections in patients with cystic fibrosis is particularly difficult since *P. aeruginosa* is the single most common pathogen encountered. Blumer et al (102) noted in a recent review of cephalosporin therapy for patients with cystic fibrosis that both cefsulodin and ceftazidime have been evaluated extensively and appear to be effective therapy for acute pulmonary exacerbations in cystic fibrosis. Thus, they felt that cephalosporin monotherapy is 'at least as effective as broad-spectrum penicillin and an aminoglycoside'. It was also noted that 'ceftazidime is the drug to which these organisms (*Pseudomonas* spp.) remain susceptible even when they are highly resistant to other β-lactam and aminoglycoside antibiotics. The experiences of several other groups stand in sharp contrast to those of Blumer and colleagues. Emergence of multiple β-lactam resistance in cystic fibrosis patients had been noted in several recent reports. Paull and Morgan (103) described 9 cystic fibrosis patients treated with ceftriaxone alone or ceftriaxone combined with tobramycin. All pre-therapy isolates were susceptible to ceftriaxone. However, after therapy, isolates from 5 patients (56%) were found to be resistant to ceftriaxone. An epidemic spread of multiresistant *P. aeruginosa* in a Danish cystic fibrosis center was recently reported by Pedersen et al (104). Cefsulodin and ceftazidime were used extensively in this center from 1978 to 1983. In March 1983 there was an increase from 5 to 42% in the monthly prevalence of multiply resistant *P. aeruginosa* among their 119 cystic fibrosis patients. It was concluded that cephalosporin monotherapy was responsible for the increased prevalence of resistant bacteria, and the authors strongly argued for combination therapy with a *Pseudomonas*-active penicillin combined with tobramycin, as well as optimal use of hygienic measures to prevent epidemic spread.

Miscellaneous infections Several clinical trials assessed the efficacy of second- and third-generation cephalosporins in non-neutropenic patients. In a study by Uwaydah et al (105), moxalactam treatment of 25 patients with typhoid fever produced defervescence of fever and amelioration of systemic symptoms in all cases. However, treatment for only 3 or 5 days resulted in relapse in 4 of 14 patients, while no relapses were observed in patients treated for 10 days. Although moxalactam was found effective, it was suggested that this antibiotic be reserved for special indications due to the potential toxic side effects of the drug. Cardenas et al (106) reported that single-dose therapy with cefalexin for acute uncomplicated urinary tract infection was effective in 87% of women who were less than 25 years of age. In contrast, cures were achieved in only 40% of women older than 40 years. The lower cure rate in the older age group may have reflected increasing anatomical changes in the urinary tract with advancing age. Frongillo et al (107) evaluated the clinical efficacy of cefamandole in the treatment of serious staphylococcal infections caused by methicillin-susceptible (MSSA) or resistant (MRSA) strains. Only 2 of 5 patients with MRSA bacteremia were cured of their infection by cefamandole, while cure was achieved in 10 of 11 patients with urinary tract and skin infections. It is possible that surgical debridement and high urine drug concentrations contributed to the high cure rate observed in patients with skin and urinary tract infections since 3 of 9 cases of septicemia, and 2 of 2 patients with endocarditis caused by MSSA failed therapy with cefamandole. The relatively poor performance of cefamandole in patients with endocarditis and septicemia underscores the warnings of Eng et al (108) and *Annual 2* (2) against the use of cefamandole for therapy of serious infections caused by MRSA or MSSA.

Surgical prophylaxis

Several recent reviews have addressed the role of the cephalosporins in prophylaxis (109, 110). However, many recent comparative studies continue to suffer from common flaws in study design and interpretations as outlined in *Annual 1* (1). Although an abundance of studies on the efficacy of expanded-spectrum cephalosporins in prophylaxis have appeared in the last year, the general concensus remains that there is still no reason to prefer second- and third-generation cephalosporins over the first-generation cephalosporins, with the possible exception of cefoxitin in colorectal surgery (1, 2, 109, 110).

Emergence of resistance during clinical use

The rapid development of resistance during therapy with many of the newer cephalosporins continues to be documented in the scientific literature (76, 83, 103, 111-117). As before, most of the organisms involved were usually those possessing inducible, chromosomal cephalosporinases (2) and resistance was associated with stable derepression of these enzymes. Also, in many patients, combination therapy did not prevent this development of resistance (76, 83, 103, 111, 112, 114, 117). Since the clinical importance of this phenomenon has now been well documented, more recent studies have focused on assessment of risk factors associated with this problem and the spread of resistant strains in the hospital environment.

The overall risk of rapid development of resistance during therapy is a subject of frequent controversy. Although many investigators have not found emergence of resistance to be a problem, this is often the result of having few patients at risk included in the study (71). The true risk of rapid development of resistance can be assessed only from studies with patients infected with organisms possessing inducible β-lactamases – for it is in this population that the risk exists. From such studies, rates of emergence of resistance between 14 and 56% have been observed (1, 2, 83, 103, 111, 117). In most studies, clinical failure was associated with resistance in the majority of patients (83, 111, 113-115, 117). To date, only 1 prospective study limited to patients infected with organisms possessing inducible β-lactamases who were treated with one of the newer cephalosporins has been performed (111). In this study, Dworzack et al (111) reported an overall occurrence of emergence of resistance in 7 of 44 (16%) patients. Emergence of resistance was more likely to occur with infections of the respiratory tract (25%) and bone or soft tissue (13%) than with infections of the urinary tract (0%). Factors other than infection occurring outside of the urinary tract that have been associated with increased risk of emergence of resistance include neutropenia, cystic fibrosis and, of course, exposure to a cephalosporin (83, 103, 104, 114, 117).

The use of cephalosporins has been associated with a number of problems which could ultimately lead to increased resistance. Burchard et al (118) examined the occurrence of *Enterobacter* bacteremia in surgical patients and found an association with prolonged cephalosporin exposure. Prevot et al (119) documented a greater risk of intestinal colonization and bacteremia with cefotaxime-resistant Enterobacteriaceae among neutropenic patients treated with cefotaxime. Chiesa et al (120) examined *Pseudomonas cepacia* recovered from patients with cystic fibrosis and found higher β-lactamase production in isolates from patients treated with ceftazidime. Weinstein (117) demonstrated a strong positive correlation between use of second- and third-generation cephalosporins and occurrence of cefotaxime-resistant *Enterobacter* in 17 medical and surgical wards over a 2-year period. He also showed that most cefotaxime-resistant *Enterobacter* initiating an infection were recovered from the urinary tract of patients who had no prior exposure to cephalosporins. This suggested nosocomial spread of these organisms (117).

89

One of the most impressive reports of nosocomial problems associated with use of the newer cephalosporins was by Bryan et al (82). These authors described an outbreak of bacteremias due to multiply resistant *Enterobacter cloacae* in a neonatal intensive care unit. This outbreak occurred only 10 weeks after switching from ampicillin/gentamicin to ampicillin/cefotaxime as empiric therapy for suspected sepsis. Surveillance stool cultures taken during this time revealed that most patients in the unit were colonized with multiply resistant *Enterobacter*. One of the most striking features of this report was the fact that significant resistance to gentamicin in this unit required 11 years to develop while resistance to cefotaxime occurred in only 10 weeks.

DOSING AND COST

The cephalosporins, and in particular those used for surgical prophylaxis, continue to account for the largest expenditure for hospital drugs in the United States. Cefoxitin and cefamandole were the top two drugs of any category in 1984 (67). Many programs have been designed and implemented to improve cephalosporin use and control cost (2, 67, 121). Education and prescription control have resulted in substantial financial savings in many institutions (122, 123). However, restriction policies are thought by many to be the best way to curb cost and reduce inappropriate use of the third-generation cephalosporins (2, 67, 122-124). Quintilliani et al (125) have recently questioned the rationale behind such programs. These authors contend that combination therapy (e.g. a penicillin and an aminoglycoside) leads to considerable hidden cost, as well as other possible problems such as drug interactions, drug competition for elimination routes, disruption of normal flora with increase in superinfections, and the need for drug serum concentration monitoring. Rahal (126) and Alford (127) disagree. Both expressed concerns about the impact of third-generation cephalosporins on infections caused by gram-negative bacteria with inducible β-lactamases, the lack of activity against many important gram-positive and cell-wall-deficient bacteria, and the lack of thoughtful assessment with individualized antibiotics when third-generation cephalosporins are automatically prescribed. As stated by Rahal (126): 'Therapy with expanded spectrum cephalosporins may prove less costly in dollars than modifiable combination therapy. The effect of cephalosporins on the microbial flora cannot be modified, however, and this will ultimately increase our true costs.'

FUTURE DIRECTIONS

Numerous new cephalosporin and cephamycin derivatives continue to be synthesized in an attempt to improve oral absorption, anti-gram-positive potency, β-lactamase stability and activity against *P. aeruginosa* (128-148). Unfortunately, few of these synthetic processes are directed at solving some of the major problems of the cephamycins and cephalosporins already extant – i.e. their ability to induce chromosomal cephalosporinases and select multiple β-lactam-resistant mutants. Although cefpirome and BMY-28142, 2 zwitterionic cephalosporins, appeared to have improved activity against stably derepressed mutants (30, 149, 150) their development beyond in vitro studies has been very slow. Nevertheless, studies of structure-activity relationships that provided these compounds with reduced affinity for chromosomal cephalosporinases and greater penetration into the cell should be pursued in an attempt to solve the ever-increasing problems posed by these enzymes. Only through such studies can the current threat to the useful lifespan of the cephamycins and cephalosporins be removed.

REFERENCES

1. Sanders CC, Sanders Jr WE (1986) The cephalosporins and cephamycins. In: Peterson PK, Verhoef J (Eds), *The Antimicrobial Agents Annual 1*, p 66. Elsevier, Amsterdam.
2. Sanders CC, Sander Jr WE (1987) The cephalosporins and cephamycins. In: Peterson PK, Verhoef J (Eds), *The Antimicrobial Agents Annual 2*, p 70. Elsevier, Amsterdam.
3. Sykes RB, Bonner DP, Swabb EA (1986) Modern beta-lactam antibiotics. *Pharmacol. Ther., 29*, 231.
4. American Society of Hospital Pharmacists (Eds) (1985) Ceftriaxone sodium. *Am. Hosp. Formul. Serv. Drug Inform., 85, Suppl B*.
5. Neu HC (1986) Beta-lactam antibiotics: structural relationships affecting in vitro activity and pharmacologic properties. *Rev. Infect. Dis., 8, Suppl 3*, S237.
6. Eichenwald HF, Schmitt HJ (1986) The cephalosporin antibiotics in pediatric therapy. *Eur. J. Pediatr., 144*, 532.
7. Fry DE (1986) Third generation cephalosporin antibiotics in surgical practice. *Am. J. Surg., 151*, 306.
8. Quintiliani R (Ed) (1986) Symposium on cefotetan. *Am. J. Obstet. Gynecol., 154*, 945.
9. Anonymous (1986) Cefotetan sodium. *Med. Lett., 28*, 70.
10. Ohashi K, Tsunoo M, Tsuneoka K (1986) Pharmacokinetics and protein binding of cefazolin and cephalothin in patients with cirrhosis. *J. Antimicrob. Chemother., 17*, 347.
11. Aronoff GR, Wolen RL, Obermeyer BD, Black HR (1986) Pharmacokinetics and protein binding of cefamandole and its 1-methyl-1H-tetrazole-5-thiol side-chain in subjects with normal and impaired renal function. *J. Infect. Dis., 153*, 1069.
12. Gonik B, Feldman S, Pickering LK, Doughtie CG (1986) Pharmacokinetics of cefoperazone in the parturient. *Antimicrob. Agents Chemother., 30*, 874.
13. Charles D, Larsen B (1986) Pharmacokinetics of cefotaxime, moxalactam and cefoperazone in the early puerperium. *Antimicrob. Agents Chemother., 29*, 873.
14. Karchmer AD (Ed) (1986) *Safety of Parenteral Cephalosporin. Natl Infectious Diseases Information Network*, Little Falls, NJ.
15. Meyers BR (1985) Comparative toxicities of third generation cephalosporins. *Am. J. Med., 79, Suppl A*, 96.
16. Drigues P, Lanau C, Combes T et al (1986) Etude de l'induction de bêta-lactamase chez *Pseudomonas aeruginosa* par le cefpiramide et trois autres céphalosporines antipyocyaniques. *Pathol. Biol., 34*, 419.

17. Shannon K, Phillips I (1986) The effects on beta-lactam susceptibility of phenotypic induction and genotypic derepression of beta-lactamase synthesis. *J. Antimicrob. Chemother.*, *18, Suppl E*, 15.

18. Livermore D, Yang Y-J (1987) Beta-lactamase lability and inducer power of newer beta-lactam antibiotics in relation to their activity against beta-lactamase inducibility mutants of *Pseudomonas aeruginosa*. *J. Infect. Dis.*, *155*, 775.

19. Sanders CC, Sanders Jr WE (1986) Type 1 beta-lactamases of gram-negative bacteria: interactions with beta-lactam antibiotics. *J. Infect. Dis.*, *154*, 792.

20. Phillips I (1986) Beta-lactamase induction and derepression. *Lancet, 1*, 801.

21. Kirkpatrick B, Ashby J, Wise R (1986) Beta-lactams and imipenem. *Lancet, 1*, 802.

22. Eng RH, Smith SM, Cherubin CE (1986) In vitro emergence of beta-lactam-resistant variants of *Pseudomonas aeruginosa*. *J. Antimicrob. Chemother.*, *17*, 717.

23. Then RL, Angehrn P (1986) Multiply resistant mutants of *Enterobacter cloacae* selected by beta-lactam antibiotics. *Antimicrob. Agents Chemother.*, *30*, 684.

24. Nicholas M-H, Honore N, Tarlier V et al (1987) Molecular genetic analysis of cephalosporinase production and its role in beta-lactam resistance in clinical isolates of *Enterobacter cloacae*. *Antimicrob. Agents Chemother.*, *31*, 295.

25. Lindberg F, Normark S (1986) Contribution of chromosomal beta-lactamases to beta-lactam resistance in Enterobacteria. *Rev. Infect. Dis.*, *8*, S292.

26. Lindberg F, Normark S (1986) Sequence of *Citrobacter freundii* OS60 chromosomal *ampC* beta-lactamase gene. *Eur. J. Biochem.*, *156*, 441.

27. Murayama SY, Yamamoto T, Suzuki I, Sawai T (1986) Mutation of *Escherichia coli* capable of expressing gene(s) for beta-lactamase production of *Citrobacter freundii*. *Antimicrob. Agents Chemother.*, *29*, 707.

28. Gates ML, Sanders CC, Goering RV, Sanders Jr WE (1986) Evidence for multiple forms of Type I chromosomal beta-lactamase in *Pseudomonas aeruginosa*. *Antimicrob. Agents Chemother.*, *30*, 453.

29. Pechinot A, Duez JM, Nordmann P et al (1986) Inhibition des céphalosporinases d'Entérobactéries par la ceftriaxone. *Pathol. Biol.*, *34*, 399.

30. Phelps DJ, Carlton DD, Farrell CA, Kessler RE (1986) Affinity of cephalosporins for beta-lactamases as a factor in antibacterial efficacy. *Antimicrob. Agents Chemother.*, *29*, 845.

31. Livermore DM, Jones CS (1986) Characterization of NPS-1, a novel plasmid mediated beta-lactamase, from two *Pseudomonas aeruginosa* isolates. *Antimicrob. Agents Chemother.*, *29*, 99.

32. Eley A, Greenwood D (1986) Characterization of beta-lactamases in clinical isolates of *Bacteroides*. *J. Antimicrob. Chemother.*, *18*, 325.

33. Cuchural GJ, Malamy MH, Tally FP (1986) Beta-lactamase-mediated imipenem resistance in *Bacteroides fragilis*. *Antimicrob. Agents Chemother.*, *30*, 645.

34. Cuchural GJ, Tally FP, Storey JR, Malamy MH (1986) Transfer of beta-lactamase-associated cefoxitin resistance in *Bacteroides fragilis*. *Antimicrob. Agents Chemother.*, *29*, 918.

35. Malouin F, Fijalkowski C, Lamothe F, Lacroix J-M (1986) Inactivation of cefoxitin and moxalactam by *Bacteroides bivius* beta-lactamase. *Antimicrob. Agents Chemother.*, *30*, 749.

36. Dougherty TJ (1986) Genetic analysis and penicillin-binding protein alterations in *Neisseria gonorrhoeae* with chromosomally mediated resistance. *Antimicrob. Agents Chemother.*, *30*, 649.

37. Faruki H, Sparling PF (1986) Genetics of resistance in a non-beta-lactamase-producing gonococcus with relatively high-level penicillin resistance. *Antimicrob. Agents Chemother., 30,* 856.

38. Bakken JS, Sanders CC, Thomson KS (1987) Selective ceftazidime resistance in *Escherichia coli* associated with outer membrane protein changes. *J. Infect. Dis., 155,* 1220.

39. Axelrod JL, Klein RM, Bergen RL, Sheikh MZ (1986) Human vitreous levels of cefamandole and moxalactam. *Am. J. Ophthalmol., 101,* 684.

40. Humbert G, Veyssier P, Fourtillan JB et al (1986) Penetration of cefmenoxime into cerebrospinal fluid of patients with bacterial meningitis. *J. Antimicrob. Chemother., 18,* 503.

41. Nahata MC, Durrell DE, Barson WJ (1986) Ceftriaxone kinetics and cerebrospinal fluid penetration in infants and children with meningitis. *Chemotherapy, 32,* 89.

42. Spector R (1986) Ceftriaxone pharmacokinetics in the central nervous system. *J. Pharmacol. Exp. Ther., 236,* 380.

43. Bliss M, Mayersohn M, Arnold T et al (1986) Disposition kinetics of cefamandole during continuous ambulatory peritoneal dialysis. *Antimicrob. Agents Chemother., 29,* 649.

44. Morse GD, Lane T, Nairn DK et al (1987) Peritoneal transport of cefonicid. *Antimicrob. Agents Chemother., 31,* 292.

45. Fillastre J-P, Fourtillan J-B, Leroy A et al (1986) Pharmacokinetics of cefonicid in uraemic patients. *J. Antimicrob. Chemother., 18,* 203.

46. Browning MJ, Holt HA, White LO et al (1986) Pharmacokinetics of cefotetan in patients with end-stage renal failure on maintenance dialysis. *J. Antimicrob. Chemother., 18,* 103.

47. Heim KL, Halstenson CE, Comty CM et al (1986) Disposition of cefotaxime and desacetyl cefotaxime during continuous ambulatory peritoneal dialysis. *Antimicrob. Agents Chemother., 30,* 15.

48. Albin H, Ragnaud JM, Demotes-Mainard F et al (1986) Pharmacokinetics of intravenous and intraperitoneal ceftriaxone in chronic ambulatory peritoneal dialysis. *Eur. J. Clin. Pharmacol., 30,* 713.

49. Sica DA, Polk RE, Kerkering TM (1986) Cefmenoxime kinetics during continuous ambulatory peritoneal dialysis. *Eur. J. Clin. Pharmacol., 30,* 713.

50. Konishi K (1986) Pharmacokinetics of cefmenoxime in patients with impaired renal function and in those undergoing hemodialysis. *Antimicrob. Agents Chemother., 30,* 901.

51. Ohkawa M, Nakashima T, Shoda R et al (1985) Pharmacokinetics of ceftazidime in patients with renal insufficiency and in those undergoing hemodialysis. *Chemotherapy, 31,* 410.

52. Midtvedt T (1986) Penicillins, cephalosporins and tetracyclines. In: Dukes MNG (Ed), *Side Effects of Drugs, Annual 10,* p. 234. Elsevier, Amsterdam.

53. Sattler F (1986) Potential for bleeding with the new beta-lactam antibiotics. *Ann. Int. Med., 105,* 924.

54. Nichols RL, Wikler MA, McDevitt JT et al (1987) Coagulopathy associated with extended-spectrum cephalosporins in patients with serious infections. *Antimicrob. Agents Chemother., 31,* 281.

55. Washida H, Tsugaya M, Hirao N et al (1986) Effect of cefmenoxime on blood coagulation in patients with urinary tract infections. *Curr. Ther. Res., 39,* 359.

56. Brown RB, Klar J, Lemeshow S et al (1986) Enhanced bleeding with cefoxitin or moxalactam. *Arch. Int. Med., 146,* 2159.
57. Agnelli G, Del Favero A, Parise P et al (1986) Cephalosporin induced hypoprothrombinemia: Is the *N*-methylthiotetrazole side chain the culprit? *Antimicrob. Agents Chemother., 29,* 1108.
58. Lipsky JJ (1984) Mechanism of the inhibition of the γ-carboxylation of glutamic acid by *N*-methylthiotetrazole-containing antibiotics. *Proc. Natl Acad. Sci., 81,* 2893.
59. Kerremans AL, Lipsky JJ, Van Loon J (1985) Cephalosporin-induced hypoprothrombinemia: possible role for thiol methylation of 1-methyltetrazole-5-thio and 2-methyl-1,3,4-thiadiazole-5-thiol. *J. Pharmacol. Exp. Ther., 235,* 382.
60. Kitson TM (1986) Inactivation of aldehyde dehydrogenase by a putative metabolite of cefamandole. *Infection, 14,* 44.
61. Freundt KJ (1986) In vitro results to explain the cefamandole-alcohol reaction in human beings. (Author's reply). *Infection, 14,* 45.
62. Turcan RG, MacDonald CM, Ings RMJ (1985) Inhibition of the rate of $^{14}CO_2$ production from (^{14}C)ethanol in rats given beta-lactam antibiotics with disulfiram-like effects. *Antimicrob. Agents Chemother., 27,* 535.
63. Murray DL, Singer DA, Singer AB (1981) Cefaclor, a cluster of adverse reactions. *N. Engl. J. Med., 303,* 1003.
64. Callahan CW, Musci MN, Santucci TF (1985) Cefaclor serum sickness-like reactions: report of a case and review of the literature. *J. Am. Osteopath. Assoc., 85,* 450.
65. Kammer RB, Short LJ (1979) Cefaclor – a summary of clinical experience. *Postgrad. Med. J., 55,* 93.
66. Levine L (1985) Quantitative comparison of adverse reactions to cefaclor vs. amoxicillin in a surveillance study. *Pediatr. Infect. Dis., 4,* 358.
67. Barriere SL (1986) Controversies in antimicrobial therapy: formulary decisions on third generation cephalosporins. *Am. J. Hosp. Pharm., 43,* 625.
68. Anonymous (1986) The choice of antimicrobial drugs. *Med. Lett., 28,* 33.
69. Anonymous (1986) Treatment of sexually transmitted diseases. *Med. Lett., 28,* 23.
70. Neu HC (1987) New antibiotics: areas of appropriate use. *J. Infect. Dis., 155,* 403.
71. Pizzo PA, Hathorne JW, Hiemenz J et al (1986) A randomized trial comparing ceftazidime alone with combination antibiotic therapy in cancer patients with fever and neutropenia. *N. Engl. J. Med., 315,* 552.
72. Donnelly JP, Marcus RE, Goldman JM et al (1985) Ceftazidime as first line therapy for fever in acute leukemia. *J. Infection, 11,* 205.
73. Verhagen CS, De Pauw B, Donnelly JP et al (1986) Ceftazidime alone for treating *Pseudomonas aeruginosa* septicemia in neutropenic patients. *J. Infect., 13,* 125.
74. Hathorne JW, Pizzo PA (1986) Is there a role for monotherapy with beta-lactam antibiotics in the initial empirical management of febrile neutropenic cancer patients? *J. Antimicrob. Chemother., 17, Suppl A,* 41.
75. Verhagen CS, De Pauw B, De Witte T et al (1987) Randomized prospective study of ceftazidime versus ceftazidime plus cephalothin in empiric treatment of febrile episodes in severely neutropenic patients. *Antimicrob. Agents Chemother., 31,* 191.
76. Schimpff SC (1986) Empiric antibiotic therapy for granulocytopenic cancer patients. *Am. J. Med., 80, Suppl 5C,* 13.
77. Kramer BS, Ramphal R, Rand KH et al (1986) Randomized comparison between two ceftazidime-containing regimens and cephalothin-gentamicin-carbenicillin in febrile granulocytopenic cancer patients. *Antimicrob. Agents Chemother., 30,* 64.

78. Klastersky J, Glauser MP, Schimpff SC et al (1986) Prospective randomized comparison of three antibiotic regimens for empirical therapy of suspected bacteremic infections in febrile granulocytopenic patients. *Antimicrob. Agents Chemother., 29,* 263.

79. Hansen SW, Fries H, Ernst P et al (1986) Latamoxef versus carbenicillin plus gentamicin or carbenicillin plus mecillinam in leukopenic, febrile patients with solid tumors. *Acta Med. Scand., 220,* 249.

80. De Jongh CA, Joshi JH, Thompson BW et al (1986) A double beta-lactam combination versus an aminoglycoside-containing regimen as empiric antibiotic therapy for febrile granulocytopenic cancer patients. *Am. J. Med. 80, Suppl 5C,* 101.

81. Young LS (1986) Empirical antimicrobial therapy in the neutropenic host. *N. Engl. J. Med., 315,* 580.

82. Bryan CS, John JF, Sharada Pai M et al (1985) Gentamicin vs cefotaxime for therapy of neonatal sepsis. *Am. J. Dis. Child., 139,* 1086.

83. Bragman S, Sage R, Booth L et al (1986) Ceftazidime in the treatment of serious *Pseudomonas aeruginosa* sepsis. *Scand. J. Infect. Dis., 18,* 425.

84. Young LS (1987) Antibiotic therapy in patients with fever and neutropenia. *N. Engl. J. Med., 316,* 411.

85. The Board of American Academy of Pediatrics (1986) Diagnosis and management of meningitis. *Pediatrics, 78, Suppl.,* 959.

86. Marks WA, Stutman HR, Marks MI et al (1986) Cefuroxime versus ampicillin plus chloramphenicol in childhood bacterial meningitis: A multicenter randomized controlled trial. *J. Pediatrics, 109,* 123.

87. Prado V, Cohen J, Banfi A et al (1986) Ceftriaxone in the treatment of bacterial meningitis in children. *Chemotherapy, 32,* 383.

88. Grimes DA, Blount JH, Patrick J (1986) Antibiotic treatment of pelvic inflammatory disease. Trends among private physicians in the United States, 1966 through 1983. *J. Am. Med. Ass., 256,* 3223.

89. Mills J, Gottlieb A, Harrison WO (1986) Treatment of gonorrhoeae with first and second generation cephalosporins and other new beta-lactam drugs. *Sex. Transm. Dis., 13,* 203.

90. Lim KB, Thirumoorty T, Lee CT et al (1986) Single dose cefoxitin in treating uncomplicated gonorrhoea caused by penicillinase producing *Neisseria gonorrhoeae* (PPNG) and non-PPNG strains. *Genitourin. Med., 62,* 224.

91. Gottlieb A, Mills J (1986) Cefuroxime axetil for treatment of uncomplicated gonorrhoea. *Antimicrob. Agents Chemother., 30,* 333.

92. Fong IW, Linton W, Simbul M et al (1986) Comparative clinical efficacy of single oral doses of cefuroxime axetil and amoxicillin in uncomplicated gonococcal infections. *Antimicrob. Agents Chemother., 30,* 321.

93. Wanas TM, Williams PEO (1986) Oral cefuroxime axetil compared with oral ampicillin in treating acute uncomplicated gonorrhoea. *Genitourin. Med., 62,* 221.

94. Laga M, Naamara W, Brunham RC et al (1986) Single-dose therapy of gonococcal ophthalmia neonatorum with ceftriaxone. *N. Engl. J. Med., 315,* 1382.

95. Bowmer MI, Mganze H, D'Costa LJ et al (1987) Single dose-ceftriaxone for chancroid. *Antimicrob. Agents Chemother., 31,* 67.

96. Hook III EW, Baker-Zander SA, Moskovitz BL (1986) Ceftriaxone therapy for asymptomatic neurosyphilis. *Sex. Transm. Dis., 13, Suppl,* 185.

97. Poindexter III AN, Sweet R, Ritter M (1986) Cefotetan in the treatment of obstetric and gynecologic infections. *Am. J. Obstet. Gynecol., 154,* 946.

98. Scalambrino S, Regallo M, Spreafico P et al (1986) Piperacillin versus cefoxitin in the treatment of infections in obstetrics and gynecology. *Curr. Ther. Res., 40,* 49.

99. Rosene K, Eschenbach DA, Tompkins LS et al (1986) Polymicrobial early postpartum endometritis with facultative and anaerobic bacteria, genital mycoplasma and *Chlamydia trachomatis:* treatment with piperacillin and cefoxitin. *J. Infect. Dis., 153,* 1028.

100. Bittner MJ, Pugsley MP, Horowitz EA et al (1986) Randomized comparison of ceftriaxone and cefamandole therapy in lower respiratory tract infections in an elderly population. *J. Antimicrob. Chemother., 18,* 621.

101. Yangco BC, Palumbo JA, Nolen T et al (1986) Comparative multicentre evaluation of the safety and efficacy of ceftazidime versus cefamandole for pneumonia. *J. Antimicrob. Chemother., 18,* 521.

102. Blumer JL, Stern RC, Yamashita TS et al (1986) Cephalosporin therapeutics in cystic fibrosis. *J. Pediatr., 108,* 854.

103. Paull A, Morgan JR (1986) Emergence of ceftriaxone-resistant strains of *Pseudomonas aeruginosa* in cystic fibrosis patients. *J. Antimicrob. Chemother., 18,* 635.

104. Pedersen S, Koch C, Hoiby N et al (1986) An epidemic spread of multiresistant *Pseudomonas aeruginosa* in a cystic fibrosis centre. *J. Antimicrob. Chemother., 17,* 505.

105. Uwaydah M, Vartivarian S, Shatila S et al (1986) Moxalactam in the treatment of typhoid fever. *Antimicrob. Agents Chemother., 30,* 338.

106. Cardenas J, Quinn EL, Rooker G (1986) Single-dose cephalexin therapy for acute bacterial urinary tract infections and acute urethral syndrome with bladder bacteriuria. *Antimicrob. Agents Chemother., 29,* 383.

107. Frongillo RF, Donati L, Federico G et al (1986) Clinical comparative study on the activity of cefamandole in the treatment of serious staphylococcal infections caused by methicillin-susceptible and methicillin-resistant strains. *Antimicrob. Agents Chemother., 29,* 789.

108. Eng RH, Corrado ML, Tillotson J et al (1985) Cefamandole for the therapy of serious *Staphylococcus aureus* infections. *J. Antimicrob. Chemother., 16,* 663.

109. Kaiser AB (1986) Antimicrobial prophylaxis in surgery. *N. Engl. J. Med., 315,* 1129.

110. DiPiro JT, Cheung RPF, Bowden TA et al (1986) Single dose systemic antibiotic prophylaxis of surgical wound infections. *Am. J. Surg., 152,* 552.

111. Dworzack DL, Pugsley MP, Sanders CC, Horowitz EA (1986) Emergence of resistance during therapy with expanded spectrum cephalosporins. In: *Abstracts, 26th Interscience Conference on Antimicrobial Agents and Chemotherapy, New Orleans, 1986,* p 188. American Society for Microbiology, Washington, DC.

112. Vuthien H, Rolland M (1986) *Citrobacter freundii:* Emergence in vivo d'un mutant résistant aux bêta-lactamines au cours d'un traitement par la ceftazidime. *Presse Méd., 15,* 1241.

113. Sorbello AF, Echols RM, Condoluci DV (1987) Clinical efficacy of once-daily ceftriaxone therapy. *Infect. Med., 4,* 69.

114. Follath F, Costa E, Thommen A, Frei R (1986) Clinical consequences of resistance development to third generation cephalosporins. In: *Abstracts, 26th Interscience Conference on Antibiotics and Chemotherapy, New Orleans, 1986,* p 288. American Society for Microbiology, Washington, DC.

115. Perronne C, Regnier B, Legrand P et al (1986) Echecs des nouvelles bêta-lactamines dans le traitement d'infections sévères à *Enterobacter cloacae. Presse Med., 15,* 1813.

116. Foord RD, Butcher ME, Williams AH (1987) The emergence of resistance of *Pseudomonas aeruginosa* in patients treated with ceftazidime. *Scand. J. Infect. Dis., 19,* 143.

117. Weinstein RA (1986) Endemic emergence of cephalosporin-resistant Enterobacter: relation to prior therapy. *Infect. Control, 7, Suppl,* 120.
118. Burchard KW, Barrall DT, Reed M, Slotman GJ (1986) *Enterobacter* bacteremia in surgical patients. *Surgery, 100,* 857.
119. Prevot M-H, Andremont A, Sancho-Garnier H, Tancrede C (1986) Epidemiology of intestinal colonization by members of the family Enterobacteriaceae resistant to cefotaxime in a hematology-oncology unit. *Antimicrob. Agents Chemother., 30,* 945.
120. Chiesa C, Labrozzi PH, Aronoff SC (1986) Decreased baseline beta-lactamase production and inducibility associated with increased piperacillin susceptibility of *Pseudomonas cephacia* isolated from children with cystic fibrosis. *Pediatr. Res., 20,* 1174.
121. DiPiro JT, Steele JCH (1987) Rational formulary selection of antimicrobials. *Am. J. Hosp. Pharmacol., 44,* 74.
122. Peterson CD, Lake KD (1985) Reducing prophylactic antibiotic costs in cardiovascular surgery: the role of the clinical pharmacist. *Drug Intell. Clin. Pharmacol., 19,* 134.
123. Moleski RJ, Andriole VT (1986) Role of the infectious disease specialist in containing cost of antibiotics in the hospital. *Rev. Infect. Dis., 8,* 488.
124. Dzierba SH, Reilly RT, Caselnova III DA (1986) Cost savings achieved through cephalosporin use review and restriction. *Am. J. Hosp. Pharm., 43,* 2194.
125. Quintiliani R, Klimek JJ, Nightingale CH (1986) Restriction policies for therapy with combination antibiotics. *J. Infect. Dis., 153,* 645.
126. Rahal JJ (1986) Comment to Richard Quintiliani. *J. Infect. Dis., 153,* 647.
127. Alford RH (1986) Comment to Richard Quintiliani. *J. Infect. Dis., 153,* 649.
128. Utsui Y, Ohya S, Magaribuchi T et al (1986) Antibacterial activity of cefmetazole alone and in combination with fosfomycin against methicillin- and cephem-resistant *Staphylococcus aureus. Antimicrob. Agents Chemother., 30,* 917.
129. Bowie WR, Shaw CE, Chan DGW et al (1986) In vitro activity of difloxacin hydrochloride (A-56619), A-56620, and cefixime (CL 284,635; FK 027) against selected genital pathogens. *Antimicrob. Agents Chemother., 30,* 590.
130. Guay DRP, Meatherall RC, Harding GK, Brown GR (1986) Pharmacokinetics of cefixime (CL 284,635; FK 027) in healthy subjects and patients with renal insufficiency. *Antimicrob. Agents Chemother., 30,* 485.
131. Lauderdale BL, Yu PKW, Washington II JA (1986) In vitro activity of an orally administered cephalosporin, LY 164846, against potentially pathogenic respiratory and dermal bacterial isolates. *Antimicrob. Agents Chemother., 29,* 560.
132. Thomas MG, Lang SDR (1986) Antimicrobial spectrum of RO 15-8074/001, a new oral cephalosporin. *Antimicrob. Agents Chemother., 29,* 945.
133. Wise R, Andrews JM, Piddock LJV (1986) In vitro activity of RO 15-8974 and RO 19-5247, two orally administered cephalosporin metabolites. *Antimicrob. Agents Chemother., 29,* 1067.
134. Leitner F, Pursiano TA, Buck RE et al (1987) BMY 28100, a new oral cephalosporin. *Antimicrob. Agents Chemother., 31,* 238.
135. Tsuji A, Hirooka H, Tamai I, Terasaki T (1986) Evidence for a carrier-mediated transport system in the small intestine available for FK 089, a new cephalosporin antibiotic without an amino group. *J. Antibiot., 39,* 1592.
136. Yamanaka H, Takasugi H, Masugi T et al (1985) Studies on beta-lactam antibiotics. VIII. Structure-activity relationships of 7-beta-[(Z)-2-carboxy-methoxyimino-2-arylacetamido]-3-cephem-4-carboxylic acids. *J. Antibiot., 38,* 1068.

137. Kawabata K, Masugi T, Takaya T (1986) Studies on beta-lactam antibiotics. XII. Synthesis and activity of new 3-ethynylcephalosporin. *J. Antibiot.*, *39*, 394.

138. Kabawata K, Yamanaka H, Takasugi H, Takaya T (1986) Studies on beta-lactam antibiotics. XIII. Synthesis and structure activity relationships of 7-beta-[(Z)-2-aryl-2-carboxymethoxyimino acetamido]-3-vinyl-cephalosporins. *J. Antibiot.*, *39*, 404.

139. Furukawa M, Arimoto M, Nakamura S et al (1986) Semisynthetic beta-lactam antibiotics. I. Synthesis and antibacterial activity of 7-beta-[2-aryl-2-(amino-acetamido)-acetamido]-cephalosporins. *J. Antibiot.*, *39*, 1225.

140. Arimoto M, Ejima A, Watanabe T et al (1986) Semisynthetic beta-lactam antibiotics. II. Synthesis and antibacterial activity of 7-beta-[2-(acylamino)-2-(2-aminothiazol-4-yl)acetamido] cephalosporins. *J. Antibiot.*, *39*, 1236.

141. Arimoto M, Hayano T, Soga T et al (1986) Semisynthetic beta-lactam antibiotics. III. Synthesis and antibacterial activity of 7-beta-[2-(2-aminothiazol-4-yl)-2-(substituted carbamoylmethoxyimino)acetamido] cephalosporins. *J. Antibiot.*, *39*, 1243.

142. Skotnicki J, Steinbaugh BA (1986) Synthesis and antibacterial activity of novel aminothiazolyl beta-lactam derivatives. *J. Antibiot.*, *39*, 372.

143. Skotnicki J, Strike DP (1986) Synthesis and antibacterial activity of C-3'-isothiazolyl and related cephalosporins. *J. Antibiot.*, *39*, 380.

144. Neu HC, Chin N-X (1986) In vitro activity and beta-lactamase stability of a new difluoro oxacephem, 6315-S. *Antimicrob. Agents Chemother.*, *30*, 638.

145. Murakami K, Doi M, Yoshida T (1986) 7-Alpha-formylamino substituent confers beta-lactamase inactivating potency on 1-oxacephalosporins. *Antimicrob. Agents Chemother.*, *30*, 447.

146. Maier R, Wetzel B, Woitun E et al (1986) Synthesis and antimicrobial activity of 7-alpha-methoxy-pyrimidinyl-ureido-cephalosporins. *Arzneim.-Forsch. Drug Res.*, *36*, 1297.

147. Fujimoto T, Otani T, Nakajima R et al (1986) In vitro activity of DQ-2556, a new cephalosporin. *Antimicrob. Agents Chemother.*, *30*, 611.

148. Hikada M, Inoue M, Mitsuhashi S (1986) In vitro antibacterial activity of L-105, a new cephalosporin. *J. Antimicrob. Agents Chemother.*, *30*, 611.

149. Naito T, Aburaki S, Kamachi H et al (1986) Synthesis and structure-activity relationship of a new series of cephalosporins, BMY-28142 and related compounds. *J. Antibiot.*, *39*, 1092.

150. Kobayashi S, Arai S, Hayashi S, Fujimoto K (1986) Beta-lactamase stability of cefpirome (HR-810), a new cephalosporin with a broad antimicrobial spectrum. *Antimicrob. Agents Chemother.*, *30*, 713.

CHAPTER 7

Chloramphenicol

JOHN G. BARTLETT

Chloramphenicol is an aromatic paranitro compound with an aliphatic side-
chain. The drug was originally isolated from *Streptomyces venezuela*, but is now
prepared primarily by chemical synthesis. The use of chloramphenicol has declined due to the evolution of resistance and the rare but almost universally lethal
complication of aplastic anemia. Despite these problems, the drug continues to
show a wide spectrum of antimicrobial activity and has lipophilicity that permits
penetration through biologic membranes. Major indications at the present time
include pediatric meningitis and typhoid fever. Chloramphenicol derivatives include thiamphenicol, fluorinated analog (SCH-25393), and substituted phenyl-bo-
ronate esters.

ACTIVITY

The major clinical indications for chloramphenicol concern infections involving
Haemophilus influenzae, Salmonella and anaerobic bacteria.

Ampicillin combined with chloramphenicol is considered the preferred drug
regimen for initial empiric treatment of meningitis in infants and children aged
3 months to 10 years according to the 1986 report of the Task Force on Diagnosis
and Management of Meningitis (1). Chloramphenicol is active in vitro against the
three major anticipated pathogens, *Neisseria meningitidis, Streptococcus pneumoniae* and *H. influenzae*; the drug is also active against most relatively penicillin-
resistant strains of *S. pneumoniae* and against most strains of *H. influenzae* that
produce β-lactamase. A study of 40 strains of *S. pneumoniae*, that were relatively
penicillin-resistant (minimum inhibitory concentration 0.12-1 μg/ml) isolated
from the nasopharynx of children showed 47.5% were also resistant to sulfametho-
xazole-trimethoprim, and 5% were resistant to rifampicin; all strains were sensitive
to chloramphenicol and vancomycin (2). Nevertheless, up to 25% of strains of *S.
pneumoniae* are allegedly resistant to chloramphenicol in selected geographic areas
such as Ibadan, Nigeria (3). Occasional strains of *H. influenzae* may also be re-

Antimicrobial Agents Annual 3
P.K. Peterson and J. Verhoef, editors
©Elsevier Science Publishers BV, 1988

sistant and rare strains were resistant to both ampicillin and chloramphenicol (4, 5). The preferred drugs for these multiply resistant strains include cefotaxime, moxalactam or ceftriaxone (1).

Another consideration with respect to the management of meningitis concerns drug interactions to provide synergy or antagonism. This has always been a controversial issue in pharmacology since it has been often difficult to show relevance in vivo of observations in vitro. Nevertheless, antagonism was demonstrated in an anecdotal case of a patient with meningitis involving *Klebsiella pneumoniae* treated with cefotaxime and chloramphenicol concomitantly (6). It might be noted that chloramphenicol is no longer considered an appropriate drug for gram-negative bacillary meningitis in general since it is bacteriostatic against these microbes and meningitis appears to be one of the few clinical settings (along with endocarditis) in which bactericidal activity is required. The reason the drug is advocated for the usual causes of meningitis is that it is bactericidal against *H. influenzae, S. pneumoniae* and *N. meningitidis*. Despite this admonition, Kim demonstrated that the combination of ampicillin and chloramphenicol was as effective as cefotaxime or imipenem in an animal model of *Escherichia coli* bacteremia and meningitis (7). Despite substantially higher bactericidal titers both in vitro and in vivo, the regimens appeared to be comparable in terms of bacterial clearance from the blood and cerebrospinal fluid (CSF).

Drug interaction between chloramphenicol and ampicillin for *H. influenzae* has been an obvious concern since this is the official recommended regimen for empiric treatment of pediatric meningitis and studies in vitro have shown both synergy and antagonism between the antibiotics. Recent studies suggest that, at least for ampicillin-susceptible and chloramphenicol-resistant strains, the chloramphenicol inhibited the bactericidal action of ampicillin to pose a potential clinical risk for the combination with such strains (8). Others have shown that ampicillin + cefotaxime is more likely to show synergy than the combination of ampicillin + chloramphenicol, at least for ampicillin-sensitive strains (9). Nevertheless, the clinical relevance of this information is obscure.

Most strains of *Salmonella* continue to show sensitivity in vitro to chloramphenicol. The major concern has been increased resistance to ampicillin and sulfonamides (10). In 1972, there was the infamous 10,000 case outbreak of typhoid fever in Central Mexico involving *S. typhi* strains resistant to all three drugs. Chloramphenicol-resistant strains of *S. typhi* were subsequently reported in various parts of the world including 16.5% of the strains isolated in California in 1971-72 (10). By 1979, only 3% of strains in the United States were resistant to either ampicillin or chloramphenicol, and no isolate was resistant to both drugs. Chloramphenicol-resistant strains of *S. typhi* still occur, but are extremely rare (10). With regard to the non-typhi strains of *Salmonella*, only about 1-2% are chloramphenicol-resistant (10). However, it is anticipated that this will increase and, furthermore, the use of antibiotics in animal feed may be an important factor in the genesis of resistant strains. In 1985, the Los Angeles County Health Department noted a 5-fold increase in the number of *S. newport* strains, most were resistant to chloramphenicol and most had a single, identical plasmid. With the use of the antibiotic sensitivity and plasmid profiles to detect multiply resistant strains, hamburger was implicated as the vehicle of transmission and the meat was subsequently traced to dairy farms where chloramphenicol had been used for growth promotion (11). It is noteworthy that the use of chloramphenicol in this fashion has never been legal in the United States, but the FDA estimates that less than 1% of the veterinary supply of chloramphenicol is actually used appropriately. Also of interest is the observation that 85% of the afflicted patients consumed only cooked hamburger and 24% had ingested penicillin or tetracycline prior to the illness. It is assumed that the antibiotics promoted disease by the reduction in colonization resistance, by selection of the resistant strains or both. The epidemic strain appeared to account for 19% of all *Salmonella* infections in California in 1985 and 87% of the 972 isolates of *S. newport*.

Anaerobic bacteria have always been considered highly susceptible to chloramphenicol. This has certainly been the case in the United States where the 8 hospital collaborative studies of over 1200 clinical isolates of the '*Bacteroides fragilis* group' were universally susceptible (12). A recent study of a heterogeneous array of 590 clinical isolates of anaerobic bacteria from 5 Canadian hospitals showed only 2 strains to be resistant to chloramphenicol (13). A recent report from Brazil also showed exceptional activity by chloramphenicol. Of 228 strains from the '*Bacteroides fragilis* group' only 2% were resistant (14). In contrast to the studies from Canada and the United States, there were exceptionally high rates of resistance to selective alternative agents in that 37% of strains were resistant to clindamycin and 21% were resistant to cefoxitin (14). The studies from the United States, Brazil, and Canada for the '*Bacteroides fragilis* group' including a combined total of approximately 1500 strains showed that all were sensitive to metronidazole and only 4 strains were resistant to chloramphenicol.

CLINICAL PHARMACOLOGY

A major concern with chloramphenicol in pediatric practices is the unpredictable metabolism of the drug in young infants. In addition, there are important drug interactions with phenobarbital, phenytoin and rifampin (1). As a consequence, the Task Force on Diagnosis and Management of Meningitis advocate monitoring of chloramphenicol serum levels as a guide to dosing regimens for both young infants and patients who receive the drugs noted above concomitantly. The therapeutic range for serum is 15-30 μg/ml.

Chloramphenicol is available for both oral and parenteral administration. The most bioavailable form is the crystalline compound for oral administration. It is also available as the palmitate ester for oral use, but the ester must be hydrolyzed prior to absorption. This may pose a problem in patients with pancreatic insufficiency including children with cystic fibrosis. The problem may be rectified with co-administration of pancreatic extract (15). The parenteral form is the succinate ester which, like chloramphenicol palmitate, lacks intrinsic biologic activity and must be hydrolyzed. After intravenous infusion about one-third of the parent ester is excreted in the urine. As a consequence, the oral crystalline form is more bio-available than the parenteral form.

CLINICAL USES

The major controversy regarding chloramphenicol usage concerns the role of alternative agents for the major disease categories in which chloramphenicol is advocated. This primarily concerns pediatric meningitis and salmonellosis, but also to some extent, anaerobic infections.

With regard to meningitis, there have been numerous studies showing that cefuroxime and several third-generation cephalosporins have potential advantages in terms of extraordinary in vitro activity against the usual pathogens, bactericidal action and extremely good penetration to provide high CSF levels. Further, there are now multiple studies to demonstrate good in vivo activity as well.

Extending the previous reports have been more recent studies to demonstrate that cefotaxime, ceftazidime and cefuroxime are the therapeutic equivalent of ampicillin combined with chloramphenicol for the treatment of pediatric meningitis (16-18). The study by Odio et al (16), concerned 85 infants and children randomized to receive cefotaxime or the 'standard therapy'. The median cerebrospinal fluid bactericidal concentration against the patients' own pathogen in the cefotaxime-treated group was 1:64 compared to 1:8 for ampicillin-chloramphenicol recipients. The two regimens were judged clinically equal according to the mean number of days of positive cerebrospinal fluid cultures, time required for defervescence, length of hospital stay, complications developing during treatment, and sequelae with long-term follow-up (16). The study by Rodriquez et al (17) concerned 100 children aged 1 month to 15 years who received ceftazidime or chloramphenicol +ampicillin. The mortality rate was 20–21% and the incidence of gross neurologic sequelae was 4-5% for both groups. The study by Marks et al (18) was a multi-centered randomized trial of 107 children given cefuroxime versus ampicillin+chloramphenicol. The CSF bactericidal concentrations versus *H. influenzae* isolates were 1:16 for each group. However, 4 of 39 patients with *H. influenzae* in the cefuroxime group had this organism recovered from the CSF culture 24–48 hours after treatment was started compared to none of 40 in the 'conventional treatment group' (this difference is not statistically significant). The overall cure rates were 95% for both groups. The authors concluded that proof of equivalence and the consequences of the delay in sterilization of CSF are unresolved issues. It should be emphasized again that the recent Task Force on Diagnosis and Management of Meningitis continues to advocate ampicillin combined with chloramphenicol as the preferred regimen for empiric treatment of pediatric meningitis in patients aged 3 months to 10 years. The alternative regimens recommended by this group include ceftriaxone, cefotaxime and ceftazidime. Recommendations are different for newborn infants where penicillin and aminoglycoside are advocated by the Task Force (1). For the infant of 1-3 months, the recommendation is for ampicillin + chloramphenicol and the alternative regimen for empiric use is ampicillin + cefotaxime (1).

The alternatives to chloramphenicol suggested for salmonellosis have traditionally been ampicillin and trimethoprim + sulfamethoxazole. There is now considerable interest in the use of third-generation cephalosporins which are highly active against virtually all strains of *Salmonella* (10). A summary of 9 published studies by Bryan et al (10) showed that the concentration necessary to inhibit 90% (MIC_{90}) of strains of *S. typhi* was less then 0.25 $\mu g/ml$ for cefotaxime, ceftriaxone, ceftazidime and moxalactam. The non-typhi strains were comparably susceptible. Clinical trials with cefoperazone, ceftazidime and ceftriaxone have been promising for both typhoid fever and non-typhoid salmonellosis. Even more active in vitro are some of the new quinolones. For example, the MIC_{90} for ciprofloxacin is 0.02-0.03 $\mu g/ml$ (10, 19). The initial clinical trials with this drug are equally impressive (19), but also anecdotal. The third-generation cephalosporins have also been successful in 12 of 13 cases of *Salmonella* meningitis and each of 5 cases of *Salmonella* osteomyelitis (10). But perhaps the most challenging therapeutic dilemma is the chronic carrier. These patients are generally treated with prolonged courses of ampicillin or trimethoprim + sulfamethoxazole with a failure rate of 30-50% (10). The alternative is cholecystectomy to eliminate chronic biliary carriage, but this is also often unsuccessful and potentially problematic with respect to the risk/benefit ratio as well as cost. Potential new approaches include the use of once-daily injections of third-generation cephalosporins that are highly active in vitro, have a long serum half-life, and are concentrated in the bile. The drugs that potentially satisfy these goals are cefoperazone and ceftriaxone; another possibly more convenient approach is prolonged oral administration of a quinolone. The conclusion regarding infections involving *Salmonella* is that chloramphenicol will continue to be considered a first-line drug for typhoid fever, that there are multiple agents that appear equally meritorious for other forms of salmonellosis, and that some of the newer drugs offer special potential advantages for the more refractory forms of infection involving this microbe (10).

FUTURE DIRECTIONS

The future of this class of antibiotics seems to be developing in two directions. One concerns analogs that are more active and/or less toxic. The second concerns the evolution of drugs that would actually supplant chloramphenicol's already rather meager place in current-day practice.

Thiamphenicol is a chloramphenicol derivative in which the nitro-group is replaced by a sulfomethyl-group. The apparent advantage is that, although this analog has been implicated in the dose-related marrow suppression side effect, it is an extremely rare cause of the most dreaded complication, aplastic anemia.

Another derivative is SCH-24893 which is the C3-fluoro analog. This substitution of the 3-hydroxyl-group means that the compound is no longer a substrate for chloramphenicol acetyltransferase. Three mechanisms of resistance to chloramphenicol have been described and include drug inactivation, reduced penetration, and resistance of intracellular targets. The most common mechanism is drug inactivation by resistance plasmids for chloramphenicol acetyltransferase. These enzymes are produced by widely divergent organisms and this represents the major, but not the exclusive, mechanism of resistance by *H. influenzae* (15).

With regard to clinical usage, there is continuing interest in the development of alternative agents for pediatric meningitis and salmonellosis. The drugs that appear to be especially promising in this regard for pediatric meningitis are the third-generation cephalosporins, and for salmonella infections the third-generation cephalosporins, monobactams and the quinolones. Chloramphenicol continues to show high activity against anaerobic bacteria despite extensive usage in many parts of the world. This experience is shared with metronidazole, and is apparently somewhat different from the experience with clindamycin and cefoxitin where there has been the evolution of resistance in at least some areas where usage has been extensive.

REFERENCES

1. Klein JO, Feigin RD, McCracken Jr GH (1986) Report of the Task Force on Diagnosis and Management of Meningitis. *Pediatrics, 78*, 959.
2. Klugman KP, Koornhaf JH, Wasas A (1986) Carriage of penicillin-resistant pneumococci. *Arch. Dis. Child., 61*, 377.
3. Nottidge VA (1985) *Haemophilus influenzae* meningitis: a 5 year study in Ibadan, Nigeria. *J. Infect. 11*, 109.
4. Campos J, Garcia-Turnel S, Gairi JM, Fabregues I (1986) Multiply resistant *Haemophilus influenzae* type b causing meningitis. *J. Pediatr., 108*, 897.
5. Coovadia YM, Coovadia HM, Van dem Eude J (1986) Meningitis due to beta-lactamase producing, chloramphenicol-resistant *Haemophilus influenzae* type b in South Africa. *J. Infect., 12*, 247.
6. Brown TH, Alford RH (1985) Failure of chloramphenicol and cefotaxime therapy in *Klebsiella* meningitis. *South. Med. J., 78*, 869.
7. Kim KS (1985) Comparison of cefotaxime, imipencin-cilastatin, ampicillin-gentamicin and ampicillin-chloramphenicol in the treatment of experimental *Escherichia coli* bacteremia and meningitis. *Antimicrob. Agents Chemother., 28*, 433.
8. MacKenzie AMR, Chan FTH (1986) Combined action of choramphenicol and ampicillin on chloramphenicol-resistant *Haemophilus influenzae. Antimicrob. Agents Chemother., 29*, 565.
9. Lapointe J-R, Lavallee C, Michaud A (1986) In vitro comparison of ampicillin-chloramphenicol and ampicillin-cefotaxime against 284 *Haemophilus* isolates. *Antimicrob. Agents Chemother., 29*, 594.
10. Bryan JP, Rocha H, Scheld WM (1986) Problems in salmonellosis: rationale for clinical trials with newer β-lactam agents and quinolones. *Rev. Infect. Dis., 8*, 189.

11. Spika JS, Waterman SH, Soo Hoo GW et al (1987) Chloramphenicol-resistant *Salmonella newport* traced through hamburger to dairy farms: a major persisting source of human salmonellosis in California. *N. Engl. J. Med., 316*, 565.

12. Tally FP, Cuchurd GJ, Jacobus NV (1985) Nationwide study of the susceptibility of the *Bacteroides fragilis* group in the U.S. *Antimicrob. Agents Chemother., 28, 675.*

13. Bourgault AM, Harding GK, Smith JA, Horsman GB, Marrie TJ, LaMothe F (1986) Survey of anaerobic susceptibility patterns in Canada. *Antimicrob. Agents Chemother., 30,* 798.

14. Eugenio A, DeAlmeida CC, Uzeda MD (1987) Susceptibility to five antimicrobial agents of strains of the *Bacteroides fragilis* group isolated in Brazil. *Antimicrob. Agents Chemother., 31,* 617.

15. Smith AL (1986) Chloramphenicol. *Assoc. Prudent Use Antibiot. Newslett., Spring,* 4.

16. Odio CM, Faingezicht I, Salas JL (1986) Cefotaxime vs. conventional therapy for the treatment of bacterial meningitis of infants and children. *Pediatr. Infect. Dis., 5,* 402.

17. Rodriquez WJ, Puig JR, Khan WH (1986) Ceftazidime vs. standard therapy for pediatric meningitis. *Pediatr. Infect. Dis., 5,* 408.

18. Marks WA, Stutman HR, Marks MI (1986) Cefuroxime versus ampicillin plus chloramphenicol in childhood bacterial meningitis: a multi-center randomized controlled trial. *J. Pediatr., 109,* 123.

19. Ramirez CA, Bran JL, Mejia CR, Garcia JF (1985) Open, prospective study of the clinical efficacy of ciprofloxacin. *Antimicrob. Agents Chemother., 28,* 128.

CHAPTER 8

Fusidic acid

DAVID GREENWOOD

Fusidic acid is the sole therapeutic representative of a family of naturally occurring tetracyclic triterpenoid antibiotics known collectively as 'fusidanes'. It has been in clinical use in Europe for over 20 years; although it is not presently available in the United States, there has been a recent awakening of American interest in the compound because of its activity against methicillin-resistant staphylococci.

Only a limited amount of new information has appeared in the literature during the last few years and little has emerged to alter the principal clinical role of fusidic acid as a useful antistaphylococcal agent.

As conventionally drawn, fusidic acid exhibits a steroid-like structure (Fig. 1). However, the stereochemistry of the molecule dictates that, in contrast to steroids, the central of the three 6-membered rings is constrained in a 'boat' configuration (1) and the compound does not possess steroid-like activity.

The antibacterial activity of fusidic acid was first detected in culture filtrates of *Fusidium coccineum*, a fungus originally isolated from monkey dung (2). Similar compounds have since been found in various fungi, including *Epidermophyton floccosum* and some other dermatophytes (3).

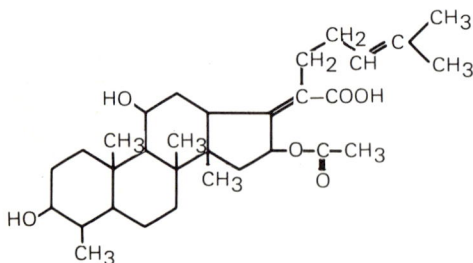

Fig. 1 Structure of fusidic acid.

Antimicrobial Agents Annual 3
P.K. Peterson and J. Verhoef, editors
© Elsevier Science Publishers BV, 1988

ACTIVITY

Spectrum of activity

Fusidic acid exhibits an idiosyncratic spectrum of activity which includes *Coryne-bacterium diphtheriae, Mycobacterium tuberculosis, Nocardia asteroides, Clostridium* species and many strains of *Bacteroides* (4–6). However, the most important

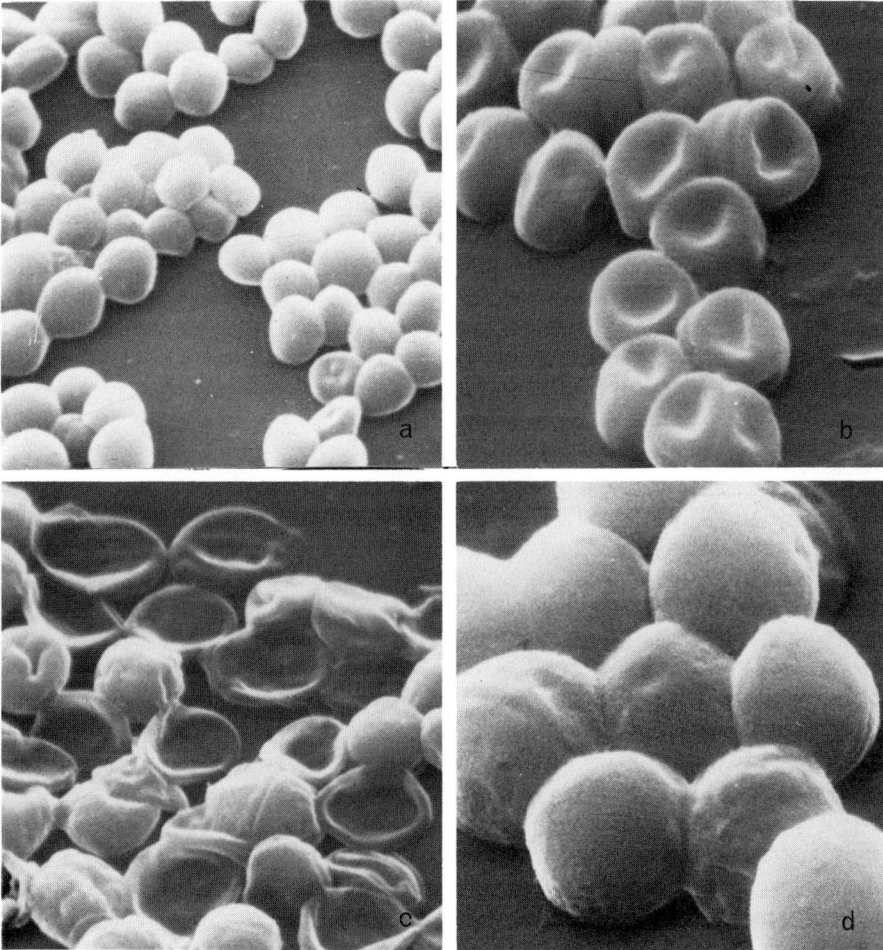

Fig. 2 Scanning electron micrographs of *Staphylococcus aureus* exposed to (a) no antibiotic, (b) 2 μg fusidic acid per ml for 1 h, (c) 2 μg fusidic acid per ml for 3 h, (d) 2 μg fusidic acid per ml + 3 μg cloxacillin per ml for 1 h. Reproduced from O'Grady and Greenwood (12, 31) by courtesy of the Editors of the *Journal of Medical Microbiology* and the *Journal of General Microbiology*.

property of the antibiotic is its high antistaphylococcal activity: most strains of *Staphylococcus aureus* and *S. epidermidis*, including methicillin-resistant strains, are inhibited by less than 0.25 μg fusidic acid per ml (4, 7). Most *S. saprophyticus* strains are, like streptococci, considerably less susceptible and gram-negative aerobic bacilli are completely resistant (4, 8).

Unexpectedly, fusidic acid has also been shown to possess some antiprotozoal activity. The compound exhibits activity at clinically achievable levels against protozoa as diverse as *Giardia lamblia* (9) and *Plasmodium falciparum* (10). Whether these results in vitro can be translated into therapeutic success remains to be established.

Mechanism of action

Fusidic acid inhibits bacterial protein synthesis. It does not bind directly to the ribosome, but achieves its effect by binding to elongation factor G (EF-G), a substance involved in translocation of the growing peptide chain during protein synthesis. In the presence of fusidic acid, one translocation event proceeds with hydrolysis of guanosine triphosphate (which provides the necessary energy) but the fusidic acid/EF-G/GDP complex remains stably bound to the ribosome and blocks further protein synthesis (11). In staphylococci, inhibition of protein synthesis is followed by collapse of the cell (Fig. 2), perhaps because cell wall autolysins continue to act in the absence of cell wall growth (12).

Resistance

Resistance to fusidic acid occurs readily. Resistance usually arises by mutations that alter factor G so that it no longer binds the drug (13). Recently, the ability to inactivate fusidic acid has been demonstrated in the nocardiform bacterium *Rhodococcus erythropolis* (14); the activity was inducible by fusidic acid and was abolished by heat.

Plasmid-mediated resistance to fusidic acid may be associated with chloramphenicol acetyltransferase (15). The enzyme does not acetylate fusidic acid, but appears to bind it efficiently (16, 17).

Naturally occurring resistance to fusidic acid in epidemic methicillin-resistant *S. aureus* remains rare, but is more common in other *S. aureus* strains (18).

Antibacterial interactions

Synergy, antagonism and indifference have all been demonstrated in staphylococci exposed to fusidic acid in combination with penicillins (12). In strains in which antagonism is seen, the presence of penicillin prevents the secondary collapse of the staphylococcal cell wall (Fig. 2d).

In a study of methicillin-resistant staphylococci from various centres in the United States, the combination of fusidic acid and rifampicin was found to display bactericidal synergy against most strains of coagulase-positive and coagulase-negative staphylococci (19). The mechanism of the interaction appeared to be mutual suppression of resistant variants.

CLINICAL PHARMACOLOGY

Fusidic acid is almost completely absorbed when administered orally, achieving concentrations in the plasma of about 30 μg/ml 2 hours after a 500 mg dose (20). More than 95% of the drug is protein-bound (21). Excretion is slow, chiefly by the biliary route, and accumulation of drug occurs so that plasma levels in excess of 100 μg/ml may be achieved during a course of treatment (22). The antibiotic is widely distributed throughout the body, penetrating in therapeutically useful concentrations into bone and synovial fluid (23), bronchial secretions (24) and heart tissue (25), but not into cerebrospinal fluid. Fusidic acid is concentrated in polymorphonuclear leukocytes and lymphocytes, at least in vitro (26).

Beeching et al (27) found that discs of acrylic bone cement impregnated with fusidic acid exhibited diffusible antibiotic activity for several weeks when tested by serial transfer on agar plates inoculated with *S. aureus*. Curiously, activity was lost much more rapidly if gentamicin was also present.

ADVERSE EFFECTS

Fusidic acid is a remarkably safe antibiotic. However, mild nausea is fairly common following oral administration, and rashes are occasionally encountered. Reversible jaundice sometimes occurs and this is more common in patients given the drug intravenously (28). Intravenous administration may be accompanied by venospasm and thrombophlebitis unless the drug is infused slowly. Intramuscular injection is not possible because of the risk of tissue necrosis.

CLINICAL USE

The use of fusidic acid is virtually restricted to the treatment of proven staphylococcal infection. Because of its good penetration into bone it has been particularly favored in the treatment of staphylococcal osteomyelitis. Since resistant variants are readily selected in vitro, it is generally considered prudent to co-administer fusidic acid with another agent, often an antistaphylococcal penicillin. Although such a combination may appear antagonistic in laboratory tests, it is unlikely that this has any clinical relevance (12). The combination of fusidic acid and rifampicin may be of value as an alternative to vancomycin in the treatment of infection caused by methicillin-resistant staphylococci (19).

In addition to its use as an antistaphylococcal agent, fusidic acid has also been suggested for the treatment of nocardiasis (5). Moreover, Cronberg et al (29) found fusidic acid as effective as vancomycin or metronidazole in the treatment of antibiotic-associated colitis caused by *Clostridium difficile* toxins.

Topical fusidic acid has been extensively used for skin infections. However, the topical use of agents which have a valuable systemic role is discouraged (30).

DOSING

Whenever possible, the oral route is preferred. Two 250 mg capsules of sodium fusidate are administered 3 times a day. Enteric-coated tablets are also available. Children may be given up to 50 mg/kg daily in 3 divided doses, as a flavored suspension.

For intravenous use, diethanolamine fusidate is administered by slow infusion. Fusidic acid ointment, cream and gel are available for topical application.

FUTURE DIRECTIONS

No naturally occurring or chemically modified congener of fusidic acid has been found that displays superior antibacterial activity, although some derivatives retain activity against fusidic-acid-resistant strains of staphylococci (2). It does not therefore appear likely that new derivatives of fusidic acid will appear in the near future. However, the antibiotic will no doubt continue to consolidate its position as an excellent antistaphylococcal agent.

REFERENCES

1. Arigoni D, Von Daehne W, Godtfredsen WO, Melera A, Vangedel S (1964) The stereochemistry of fusidic acid. *Experientia, 20,* 344.
2. Von Daehne W, Godtfredsen WO, Rasmussen PR (1979) Structure-activity relationships in fusidic acid-type antibiotics. *Adv. Appl. Microbiol., 25,* 95.
3. Perry MJ, Hendricks-Gittins A, Stacey LM, Adlard MW, Noble WC (1983) Fusidane antibiotics produced by dermatophytes. *J. Antibiot., 36,* 1659.
4. Godtfredsen WO, Roholt K, Tybring L (1962) Fucidin, a new orally active antibiotic. *Lancet, 1,* 928.
5. Black WA, McNellis DA (1971) Comparative in-vitro sensitivity of *Nocardia* species to fusidic acid. *J. Med. Microbiol., 4,* 293.
6. Steinkraus GE, McCarthy LR (1979) In vitro activity of sodium fusidate against anaerobic bacteria. *Antimicrob. Agents Chemother., 16,* 120.
7. Guenthner SH, Wenzel RP (1984) In vitro activities of teichomycin, fusidic acid, flucloxacillin, fosfomycin and vancomycin against methicillin-resistant *Staphylococcus aureus. Antimicrob. Agents Chemother., 26,* 268.

8. Richardson JF, Marples RR (1980) Differences in antibiotic susceptibility between *Staphylococcus epidermidis* and *Staphylococcus saprophyticus*. *J. Antimicrob. Chemother., 6*, 499.

9. Farthing MJG, Inge PMG (1986) Antigiardial activity of the bile salt-like antibiotic sodium fusidate. *J. Antimicrob. Chemother., 17*, 165.

10. Black FT, Wildfang IL, Borgbjerg K (1985) Activity of fusidic acid against *Plasmodium falciparum* in vitro. *Lancet, 1*, 578.

11. Cundliffe E (1972) The mode of action of fusidic acid. *Biochem. Biophys. Res. Commun., 46*, 1794.

12. O'Grady F, Greenwood D (1973) Interactions between fusidic acid and penicillins. *J. Med. Microbiol., 6*, 441.

13. Bernardi A, Leder P (1970) Protein biosynthesis in *Escherichia coli*. *J. Biol. Chem., 345*, 4263.

14. Dabbs ER (1987) Fusidic acid resistance in *Rhodococcus erythropolis* due to an inducible extracellular inactivating enzyme. *FEMS Microbiol. Lett., 40*, 135.

15. Völker TA, Iida S, Bickle TA (1982) A single gene coding for resistance to both fusidic acid and chloramphenicol. *J. Mol. Biol., 154*, 417.

16. Bennett AD, Shaw WV (1983) Resistance to fusidic acid in *Escherichia coli* mediated by the type I variant of chloramphenicol acetyl-transferase: a plasmid-encoded mechanism involving antibiotic binding. *Biochem. J., 215*, 29.

17. Proctor GN, McKell J, Rownd RH (1983) Chloramphenicol acetyltransferase may confer resistance to fusidic acid by sequestering the drug. *J. Bacteriol., 155*, 937.

18. Report (1985) Workshop on methicillin-resistant *Staphylococcus aureus* held at the headquarters of the Public Health Laboratory Service on 8 January 1985. *J. Hosp. Infect., 6*, 342.

19. Farber BF, Yee YC, Karchmer AW (1986) Interaction between rifampin and fusidic acid against methicillin-resistant coagulase-positive and -negative staphylococci. *Antimicrob. Agents Chemother., 30*, 174.

20. Wise R, Pippard M, Mitchard M (1977) The disposition of sodium fusidate in man. *Br. J. Clin. Pharmacol., 4*, 615.

21. Bannatyne RM, Cheung R (1982) Protein binding of fusidic acid. *Curr. Ther. Res. Clin. Exp., 31*, 159.

22. Hierholzer G, Knothe H, Rehn J, Koch F (1966) Fusidinsäure-Konzentrationen in chronisch entzündetem Gewebe: Untersuchungen zur chronischen posttraumatischen Osteomyelitis. *Arzneim. Forsch., 16*, 1549.

23. Hierholzer G, Rehn J, Knothe H, Masterson J (1974) Antibiotic therapy of post-traumatic osteomyelitis. *J. Bone Jt Surg., 56B*, 721.

24. Kraemer R, Schaad UB, Lebek G, Rüdeberg A, Rossi E (1982) Sputum penetration of fusidic acid in patients with cystic fibrosis. *Eur. J. Pediatr., 138*, 172.

25. Bergeron MG, Desaulniers D, Lessard C, Lemieux M, Després J-P, Métras J, Raymond G, Brochu G (1985) Concentrations of fusidic acid, cloxacillin, and cefamandole in sera and atrial appendages of patients undergoing cardiac surgery. *Antimicrob. Agents Chemother., 27*, 928.

26. Forsgren A, Bellahsène A (1985) Antibiotic accumulation in human polymorphonuclear leucocytes and lymphocytes. *Scand. J. Infect. Dis., Suppl 44*, 16.

27. Beeching NJ, Thomas MG, Roberts S, Lang SDR (1986) Comparative in-vitro activity of antibiotics incorporated in acrylic bone cement. *J. Antimicrob. Chemother., 17*, 173.

28. Humble MW, Eykyn SJ, Phillips I (1980) Staphylococcal bacteraemia, fusidic acid and jaundice. *Br. Med. J., 280*, 1495.

29. Cronberg S, Castor B, Thorén A (1984) Fusidic acid for the treatment of antibiotic-associated colitis induced by *Clostridium difficile. Infection, 12*, 276.

30. *British National Formulary, Number 14* (1987) Anti-infective skin preparations (p 375). British Medical Association and the Pharmaceutical Society of Great Britain, London.

31. Greenwood D, O'Grady F (1972) Scanning electron microscopy of *Staphylococcus aureus* exposed to some common anti-staphylococcal agents. *J. Gen. Microbiol., 70*, 263.

CHAPTER 9

Lincosamides

PAUL E. HERMANS

Clindamycin maintains its position as one of the important agents to treat anaerobic infections. It also continues to be an effective agent against *Staphylococcus
aureus*, although semisynthetic penicillinase-resistant penicillins and first-generation cephalosporins are favored for infections in which a bactericidal effect is desired, such as endocarditis. There is no important new information on dosing and
pharmacokinetics. Among various well-known side effects, pseudomembranous
ileocolitis is the most important one, but is treatable.

ACTIVITY

Mechanism of action

Ability of Bacteroides fragilis after exposure to clindamycin to form abscesses   Pre-
treatment of *B. fragilis* with subinhibitory concentrations of clindamycin did not
affect the ability of live or heat-killed organisms to produce intra-abdominal abscesses in a mouse model (1). As in previous studies, this animal model requires
mixing with sterile cecal contents.

*Subinhibitory concentration of clindamycin influences the effect of Bacteroides fragi-
lis on phagocytosis*   Evidence is provided that the known inhibitory effect of *B.
fragilis* on human polymorphonuclear leukocyte bactericidal activity against
Escherichia coli is due to utilization of the third component of the complement
system (2). When *B. fragilis* and serum are pre-incubated with a subinhibitory
concentration of clindamycin ($^1/_2$ MIC) subsequent phagocytosis of *E. coli* is increased.

Clindamycin effect on chemotaxis and phagocytosis of leukocytes   The effect of
several antimicrobial agents on chemotaxis and chemiluminescence (a measure of
phagocytosis) of human polymorphonuclear leukocytes was evaluated (3). Pipera-

Antimicrobial Agents Annual 3
P.K. Peterson and J. Verhoef, editors
© Elsevier Science Publishers BV, 1988

cillin and clindamycin had a positive effect on both functions. Cefoxitin and cefotaxime decreased both functions. Tobramycin, gentamicin and netilmicin did not affect either chemotaxis or phagocytosis.

Influence of subinhibitory concentrations of clindamycin on phagocytosis of Staphylococcus aureus in relation to protein A   Evidence was provided that the enhanced uptake of *S. aureus* strains by polymorphonuclear leukocytes after incubation in subinhibitory concentrations of clindamycin is due, in part, to a reduction in the amount of protein A at the bacterial cell surface (4). The study was done with 4 protein-A-rich strains and 3 protein-A-poor strains of *S. aureus*. Incubation was in concentrations of clindamycin that were 0.25 and 0.5 times the MIC of clindamycin and without the antibiotic. The effect of trypsin on uptake and detectable protein A was intermediate between the effect of the two above concentrations of clindamycin.

Failure of clindamycin to facilitate intracellular killing by leukocytes   Entry of antimicrobial agents into phagocytes is a prerequisite for activity against intracellular bacteria. On the other hand, accumulation of an antimicrobial agent does not necessarily imply that intracellular killing of a micro-organism will be facilitated. This was demonstrated for a strain of *S. aureus* and human polymorphonuclear leukocytes (5). Following phagocytosis clindamycin and erythromycin, which achieved high intracellular levels, failed to reduce the number of viable intracellular staphylococci significantly during 3 hours of antibiotic exposure. Rifampin also achieved high intracellular levels and increased intracellular killing occurred. Gentamicin and penicillin G penetrated leukocytes poorly, but gentamicin was associated with rapid intracellular killing, whereas penicillin was not.

Spectrum of activity

Susceptibility of staphylococcal species   Studies in vitro of the susceptibility of 3 species of coagulase-negative staphylococci (*S. epidermidis, S. haemolyticus* and *S. hominis*) confirm that clindamycin is not a therapeutic option, unless susceptibility can be clearly demonstrated (6). However, all 49 strains of a fourth species (*S. saprophyticus*) were susceptible to clindamycin, but also to penicillin, oxacillin and many other antimicrobial agents. *S. saprophyticus* is a cause of urinary tract infections in otherwise healthy individuals. Methicillin-resistant staphylococci were uniformly susceptible in vitro to vancomycin, rifampin and ciprofloxacin. There was variable susceptibility to gentamicin and the combination of trimethoprim + sulfamethoxazole.

Comparison of imipenem with clindamycin with regard to anaerobes   It is important that information about the activity of new antimicrobial agents include a comparison with older agents known to be effective. The use of a newer agent cannot be solely based on a comparison of in vitro data such as MICs. Yet such infor-

Table 1 *Percent of strains resistant*

No. of strains tested	Bacteroides fragilis group (260)	Bacteroides species (35)	Clostridium perfringens (78)	Clostridium species (109)	Fusobacterium species (7)	Peptococcus species (50)	Peptostreptococcus species (13)	Propionibacterium species (8)	Veillonella species (7)
Penicillin (16 and 32 µg/ml)	37 (15)	11 (0)	0 (0)	7 (7)	R	0 (0)	none	none	R
Cefoxitin (16 and 32 µg/ml)	21 (2)	14 (6)	0 (0)	19 (17)	none	0 (0)	none	none	none
Moxalactam (16 and 32 µg/ml)	15 (12)	17 (14)	0 (0)	23 (17)	R	12 (4)	none	none	R
Ticarcillin (64 and 128 µg/ml)	13 (12)	0 (0)	0 (0)	8 (7)	R	0 (0)	none	none	R
Clindamycin (4 and 8 µg/ml)	0.7 (0.3)	0 (0)	1 (1)	13 (8)	R	10 (8)	none	none	none
Chloramphenicol (8 and 16 µg/ml)	0 (0)	0 (0)	1 (1)	1 (1)	none	0 (0)	none	none	none
Metronidazole (8 and 16 µg/ml)	0 (0)	0 (0)	0 (0)	1 (1)	none	16 (16)	R	all	none

Under each antibiotic the lower and higher breakpoints are given. Under each group of micro-organisms are listed the % of strains that are resistant at the lower and higher (between parentheses) breakpoint. When the no. of strains tested was too small to express resu'ts in %, 'none' means no resistant strains, 'R' means resistant were found and 'all' means all tested strains were resistant.

Table 2   *Percent of strains resistant*

	Bacteroides fragilis (153)	Bacteroides thetaiotaomicron (35)	Bacteroides ovatus (27)	Bacteroides vulgatus (22)	Bacteroides distasonis (18)	Bacteroides uniformis (5)
Penicillin (16 and 32 μg/ml)	29 (18)	65 (12)	65 (8)	9 (9)	44 (22)	none
Cefoxitin (16 and 32 μg/ml)	7 (0)	82 (9)	35 (8)	0 (0)	33 (0)	none
Moxalactam (16 and 32 μg/ml)	3 (3)	35 (29)	35 (27)	0 (0)	61 (50)	none
Ticarcillin (64 and 128 μg/ml)	16 (14)	6 (6)	8 (8)	14 (5)	17 (17)	none
Clindamycin (4 and 8 μg/ml)	0.6 (0.6)	0 (0)	0 (0)	0 (0)	0 (0)	none
Chloramphenicol (8 and 16 μg/ml)	0 (0)	0 (0)	0 (0)	0 (0)	0 (0)	none
Metronidazole (8 and 16 μg/ml)	0 (0)	0 (0)	0 (0)	0 (0)	0 (0)	none

For explanation, see legend, Table 1.

mation is basic to the initiation of therapeutic trials. In a comparative study of the MIC_{90} the carbapenem, imipenem, was found to be consistently the most active antibiotic and also more active than clindamycin against the *B. fragilis* group, *Bacteroides* species, *Fusobacterium* species, anaerobic cocci, *Clostridium perfringens*, other *Clostridium* species and certain other non-spore-forming gram-positive rods (7). Amoxicillin+clavulanic acid also appears to be a reasonable therapeutic option in most anaerobic infections, based on in vitro data.

Susceptibility patterns of anaerobes   A survey of anaerobic susceptibility patterns in Canada was done against 590 anaerobic isolates during 1984 (8). Cefoxitin, clindamycin, chloramphenicol and metronidazole continue to be very active against most isolates (see Tables 1 and 2). Major regional differences in susceptibility patterns were not observed.

Susceptibility of Capnocytophaga species   The in vitro susceptibility of 41–120 strains of *Capnocytophaga* species to 29 antimicrobial agents was determined (9). The sources of the clinical isolates were mainly from the respiratory tract, oral ulcerations and blood in compromised patients and from periodontal pockets, gingival scrapings, and the respiratory tract in non-compromised patients. The MIC at which 90% of the strains were inhibited were as follows in order of decreasing activity: clindamycin 0.03 μg/ml, BMY-28142 0.06 μg/ml, cefpirome 0.12 μg/ ml, ciprofloxacin 0.26 μg/ml, ofloxacin 0.50 μg/ml, imipenem 0.50 μg/ml and the third-generation cephalosporins cefotaxime, ceftazidime and ceftriaxone 0.50 μg/ ml. The MICs of these fastidious organisms were determined by an agar dilution method with hemoglobin supplementation. On the basis of this study, penicillin, ampicillin, first- and second-generation cephalosporins, aztreonam, moxalactam, norfloxacin, ticarcillin, aminoglycosides, vancomycin and trimethoprim are not recommended for the treatment of infections caused by *Capnocytophaga* species.

Resistance mechanisms

Multiply resistant Streptococcus pneumoniae strains   Several isolates of *S. pneumoniae* from patients in Brooklyn were 'antibiotic resistant'. These isolates were serotype 19A strains. They were resistant to β-lactam antibiotics, tetracycline, chloramphenicol and trimethoprim+sulfamethoxazole. They were susceptible to erythromycin, clindamycin, vancomycin and rifampin (10).

Clindamycin-resistant strains of Streptococcus pneumoniae   A report from South Africa emphasizes the seriousness of pneumonia due to multiply-resistant pneumococci. These strains are also resistant to clindamycin (11). The authors suggest that the need may arise for routine antibiotic-sensitivity testing of all cultured isolates of *S. pneumoniae*.

Resistance of species of the Bacteroides fragilis group   Two hundred and forty-six clinical isolates belonging to the *B. fragilis* group collected from 1977 to 1982 at the Wadsworth Veterans Administration Medical Center in Los Angeles were tested for susceptibility to clindamycin and cefoxitin (12). There was no significant change in resistance to either clindamycin (breakpoint 8 μg) or cefoxitin (breakpoint 32 μg) over the 6-year survey for any individual species or the *B. fragilis* group in total. However, there were strong differences in susceptibility among species of the *B. fragilis* group. *B. thetaiotaomicron, B. distasonis*, and *B. ovatus* are more resistant to cefoxitin than *B. fragilis* and *B. vulgatus*. The first two species are also more resistant to clindamycin than are other species of the *B. fragilis* group.

MLS-type of resistance of Staphylococcus aureus strains   Not long after the introduction of erythromycin in 1952 resistant strains of *S. aureus* were reported from several parts of the world. One type of resistance – the MLS resistance – is inducible and depends on biochemical modification of the 50S ribosome subunit. This modification confers resistance to macrolides, lincosamides and streptogramin (the MLS group). This interesting phenomenon has recently been reviewed (13).

Emergence of resistant anaerobic organisms during treatment with clindamycin   An interesting survey was done to determine the emergence of clindamycin-resistant anaerobic micro-organisms after therapy with clindamycin in women with pelvic soft-tissue infections (14). Only 5 (0.7%) of 685 isolates tested from 100 women who had endometrial cultures prior to antibiotic therapy were resistant to clindamycin. From 100 endometrial cultures taken immediately after clindamycin therapy, 28 cultures yielded 57 anaerobic bacteria. Of the 40 anaerobic organisms for which MICs of clindamycin were determined, 25 organisms or 62.5% were resistant to clindamycin. An organism was considered resistant to clindamycin, when its MIC was $\geq$ 8 μg/ml. All organisms that were resistant to clindamycin had MICs of >64 μg/ml, except two. The most common isolates after therapy were anaerobic gram-positive cocci. However, 4 of 7 *Bacteroides* species isolated were also resistant to clindamycin. Nine cultures were repeated 1–9 weeks after treatment and yielded 18 anaerobic isolates of which 55% were resistant. Although the clinical significance of these findings is not known, it would seem prudent for physicians to consider that patients who had recent clindamycin exposure may harbor resistant anaerobic micro-organisms.

CLINICAL PHARMACOLOGY

There are few reports on concentrations of antibiotics in human lung tissues. The concentrations of clindamycin in human lung tissue were determined in 11 patients with lung tumors who were treated with the antibiotic (15). After a 600 mg drip infusion for 1 hour, the concentrations of clindamycin in lung tissue were 24 and 23 μg/g, 2 and 3 hours after the start of drip infusion, respectively. In the case of 1200 mg drip infusion, the value reached 47 μg/g in 2 hours and 39 μg/g in 33 hours. The concentrations in lung tissue were about 4–5 times higher than in blood.

CLINICAL USES

Shift from clindamycin to vancomycin in peritonitis that occurs with peritoneal dialysis   Until recently the first-line treatment of peritonitis in patients on continuous ambulatory peritoneal dialysis consisted of gentamicin with clindamycin. The emergence of multiply resistant strains of *Staphylococcus epidermidis* among such patients has led to the introduction of antibiotic regimens in which vancomycin is substituted for clindamycin and administered by peritoneal lavage (16).

Comments on clinical trials in intra-abdominal and pelvic infections   A large number of studies involving the use of newer antimicrobial agents singly or in combination with older agents in the treatment of abdominal and pelvic infections have been published. These studies are very difficult to evaluate. They often have a bottomline of about 70% efficacy, suggesting that any reasonable choice of antimicrobial agents will be more or less equally effective. Most of these studies are published in special issues of clinical journals and are sponsored by potentially self-interested groups. Often they are reviews of symposia that were held in desirable vacation settings, in luxurious hotels, with gourmet meals for active and passive participants. This reviewer is critical of this type of evaluation of new therapeutic agents. Besides the problem of possible decrease of objectivity in such settings, there are also intrinsic scientific problems. Most studies are not well controlled and the extremely important role of surgical drainage or corrective intervention cannot be evaluated. Most importantly, it is almost never possible to determine why patients were enrolled and who made decisions to enroll or not enroll a potential candidate for treatment. From our own observations, patients are derived from a number of surgical and medical services. These services often have different attitudes with regard to participation in protocol studies. Most important is the impression that physicians have a tendency to 'protect' their very ill patients from therapeutic trials and prefer standard treatment programs they are familiar with. Therefore, detailed data on the type of patients that were not entered in the study should be available.

DOSING

There continues to be some interest in determining compatibility of certain antibiotic mixtures, because of the potential of reducing preparation and administration costs. In this connection stability of clindamycin phosphate when mixed with ceftizoxime sodium, cefamandole naftate and cefazolin sodium in either 5% dextrose or 0.9% sodium chloride for 48 hours was demonstrated (17). Clindamycin was also stable with ceftizoxime sodium in 0.9% sodium chloride for 24 hours (17).

FUTURE DIRECTIONS

Antimicrobial agents such as the combination of *N*-formimidoylthienamycin cilastatin (imipenem) will be a serious challenge to the 3 main agents for use in anaerobic infections: chloramphenicol, clindamycin and metronidazole. It will take considerable time and effort to define specific uses for the increasing number of available agents.

REFERENCES

1. Zaleznik DF, Zhang Z, Onderdonk AB, Kasper DL (1986) Effect of subinhibitory doses of clindamycin on the virulence of *Bacteroides fragilis*: role of lipopolysaccharide. *J. Infect. Dis., 154*, 40.
2. Namavar F, Kaan JA, Verweij-Van Vught AMJJ, Vel WAC, Bal M, Kester ADM, MacLaren DM (1986) Effect of *Bacteroides fragilis* grown in the presence of clindamycin, metronidazole and fusic acid on opsonization and killing of *Escherichia coli. Eur. J. Clin. Microbiol., 5*, 324.
3. Ford LC, Quan WL, Lagasse LD (1986) Recommendations for the use of antibiotics in gynaecological oncology. *J. Obstet. Gynaecol., 6 (S1)*, 42.
4. Veringa EM, Verhoef J (1986) Influence of subinhibitory concentrations of clindamycin on opsonophagocytosis of *Staphylococcus aureus*, a protein-A-dependent process. *Antimicrob. Agents Chemother., 30*, 796.
5. Hand WL, King-Thompson NL (1986) Contrast between phagocyte antibiotic uptake and subsequent intracellular bactericidal activity. *Antimicrob. Agents Chemother., 29*, 135.
6. Fass RJ, Helsel VL, Barnishan J, Ayers LW (1986) In vitro susceptibility of four species of coagulase-negative staphylococci. *Antimicrob. Agents Chemother., 30*, 545.
7. Goldstein EJC, Citron DM (1986) Comparative in vitro activities of amoxicillin-clavulanic acid and imipenem against anaerobic bacteria isolated from community hospitals. *Antimicrob. Agents Chemother., 29*, 158.
8. Bourgault AM, Harding GK, Smith JA, Horsman GB, Marrie TJ, Lamothe F (1986) Survey of anaerobic susceptibility patterns in Canada. *Antimicrob. Agents Chemother., 30*, 798.
9. Rummens JL, Gordts B, Van Landuyt HW (1986) In vitro susceptibility of *Capnocytophaga* species to 29 antimicrobial agents. *Antimicrob. Agents Chemother., 30*, 739.
10. Simberkoff MS, Lakaszewski M, Cross A et al (1986) Antibiotic-resistant isolates of *Streptococcus pneumoniae* from clinical specimens: a cluster of serotype 19A organisms in Brooklyn, New York. *J. Infect. Dis., 153*, 78.
11. Feldman C, Kellenbach JM, Miller SD et al (1985) Community-acquired pneumonia due to penicillin-resistant pneumococci. *N. Engl. J. Med., 313*, 615.
12. Wexler HM, Harris B, Carter WT, Finegold SM (1986) Six year retrospective survey of the resistance of *Bacteroides fragilis* group species to clindamycin and cefoxitin. *Di-*

agn. Microbiol. Infect. Dis., 4, 247.

13. Weisblum B (1985) Inducible resistance to macrolides, lincosamides, and streptogramin B antibiotics: the resistance phenotype, its biological diversity, and structural elements that regulate expression: a review. *J. Antimicrob. Chemother., 16, Suppl*, 63.

14. Ohm-Smith MJ, Sweet RL, Hadley WK (1986) Occurrence of clindamycin-resistant anaerobic bacteria isolated from cultures taken following clindamycin therapy. *Antimicrob. Agents Chemother., 30*, 11.

15. Ikeda T, Sakai T, Kikuchi K, Suito T (1985) Concentrations of clindamycin phosphate in lung tissue. *Jpn. J. Antibiot., 38*, 3477.

16. Brauner L, Kahlmeter G, Lindholm T, Simonsen O (1985) Vancomycin and netilmicin as first line treatment of peritonitis continuous ambulatory peritoneal dialysis patients. *J. Antimicrob. Chemother., 15*, 751.

17. Bosso JA, Townsend RJ (1985) Stability of clindamycin phosphate and ceftizoxime sodium, cefoxitin sodium, cefamandole naftate or cefazolin sodium in two intravenous solutions. *Am. J. Hosp. Pharm., 42*, 2211.

CHAPTER 10

Macrolides

R.W. AUCKENTHALER, A. ZWAHLEN and F.A. WALDVOGEL

In the last 3 decades, macrolide antimicrobial agents have been widely used in the treatment of infections caused by susceptible gram-positive organisms. Macrolides were mainly administered as second-choice antibiotics to patients allergic to penicillins and their derivatives, and to outpatients with respiratory tract infections. Today erythromycin has, in addition, become standard therapy for infections caused by *Mycoplasma pneumoniae, Legionella* species, *Bordetella pertussis* and *Campylobacter* species, and for eradication of *Corynebacterium diphtheriae* from the nasopharynx; it is accepted for the treatment of acne, soft tissue and skin infections, otitis media, bronchitis, and sexually transmitted disease, particularly if caused by *Chlamydia* species (1–3). Spiramycin, with an antimicrobial activity similar to, but with less potency than erythromycin, has become a possible alternative to pyrimethamine and sulfonamide combinations in the treatment of toxoplasmosis. Since 1977, macrolides have recaptured interest through the development of totally or semisynthetic macrolide antibiotics (4). Particularly larger molecules such as 16- or 18-membered macrolides show increased antibacterial potency, a larger spectrum including various antiviral, antifungal or even antiparasitic activity and better pharmacological properties (5–8). In contrast to aminoglycosides or β-lactam antibiotics, these antibiotics achieve very high tissue and intracellular concentrations (9–11). This property might contribute to their clinical efficacy, despite the fact that they are mainly bacteriostatic.

Macrolide antibiotics were originally isolated from various *Streptomyces* species and can be synthesized by condensation of acetate, propionate and, in some cases, butyrate units. The final structure is characterized by a macrocyclic lactone ring attached to two or more sugar moieties. Fourteen-membered macrolides include the classical erythromycins A, B, C and D (12), oleandomycin, trioleandomycin and more recent compounds such as albocycline (13), megalomycin (14), lankamycin (14) and RU-28965 (11, 15–17). Sixteen-membered macrolides include the traditional spiramycin (18, 19) and its derivatives (20, 21), tylosin (22), josamycin (23), rosaramicin (24), turimycin (25) and miocamycin (midecamycin) with toxicological and very few clinical studies (26–29). In general, the spectrum and

Antimicrobial Agents Annual 3
P.K. Peterson and J. Verhoef, editors
© Elsevier Science Publishers BV, 1988

antimicrobial activity of these drugs are similar to erythromycin, but improved pharmacological properties are observed for certain derivatives.

ACTIVITY

Mechanism of action

Macrolides inhibit RNA-dependent protein synthesis by stimulating the dissociation of peptidyl tRNA from ribosomes. They reversibly bind to the 50S ribosomal subunit and block the P-site, resulting in impaired transpeptidation and/or translocation. The affinity for the P-site can be modified by various purine moieties, an observation which could explain the synergism observed between rosaramicin and puromycin (30, 31). The competition for binding sites in the presence of chloramphenicol or lincomycin is antagonistic for the activity of macrolides. Depending on drug concentration, microbial species, phase of growth and inoculum density, macrolides are bacteriostatic or bactericidal. Probably because of the better penetration of non-ionized drug through the bacterial cell wall, the activity of the weak-base macrolides is increased in alkaline pH.

Spectrum of activity

The antimicrobial activity of erythromycin is directed mainly against gram-positive bacteria including staphylococci, streptococci, corynebacteria, *Listeria monocytogenes*, some *Erysipelothrix rhusiopathiae* (32), *Bacillus* species and certain species of *Clostridium*, *Actinomyces* and *Mycobacterium* (33). Their gram-negative spectrum includes *Neisseria gonorrhoeae*, *N. meningitidis*, *Brucella suis*, *B. melitensis*, *Bacteroides* species, *Campylobacter* species, *Branhamella catarrhalis* (31) and *Chlamydia* species. None of the newer compounds has an expanded spectrum against Enterobacteriaceae or *Pseudomonas* species and anaerobes (1–3, 15). Spiramycin has a major activity against toxoplasmosis and possibly cryptosporidiosis (35, 36). Newer compounds, particularly if they contain more than 16-membered lactone rings, have a larger spectrum with activity against fungi, virus or parasites (5–8). Determination of minimal inhibitory concentrations is standardized for most of the organisms mentioned above (34), and comparative studies confirm minimal differences of activity between macrolide compounds (16, 38, 40). Testing Legionellaceae, however, presents a real problem: better standardization is necessary because certain antibiotics are inactivated by the ingredients contained in the agar promoting the growth of the organisms tested (41).

Resistance mechanisms

Resistance to macrolides may result from decreased permeability of the cell wall in Enterobacteriaceae, alteration of the target site or drug inactivation. Alteration of 23S ribosomal RNA of the 50S subunit by N^6-demethylation of adenine confers resistance to macrolides (M), lincosamines (L) and streptogramin type B (MLS_B) by reducing the affinity between the antibiotics and the ribosome. This alteration is expressed either in an inducible mode, in the presence of subinhibitory concentrations of the antibiotic, with dissociated resistance, or, constitutively with resistance of the entire bacterial population or zonally. Similarly to methicillin-resistant *Staphylococcus aureus*, the expression of the resistance has been shown to be temperature-dependent (42). MLS_B resistance has been described for a variety of bacteria such as *Staphylococcus* species, *Streptococcus* species including *S. pneumoniae, Corynebacterium diphtheriae, Bacteroides fragilis, Clostridium perfringens, Lactobacillus casei, Streptomyces erythreus, Listeria* species and recently *Legionella* species (43–46). As a rule, the resistance is plasmid-mediated, transposable in staphylococci or streptococci, and rarely occurs on the chromosome (47–56). Four distinct classes of MLS_B-resistance determinants have been defined, 2 for gram-positive cocci, and 1 each for *Bacillus licheniformis* and *Bacteroides fragilis* (50) and the molecular genetics of resistance have been described in detail (51). The complete nucleotide sequence of *ermA*, the prototype MLS_B-resistance gene from *Staphylococcus aureus*, has been determined (57, 58). In addition to MLS_B resistance, another mechanism involving inactivation of macrolides has been described in gram-positive organisms and even in *Escherichia coli*, conferring resistance on either M and/or L and/or S or S_A or S_B antibiotics (59, 60).

CLINICAL PHARMACOLOGY

Adequate assay techniques are essential for the correct interpretation of pharmacokinetic data: classical agar-diffusion microbiological assay methods are still in use. In addition, high-pressure liquid chromatography (61–63), complex formation with bromcresol purple (64), and tissue uptake measured with radioactive labeled antibiotics can be used (65, 66).

The pharmacokinetics of erythromycin have been extensively reviewed (1, 3, 67, 68). Serum half-life varies from 1.2–2.6 h for erythromycin (3), 3.3–4.8 h for rosaramicin (24), 0.9–1.5 h for josamicin (69) and 3–4 h for spiramycin (70). The elimination half-life of erythromycin is similar in hemodialyzed patients, thus making dosage adjustment unnecessary for patients receiving less than 1.5 g/d (71). Erythromycin is primarily bound to α-globulin and because of impaired α-globulin production high concentrations of the free fraction of erythromycin can be measured in cirrhotic patients (72). Macrolides are mainly eliminated in active form through the bile, leading to high stool concentrations (3, 24). Partial deactivation by demethylation takes place in the liver, yielding various metabolites (1, 3, 24, 69).

Excellent tissue and body fluid penetration is the hallmark of macrolides, except for cerebrospinal fluid. High concentrations are achieved in the upper and lower respiratory tract (70, 74–76), particularly by josamycin (77, 78). An interesting aspect of macrolides is their ability to penetrate into phagocytes as measured by microscope-autoradiography with ^{3}H-labeled erythromycin, and hopefully to kill intracellular micro-organisms (79–82). They also seem to have immunostimulatory properties by inhibiting the release of prostaglandin subclasses (83). Compared to extracellular fluid the intracellular concentration of erythromycin is 9–23 times higher in alveolar macrophages (84), 4–12 times higher in various tissue culture cells of human organs (65), and 10–13 times higher in polymorphonuclear leukocytes (80, 85). Even if high concentrations are achieved intracellularly, the antimicrobial activity of the antibiotic against phagocytosed bacteria is difficult to prove and remains controversial. In an elegant study using a functional test with a semiautomated photometric method, erythromycin was shown to be active intracellularly only at very high concentrations (86).

ADVERSE EFFECTS AND DRUG INTERACTIONS

Adverse effects

Although macrolide antibiotics have few severe side-effects, one of their main limitations is gastrointestinal intolerance. Abdominal cramps, nausea and vomiting occurred in 45% of children given erythromycin ethylsuccinate and in 14% of those receiving erythromycin estolate (87), resulting in a high incidence of discontinuation of the medication. Similarly, intravenous infusion of erythromycin lactobionate (1 g in 30 min) in healthy young adults produced an unexpectedly high incidence of complications (68%) with pronounced systemic and gastrointestinal effects (88). The untoward effects seemed more frequent in young than in older patients, suggesting a possible age-related susceptibility of smooth muscle to the drug. The gastrointestinal motility-stimulating activity of macrolide antibiotics seems to be closely related to their chemical configuration (89–91). In dogs 14-membered macrolides such as erythromycin and oleandomycin induce strong slow phasic and unco-ordinated contractions of the stomach, duodenum and upper jejunum. The contractions of gastrointestinal smooth muscles are dose-dependent and can be blocked by atropine. In contrast, 16-membered macrolides (acetylspiramycin, tylosin, kitasamycin) have no such effects (89). The mechanisms by which 14-membered macrolides interfere with the physiological and consistent motility pattern migrating from the stomach to the terminal ileum is unknown.

Reversible cholestatic hepatitis has been observed in adults treated with erythromycin estolate. The analysis by Inman and Rawson (92) using prescription-event monitoring, suggests that erythromycin-associated hepatitis is less frequent than previously thought and occurs in less than 1 in 1000 cases. French authors reviewed their experience of erythromycin hepatitis and showed that it does occur in children, although less frequently than in adults (89). The estolate salt was responsible for 80–90% of the erythromycin-induced hepatitis, but hepatitis has also been observed in patients treated with the ethylsuccinate, propionate and stearate salts of erythromycin respectively (94–97). In vitro, erythromycin estolate and its sodium lauryl moiety are more toxic for isolated rat hepatocytes than erythromycin ethylsuccinate (98). The exact mechanism for the hepatotoxicity of macrolides remains unknown. However, there is evidence both for toxicity and for allergic mechanisms (99, 100). In-vivo and in-vitro studies show minor ultrastructural lesions of the hepatocytes, which might be related to the 14-membered macrolides forming unstable nitrosoalkanes and metabolites reactive with glutathione or cysteine. In addition, necrosis of a few hepatocytes could liberate plasma membrane proteins into the circulation, which are modified by the covalent binding of the reactive metabolites. Such modified liver antigens might trigger an immune response with an allergic type of hepatitis associated with jaundice. Rapid recurrence of hepatitis in patients with previous drug-induced jaundice retreated with erythromycin strongly suggests a hyperergic mechanism. In contrast to tetracycline, erythromycin does not seem to exert selection pressure on the intestinal flora (101).

Transient hearing impairment due to cranial nerve toxicity of erythromycin is rare and might be related to pre-existing renal or hepatic disease, particularly in elderly women (96, 97, 102). The meaning of ophthalmological alterations of the fundus observed in dogs treated with rosaramicin is unclear (98).

Recurrent ventricular tachycardia and QT-prolongation after mitral valve replacement have been associated with erythromycin administration (103). Erythromycin has an important impact on the gut microflora and decreases the number of aerobic and anaerobic bacteria by more than $5 \log_{10}$ (104). However, antibiotic-associated colitis due to erythromycin is extremely rare. Erythromycin reduces greatly the numbers of *Streptococcus salivarius* in the oropharyngeal secretions (105), which might impair resistance to colonization with Group A streptococci.

Drug interactions

Macrolides have the potential to interfere with the hepatic metabolism of other drugs (109, 111). They induce the production of cytochrome P-450 isoenzymes with varying affinity for macrolides. These induced isoenzymes actively demethylate and oxidize the macrolides into nitrosoalkanes which form a stable inactive complex with the iron of cytochrome P-450. This complex decreases metabolism for other drugs and may produce drug interactions (99, 109, 110). Josamicin and midecamycin, two of the 16-membered macrolides, do not bind to cytochrome P-450 and have less interaction with other drugs (109, 111). Human subjects treated with erythromycin or troleandomycin have 20–30% decreased clearance of antipyrine (phenazone), methylprednisolone and theophylline (112–114). Although the clinical significance of these interactions has been questioned (115), the administration of erythromycin has been associated with increased theophylline toxicity (113), signs of carbamazepine overdosage (116), and increased sensitivity to ergotamine (106). In addition, erythromycin can potentiate warfarin-induced hypoprothrombinemia by slowing warfarin clearance (117–119). Erythromycin also increases the bioavailability of digoxin, apparently through alteration of the gut microflora which forms digoxin metabolites (106). Sixteen-membered macrolides such as josamycin, spiramycin and midecamycin are rarely, if ever, involved in drug interactions (111).

CLINICAL USES

Erythromycin remains an alternative to penicillins for the treatment of infections caused by susceptible micro-organisms and is the drug of choice for some infectious diseases due to *Mycoplasma pneumoniae* and *Legionella* species.

Respiratory infections

Oral administration of erythromycin has been used for eradication of Group A streptococci from the throat. Its varying clinical efficacy might be related to variables such as bioavailability of formulations, compliance, tissue concentrations and modified phagocytosis in the presence of subinhibitory concentrations (67, 87, 93, 120). The utility of treating otitis media with antibiotics has been recently questioned (121). Nonetheless, erythromycin alone (122) or in association with a sulfonamide (1) seems as efficient as other drug regimens. As mentioned above, penetration of erythromycin into secretions of the middle ear, paranasal sinuses and bronchi is slow but, in the steady state, the drug levels are equal to or greater than the serum concentrations (74). Sufficient levels are reached to inhibit in vitro the growth of most pathogens involved in respiratory tract infections with the exception of strains of *Haemophilus influenzae*.

Erythromycin is the standard therapy for *Mycoplasma pneumoniae* infections: it significantly shortens the duration of fever, and accelerates clearing of chest roentgenograms but has no influence on bacterial shedding; in children, no significant effects of treatment were noted on pulmonary function alterations attributed to *Mycoplasma* infections (123, 124).

Treating moderate and severe *Legionella* species infection with high doses of erythromycin in association with rifampin is widely accepted (1, 125). Erythromycin uptake and accumulation by human polymorphonuclear leukocytes (80) and by alveolar macrophages (84) probably result in efficient killing of intracellular *Legionella*. However, treatment failures have also been reported (126).

Endocarditis prophylaxis

Erythromycin stearate, given as a single dose of 1.5 g orally 1 hour before dental extraction, decreased the incidence of bacteremia from 43% to only 15%. In addition, bacteremia in erythromycin-treated patients was observed with low serum concentrations (127, 128). In addition, resistant streptococci have been cultured over 43 weeks after 1 or 2 doses of erythromycin and thus make questionable the recommended prophylaxis for repeated dental procedures (129).

Sexually transmitted disease

Erythromycin or tetracycline is the drug of choice for the treatment of urethral, endocervical and rectal infections due to *Chlamydia trachomatis* including lympho-granuloma venereum. Erythromycin is also active against *Neisseria gonor-rhoeae, Treponema pallidum* and *Haemophilus ducreyi* (1). Single-dose therapy combining rifampicin and erythromycin was found to be efficacious for uncompli-cated gonorrhea in women, although this regimen failed to eradicate *Chlamydia trachomatis* (130). Prophylactic erythromycin treatment for 7 days given at 36 weeks' gestation in infected mothers protects the newborn from chlamydial infec-tions (131). Eye ointment at 0.5% is efficacious against ophthalmia neonatorum (132).

Chronic prostatitis

The high levels of erythromycin concentrations achieved in prostatic secretions justify consideration of this antibiotic for chronic prostatitis especially when infec-tions due to *Chlamydia* are suspected (133).

Prophylaxis of fever and infection in cancer patients

Comparison of trimethoprim-sulfamethoxazole plus erythromycin versus placebo as prophylaxis for bacterial infection in neutropenic patients showed no signifi-cant reduction in fever episodes. However, adverse reactions due to the prophyla-xis were so frequent that they resulted in very poor compliance (134).

Gastrointestinal infections

A 5-day course of erythromycin stearate (500 mg twice daily) to patients with in-fectious diarrhea due to *Campylobacter jejuni* had no effect on the mean duration of symptoms but significantly shortened bacterial shedding (135, 137). Patients with the acquired immunodeficiency syndrome (AIDS) frequently present debili-tating diarrhea due to *Cryptosporidium* species. In one study spiramycin adminis-tration resulted in complete resolution of diarrhea in half of the patients and in symptomatic improvement of the others (36, 138); however, these studies need fur-ther confirmation. The role of macrolides in the prophylaxis of traveller's diarrhea has not been clarified (139).

Toxoplasmosis

Spiramycin has been used for several years, mainly in France, for the treatment of extracranial toxoplasmosis. The efficacy of the 16-membered macrolides cannot yet be generalized, since josamycin has been shown to be inefficient in experimen-tal toxoplasmosis in mice (140).

Reactions to BCG vaccination

In patients with reactions to BCG vaccination, erythromycin and isoniazide had similar effects on the size of ulceration (141), although a placebo-controlled trial of each drug is now necessary before further recommendations can be made.

DOSING

According to the literature, various erythromycin formulations or 16-membered macrolides will achieve different serum levels after a given oral dose (1–3, 68). It is difficult to evaluate fully the clinical relevance of these findings, because similar studies performed by different investigators have produced opposite results depending on food intake, single or multiple dosage etc. (142, 143). Nonetheless, all the available preparations are sufficiently absorbed to result in serum concentrations above the minimal inhibitory concentration of the susceptible pathogens discussed previously. The recommended dosage of erythromycin is usually 250–500 mg q.i.d. Moderate or severe infections caused by *Legionella* species should be treated with 4 g i.v. and rifampicin 1200 mg (125). Patients treated with erythromycin for less than 3 weeks have a higher relapse rate than those treated for a longer period (1). For other macrolides at present in use the recommended dosage is similar. No data are available for RU-28965 or rosaramicin since these drugs are not yet commercially available.

FUTURE DIRECTIONS

Macrolides have been used in clinical medicine for 3 decades now and remain a cornerstone of antimicrobial therapy. The pharmacological properties of the 14-membered macrolides have been improved, however, and they may be replaced in the future by 16-membered macrolides which are almost free from side-effects. Attempts to derive new compounds semisynthetically and to develop 18-membered macrolides will possibly expand the spectrum of activity against viruses, fungi or parasites. Their excellent tissue penetration, intracellular activity and possible non-specific immunostimulatory properties, such as improved migration and phagocytosis by polymorphonuclear leukocytes (144), will maintain interest in the development of new macrolides.

REFERENCES

1. Washington II JA, Wilson WR (1984) Erythromycin: a microbial and clinical perspective after 30 years of clinical use. I. II. *Mayo Clin. Proc., 60,* 189, 271.
2. Steigbigel NH (1984) Erythromycin, lincomycin, and clindamycin. In: Mandell GL,

Douglas RG, Bennett JE (Eds), *Principles and Practice of Infectious Diseases, 2nd ed*, p 224. Wiley, New York.

3. Chow AW (1984) Erythromycin. In: Ristuccia AM, Cunha BA (Eds), *Antimicrobial Therapy*, p 209. Raven Press, New York.

4. Paterson I, Mansuri MM (1985) Recent developments in the total synthesis of macrolide antibiotics. *Tetrahedron, 41*, 3569.

5. Omura S, Nakagawa A, Imamura N et al (1985) Structure of a new macrolide antibiotic X-14952B. *J. Antibiot., 38*, 674.

6. Werner G, Hagenmaier H (1984) Metabolic products of microorganisms: Bafilomycin, a new group of macrolide antibiotics – production, isolation, chemical structure and biological activity. *J. Antibiot., 37*, 110.

7. Kinoshita K, Satoi S, Hayashi M (1985) Mycinamicins, new macrolide antibiotics. VIII. Chemical degradation and absolute configuration of mycinamicins. *J. Antibiot., 38*, 522.

8. Goetz MA, McCormick PA, Monaghan RL, Ostlind DA (1985) L-155, 175: a new antiparasitic macrolide – fermentation, isolation, structure. *J. Antibiot., 38*, 161.

9. Fuchs PC, Thornsberry C, Barry AL et al (1979) Rosamicin: in vitro activity comparison with erythromycin and other antibiotics against clinical isolates from the genitourinary tract and *Neisseria meningitidis J. Antibiot., 32*, 920.

10. Strausbaugh LJ, Bolton WK, Dilworth JA et al (1976) Comparative pharmacology of josamycin and erythromycin stearate. *Antimicrob. Agents Chemother., 10*, 450.

11. Tremblay D, Bryskier A, Vuckovic M et al (1985) RU 28965, nouveau macrolide semi-synthétique: biodisponibilité et profil pharmacocinétique après administration par voie orale. *Pathol. Biol., 33*, 502.

12. Kibwage IO, Hoogmartens J, Roets E et al (1985) Antibacterial activities of erythromycins A, B, C, and D, and some of their derivatives. *Antimicrob. Agents Chemother., 28*, 630.

13. Harada K, Nishida F, Takagi H, Suzuki M (1984) Studies on an antibiotic, albocycline. VII. Minor components of albocycline. *J. Antibiot., 37*, 1876.

14. Allen NE (1977) Macrolide resistance in *Staphylococcus aureus* inducers of macrolide resistance. *Antimicrob. Agents Chemother., 11*, 669.

15. Barlam T, Neu HC (1984) In vitro comparison of the activity of RU 28965, a new macrolide, with that of erythromycin against aerobic and anaerobic bacteria. *Antimicrob. Agents Chemother., 25*, 529.

16. Jones RN, Barry AL, Thornsberry C (1983) In vitro evaluation of the three new macrolide antimicrobial agents, RU 28965, RU 29065, and RU 29702, and comparisons with other orally administered drugs. *Antimicrob. Agents Chemother., 24*, 209.

17. Rolston KVI, LeBlanc B, Ho DH (1986) In-vitro activity of RU-28965, a new macrolide, compared to that of erythromycin. *J. Antimicrob. Chemother., 17*, 161.

18. Sano H, Sunazuka T, Tanaka H et al (1984) Chemical modification of spiramycins. III. Synthesis and antibacterial activities of 4″-sulfonates and 4″-alkylethers of spiramycin I. *J. Antibiot., 37*, 750.

19. Sano H, Sunazuka T, Tanaka H et al (1984) Chemical modification of spiramycins. IV. Synthesis and in vitro and in vivo activities of 3″,4″-diacylates and 3,3″,4″-triacylates of spiramycin I. *J. Antibiot., 37*, 760.

20. Sano H, Inoue M, Omura S (1984) Chemical modification of spiramycins. II. Synthesis and antimicrobial activity of 4′-deoxy derivatives of neospiramycin I and their 12-(Z)-isomers. *J. Antibiot., 37*, 738.

21. Sano H, Tanaka H, Yamashita K et al (1985) Chemical modification of spiramycins. V. Synthesis and antibacterial activity of 3′ or 4‴-de-*N*-methylspiramycin I and their *N*-substituted derivatives. *J. Antibiot., 38*, 186.

22. Omura S, Tanaka Y, Mamada H, Masuma R (1984) Effect of ammonium ion, inorganic phosphate and amino acids on the biosynthesis of protonolide, a precursor of tylosin aglycone. *J. Antibiot., 37*, 494.

23. Wildfeuer A, Vanek E (1984) Aktivität von Josamycin gegen *Staphylococcus aureus* in vitro. *Therapiewoche, 34*, 6969.

24. Lin CC, Chung M, Gural R et al (1984) Pharmacokinetics and metabolism of rosaramicin in humans. *Antimicrob. Agents Chemother., 26*, 522.

25. Hesse G, Hoffmann H, Fricke H, Fleck WF (1983) Protein binding of the macrolide antibiotic turimycin: methodological effects on results. *Pharmazie, 38*, 740.

26. Yokota M, Takeda U, Odaki M (1984) Toxicological studies on a new macrolide antibiotic, midecamycin acetate (miocamycin). IV-1-9. Toxicity of metabolites of miocamycin. *Jpn. J. Antibiot., 37*, 1488.

27. Moriguchi M, Takedu U, Hata T (1984) Effects of midecamycin acetate (miocamycin), a new macrolide antibiotic, on reproductive performances in rats and rabbits. *Jpn. J. Antibiot., 37*, 1572.

28. Watanabe T, Miyauchi K, Kazuno Y (1984) In vitro and in vivo activity of miocamycin and a metabolite, Mb-12, against *Mycoplasma pneumoniae. Drugs Exp. Clin. Res., 10*, 371.

29. Rimoldi R, Fioretti M, Bandera M (1985) Clinical experience with miocamycin in the treatment of respiratory tract infections. *Drugs Exp. Clin. Res., 11*, 263.

30. Siegrist S, Velitchkovitch S, Moreau N, Le Goffic F (1984) Effect of P and A site substrates on the binding of a macrolide to ribosomes: analysis of the puromycin-induced stimulation. *Eur. J. Biochem., 143*, 23.

31. Tejedor F, Ballesta JPG (1985) Components of the macrolide binding site on the ribosome. *J. Antimicrob. Chemother., 16, Suppl A*, 53.

32. Takahashi T, Sawada T, Ohmae K et al (1984) Antibiotic resistance of *Erysipelothrix rhusiopathiae* isolated from pigs with chronic swine erysipelas. *Antimicrob. Agents Chemother., 25*, 385.

33. Power JT, Stewart IC, Ross JD (1984) Erythromycin in the management of troublesome BCG lesions. *Br. J. Dis. Chest, 78*, 192.

34. Ahmad F, McLeod DT, Croughan MJ, Calder MA (1984) Antimicrobial susceptibility of *Branhamella catarrhalis* isolated from bronchopulmonary infections. *Antimicrob. Agents Chemother., 26*, 424.

35. Nye F (1979) Treating toxoplasmosis. *J. Antimicrob. Chemother., 5*, 244.

36. Collier AC, Miller RA, Meyers JD (1984) Cryptosporidiosis after marrow transplantation: person-to-person transmission and treatment with spiramycin. *Ann. Intern. Med., 101*, 205.

37. National Committee for Clinical Standards (1979) *Performance Standard for Antimicrobic Susceptibility Tests.* Approved Standards, American Society for Microbiology, Washington, DC.

38. Wang WL, Reller LB, Blaser MJ (1984) Comparison of antimicrobial susceptibility patterns of *Campylobacter jejuni* and *Campylobacter coli. Antimicrob. Agents Chemother., 26*, 351.

39. Lacey RW, Lord VL, Howson GL (1984) In-vitro evaluation of miokamycin: bactericidal activity against streptococci. *J. Antimicrob. Chemother., 13*, 5.

40. Goossens H, De Mol P, Coignau H et al (1985) Comparative in vitro activities of az-treonam, ciprofloxacin, norfloxacin, ofloxacin, HR 810 (a new cephalosporin), RU28965 (a new macrolide), and other agents against enteropathogens. *Antimicrob. Agents Chemother., 27,* 388.

41. Bornstein N, Roudier C, Fleurette J (1985) Determination of the activity on *Legionella* of eight macrolides and related agents by comparative testing of three media. *J. Antimicrob. Chemother., 15,* 17.

42. Welch WD, Southern PM (1984) Unusual susceptibility of methicillin-resistant *Staphylococcus aureus* to erythromycin, clindamycin, gentamicin, and tetracycline at 30 degr. C but not at 35 degr. C. *J. Clin. Microbiol., 19,* 831.

43. Dowling JN, McDevitt DA, Pasculle WA (1985) Isolation and preliminary characterization of erythromycin-resistant variants of *Legionella micdadei* and *Legionella pneumophila. Antimicrob. Agents Chemother., 27,* 272.

44. Buu-Hoi A, Bieth G, Horaud T (1984) Broad host range of streptococcal macrolide resistance plasmids. *Antimicrob. Agents Chemother., 25,* 289.

45. Rollins LD, Lee LN, LeBlanc DJ (1985) Evidence for a disseminated erythromycin resistance determinant mediated by Tn917-like sequences among Group D streptococci isolated from pigs, chickens, and humans. *Antimicrob. Agents Chemother., 27,* 439.

46. Duval J (1985) Evolution and epidemiology of MLS resistance. *J. Antimicrob. Chemother., 16, Suppl A,* 137.

47. Callihan DR, Young FE, Clark VL (1984) Presence of two unique genes encoding macrolide-lincosamide-streptogramin resistance members of the *Bacteroides fragilis* group as determined by DNA-DNA homology. *J. Antimicrob. Chemother., 14,* 329.

48. Nakajima Y, Abe H, Endou K, Matsuoka M (1984) Resistance to macrolide antibiotics in *Staphylococcus aureus* susceptible to lincomycin and mikamycin B. *J. Antibiot., 37,* 675.

49. Weisblum B (1984) Inducible erythromycin resistance in bacteria. *Br. Med. Bull., 40,* 47.

50. Courvalin P, Ounissi H, Arthur M (1985) Multiplicity of macrolide-lincosamide-streptogramin antibiotic resistance determinants. *J. Antimicrob. Chemother., 16, Suppl A,* 91.

51. Horaud T, Le Bouguenec C, Pepper K (1985) Molecular genetics of resistance to macrolides, lincosamides and streptogramin B (MLS) in streptococci. *J. Antimicrob. Chemother., 16, Suppl A,* 111.

52. Murphy E, Lofdahl S (1984) Transposition of Tn554 does not generate a target duplication. *Nature (London), 307,* 217.

53. Tally FP, Biieluch VM, Cuchural GJ, Malamy MH (1984) Antibacterial resistance in bacteroides. *Drugs Exp. Clin. Res., 10,* 149.

54. Tally FP, Cuchural GJ, Malamy MH (1984) Mechanisms of resistance and resistance transfer in anaerobic bacteria: factors influencing antimicrobial therapy. *Rev. Infect. Dis., 6, Suppl,* 260.

55. Smith CJ, Macrina FL (1984) Large transmissible clindamycin resistance plasmid in *Bacteroides ovatus. J. Bacteriol., 158,* 739.

56. Banai M, LeBlanc DJ (1984) *Streptococcus faecalis* R plasmid pJH1 contains an erythromycin resistance transposon (Tn3871) similar to transposon Tn917. *J. Bacteriol., 158,* 1172.

57. Murphy E (1985) Nucleotide sequence of *ermA,* a macrolide-lincosamide-streptogramin B determinant in *Staphylococcus aureus. J. Bacteriol., 162,* 633.

58. Weisblum B (1985) Inducible resistance to macrolides, lincosamides and streptogramin type B antibiotics: the resistance phenotype, its biological diversity and structural elements that regulate expression – a review. *J. Antimicrob. Chemother., 16, Suppl A*, 63.

59. Barthélémy P, Autissier D, Gerbaud G, Courvalin P (1984) Enzymic hydrolysis of erythromycin by a strain of *Escherichia coli*. *J. Antibiot., 37*, 1692.

60. Ounissi H, Courvalin P (1985) Nucleotide sequence of the gene *ereA* encoding the erythromycin esterase in *Escherichia coli. Gene, 35*, 271.

61. Duthu GS (1984) Assay of erythromycin from human serum by high performance liquid chromatography with electrochemical detection. *J. Liquid Chromatogr., 7*, 1023.

62. Chen ML, Chiou WL (1983) Analysis of erythromycin in biological fluids by high performance liquid chromatography with electrochemical detection. *J. Chromatogr., 278*, 91.

63. Ducci M, Scalori V (1984) A rapid and sensitive high-pressure liquid chromatographic method for monitoring josamycin levels in plasma. *Int. J. Clin. Pharmacol. Res., 4*, 195.

64. Dabrowska D, Regosz A, Tamkun L, Kaminska E (1984) Methods of determination of erythromycin. II. Studies on the complex formation between erythromycin and bromcresol purple and its application to the determination of erythromycin in pharmaceutical preparations. *Sci. Pharm., 52*, 220.

65. Martin JR, Johnson P, Miller MF (1985) Uptake, accumulation, and egress of erythromycin by tissue culture cells of human origin. *Antimicrob. Agents Chemother., 27*, 314.

66. Pike VW, Polmer AJ, Horlock PL et al (1984) Semi-automated preparation of a ^{11}C-labelled antibiotic (*N*-methyl ^{11}C) erythromycin A lactobionate. *Int. J. Appl. Radiat. Isotopes, 35*, 103.

67. Piccolo J, Sakr A (1984) Influence of crystalline state and particle size on the dissolution rate of erythromycin estolate. *Pharm. Ind., 46*, 1277.

68. Osono T, Umezawa H (1985) Pharmacokinetics of macrolides, lincosamides and streptogramins *J. Antimicrob. Chemother., 16, Suppl A*, 151.

69. Nicoletti P, Novelli A, Mazzei T et al (1983) Clinical pharmacokinetic and antimicrobial evaluation of josamycin in comparison with other macrolide antibiotics. In: Spitzy KH, Karrer K (Eds), *Proceedings, 13th International Congress of Chemotherapy, Vienna, 1983, Part 36*, p 29. Egermann, Vienna.

70. Fournier JP, Loiseau P (1981) Les macrolides antibiotiques. *Actual. Pharm., 176*, 50.

71. Iliopoulou A, Downey K, Chaput de Saintonge DM, Turner P (1982) Should erythromycin dose be altered in haemodialysis patients? *Eur. J. Clin. Pharmacol., 23*, 435.

72. Barre J, Houin G, Rosenbaum J et al (1984) Decreased alpha 1-acid glycoprotein in liver cirrhosis: consequences for drug protein binding. *Br. J. Clin. Pharmacol., 18*, 652.

73. Fourtillan JB, Lefèbvre MA, Ghanassia JP (1983) Pharmacokinetic handling of josamycin and its metabolites during oral repeated dosings in man. In: Spitzy KH, Karrer K (Eds), *Proceedings, 13th International Congress of Chemotherapy, Vienna, 1983, Part 36*, p 11. Egermann, Vienna.

74. Walstad RA, Hellum KB (1984) Penetration of erythromycin in respiratory tract infections. *Acta Oto-Laryngol., 98, Suppl*, 50.

75. Brzezinska H, Brozik H, Mikucki J et al (1984) Concentrations of cloxacillin and erythromycin in the tonsils of children after administration of therapeutic doses. *Int. J. Pediatr. Otorhinolaryngol., 7*, 51.

76. Gibson DH, Fitzgeorge RB (1983) Persistence in serum and lungs of guinea pigs of erythromycin, gentamicin, chloramphenicol and rifamicin and their in-vitro activities against *Legionella pneumophila. J. Antimicrob. Chemother., 12,* 235.

77. Wildfeuer A, Lemme JD (1985) Zur Pharmakokinetik von Josamycin. *Arzneim.-Forsch./Drug Res., 35,* 639.

78. Wildfeuer A, Seibold H, Lemme JD (1985) Antimikrobielle Aktivität von Josamycin im Respirationstrakt. *Fortschr. Med., 103,* 155.

79. Miller MF, Martin JR, Levy NL (1984) Intracellular killing of *Legionella* by erythromycin. *Lancet, 1,* 348.

80. Miller MF, Martin JR, Johnson P et al (1984) Erythromycin uptake and accumulation by human polymorphonuclear leukocytes and efficacy of erythromycin in killing ingested *Legionella pneumophila. J. Infect. Dis., 149,* 714.

81. Laufen H, Wildfeuer W, Räder K (1985) Uptake of antimicrobial agents by human polymorphonuclear leukocytes. *Arzneim.-Forsch./Drug Res., 35,* 1097.

82. Pocidalo JJ, Albert F, Desnottes JF, Kernbaum S (1985) Intraphagocytic penetration of macrolides: in-vivo comparison of erythromycin and spiramycin. *J. Antimicrob. Chemother., 16, Suppl A,* 167.

83. Anderson R, Fernandes AC, Eftychis HE (1984) Studies on the effects of ingestion of a single 500 mg oral dose of erythromycin stearate on leucocyte motility and transformation and on release in vitro of prostaglandin Esub2 by stimulated leucocytes. *J. Antimicrob. Chemother., 14,* 41.

84. Hand WL, Corwin RW, Steinberg TH, Grossman GD (1984) Uptake of antibiotics by human alveolar macrophages. *Am. Rev. Resp. Dis., 129,* 933.

85. Prokesch RC, Hand WL (1982) Antibiotic entry into human polymorphonuclear leukocytes. *Antimicrob. Agents Chemother., 21,* 373.

86. Vosbeck K, James PR, Zimmermann W (1984) Antibiotic action on phagocytosed bacteria measured by a new method for determining viable bacteria. *Antimicrob. Agents Chemother., 25,* 735.

87. Ginsburg CM, McCracken GH, Crow SD et al (1984) Erythromycin therapy for group A streptococci pharyngitis: results of a comparative study of the estolate and ethylsuccinate formulations. *Am. J. Dis. Child., 138,* 536.

88. Putzi R, Blaser J, Luthy R et al (1983) Side-effects due to the intravenous infusion of erythromycin lactobionate. *Infection, 11,* 161.

89. Itoh Z, Suzuki T, Nakaya M, Inoue M, Mitsuhashi S (1984) Gastrointestinal motor-stimulating activity of macrolide antibiotics and analysis of their side effects on the canine gut. *Antimicrob. Agents Chemother., 26,* 863.

90. Itoh Z, Suzuki T, Nakaya M et al (1985) Structure-activity relation among macrolide antibiotics in initiation of interdigestive migrating contractions in the canine gastrointestinal tract. *Am. J. Physiol., 11,* G320.

91. Zara GP, Thompson HH, Pilot MA, Ritchie HD (1985) Effects of erythromycin on gastrointestinal tract motility. *J. Antimicrob. Chemother., 16, Suppl A,* 175.

92. Inman WHW, Rawson NSB (1983) Erythromycin estolate and jaundice. *Br. Med. J., 286,* 1954.

93. Funck-Brentano C, Pessayre D, Benhamou JP (1983) Hépatites dues à divers dérivés de l'erythromycine. *Gastroentérol. Clin. Biol., 7,* 362.

94. Diehl AM, Latham P, Boitnott JK et al (1984) Cholestatic hepatitis from erythromycin ethylsuccinate: report of two cases. *Am. J. Med., 76,* 931.

95. Richelmio P, Baldi C, Manzo L et al (1984) Erythromycin estolate impairs the mito-

chondrial and microsomal calcium homeostasis: correlation with hepatotoxicity. *Arch. Toxicol., Suppl 7*, 298.

96. Snavely SR, Hodges GR (1984) The neurotoxicity of antibacterial agents. *Ann. Intern. Med., 101*, 92.

97. Hugues FC, Laccourreye A, Lasserre MH, Toupet M (1984) Recherche d'une toxicité cochléaire chez le malade âgé. *Thérapie, 39*, 591.

98. Massa T, Davis GJ, Schiavo D et al (1984) Tapetal changes in beagle dogs. II. Ocular changes after intravenous administration of a macrolide antibiotic: rosaramycin. *Toxicol. Appl. Pharmacol., 72*, 195.

99. Pessayre D, Larrey D, Funck-Brentano C, Benhamou JP (1985) Drug interactions and hepatitis produced by some macrolide antibiotics. *J. Antimicrob. Chemother., 16, Suppl A*, 181.

100. Lavarenne J, Dumas R, Maradeix B, Fialp J (1984) Hépatitis en cours de l'antibiothérapie. *Thérapie, 39*, 517.

101. Adams SJ, Cunliffe WJ, Cooke EM (1985) Long-term antibiotic therapy for acne vulgaris: effects on the bowel flora of patients and their relatives. *J. Invest. Dermatol., 85*, 35.

102. Haydon RC, Thelin JW, Davis WE (1984) Erythromycin ototoxicity: analysis and conclusions based on 22 case reports. *Otolaryngol. Head Neck Surg., 92*, 678.

103. McCombe JM, Campbell NPS, Cleland J (1984) Recurrent ventricular tachycardia associated with QT prolongation after erythromycin. *Am. J. Cardiol., 54*, 922.

104. Nord CE, Kagar L, Heimdahl A (1984) Impact of antimicrobial agents on the gastrointestinal microflora and the risk of infections. *Am. J. Med., 76(5a)*, 99.

105. Heimdahl A, Nord CE, Borthen L (1984) Impact of phenoxymethylpenicillin, erythromycin, clindamycin and doxycyclin on *Streptococcus salivarius* in the oropharynx. *J. Antimicrob. Chemother., 13*, 505.

106. Ludden TM (1985) Pharmacokinetic interactions of the macrolide antibiotics. *Clin. Pharmacokinet., 10*, 63.

107. Baldit C, Albin H (1985) Interactions médicamenteuses avec les macrolides. *Méd. Mal. Infect., No. Spéc.*, 41.

108. Descotes J, André P, Evreux JC (1985) Pharmacokinetic drug interactions with macrolide antibiotics. *J. Antimicrob. Chemother., 15*, 659.

109. Larrey D, Tinel M, Pessayre D (1983) Formation of inactive cytochrome P-450 Fe(II)-metabolite complexes with several erythromycin derivatives but not with josamycin and midecamycin in rats. *Biochem. Pharmacol., 39*, 1487.

110. Wrighton SA, Schuetz EG, Watkins PB et al (1985) Demonstration in multiple species of inducible hepatic cytochromes P-450 and their mRNAs related to the glucocorticoid-inducible cytochrome P-450 of the rat. *Mol. Pharmacol., 28*, 312.

111. Bartolucci L, Gradoli C, Vincenzi V et al (1984) Macrolide antibiotics and serum theophylline levels in relation to the severity of respiratory impairment: a comparison between the effects of erythromycin and josamycin. *Chemiotherapia, 3*, 286.

112. Pessayre D (1983) Effects of macrolide antibiotics on drug metabolism in rats and humans. *Int. J. Clin. Pharmacol. Res., 3*, 449.

113. Reisz G, Pingleton SK, Melethil S, Ryan PB (1983) The effect of erythromycin on theophylline pharmacokinetics in chronic bronchitis. *Am. Rev. Resp. Dis., 127*, 581.

114. LaForce CF, Szefler SJ, Miller MF et al (1983) Inhibition of methylprednisolone elimination in the presence of erythromycin therapy. *J. Allergy Clin. Immunol., 72*, 34.

115. Hildebrandt R, Gundert-Rémy U, Moeller H, Weber E (1984) Lack of clinically im-

portant interaction between erythromycin and theophylline. *Eur. J. Clin. Pharmacol., 26*, 485.

116. Wong YY, Lundden TD, Bell RD (1983) Effect of erythromycin on carbamazepine kinetics. *Clin. Pharmacol. Ther., 33*, 460.

117. Bachmann K, Schwarz JI, Forney Jr R et al (1984) The effect of erythromycin on the disposition kinetics of warfarin. *Pharmacology, 28*, 171.

118. Schwartz JI, Bachmann K (1984) Erythromycin – warfarin interaction. *Arch. Intern. Med., 144*, 2094.

119. Sato RI, Gray DR, Brown SE (1984) Warfarin interactions with erythromycin. *Arch. Intern. Med., 144*, 2413.

120. Lam C, Basalka E (1985) Effect of subinhibitory concentrations of josamycin on the expression of M protein by group A streptococci. *Eur. J. Clin. Microbiol., 4*, 279.

121. Van Buchem FL, Peeters MF, Van 't Hof MA (1985) Acute otitis media: a new treatment strategy. *Br. Med. J., 290*, 1033.

122. Ernstson S, Sundberg L (1984) Erythromycin in the treatment of otitis media with effusion (OME). *J. Laryngol. Otol., 98*, 767.

123. Sabato AR, Martin AJ, Marmion BP et al (1984) *Mycoplasma pneumoniae*; acute illness, antibiotics, and subsequent pulmonary infection. *Arch. Dis. Child., 19*, 1034.

124. Shanson DC, McNabb WR, Williams TDM, Lant AF (1984) Erythromycin compared with a combination of ampicillin plus floxacillin for the treatment of community acquired pneumonia in adults. *J. Antimicrob. Chemother., 14*, 75.

125. Meyer RD (1983) *Legionella* infections: a review of five years of research. *Rev. Infect. Dis., 5*, 258.

126. Rudin JE, Evans TL, Wing EJ (1984) Failure of erythromycin in treatment of *Legionella micdadei* pneumonia. *Am. J. Med., 76*, 318.

127. Shanson DC, Akash S, Harris M, Tadayon M (1985) Erythromycin stearate, 1.5 g, for the oral prophylaxis of streptococcal bacteremia in patients undergoing dental extraction: efficacy and tolerance. *J. Antimicrob. Chemother., 15*, 83.

128. Josefsson K, Heimdahl A, Von Konow L, Nord CE (1985) Effect of phenoxymethyl-penicillin and erythromycin prophylaxis on anaerobic bacteraemia after oral surgery. *J. Antimicrob. Chemother., 26*, 243.

129. Harrison GAJ, Stross WP, Rubin MP et al (1985) Resistance in oral streptococci after repeated three-dose erythromycin prophylaxis. *J. Antimicrob. Chemother., 15*, 471.

130. Boakes AJ, Loo PSL, Ridgway GL et al (1984) Treatment of uncomplicated gonorrhoea in women with a combination of rifampicin and erythromycin. *Br. J. Ven. Dis., 60*, 309.

131. Schachter J, Sweet RL, Grossman M et al (1986) Experience with the routine use of erythromycin for chlamydial infections in pregnancy. *N. Engl. J. Med., 314*, 276.

132. Oriel JD (1984) Ophthalmia neonatorum: relative efficacy of current prophylactic practices and treatment. *J. Antimicrob. Chemother., 14*, 209.

133. Madsen PO, Jensen KME, Iversen P (1983) Chronic bacterial prostatitis: theoretical and experimental considerations. *Urol. Res., 11*, 1.

134. Kramer BSD, Carr DJ, Rand KH et al (1984) Prophylaxis of fever and infection in adult cancer patients: a placebo-controlled trial of oral trimethoprim-sulfamethoxazole plus erythromycin. *Cancer, 53*, 329.

135. Pai CH, Gilles F, Tuomanen E, Marks MI (1983) Erythromycin in treatment of *Campylobacter* enteritis in children. *Am. J. Dis. Child., 137*, 286.

136. Mandal BK, Ellis ME, Dunbar EM, Whale K (1984) Double-blind placebo-controlled

trial of erythromycin in the treatment of clinical *Campylobacter* infection. *J. Antimicrob. Chemother., 13*, 619.

137. Burridge R, Warren C, Phillips I (1986) Macrolide, lincosamide and streptogramin resistance in *Campylobacter jejuni/coli. J. Antimicrob. Chemother., 17*, 315.

138. Portnoy D, Whiteside ME, Buckley III E, MacLeod CL (1984) Treatment of intestinal cryptosporidiosis with spiramycin. *Ann. Intern. Med., 101*, 202.

139. Roue R, Ghanassia JP, d'Enfert J, Modai J (1985) Utilisation de la josamycine dans la prévention de la diarrhée des voyageurs. *Med. Mal. Infect., No. Spéc.*, 84.

140. Terragna A, Canessa A, Terragna FM (1985) Effect of josamycin on experimental toxoplasmosis in mice. *IRCS Med Sci., 13*, 310.

141. Hanley SP, Gumb J, MacFarlane JT (1985) Comparison of erythromycin and isoniazid in treatment of adverse reactions to BCG vaccination. *Br. Med. J., 290*, 970.

142. Schreiner A, Digranes A (1984) Absorption of erythromycin stearate and enteric-coated erythromycin base after a single oral dose immediately before breakfast. *Infection 12*, 345.

143. Tjandramaga TB, Van Hecken A, Mullie A et al (1984) Relative bioavailability of enteric coated pellets, stearate and ethylsuccinate formulations of erythromycin. *Pharmacology, 29*, 305.

144. Fernandes AC, Anderson R, Theron AJ et al (1984) Enhancement of human polymorphonuclear leukocyte motility by erythromycin in vitro and in vivo. *S. Afr. Med. J., 66*, 173.

CHAPTER 11

Metronidazole

DALE N. GERDING

Studies of metronidazole, an older antimicrobial agent, continue to focus on the area of clinical applications of this unique compound, particularly in colon surgery prophylaxis and a variety of gynecologic infections. Metronidazole alone has been shown to be inferior to moxalactam alone and to a combination of metronidazole plus cefuroxime in colon surgery prophylaxis (1, 2). The addition of oral neomycin to intravenous metronidazole resulted in comparable infection rates as with moxalactam alone (3). The long-standing standard regimen of oral neomycin plus oral erythromycin was found inferior to a combination of intravenous metronidazole plus ceftriaxone in still another study of prophylaxis in colon-rectal surgery (4). Use of mechanical (mannitol) bowel cleansing alone or with intravenous metronidazole, oral neomycin, or all 8 showed a statistically significantly lower postoperative infection rate for the use of all 3 modalities (5).

Continued studies of metronidazole in gynecologic infections show that bacterial vaginosis can be effectively treated with either oral or vaginal metronidazole, and that single dose (2 g) oral therapy is as effective as 400 mg twice a day for 5 days (6, 7). Inhibition of adhesion of *Gardnerella vaginalis* to vaginal epithelium may be the mechanism of successful metronidazole therapy in bacterial vaginosis (8). In the treatment of pelvic inflammatory disease various combinations of metronidazole combined with penicillin, mezlocillin and ampicillin have shown variable rates of success, largely dependent upon the number of failures due to *Chlamydia trachomatis* (9–11). Resistant *Trichomonas vaginalis* has been successfully treated with the use of higher doses of metronidazole (12).

Metronidazole [1(2-hydroxyethyl)-2-methyl-5-nitroimidazole] was marketed in 1960 as the first systemic antitrichomonal agent after syntheses in the Rhone-Poulenc Laboratories in France in 1956 following systematic screening of some 150 nitroheterocyclic compounds for in vivo and in vitro activity.

Antimicrobial Agents Annual 3
P.K. Peterson and J. Verhoef, editors
© Elsevier Science Publishers BV, 1988

ACTIVITY

In addition to activity against *Trichomonas vaginalis*, metronidazole is also active against the protozoans *Giardia lamblia, Entamoeba histolytica,* and *Balantidium coli*, but not *Pneumocystis carinii*. For obligate anaerobic bacterial organisms, in particular, *Bacteroides fragilis* and *Clostridium perfringens*, the compound is bactericidal and susceptibility to metronidazole in Canada and France among 590 and 165 obligate anaerobic clinical isolates, respectively, showed only one resistant organism among *Bacteroides* and *Clostridium* species (13, 14). About 15% of peptococci and peptostreptococci were resistant as were 100% of *Propionibacterium acnes*, a common skin organism with very low pathogenicity (14). One recent anecdotal report described a single *B. fragilis* isolate resistant to metronidazole (and imipenem), an extremely rare occurrence, but one which bears watching (15). One report suggests that metronidazole susceptibility is correlated with the presence of the enzyme pyruvate: ferredoxin oxidoreductase which is found in all susceptible obligate anaerobes, but not in facultative anaerobes, *P. acnes*, and *Actinomyces israelii* which are resistant to metronidazole (16). Metronidazole is comparable in vitro to newer combinations of ticarcillin or amoxicillin and clavulanic acid against *B. fragilis* group organisms (17).

   T. vaginalis organisms resistant to metronidazole remain rare; however, data on clinical metronidazole treatment of patients with resistant *T. vaginalis* infection have been assembled for 31 cases from the United States and Canada. These data indicate that 27 of 31 cases were cured by increasing the metronidazole dosage from 2.1 g/d for 8 days (highest average failure dose), to 2.6 g/d for 9 days (12). As in bacterial organisms, ferredoxin-mediated reduction of metronidazole nitrogroups is proposed to be the mechanism of the trichomonacidal activity (18).

CLINICAL PHARMACOLOGY

Serum half-life of metronidazole ranges from 6.1 to 7.1 hours after intravenous, oral or rectal suppository administration and is unchanged to slightly prolonged in the presence of renal insufficiency (19, 20). About 25% of metronidazole and its metabolites are removed from serum by hemodialysis; however, supplemental dosing following dialysis is recommended only in seriously ill patients due to the normally high therapeutic ratio (21).

   Metronidazole is metabolized by the liver and secreted into bile, but several recent studies failed to detect metronidazole in the stool samples of patients without diarrhea (22, 23). In patients with *Clostridium difficile* diarrhea, metronidazole and hydroxymetronidazole were detected in diarrhea stool samples in therapeutic concentrations following both oral and intravenous metronidazole, but were undetectable once diarrhea had subsided. These observations suggest that intravenous metronidazole may be an effective means of administration for patients with *C. difficile* diarrhea or colitis who are unable to take oral medications.

139

Wide variability in the concentration of metronidazole in vaginal fluid may account for variation in the successful therapy of vaginitis (24).

ADVERSE EFFECTS AND DRUG INTERACTIONS

Gastrointestinal symptoms (nausea, vomiting, metallic taste, anorexia and diarrhea) are the most common (5–10%) side effect of metronidazole, but central nervous system (CNS) toxicity is the most serious adverse reaction. CNS symptoms include peripheral neuropathy, ataxia, vertigo, headaches, confusion and convulsions. Symptoms usually occur with high dosage, prolonged administration, or concomitant hepatic failure leading to drug accumulation (25, 26). The occurrence of an antabuse effect in approximately 10% of patients who take metronidazole and consume ethanol has been re-emphasized (27). Concerns remain over the safety of long-term administration, both because of neurologic sequelae (sensory neuropathy) and animal evidence of carcinogenicity.

CLINICAL USES

Progress continues in the use of metronidazole for wound infection prophylaxis in colon and rectal surgery. The need for agents active against both anaerobic and facultatively aerobic bacteria has been re-emphasized and traditional oral agent prophylactic regimens have been challenged. Intravenous metronidazole and ceftriaxone were superior to oral neomycin and erythromycin (3/31 *vs* 12/29 infections, P < 0.01) (4). Metronidazole (500 mg i.v.) was inferior to moxalactam (2 g i.v.) (26.3% *vs* 11.1% infection rates) leading to cessation of the study because of the high infection rate with metronidazole alone (1). However, another trial showed that oral neomycin plus metronidazole i.v. was as effective as moxalactam i.v. (3). In a somewhat different protocol, cefuroxime (1.5 g i.v. q 8 h × 2 d) was added postoperatively to preoperative metronidazole prophylaxis on the basis of semiquantitative aerobic cultures of peritoneal fluid during surgery. Infection rates were reduced from 41.2% in patients with > 5 colony-forming units per ml of bacteria, to 8.3% (P < 0.003) by the addition of cefuroxime (2). In a small study, the use of mechanical (hypertonic solution) bowel cleansing combined with oral neomycin, metronidazole, or both, revealed that infection rates of 40 to 46% with the first 3 regimens were reduced to 6% (P < 0.05) with the use of all 3 modalities together (5). Similarly, the benefit of 10% mannitol mechanical bowel preparation plus oral neomycin was enhanced significantly by the addition of intravenous metronidazole (8/37 *vs* 0/31 infections, P < 0.02) (28).

In gynecologic infections there is increased evidence that 2 g metronidazole single-dose is as effective as 400 mg twice daily for 5 days when treating bacterial (*Gardnerella*) vaginosis (89% *vs* 90% cure rate), although recurrence (relapse or reinfection?) may be higher with the single-dose regimen (7). Acceptability, lack of side effects and compliance all make single-dose treatment preferable, especially since treatment of *T. vaginalis*, a frequent accompanying organism, is also effective with the single-dose regimen. Vaginal suppositories (500 mg/d) are as effective as oral therapy for bacterial vaginosis (6). Adherence of *G. vaginalis* to vaginal epithelial cells is inhibited by subinhibitory concentrations of metronidazole, a possible explanation for the clinical efficacy of metronidazole in *Gardnerella* vaginosis (8).

Treatment of pelvic inflammatory disease (PID) remains difficult due to the multiple potential pathogens including *Chlamydia trachomatis, Neisseria gonorrhoeae*, obligate anaerobic bacteria, gram-negative aerobic bacilli, staphylococci and streptococci. A comparative trial of penicillin plus metronidazole and doxycycline plus metronidazole revealed a significantly better response rate for the latter regimen (81% *vs* 47%, P < 0.04) (9). Failure rates for chlamydial infections were particularly high. In another PID study, sulbactam + ampicillin cured 19/20 patients compared to 16/19 cured with metronidazole + gentamicin (11). Failures were associated with isolation of *C. trachomatis*. The combination mezlocillin + metronidazole was found to be effective in 62/63 PID patients treated in a noncomparative trial in which *C. trachomatis* was not isolated (10).

Efficacy of metronidazole for the treatment of *Clostridium difficile* toxin-associated colitis has been confirmed to be as efficacious as vancomycin in a retrospective study (29). Metronidazole may be effective for pseudomembranous colitis when administered by the intravenous route, although more data are needed (22). Use of metronidazole treatment of *C. difficile* toxin-positive patients failed to eradicate an endemic problem on the hospital ward of a long-term care facility (30). Failure may have been due to the lack of detectable metronidazole in the stool of patients who did not have diarrhea (22).

DOSING

Oral usage of metronidazole predominates due to its excellent bioavailability and lower cost of administration. Bioavailability is about 80–84% for oral administration compared to only about 50% for rectal suppositories for which peak blood levels are much more variable. Usual daily dose ranges from 750 mg to 3 g depending upon the disease being treated.

FUTURE DIRECTIONS

Use of metronidazole is likely to continue to expand as an antibacterial agent for anaerobic infection. Further controlled studies of the use of this agent in combination with antiaerobic antibiotics for the treatment as well as prophylaxis of abdominal infection are still needed to evaluate efficacy and toxicity, particularly the frequency of *Clostridium difficile* diarrhea as a complication of therapy. Substitu-

tion of metronidazole for clindamycin has been shown to be economically beneficial in hospitals (31), but care should be taken to insure that adequate therapy
for aerobic organisms is provided in mixed aerobic and anaerobic infections.
Questions regarding neurologic toxicity and possible risk of malignancy with metronidazole use remain to be answered.

REFERENCES

1. Raetzel G, Harnoss B-M, Gortz G et al (1986) Systemic antibiotic prophylaxis with
   metronidazole in elective colon and rectal surgery: results of a controlled clinical study
   and critical literature review. *Arzneim. Forsch./Drug Res., 36,* 976.
2. Claesson BEB, Filipsson S, Holmlund DEW et al (1986) Selective cefuroxime prophylaxis following colorectal surgery based on intraoperative dipslide culture. *Br. J.
   Surg., 73,* 953.
3. Hinchey EJ, Richards GK, Lewis R et al (1987) Moxalactam as single-agent prophylaxis in the prevention of wound infection following colon surgery. *Surgery, 101,* 15.
4. Weaver M, Burdon DW, Youngs DJ, Keighley MRB (1986) Oral neomycin and
   erythromycin compared with single-dose systemic metronidazole and ceftriaxone prophylaxis in elective colorectal surgery. *Am. J. Surg., 151,* 437.
5. Adeyemi SD, Da Rocha-Afodu JT (1986) Clinical studies of 4 methods of bowel preparation in colorectal surgery. *Eur. Surg. Res., 18,* 331.
6. Bistoletti P, Fredricsson B, Hagstrom B, Nord C-E (1986) Comparison of oral and
   vaginal metronidazole therapy for non-specific vaginosis. *Gynecol. Obstet. Invest., 21,*
   144.
7. Mohanty KC, Deighton R (1985) Comparison of two different metronidazole regimens in the treatment of *Gardnerella vaginalis* infection with or without trichomoniasis. *J. Antimicrob. Chemother., 16,* 799.
8. Peeters M, Piot P (1985) Adhesion of *Gardnerella vaginalis* to vaginal epithelial cells:
   variables affecting adhesion and inhibition by metronidazole. *Genitourin. Med., 61,*
   391.
9. Heinonen PK, Teisala K, Punnonen R (1986) Treating pelvic inflammatory disease
   with doxycycline and metronidazole or penicillin and metronidazole. *Genitourin Med.,
   62,* 235.
10. Mendling W, Krasemann C (1986) Bacterial findings and therapeutic consequences
    in adnexitis. *Geburtshilfe Framenheilkd., 46,* 462.
11. Crombleholme W, Landers D, Ohm-Smith M (1986) Sulbactam/ampicillin versus me-
    tronidazole/gentamicin in the treatment of severe pelvic infections. *Drugs, 31, Suppl
    2,* 11.
12. Lossick JG, Muller M, Gorell TE (1986) In vitro drug susceptibility and doses of me-
    tronidazole required for cure in cases of trichomoniasis. *J. Infect. Dis., 153,* 948.
13. Derriennic M, Reynaud A, Launay C, Courtieu AL (1986) The in vitro activity of
    piperacillin, amoxicillin, cefoxitin, and metronidazole against obligate anaerobic bac-
    teria. *Presse Méd., 15,* 2279.
14. Bourgault A-M, Harding GK, Smith JA et al (1986) Survey of anaerobic susceptibility
    patterns in Canada. *Antimicrob. Agents Chemother., 30,* 798.
15. Lamothe F, Fijalkowski C, Malouin F et al (1986) *Bacteroides fragilis* resistant to
    both metronidazole and imipenem. *J. Antimicrob. Chemother., 18,* 642.

16. Marikawa S (1986) Distribution of metronidazole susceptibility factors in obligate anaerobes. *J. Antimicrob. Chemother., 18,* 565.
17. Bourgault A-M, Lamothe F (1986) In vitro activity of amoxicillin and ticarcillin in combination with clavulanic acid compared with that of new beta-lactam agents against species of the *Bacteroides fragilis* group. *J. Antimicrob. Chemother., 17,* 593.
18. Moreno SNJ, Docampo R (1985) Mechanism of toxicity of nitro compounds used in the chemotherapy of trichomoniasis. *Environ. Health Perspect., 64,* 199.
19. Bergan T, Thorsteinsson SB (1985) Pharmacokinetics of metronidazole and its metabolites in reduced renal function. *Chemotherapy (Basel), 32,* 305.
20. Somogyi AA, Kong CB, Gurr FW et al (1984) Metronidazole pharmacokinetics in patients with acute renal failure. *J. Antimicrob. Chemother., 13,* 183.
21. Lau AH, Chang CW, Sabatini S (1986) Hemodialysis clearance of metronidazole and its metabolites. *Antimicrob. Agents Chemother., 29,* 235.
22. Bolton RP, Culshaw MA (1986) Faecal metronidazole concentrations during oral and intravenous therapy for antibiotic associated colitis due to *Clostridium difficile. Gut, 27,* 1169.
23. Hoverstad T, Carlsted-Duke B, Lingaas E et al (1986) Influence of ampicillin, clindamycin and metronidazole on faecal excretion of short-chain fatty acids in healthy subjects. *Scand. J. Gastroenterol., 21,* 621.
24. Larsen B, Hunter Wilson A, Glover DD, Charles D (1986) Implications of metronidazole pharmacodynamics for therapy of trichomoniasis. *Gynecol. Obstet. Invest., 21,* 12.
25. Halloran TJ (1982) Convulsions associated with high cumulative doses of metronidazole. *Drug Intell. Clin. Pharm., 16,* 409.
26. Alvarez RS, Richardson DA, Bent AE, Ostergard DR (1983) Central nervous system toxicity related to prolonged metronidazole therapy. *Am. J. Obstet. Gynecol., 145,* 640.
27. Alexander I (1985) 'Alcohol-antabuse' syndrome in patients receiving metronidazole during gynaecological treatment. *Br. J. Clin. Pract., 39,* 292.
28. Jagelman DG, Fazio VW, Lavery IC, Weakley FL (1985) A prospective, randomized, double-blind study of 10% mannitol mechanical bowel preparation combined with oral neomycin and short-term, perioperative, intravenous Flagyl as prophylaxis in elective colorectal resections. *Surgery, 98,* 861.
29. Talbot RW, Walker RC, Beart Jr RW (1986) Changing epidemiology, diagnosis, and treatment of *Clostridium difficile* toxin-associated colitis. *Br. J. Surg., 73,* 457.
30. Bender BS, Laughon BE, Gaydos C (1986) Is *Clostridium difficile* endemic in chronic-care facilities? *Lancet, 2,* 11.
31. Greene SA, Record KE, Rapp RP et al (1986) Pharmacy initiatives to reduce clindamycin use. *Am. J. Hosp. Pharm., 43,* 1210.

CHAPTER 12

Nitrofurantoin

KENNETH L. VOSTI

Since publication of *The Antimicrobial Agents Annual 2* nothing of significance has appeared in the literature and the discussion which follows continues to represent a current perspective regarding nitrofurantoin.

Although nitrofurans have been recognized for many years prior to their work, Dodd and Stillman in 1944 were the first to report studies of antimicrobial activity among 42 furan derivatives. Among the various nitrofurans studied, nitrofurantoin has emerged as the most extensively used in human subjects. Its properties, pharmacokinetics, and clinical experience have been detailed extensively in previous reviews (1, 2). The microcrystal (Furadantin) and the macrocrystal (Macrodantin) preparations of nitrofurantoin continue to be popular drugs in the treatment of infections of the urinary tract because of their demonstrated clinical efficacy, low incidence of serious toxicity and the infrequent development of bacterial resistance. The additional clinical utility of these compounds is seen in recent reports of the use of a single dose of nitrofurantoin to treat uncomplicated infections of the urinary tract in women (3) and of a combination of nitrofurantoin and sulfadiazine to treat patients with recurrent infections of the urinary tract (4). Furazolidone, another nitrofuran, has become useful in the treatment of traveller's diarrhea (5). On the other hand, potential problems associated with the use of a nitrofurantoin are underscored in a recent comprehensive review of its toxicity (6).

The adhydrous micro- and macrocrystals of nitrofurantoin are synthetic derivatives of a group of compounds called 'nitrofurans'. Anhydrous nitrofurantoin has a molecular weight of 238.16 and a basic formula of $C_8H_6N_4O_5$. It is prepared as a yellow powder of micro- or macrocrystals and is a weak acid with a pKa of 7.2. It has low solubility in water but is highly soluble in alkaline solutions.

ACTIVITY

The antimicrobial activity of the furan derivatives appears to depend upon the presence of a nitro-group in the 5-position and in many variations of the sidechain

Antimicrobial Agents Annual 3
P.K. Peterson and J. Verhoef, editors
© Elsevier Science Publishers BV, 1988

Furan   Nitrofurantoin

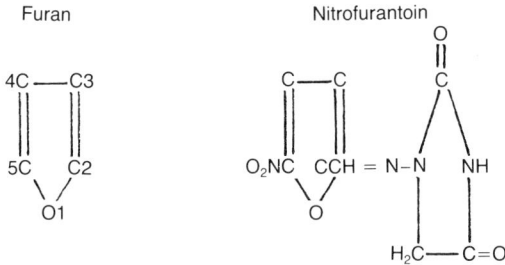

Fig. 1   The structure of furan and its derivative, nitrofurantoin.

at the 2-position (Fig. 1). The mechanism of action of nitrofurantoin still remains to be completely defined; however, it is thought to be related to its ability to inhibit a number of microbial enzymes important to their growth and survival. The antimicrobial spectrum of activity includes many species of both gram-negative and gram-positive bacteria. Generally more than 90% of isolates of *Escherichia coli* and approximately 70% of isolates of *Klebsiella* and *Enterobacter* species are sensitive to nitrofurantoin. Little or no activity is exhibited for isolates of *Proteus* species and *Pseudomonas aeruginosa*. The minimum inhibitory concentrations of sensitive organisms are generally less than 10 μg/ml and the minimum bactericidal concentrations are usually within one or two 2-fold dilutions of the minimum inhibitory concentrations.

The selection of resistant mutants is unusual during treatment with nitrofurantoin. Although resistance is rare among clinical isolates, some concern is raised by the recent in-vitro studies with an isolate of *E. coli* containing an R-plasmid conferring resistance on gentamicin, kanamycin and other antibiotics, including chloramphenicol (7). The induction of a mutant with a high level of resistance to nitrofurantoin resulted in an increased production of 3-*N*-acetyltransferase activity and increased resistance to the two aminoglycosides but not to chloramphenicol. The mechanism of resistance to this compound is not known and does not appear to be transferable by plasmids.

CLINICAL PHARMACOLOGY

Oral doses of nitrofurantoin are rapidly and completely absorbed from the gastrointestinal tract; the macrocrystal form of the drug is absorbed and excreted more slowly than the micro-form. Serum levels in excess of the minimum inhibitory concentrations for most organisms are generally not attained with standard doses; however, average urinary concentrations of approximately 200 μg/ml are readily attained. The blood or plasma elimination half-life ($t^{1}/_{2}$) is approximately 30 minutes. The rate of excretion parallels the creatinine clearance and thus in patients with significant renal failure there may be decreased antimicrobial activity in urine as well as an increased potential for toxicity (8, 9). Although significant renal tubular and interstitial accumulations of nitrofurantoin are found normally, the penetration of nitrofurantoin into other body tissues, including the prostate, is poor.

The excretion of nitrofurantoin is dependent upon glomerular filtration, tubular secretion, and tubular reabsorption. Tubular reabsorption is affected significantly by pH, with alkaline conditions causing a reduced tubular reabsorption and a consequent greater concentration of nitrofurantoin in urine. On the other hand, acid conditions enhance tubular reabsorption of nitrofurantoin and appear to increase kidney tissue levels as reflected by increased renal lymph concentrations. A major portion of the administered dose is probably eliminated by enzymatic degradation since most mammalian tissues are capable of degrading the drug. Although many enzymes have been demonstrated to inactivate nitrofurantoin in vitro, the precise in vivo metabolic pathways for inactivating nitrofurantoin have not been identified.

ADVERSE EFFECTS AND DRUG INTERACTIONS

Adverse effects

Adverse reactions to nitrofurantoins may affect a variety of organ systems (6). The most common forms involve the gastrointestinal tract and consist of nausea, vomiting and sometimes diarrhea; late, serious reactions may involve the lung, liver, and central nervous system and may result in irreversible damage.

Gastrointestinal   Nausea and vomiting are the most common reactions and may be dose-related; they may be prevented by taking the dosage with milk or food and appear to occur less frequently with the macrocrystalline form of the drug (10). Liver function abnormalities include both hepatocellular damage and cholestasis. A rare but serious abnormality is the development of chronic active hepatitis (11). The mechanisms for toxic reactions in the liver are not known, although they are presumed to represent either a hypersensitivity or toxic reaction to nitrofurantoin or one of its metabolic degradation products.

Pulmonary   Acute, subacute and chronic pulmonary reactions may occur. Acute reactions generally are characterized by the abrupt onset of fever, chills, cough, dyspnea and chest pain (12). Pulmonary infiltrates and pleural effusions may occur (12, 13). Peripheral and local eosinophilia may also be found. This reaction characteristically occurs early during the administration of the drug and clears quickly with discontinuance of therapy. The subacute form is more subtle in presentation and therefore symptoms may not be recognized as being drug-related as quickly as with the acute form. Similarly the resolution of signs may be more protracted after the cessation of the drug. The chronic form of the pulmonary reaction is associated with the insidious onset of malaise, dyspnea and cough. Chest films may reveal a diffuse interstitial pneumonitis and/or fibrosis (14, 15). Pulmonary function may be altered and the abnormalities may be permanent. This syndrome is more likely to occur in patients receiving prolonged continuous treatment or prophylaxis with nitrofurantoin. The severity of the reaction, the speed of resolution, and the risk of permanent impairment all appear to be related to the speed of recognition of the existence of a drug reaction and therefore to the need for early discontinuance of the drug.

The mechanism resulting in pulmonary reactions to nitrofurantoin is not certain. The clinical features of the acute reaction suggest a hypersensitivity reaction. Other observations demonstrate that lung cell injury due to nitrofurantoin demonstrate that lung cell injury due to nitrofurantoin is caused by an oxidant mechanism (16). Whether each alone or both in combination explain the various pulmonary reactions remains to be determined.

Skin Reactions are rare and include macropapular, erythematous or eczematous eruptions, pruritus, urticaria, angioedema, exfoliative dermatitis, and erythema multiforme.

Hematological A variety of hematological reactions have been reported and include hemolytic anemia, granulocytopenia, agranulocytosis, leukopenia, thrombocytopenia, eosinophilia, and megaloblastic anemia. These abnormalities are usually reversible following withdrawal of the drug. Rare reports of aplastic anemia exist.

The mechanism by which nitrofurantoin induces hemolysis may be related to its intracellular metabolic effects which result in certain enzyme deficiencies, particularly in reduced glutathione, and in an increased conversion of erythrocytes to echinocytes (17). Since these changes in vitro do not in themselves lead to hemolysis, it is postulated that they result in membrane damage which in turn leads to their increased clearance and destruction by the reticuloendothelial system. How nitrofurantoin induces other hematological abnormalities is even more uncertain.

Central nervous system Nystagmus and vertigo have been noted occasionally and clear on discontinuance of the drug. Of a more serious nature is the occasional occurrence of a polyneuropathy which in its most serious form may be associated with irreversible demyelination and degeneration of peripheral nerves (18). In most cases the symptoms begin within the first 45 days of treatment. The degree of recovery tended to be inversely related to the severity of symptoms.

The mechanism mediating neurotoxicity is not clear, but it has been postulated that it may be due to the accumulation of toxic, metabolic products in patients with concomitant renal insufficiency or to interference with intermediary metabolism in the neuron.

Other reactions   Anaphylaxis and attacks of bronchospasm in patients known to have asthma have been reported rarely. Drug fever, general malaise, and arthralgias have been reported occasionally.

Drug interactions

The effect of food in delaying the absorption of nitrofurantoin has been noted already. Certain of the magnesium salts, but not the aluminum salts, have been shown to decrease the absorption of single doses of nitrofurantoin, presumably as a result of adsorption (19). This may lead to inadequate concentrations of drug in the urine. A single case has been reported suggesting an interaction of drug in the urine. A single case has been reported suggesting an interaction of nitrofurantoin with diphenylhydantoin (20). This reaction resulted in decreased plasma levels of diphenylhydantoin with a subsequent increase in the frequency of seizure activity. The effect was reversed rapidly by the discontinuance of nitrofurantoin. Because of the availability of a number of other effective drugs to treat infections of the urinary tract, the simplest way to avoid such adverse interactions is to use other antimicrobial agents.

CLINICAL USES

Nitrofurantoin has a long and effective history in the treatment of uncomplicated infections of the lower urinary tract. This drug has also been used effectively to prevent infections of the urinary tract. Under these circumstances the drug may be administered as either an a.m. and p.m., single p.m. (21, 22) or single post-intercourse dose (23). As discussed above, such patients should be monitored carefully for the possibility of developing significant adverse reactions. A recent report has suggested the efficacy of a single oral dose of 200 mg of an unspecified nitrofurantoin in treating symptomatic lower urinary tract infections in women (3). A cure rate of 95% with single-dose therapy was comparable to that attained giving 50 mg orally q.i.d. of the same nitrofurantoin for 10 days, but serious adverse reactions were significantly less frequent in patients treated with single-dose therapy. In another study of patients with recurrent infections of the urinary tract, the efficacy of the concurrent administration of nitrofurantoin (100 mg) and sulfadiazine (300 mg), given orally q. 12 hours for 7 days, was assessed. The cure rate achieved was comparable to those attained with some of the newer and more expensive agents. The relatively common occurrence of side-effects (37%), although mild, limits the usefulness of the concurrent administration of these two drugs.

Contraindications

Nitrofurantoin should not be used in patients with known hypersensitivity to the drug. This agent is also contraindicated in patients with serious impairment in renal function (creatinine clearances of less than 40 ml/min). The increased risk of serious toxicity in these patients is discussed above.

The drug should not be used in pregnant patients near or at term, in newborns and neonates under 1 month of age, and in patients known to have a glucose-6-phosphate dehydrogenase deficiency in their red blood cells because of the likelihood of developing a hemolytic anemia.

DOSING

The two available preparations are nitrofurantoin USP (Furadantin) 50 and 100 mg tablets and nitrofurantoin macrocrystals (Macrodantin) 25, 50 and 100 mg capsules. A Furadantin suspension, containing 25 mg/5 ml, is available for pediatric usage.

All forms of the drug are administered orally. In adults, conventional therapy has consisted of the administration of 50–100 mg q.i.d. of either Furadantin or Macrodantin for 5–10 days. A recent study has suggested that a comparable cure rate with less toxicity may be attained with a single dosage of 200 mg. The long-term administration of these agents generally consist of 50–100 mg b.i.d. or a single dose p.m. or post-intercourse.

Suggested dosage for children is 5–7 mg/kg of body weight in 4 equally divided doses every 24 hours. A longer duration of therapy may be required for children than for adults. No experience with single-dose therapy in children has yet been reported.

FUTURE DIRECTIONS

Primary objectives for future developments include better definition of the mechanism of action and the metabolic pathways of degradation of nitrofurantoin. Similarly, a better understanding of the mechanisms involved in adverse reactions would be welcome, particularly if they would allow the identification of at-risk populations of patients. The usefulness of other nitrofurans (e.g. furazolidone) in the prevention and treatment of traveller's diarrhea should be investigated further.

REFERENCES

1. Introduction to the nitrofurans. In: *The Nitrofurans*, p 1. Eaton Laboratories, Norwich, 1958.
2. Conklin JD (1978) The pharmacokinetics of nitrofurantoin and its related bioavailability. *Antibiot. Chemother., 25*, 233.
3. Gossius G (1984) Single-dose nitrofurantoin therapy for urinary tract infections in women. *Curr. Ther. Res., 35*, 925.

4. Brumfitt W, Hamilton-Miller JMT (1984) Treatment of recurrent urinary infections with a combination of nitrofurantoin and sulfadiazine. *Chemotherapy, 30*, 270.

5. Dupont HL, Ericsson CD, Galendo E et al (1984) Furazolidone versus ampicillin in the treatment of traveller's diarrhea. *Antimicr. Agents Chemother., 26*, 160.

6. D'Arcy PF (1985) Nitrofurantoin. *Drug Intel. Clin. Pharm., 18*, 540.

7. Breeze AS, Obaseiki-Ebor EE (1984) The enhancement of R-plasmid mediated resistance to aminoglycoside antibiotics by mutations to nitrofurantoin resistance in *Escherichia coli. J. Antimicrob. Chemother., 14*, 477.

8. Sachs J, Taggart G, Noel P, Kunin CM (1968) Effect of renal function on urinary recovery of orally administered nitrofurantoin. *N. Engl. J. Med., 278*, 1032.

9. Felts J, Hayes DM, Gergen JA, Toole JF (1971) Neural, hematologic and bacteriologic effects of nitrofurantoin in renal insufficiency. *N. Engl. J. Med., 51*, 331.

10. Kalowski S, Radford N, Kincaid-Smith P (1974) Crystalline and macrocrystalline nitrofurantoin in the treatment of urinary tract infections. *N. Engl. J. Med., 290*, 385.

11. Tolman KG (1980) Nitrofurantoin and chronic active hepatitis. *Ann. Intern. Med., 92*, 119.

12. Murray MJ, Kronenberg R (1965) Pulmonary reactions simulating cardiac pulmonary edema caused by nitrofurantoin. *N. Engl. J. Med., 273*, 1185.

13. Hailey FJ, Glascock HW, Hewitt WF (1969) Pleuropneumonic reactions to nitrofurantoin. *N. Engl. J. Med., 281*, 1087.

14. Rosenow EC, DeRemee RA, Dines DE (1968) Chronic nitrofurantoin pulmonary reaction. *N. Engl. J. Med., 279*, 1258.

15. Bone RC, Wolfe J, Sobonya RE et al (1976) Desquamative interstitial pneumonia following long term nitrofurantoin therapy. *Am. J. Med., 60*, 697.

16. Martin WJ (1983) Nitrofurantoin: evidence for the oxidant injury of lung parenchymal cells. *Ann. Rev. Resp. Dis., 127*, 482.

17. Dershwitz M, Ts'ao C-H, Novaak RF (1985) Metabolic and morphologic effects of the antimicrobial agent nitrofurantoin on human erythrocytes in vitro. *Biochem. Pharmacol., 34*, 1963.

18. Toole JF, Parish ML (1973) Nitrofurantoin polyneuropathy. *Neurology, 23*, 554.

19. Naggar VF, Khalil SA (1979) Effect of magnesium trisilicate on nitrofurantoin absorption. *Clin. Pharmacol. Ther., 25*, 857.

20. Heipertz R, Pilz H (1978) Interaction of nitrofurantoin with diphenylhydantoin. *J. Neurol., 218*, 297.

21. Lohr JA, Nunley DH, Howards SS, Ford RF (1977) Prevention of recurrent urinary tract infections in girls. *Pediatrics, 59*, 562.

22. Stamey TA, Condy M, Mihara G (1977) Prophylactic efficacy of nitrofurantoin macrocrystals and trimethoprim-sulfamethoxazole in urinary infections. *N. Engl. J. Med., 296*, 780.

23. Vosti KL (1975) Recurrent urinary tract infections: prevention by prophylactic antibiotics after sexual intercourse. *J. Am. Med. Assoc., 231*, 934.

CHAPTER 13

Imipenem/cilastatin

S. RAGNAR NORRBY

This review will concentrate on new information gathered during the past year when the fixed 1:1 combination of the two drugs was introduced for clinical use in several countries, including the United States. For older information the reader is referred to *Annuals 1 and 2* (1, 2).

ACTIVITY

Aminopenicillins, cephalosporins and monobactams exert their antibacterial effect on gram-negative bacteria by binding to penicillin-binding proteins (PBPs) 1 and 3. Aminopenicillins (mecillinam) bind only to PBP-2 which results in the formation of large spheroplasts which lyse at antibiotic concentrations which are considerably higher than the minimal inhibitory concentrations. Imipenem, on the other hand, binds with highest affinity to PBP-2 and then to PBP-1. This leads to the formation of spheroplasts which rapidly lyse and bactericidal concentrations are similar to inhibitory concentrations. Contrary to β-lactams which bind to PBP-3, no filaments are formed.

These differences in mode of action between imipenem and other β-lactams may explain the observation that imipenem, contrary to penicillins and cephalosporins, has a post-antibiotic effect (PAE) when used against gram-negative bacteria. This means that when a bacterial culture is exposed to imipenem, which is then removed, growth will not resume until after a lag-period (3–5). Baquero et al (5) showed that imipenem exposure resulted in a considerable PAE when tested against *Escherichia coli, Enterobacter cloacae, Pseudomonas aeruginosa, Acinetobacter calcoaceticus, Staphylococcus aureus*, and *Streptococcus faecalis* (Table 1). A possible explanation for these findings may be that when a culture of gram-negative bacteria is exposed to penicillins or cephalosporins, which are then removed, large numbers of cells will be formed from each filament. With imipenem, on the other hand, each bacterial cell is a single entity. In agreement with this, the PAE of gentamicin (an antibiotic which also does not induce filament formation) is similar to that of imipenem. Moreover, penicillins and cephalosporins do

---

Antimicrobial Agents Annual 3
P.K. Peterson and J. Verhoef, editors
© Elsevier Science Publishers BV, 1988

TABLE 1   *Postantibiotic effect (PAE) of imipenem and other β-lactam antibiotics*

Species tested	PAE (min) when exposed to:					
	IMI	CAZ	CTX	PIP	AMP	GEN
Escherichia coli	135	10	0	15	NT	205
Enterobacter cloacae	130	33	114	0	NT	272
Klebsiella pneumoniae	61	38	35	10	NT	47
Pseudomonas aeruginosa	72	2	32	0	NT	88
Acenetobacter calcoaceticus	> 300	25	142	0	NT	> 300
Streptococcus faecalis	168	NT	NT	121	187	NT
Staphylococcus aureus	206	NT	117	52	NT	290

Each antibiotic was tested at two concentrations; data given are the highest observed. IMI = imipenem; CAZ = ceftazidime; CTX = cefotaxime; PIP = piperacillin; AMP = ampicillin; GEN = gentamicin; NT = not tested. Data from Baquero et al (5).

not differ markedly from imipenem in their PAE against gram-positive organisms, which do not form filaments when exposed to β-lactams. The clinical relevance of PAE is difficult to evaluate; if relevant, it would enable the use of longer dose intervals even if the drug concentration at the site of infection falls below inhibitory levels. In a small study Gudmundsson et al (6) demonstrated that imipenem, but not cefoperazone, gave a PAE in mice infected with *P. aeruginosa*. Thus, the PAE of imipenem may be a clinically relevant phenomenon.

As reviewed previously (1, 2), imipenem has a very high degree of β-lactamase stability and is hydrolyzed only by zinc-containing enzymes which are commonly produced by *Pseudomonas maltophilia* and has been reported in one isolate of *Bacteroides fragilis*. An enzyme active against imipenem has also been found in *Aeromonas hydrophilia* (7). In a recent study, Labia et al (8) confirmed the high degree of β-lactamase stability and also showed that imipenem has a moderate affinity for a wide range of enzymes tested. Despite its high degree of β-lactamase stability, imipenem is one of the most potent inducers of β-lactamase in species which have the *amp*C gene (9), e.g. *Pseudomonas, Enterobacter* and *Citrobacter* (10, 11). However, contrary to many cephalosporins, imipenem does not cause a genotypic derepression of β-lactamase synthesis nor is it hydrolyzed by the enzyme produced (11). Thus, when an organism containing the *amp*C gene is exposed to imipenem, it is likely to produce large amounts of enzyme and become resistant to most cephalosporins and penicillins; however, when imipenem is removed, it will return to a state of low enzyme production.

As reviewed in *Annual 2*, resistance to imipenem may emerge in *Pseudomonas* species (2). In many clinical studies, especially those on treatment of respiratory tract infections, such resistance has been reported. However, in most cases the resistant strains have retained their susceptibility to other β-lactams. It has been postulated that this is due to imipenem utilizing different porins from other β-lactams for its penetration through the outer membrane of *Pseudomonas* cells. Resistance should then be the result of chromosomally coded alterations of outer membrane proteins, rendering the bacteria impermeable to imipenem but not to other β-lactams (Kahan FM, personal communication).

The physiologic role of dehydropeptidase-I, the renal enzyme which hydrolyses imipenem and is inhibited by cilastatin, still remains unclear. It has been suggested by Welch and Campbell (12) that dehydropeptidase-I salvages amino acids from peptides appearing in catabolic stages. As reviewed by Birnbaum et al (13), no negative effects of cilastatin have yet been demonstrated in animals or man.

CLINICAL PHARMACOLOGY

The complex kinetics of imipenem and cilastatin, alone or in combination, were reviewed in *Annuals 1 and 2* (1, 2). A majority of previous studies were performed in healthy male subjects. MacGregor et al (14) have studied the kinetics in patients with serious infections treated with imipenem/cilastatin. The renal function of the patients was normal or moderately decreased. Kinetic parameters for imipenem were similar to those found in healthy volunteers. The mean plasma half-life in patients was 80 min compared to 60 min reported in volunteers, i.e. a moderate prolongation. The urinary recovery of active imipenem was about 10% lower in patients than in healthy subjects. This could have been due to less frequent urine sampling, resulting in loss of activity in bladder urine due to non-specific degradation of imipenem. In the same study, penetration of imipenem into wound drainage fluid, sputum and bone tissue was measured. Concentrations of imipenem varied but were generally high in wound drainage and sputum but rather low in bone tissue when sampled 15–120 min after administration of a 1 g dose of imipenem. Concentrations in saliva, nasogastric tube aspirate, gastric fluid, duodenal fluid and ileum fluid were generally very low. The low ileum fluid concentrations were in agreement with a previous study which showed that imipenem is not or only minimally excreted via the bile (15). In another study, Wise et al (16) found high imipenem levels in cantharide-induced blister fluid and peritoneal fluid from patients without peritonitis. High levels of both components were found in children with bacterial meningitis (17). Finch et al (18) studied the kinetics of imipenem and cilastatin in elderly and found that the half-lives were 1.6 and 2.1 hours, respectively, compared to about 1 hour for both compounds in healthy young volunteers. These data are similar to those found in patients with renal failure; the imipenem half-life increases only marginally and not above 3 hours in severe renal impairment while the increase in the cilastatin half-life is more marked (19). This is probably due to a more rapid extrarenal metabolism of imipenem than of cilastatin. As a consequence of these differences in the kinetics of imipenem and cilastatin in patients with renal failure, accumulation of cilastatin may occur if therapeutic levels of imipenem are maintained in such patients.

CLINICAL USES

With its unusually broad antibacterial spectrum, imipenem/cilastatin has its main indications in infections caused by a mixed aerobic/anaerobic flora or by multiresistant hospital-acquired pathogens. Species against which the efficacy of imipenem/cilastatin has been questioned are methicillin-resistant staphylococci (*S. aureus* and coagulase-negative staphylococci). In a small but well-performed study, Fan et al (20) treated patients with infections caused by methicillin-sensitive or methicillin-resistant strains of *S. aureus* and achieved clinical cure in 10/11 patients with methicillin-resistant strains and in 11/12 with methicillin-susceptible-strains. In one patient with a cellulitis caused by a methicillin-resistant strain the staphylococci persisted despite clinical cure; in all other patients bacteriologic elimination was achieved. Another situation in which imipenem is currently being studied is infections in neutropenic patients. In an uncontrolled study Bodey et al (21) treated 71 neutropenic patients with 79 febrile episodes. Of patients with verified infections, 15/19 with septicemia, 8/13 with pneumonia, 6/6 with soft tissue infections, 3/3 with head and neck infections and 2/4 with other infections responded favorably to imipenem/cilastatin. During treatment, 4 patients developed microbiologically verified superinfections: 1 case of *Candida* septicemia, 1 of *Aspergillus* pneumonia, 1 of *P. aeruginosa* soft tissue infections (imipenem-susceptible strain) and 1 of *P. maltophilia* septicemia (imipenem-resistant strain).

ADVERSE EFFECTS AND INTERACTIONS

Table 2 summarizes adverse reactions to imipenem/cilastatin reported in 3470 patients (22). Upper gastrointestinal reactions are common with imipenem/cilastatin and depend to a large extent on the rate of infusion, in most patients the reactions subside when the infusion time is increased. The relatively high frequency of seizures has caused some concern. Of the 37 patients who were reported to have had seizures, 7 had had grand mal seizures, focal seizures or myoclonus considered by the investigators to be probably or definitely drug-related. These patients had all received high imipenem/cilastatin doses relative to their body weight and renal function. In addition to these patients another 15 patients with seizures were noted in the case-report forms but were not registered as having had adverse reactions. A review of the case-records showed that seizures had occurred in another 25 patients included in trials of imipenem/cilastatin, but those reactions were not mentioned in the case-report forms. In the 62 patients with seizures, central nervous system (CNS) disorders could be identified in 50 patients and other contributing factors in all remaining patients. This indicates that the risk of neurotoxic reactions to imipenem/cilastatin is related to underlying CNS disorders and/or overdosing of the drug.

Due to the broad antibacterial spectrum of imipenem, fears have been expressed that imipenem will cause ecologic disturbances. Several studies have been per-

TABLE 2   *Frequency of adverse reactions reported in 3470 patients included in clinical trials of imipenem/cilastatin*

Type of reaction	Frequency (%)
Local reactions at sites of infusion	3.9 (2.7)
Skin reactions – all types	3.0 (2.3)
Unspecified rash	2.3 (1.8)
Pruritus	0.4 (0.4)
Urticaria	0.3 (0.2)
Diarrhea – all types	2.9 (1.8)
Pseudomembranous colitis	0.1 (0.1)
Nausea	2.7 (2.4)
Vomiting	1.6 (1.4)
Seizures	1.1 (0.5)
Fever or drug fever	0.5 (0.3)
Other clinical reactions*	1.9 (1.2)
Increased AST	5.8 (3.6)
Increased ALT	5.3 (3.4)
Increased alkaline phosphatase	5.2 (2.9)
Eosinophilia	3.7 (3.0)
Thrombocytosis	2.6 (1.6)
Positive direct Coombs' test	1.8 (1.6)
Increased serum creatinine	1.7 (0.5)
Increased BUN	1.4 (0.3)
Increased bilirubin	1.3 (0.5)
Decreased white blood cell count	1.2 (0.9)
Hypoprothrombinemia	1.0 (0.3)
Neutropenia	0.9 (0.6)
Leukocyturia	0.9 (0.2)
Thrombocytopenia	0.8 (0.4)
Abnormal potassium	0.7 (0.1)

*Reactions occurring in 0.4% or less of the patients.
Note that several patients had more than one experience. Figures within brackets indicate reactions classified by the investigators as definitely, probably or possibly related to imipenem/cilastatin. Data from Calandra et al (21).

formed on the effects of imipenem/cilastatin on the normal fecal flora (23–25). In all of them the changes found were moderate. Imipenem seems to cause no serious adverse ecologic effects, which is also indicated by the low frequency of pseudo-membranous colitis (Table 2).

Data on interactions between imipenem/cilastatin and other drugs are lacking. Due to the possible risk of induction of β-lactamase production in certain gram-negative species, combinations with other β-lactam antibiotics should be avoided.

FUTURE DIRECTIONS

Some possible indications for imipenem/cilastatin have still to be carefully evaluated. Examples are infections in neutropenic patients, children and neonates. Two unpublished studies clearly demonstrate that in patients with severe neutropenia the efficacy of imipenem/cilastatin monotherapy is comparable to that of a combination of amikacin and piperacillin (Norrby et al; Wade et al). There is also a continuous search for new carbapenems which are not metabolized in the kidneys and which could be given alone without cilastatin. Another goal is to find a carbapenem which is absorbed after oral administration. Such a development might, however, lead to a too widespread use of this valuable group of antibiotics with subsequent risk of increased frequency of resistance. Intensive research is also ongoing in the field of the penems which have many similarities to the carbapenems but lack activity on *Pseudomonas* and enterococci.

REFERENCES

1. Norrby SR (1986) Penems and carbapenems. In: Peterson PK, Verhoef J (Eds), *The Antimicrobial Agents Annual 1*, p 138, Elsevier, Amsterdam.
2. Norrby SR (1987) Imipenem/cilastatin. In: Peterson PK, Verhoef J (Eds), *The Antimicrobial Agents Annual 2*, p 144, Elsevier, Amsterdam.
3. Bustamte CI, Drusano GL, Cohn DI, Standiford HC (1984) Postantibiotic effect of imipenem on *Pseudomonas aeruginosa*. *Antimicrob. Agents Chemother., 26*, 678.
4. McDonald PJ, Hakendorf P, Pruul H (1982) Recovery period of bacteria after brief exposure to *N*-formimidoyl thienamycin and other antibiotics. In: Periti P, Grassi GG (Eds), *Current Chemotherapy and Immunotherapy*, p 741, American Society for Microbiology, Washington, DC.
5. Baquero F, Culebras E, Patrón C, Pérez-Díaz JC, Medrano JC, Vicente MF (1986) Postantibiotic effect of imipenem on Gram-positive and Gram-negative micro-organisms. *J. Antimicrob. Chemother., 18, Suppl E*, 47.
6. Gudmundsson S, Vogelman B, Craig WA (1986) The in-vivo postantibiotic effect of imipenem and other new antimicrobials. *J. Antimicrob. Chemother., 18, Suppl E*, 67.
7. Shannon K, King A, Phillips I (1986) β-Lactamases with high activity against imipenem and Sch 34343 from *Aeromonas hydrophilia*. *J. Antimicrob. Chemother., 17*, 45.
8. Labia R, Morand A, Guionie M (1986) β-Lactamase stability of imipenem. *J. Antimicrob. Chemother., 18, Suppl E*, 1.
9. Lindberg F, Normark S (1986) Contribution of chromosomal β-lactamases to β-lactam resistance in enterobacteria. *Rev. Infect. Dis., 8, Suppl 3*, S292.
10. Livermore DM (1986) Beta-lactamase induction in *Pseudomonas aeruginosa* by imipenem and its influence on susceptibility tests. In: Ishigami J (Ed), *Current Chemotherapy and Immunotherapy*, p 1193. American Society for Microbiology, Washington DC.
11. Shannon K, Phillips I (1986) The effects on β-lactam susceptibility of phenotypic induction and genotypic derepression of β-lactamase synthesis. *J. Antimicrob. Chemother., 18, Suppl E*, 15.

12. Welch CL, Campbell BJ (1978) Uptake of tritiated glycine from L-alanyl tritiated glycine into kidney cortex brush border vesicles: role of renal dipeptidases. *Fed. Proc.,* *37*, 1533.

13. Birnbaum J, Kahan FM, Kropp H, MacDonald JS (1985) Carbapenems, a new class of beta-lactam antibiotics: discovery and development of imipenem/cilastatin. *Am. J.* *Med., 78, Suppl 6A*, 3.

14. MacGregor RR, Gibson GA, Bland JA (1986) Imipenem pharmacokinetics and body fluid concentrations in patients receiving high-dose treatment for serious infections. *Antimicrob. Agents Chemother., 29*, 188.

15. Norrby SR, Rogers JD, Ferber F et al (1984) Disposition of radiolabeled imipenem and cilastatin in normal human volunteers. *Antimicrob. Agents Chemother., 26*, 707.

16. Wise R, Donovan IA, Lockley MR, Drumm J, Andrews JM (1986) The pharmacokinetics and tissue penetration of imipenem. *J. Antimicrob. Chemother., 18, Suppl E*, 93.

17. Jacobs RF, Kearns GL, Brown AL, Congee DC (1986) Cerebrospinal fluid penetration of imipenem and cilastatin (Primaxin) in children with central nervous system infections. *Antimicrob. Agents Chemother., 9*, 670.

18. Finch RG, Craddock C, Kelly J, Deaney NB (1986) Pharmacokinetic studies of imipenem/cilastatin in elderly patients. *J. Antimicrob. Chemother., 18, Suppl E*, 103.

19. Verbist L, Verpooten GA, Giuliano RA et al (1986) Pharmacokinetics and tolerance after repeated doses of imipenem/cilastatin in patients with severe renal failure. *J.* *Antimicrob. Chemother., 18, Suppl E*, 115.

20. Fan W, Del Busto R, Love M et al (1986) Imipenem-cilastatin in the treatment of methicillin-sensitive and methicillin-resistant *Staphylococcus aureus* infections. *Antimicrob. Agents Chemother., 29*, 26.

21. Bodey GP, Alvarez ME, Jones PG, Rolston KI, Steelhammer L, Fainstein V (1986) Imipenem-cilastatin as initial therapy for febrile cancer patients. *Antimicrob. Agents* *Chemother., 30*, 211.

22. Calandra GB, Wang C, Aziz M, Brown KR (1986) The safety profile of imipenem/cilastatin: worldwide clinical experience based on 3470 patients. *J. Antimicrob. Chemother., 18, Suppl E*, 193.

23. Nord CE, Kager L, Philipson A (1985) Effect of imipenem/cilastatin on the colonic microflora. *Rev. Infect. Dis., 7*, S432.

24. Wexler HM, Finegold SM (1985) Impact of imipenem/cilastatin therapy on normal fecal flora. *Am. J. Med., 78, Suppl 6A*, 41.

25. Welkon CJ, Long SS, Gilligan PH (1986) Effect of imipenem-cilastatin therapy on fecal flora. *Antimicrob. Agents Chemother., 29*, 741.

CHAPTER 14

Penicillins

GEORGE M. ELIOPOULOS

Although work continues on the development of new penicillins, as illustrated by the publication of several papers which assess the in-vitro activity of foramidocillin (BRL-36650), a new β-lactamase-stable penicillin with antipseudomonal activity (1), and by description of BRL-20330, an oral prodrug of temocillin (1), the most significant papers of 1986 have dealt with studies which expand our understanding of the mechanisms of action of and resistance to β-lactam antibiotics.

Substantial attention has been directed to studies of tolerance to the bactericidal action of penicillins, with special emphasis on the need to develop a uniform definition of this phenomenon. New techniques have been applied to the examination of penicillin-binding proteins (PBPs), including studies of immunologic relatedness of those proteins, and more detailed comparisons of PBPs using fluorography following proteolytic digestion. Most significantly, several non-β-lactam agents have now been described which bind to PBPs. While this work is in its infancy, development of these agents not only provides unique opportunities to study mechanisms of inhibition of bacterial cell growth but may also extend enormously possible options for synthesis of new chemotherapeutic agents.

Clinical studies continue to be important, not only to determine optimal regimens for therapy in specific situations and to assess new agents, but also to show comparable effectiveness of presently available agents – a very important undertaking in the highly competitive market for β-lactam antibiotics. A significant number of the studies published in 1986 deal with aztreonam, ticarcillin + clavulanic acid, or new cephalosporins, and these will be discussed elsewhere in this volume. This Chapter will deal with such studies only when comparisons bear directly on understanding of the clinical role of penicillins.

STRUCTURE, DERIVATION

With the virtual explosion of new β-lactam antibiotics over the last few years, it has become increasingly difficult to maintain an accurate perspective on the com-

Antimicrobial Agents Annual 3
P.K. Peterson and J. Verhoef, editors
© Elsevier Science Publishers BV, 1988

parative properties of members of this class of antibiotics. Rolinson (2) has undertaken the important task of providing a catalog of these agents which describes representative antimicrobial activities and pertinent pharmacokinetic properties. Neu (3) has recently reviewed structure-function relationships of β-lactam antibiotics, including the newer penicillins such as temocillin, a 6α-methoxy derivative of ticarcillin, and foramidocillin (BRL-36650). Properties of these β-lactamase-stable penicillins are described in *Annual 2* (1).

The relative contributions of R- and S-epimers to the antibacterial activity of temocillin have been examined; the former was found to possess the greater antimicrobial potency and to account in large part for the activity of the natural mixture (4). An *o*-methylphenyl ester of temocillin (BRL-20330) appears promising as an orally administered prodrug of the parent compound (5). The ester is rapidly converted to temocillin upon enteral adsorption. In doses employed (equivalent to 400–800 mg temocillin), the drug appeared to be well-tolerated and resulted in maximum mean serum concentrations of 9.8–15.8 μg/ml. The long serum elimination half-life of temocillin, approximately 5–6 hours, and high achievable urinary concentrations suggest that BRL-20330 may be an attractive oral drug if clinical studies confirm its efficacy.

Several new compounds with antipseudomonal activity have been synthesized. One group comprises a number of 6α-methoxysulbenicillin analogs which demonstrate poor activity against gram-positive organisms but inhibit a range of gram-negative bacteria, including strains of *Pseudomonas aeruginosa* resistant to ticarcillin and piperacillin (6). The second group consists of several ureidopenicillins containing catechol moieties (which are felt to facilitate activity against gram-negative bacilli) (7). One representative compound inhibited a carbenicillin-resistant strain of *P. aeruginosa* at a concentration of 0.2 μg/ml, and proved effective in an experimental mouse infection. While interesting, these compounds are at too early a stage in development to permit assessment of their potential utility.

ACTIVITY – MECHANISMS OF ACTION AND RESISTANCE

In vitro activity   Several papers extend previous data pertaining to the in vitro activity of BRL-36650, which is now called 'foramidocillin' (8–10). Representative activities are shown in Table 1. This drug shows good activity against gram-negative organisms, including *P. aeruginosa*, but no useful activity against gram-positive bacteria or anaerobes. It was found to be a poor inducer of chromosomal β-lactamases, to be resistant to hydrolysis by a variety of plasmid-mediated and chromosomal β-lactamases, and to have poor affinity for the chromosomally mediated enzymes of *P. aeruginosa* (9). Against organisms resistant to third-generation cephalosporins, minimal inhibitory concentrations (MICs) of foramidocillin tend to be slightly higher than those demonstrated for susceptible strains, but most remain susceptible to the new agent (11).

TABLE 1   In vitro activity of foramidocillin (BRL-36650)

Organism	MIC$_{90}$ (µg/ml)				MIC range (µg/ml)		
	Ref. 8	Ref. 9	Ref. 10		Ref. 8	Ref. 9	Ref. 10
Pseudomonas aeruginosa	0.5	4	3.12		0.12–1.0	0.06–16	0.78–25
Escherichia coli	0.25	0.5	3.12		≤0.03–0.5	0.03–2	0.39–25
Klebsiella pneumoniae	0.5	—	6.25		≤0.03–1.0	—	0.39–12.5
Klebsiella spp.	—	1.0	—		—	0.03–16	—
Serratia marcescens	1.0	0.5	3.12		≤0.03–8	0.25–16	0.78–3.12
Enterobacter cloacae	2	—	6.25		≤0.03–8	—	1.56–>50
Enterobacter spp.	—	2	—		—	0.06–16	—

Penicillin-binding proteins (PBPs) Studies of the target sites of penicillin action continue to play an important part in the elucidation of mechanisms by which bacteria are inhibited by β-lactams (12, 13), and increasingly more sophisticated techniques have been applied to this endeavor. Detailed kinetic analysis of PBP-[³H]penicillin interactions in penicillin-resistant transformant pneumococcal strains has provided evidence that resistance results from both diminished affinity of PBPs for penicillin and decreased absolute quantities of specific PBPs present, but not from altered deacylation rates of penicilloyl-PBP complexes (14). Recent investigations have also included analysis of peptide patterns following partial proteolysis of PBPs, as well as application of immunologic methods to examine the relatedness of PBPs from resistant strains to those of susceptible isolates. In pneumococci, the high-molecular-weight PBPs found in resistant strains indeed appear to be immunologically related to those of penicillin-susceptible strains, while distinct patterns detected by fluorography following partial proteolytic digestion of these PBPs indicate that genetic events leading to penicillin resistance result in alterations at or near the 'active center' of the proteins (15). Antisera against highly purified PBPs of *Haemophilus influenzae* have been used to study the immunologic relatedness not only of PBPs of this species, but also those of other species of the families Pasteurellaceae and Enterobacteriaceae (16).

Considerable attention has also been given to mechanisms of methicillin (β-lactam) resistance in staphylococci. Analysis of PBPs following partial proteolytic digestion described above has been applied to these organisms as well. Such studies confirm the occurrence of a low-affinity PBP (2a or 2″) in several independent isolates of methicillin-resistant *Staphylococcus aureus* (17) and suggest a relatedness between this protein and PBP-2 of methicillin-susceptible strains (18). Reynolds and Brown (19) reported that greater amounts of PBP-2″ were observed in strains grown in subinhibitory concentrations of methicillin or in media with high salt content incubated at 30°C (conditions which favor detection of methicillin-resistant organisms). Nevertheless, while it is widely assumed that expression of this PBP is responsible for methicillin resistance in *S. aureus*, studies by Hartman and Tomasz (20) suggest that the situation may be far more complex. Working with strains that demonstrated homogeneous, heterogeneous or thermosensitive (resistant at 30°C, susceptible at 37°C) heterogeneous resistance to methicillin, these authors detected PBP-2a production in the latter groups regardless of growth temperature and resulting phenotypic susceptibility pattern. Thus, it appears that in heterogeneously methicillin-resistant *S. aureus* the presence of PBP-2a (as detected by binding of radiolabeled penicillin) is not sufficient to convey phenotypic resistance. Additional papers pertaining to the genetics of penicillin resistance and physiologic properties of PBPs will not be discussed here (21–26).

A crucial development to which attention should be called has been the discovery of non-β-lactam antimicrobial compounds which bind to PBPs. Boyd et al (27, 28) have described the synthesis of γ-lactam penems and carbapenems with antibacterial activity. In addition, Nozaki et al (29) have discovered a natural dicyclic dipeptide which binds to PBPs, inhibits peptidoglycan synthesis, and is susceptible

161

to hydrolysis by β-lactamases. Clearly, these reports are of enormous significance, not only in terms of potential for new drug development, but also in view of the possible role of these agents as tools for a better understanding of mechanisms of action of and resistance to the β-lactam antibiotics.

β-Lactamases Production of β-lactamases remains the most important mechanism of resistance to penicillins among clinical bacterial isolates. Classification of these enzymes has been recently reviewed in depth by Bauernfeind (30). Given the wide variation in methods currently used in reports of newly described enzymes as well as in papers defining the β-lactamase stability of new β-lactams, a need has been perceived to establish guidelines for methodologies appropriate to these studies. Bush and Sykes (31) have recently proposed such guidelines.

Several new plasmid-mediated β-lactamases have been described; other papers extend previous investigations of recently detected enzymes (Table 2). Livermore et al (38) discussed the differential susceptibilities of TEM-1 producing *Escherichia coli* to various (β-lactamase hydrolyzable) aminopenicillins. Transconjugants possessing the TEM-1 enzyme demonstrated substantially greater resistance to ampicillin compared with the enzyme-free parent strain, with more modest increases in resistance to mezlocillin. While the velocity (V_{max}) of mezlocillin hydrolysis was rapid, the physiologic efficiency (V_{max}/K_m) of the reaction was lower than that found for ampicillin or azlocillin, providing at least a partial explanation for the observed differences in susceptibility.

In recent years, considerable attention has been directed to the role of chromosomally mediated, inducible β-lactamases of gram-negative bacteria in mediating resistance to extended-spectrum penicillins and third-generation cephalosporins. Derepression of β-lactamase production accounts for β-lactam resistance in some clinical isolates retrieved from patients previously treated with these agents (39); however, in other strains, alterations in permeability barriers are the major factor in development of resistance (40). It is well known that β-lactam antibiotics vary widely in their potential to act as 'inducers' of the chromosomally mediated enzymes (41, 42), and low activity as an inducer of β-lactamase has been assumed to be a favorable characteristic of an antibiotic. A concept which has more recent-

TABLE 2 *Some recently described plasmid-mediated β-lactamases*

Enzyme	Mol. wt	pI	Source	Ref. No.
CARB-4	22 000	4.3	*Pseudomonas aeruginosa*	32
NPS-1	25 000	6.5	*Pseudomonas aeruginosa*	33
OHIO-1	22 000	7.0	Enterobacteriaceae	34
OXA-4	23 000	7.45	*Pseudomonas aeruginosa*	35
ROB-1	—	8.1	*Haemophilus influenzae*	36
SAR-1	33 700	4.9	*Vibrio cholerae*	37

ly emerged is that β-lactams may, in addition, differ in their abilities to act as 'selectors' of stably derepressed mutants (42, 43). The effectiveness of an agent as a selector does not necessarily correlate with its capacity to act as an inducer. The various factors which determine the net activity of β-lactam antibiotics against gram-negative bacteria are discussed in detail by Sanders and Sanders (42). Studies with laboratory mutants of *P. aeruginosa* demonstrating sequential stages of β-lactamase derepression have now provided evidence for the existence of multiple forms of Type I enzyme in this species (44).

Bactericidal activity   Investigations of mechanisms by which certain susceptible micro-organisms evade killing upon exposure to penicillins as well as comparative studies of the relative bactericidal activities of new agents have been complicated both by inconsistent definitions of 'tolerance' and by various technical factors which influence determination of accurate bactericidal end-points. Fortunately, this topic has recently received increasing and well-deserved attention. Distinction has been drawn between genotypic tolerance, a property characteristic of a particular isolate, and phenotypic tolerance which describes behavior influenced by the growth conditions employed (45, 46). Analyses of bactericidal activity must also differentiate between tolerance (as defined by diminished rates of killing upon exposure to an antibiotic, relative to some standard), the existence of persisters (incomplete killing due to subpopulations in a resting state), and paradoxical effects (47). To date, studies of tolerance to the bactericidal effects of penicillins have been hampered by the lack of suitable standard reference strains. Recently, construction of a stable, penicillin-tolerant mutant strain of *S. aureus* has been described, which may serve this purpose (48).

Antibiotic combinations   Interactions between penicillins and aminoglycosides have been examined by several groups. Yee et al (49) studied mechanisms of penicillin-streptomycin synergism against viridans streptococci and concluded that, as in the case of enterococci, penicillin stimulated the intracellular uptake of radiolabelled aminoglycoside. Other investigators have suggested that important differences in penicillin-streptomycin interactions may exist between viridans streptococci and enterococci (50). Enhanced uptake of streptomycin in the presence of oxacillin was also demonstrated in *S. aureus* (51). This effect was dependent upon the concentrations of antibiotics used and resulted in synergistic killing only in the absence of high-level resistance to streptomycin. These authors proposed that release of teichoic acids upon exposure to the penicillin facilitated the penetration of streptomycin through the charged surface coat. Other reports utilized animal models to explore the effects of streptomycin dosage in treatment of enterococcal endocarditis (52) and to examine penicillin + streptomycin combinations in therapy of Group B streptococcal endocarditis (53). Further information has also been provided pertaining to the in vitro (54, 55) and in vivo (55) activities of the extended-spectrum penicillins against *P. aeruginosa*.

The role of PBPs in mediating cell lysis in *E. coli* was examined by Gutmann et al (56), using both thermosensitive PBP mutants and combinations of β-lactams with affinities for specific target proteins. Combinations of drugs which inhibited either PBP-1+2 or PBP-2+3 (or a single drug inhibiting one of those PBPs preferentially under conditions at which the complementary protein was not expressed) resulted in rapid cell lysis while either drug alone demonstrated primarily a bacteriostatic effect. Although it is widely believed that active cell growth is required for penicillins to exert a lytic bactericidal effect, this may not always be the case. In studies carried out with *E. coli* under conditions of amino acid deprivation which prevented growth, ampicillin-induced cell lysis was observed in the presence of any one of several inhibitors of ribosomal protein synthesis which, by disrupting normal control mechanisms, permitted continued peptidoglycan synthesis (57). These intriguing observations clearly merit further investigation.

Another report called attention to the fact that combinations of ampicillin with chloramphenicol may be antagonistic against chloramphenicol-resistant strains of *H. influenzae* (58). Antagonism of the bactericidal activity of ampicillin by clinically achievable concentrations of chloramphenicol was found against 3 strains resistant to the latter agent (MIC = 10 μg/ml), by both checkerboard titrations and time-kill studies. In the course of development of the fluoroquinolone antimicrobial agents, combinations of these agents with cell-wall-active antibiotics have also been evaluated. The effectiveness of azlocillin + ciprofloxacin combinations against *P. aeruginosa* infections was studied in an infected subcutaneous chamber model in rabbits (59) and in a neutropenic mouse model (60). A beneficial effect of the combination compared with the individual agents was seen in each case. Although in vitro synergism by this combination could be demonstrated against some isolates (60), it seems likely that suppression of the emergence of resistant subpopulations would be an important factor in the outcome of such studies. One observation which must be appreciated in assessing animal studies with this combination is that administration of azlocillin often results in higher serum levels of ciprofloxacin than those obtained when the latter drug is given alone (59).

Intracellular activity   Extending previous work which demonstrated the efficacy of liposome-entrapped ampicillin in a mouse model of *Listeria monocytogenes* infection, Bakker-Woudenberg et al (61) found that use of liposomes resulted in increased intracellular delivery of ampicillin to mouse peritoneal macrophages, where the drug exerted a significant bactericidal effect. Two studies demonstrated enhanced bactericidal efficacy of penicillins against pre-opsonized *S. aureus* within human blood monocytes compared with that observed in culture medium, even at conditions under which intrinsic monocyte antibacterial mechanisms were inoperative (62, 63). Two other papers, however, reported poor bactericidal activity of benzylpenicillin against *S. aureus* within normal polymorphonuclear leukocytes (64) or of amoxicillin against staphylococci in neutrophils pulsed with sodium fluoride (to inactivate oxygen-dependent antimicrobial systems) or in cells derived from patients with chronic granulomatous disease (65).

Other effects Mechanisms by which penicillins exert a protective effect against development of endocarditis during transient viridans streptococcal bacteremia were examined by Moreillon et al (66). Using a strain of *Streptococcus intermedius* which was inhibited but not killed by clinically attainable concentrations of amoxicillin, these authors first confirmed earlier observations that amoxicillin reduces the adherence of bacteria to platelet-fibrin clots in vitro. Extending this work to a rat model of aortic valve endocarditis, two further observations were made: (a) administration of penicillinase 30 min following bacteremia reversed the prophylactic effects of amoxicillin; (b) when high bacterial inocula were employed, multiple doses of amoxicillin were required to achieve a significant reduction in the occurrence of endocarditis. Reasons why such a prolonged bacteriostatic effect would be required to diminish the likelihood of infection are at present not completely understood.

The effects of ampicillin at subinhibitory concentrations on the binding of *H. influenzae* type b to human buccal epithelial cells were studied in vitro (67). Exposure of either bacteria or epithelial cells to antibiotic reduced bacterial adhesion. In addition, binding could be reversed if cells with adherent bacteria were exposed to antibiotic. These results suggest direct interactions between antibiotics and binding sites on both bacteria and human cells.

CLINICAL PHARMACOLOGY

The pharmacokinetics of foramidocillin (BRL-36650) were examined in 10 volunteers (68). Following intravenous infusion of 1 g single doses of drug, serum concentrations of approximately 100 μg/ml were attained at 30 min. Concentrations decreased to approximately 60 μg/ml at 1 hour, and to 10 μg/ml at 4 hours. Peak serum bactericidal titers achieved ranged from $\geq$ 1:2048 against *E. coli* to 1:32 against piperacillin-susceptible *P. aeruginosa* and 1:4 against piperacillin-resistant strains of this species.

Another new agent under investigation is lenampicillin (KBT-1585), an ampicillin prodrug which upon absorption is hydrolyzed to parent compound and acetoin. Comparison of orally administered ampicillin and lenampicillin in the fasting state demonstrated that peak serum ampicillin levels attained with the ester were approximately twice those achieved with oral ampicillin (69). Administration of lenampicillin with food did not affect the absolute bioavailability of drug, but did result in decreased peak serum levels.

Several published reports further evaluated the pharmacokinetics of antipseudomonal penicillins. Akbaraly et al (70) reviewed the kinetics of apalcillin in pediatric patients, including premature infants and newborns, and suggested dosage recommendations based on age. Single-dose studies at two dosage levels of ticarcillin failed to detect evidence of dose-dependent pharmacokinetics for this antibiotic (71). Dose-dependent pharmacokinetics were confirmed, however, in comparisons between 4 g and 5 g multiple doses of mezlocillin. While statistically significant, the differences detected in total body clearances of the drug at these comparative doses were small in practical terms (72). Comparative pharmacokinetics between 4 g doses of azlocillin and piperacillin were examined using a randomized, cross-over design (73). Serum concentrations of the former exceeded those of the latter at the peak level, and remained greater through 4 hours of sampling. Renal clearance of azlocillin (61 ml/min) was significantly lower than that of piperacillin (81 ml/min). The therapeutic implications of such observations are speculative. Van Laethem and Klastersky (74) have reported serum bactericidal titers against *Klebsiella pneumoniae* and *P. aeruginosa* achieved following administration of mezlocillin, alone or in combination with amikacin, in comparison with those obtained with ceftazidime.

A cross-over design was employed to assess the comparative bioavailabilities of orally administered flucloxacillin and cloxacillin. The bioavailability of the newer drug was felt to be superior to that of the older; in addition, serum half-life of flucloxacillin (1.5 h) was significantly greater than that of cloxacillin (0.9 h) (75). The pharmacokinetics of flucloxacillin were examined in another study, with particular attention to penetration into extravascular sites in view of the high degree of protein binding (96%) of the antibiotic (76). Following administration of a 2 g dose intravenously, mean peak serum concentrations of 155 μg/ml were obtained. The drug was eliminated with a terminal half-life of approximately 2 hours, following a long distribution phase. Comparisons of 'area under the curve' for serum and lymphatic fluid suggested a penetration ratio of approximately 20%; however, peak concentrations attainable in lymph and suction skin blister fluid were substantially below those in serum.

Because of the poor penetration of antibiotics into the posterior chamber of the eye, treatment of bacterial endophthalmitis generally requires the intravitreal injection of one or more antibiotics and, even then, results are often unsuccessful. Barza et al (77) report the experimental use of transscleral iontophoresis to enhance delivery of antibiotics into the vitreous humor of rabbit eyes. Intravitreal levels of ticarcillin as high as 94 μg/ml could be achieved following a 10-min application of electric current through an antibiotic-filled cylinder placed on the sclera. Although the procedure produced histologic damage immediately adjacent to the application site, it was felt that this degree of injury was not substantially greater than that created by puncture of the globe for direct antibiotic injection. Even taking into account differences between rabbit and human eyes, the authors felt that iontophoresis held promise as a method for delivery of antibiotics in ophthalmic infections.

ADVERSE EFFECTS AND DRUG INTERACTIONS

The incidence of skin rashes after exposure to penicillins was assessed in a review of approximately 20,000 records of hospitalized patients in Switzerland (78). Rashes occurred in approximately 8% of patients receiving aminopenicillins, in 4.7%

of those receiving other penicillins, and in 1.9% of cephalosporin-treated patients. To what extent these results were influenced by differences in duration of various therapeutic regimens is not clear. This study did not confirm previous reports of an increased risk for the development of rashes in patients simultaneously treated with a penicillin and allopurinol. Another study of 90 patients with skin reactions attributed to penicillins likewise found that late reactions (rash) were seen more commonly with aminopenicillins than with penicillin G; early-onset reactions (urticaria, Arthus-like reactions at injection sites) occurred more commonly with the latter drug (79). Wendel et al (80) reported successful desensitization of 15 pregnant penicillin-allergic women with oral penicillin V. All had histories of allergic reactions to penicillins and positive intradermal skin tests. Pruritus and urticaria were encountered, but did not prevent completion of desensitization and subsequent administration of penicillin G. One patient with infection due to *Listeria monocytogenes* aborted. The topic of cross-sensitivity to cephalosporins among penicillin-allergic patients is discussed by Anderson (81). References pertaining to penicillin-induced hypersensitivity vasculitis are provided in a general review of drug-related causes of this entity (82).

Potential bleeding complications associated with the use of β-lactam antibiotics are discussed by Sattler et al (83). In that paper, mechanisms by which such complications may occur and risks associated with specific agents are examined. Fletcher et al (84) found that each of several penicillins tested, including benzylpenicillin and nafcillin in addition to carboxy- and ureido-penicillins, inhibited platelet aggregation in vitro in a dose-dependent and reversible manner. The applicability of these data is uncertain, however, given the high drug concentrations used.

Other reports present cases of benzylpenicillin-induced neutropenia (85) and cholestatic hepatitis following exposure to dicloxacillin (86). In vitro inactivation of aminoglycosides by apalcillin in a time- and concentration-dependent manner has been demonstrated (87).

CLINICAL USES

The rationale for use of antibiotic prophylaxis against endocarditis was examined by Kaye (88), in light of American Heart Association guidelines. Updated regimens which include greater use of penicillin V or amoxicillin in selected circumstances should facilitate administration of appropriate prophylaxis. Relapse of secondary syphilis in a patient 5 months following therapy with 2.4 million units of benzathine penicillin was reported by Markovitz et al (89). The patient had alleged sexual abstinence during this interval. The authors concluded that, given the very low failure rate of standard penicillin regimens in early syphilis, isolated reports of this type do not necessarily warrant major changes in therapeutic approaches to this disease.

The impact of adding metronidazole to phenoxymethylpenicillin in the treatment of peritonsillar abscess was examined in a double-blind study which enrolled

20 patients in the group receiving the combination while an equal number received penicillin V alone (90). Aspiration of abscess contents and surgical incision/drainage were performed according to standard practice. While some β-lactamase-producing anaerobes persisted with the latter regimen, Group A streptococci were eradicated effectively by either regimen, and overall clinical responses were equivalent. Failure to eradicate Group A streptococci from the pharynx following treatment of pharyngitis with penicillin is not uncommon. The question of whether tolerance to the bactericidal effect of penicillin plays a role in such cases was explored by Kim and Kaplan (91). Strains were screened for tolerance by a gradient-replica plate technique; tolerance was confirmed by time-kill studies. Tolerant strains were found in none of 48 successfully treated patients, but were present prior to therapy in 9 of 37 patients who failed to clear the organisms from the pharynx. Interestingly, 5 patients with non-tolerant strains at the initial visit were found to harbor tolerant isolates following treatment. While penicillin therapy may have only favored recolonization with tolerant strains, it is also possible that exposure to the antibiotic may have favored selection of tolerant subpopulations or mutant colonies, as has been suggested for other bacteria (48).

The clinical efficacies of cyclacillin and amoxicillin, each at 500 mg thrice daily, in the treatment of acute maxillary sinusitis were compared in a study which enrolled 80 patients (92). All patients underwent aspiration of sinus fluid with quantitative cultures. An overall clinical cure rate of 91% was achieved, with no significant differences between the two treatment groups. Rash was seen more often in amoxicillin-treated patients (4 *vs* 1), but this result was not statistically significant. Diarrhea occurred in 1 patient of each group. Amoxicillin at a lower dose (250 mg every 8 hours) and minocycline (100 mg twice daily) were compared in another randomized study of acute maxillary sinusitis (93). Twenty-one of 22 amoxicillin-treated patients versus all of 25 minocycline-treated patients were cured or improved. Minor adverse reactions were noted during 10% of amoxicillin courses.

The activities of ampicillin and ceftriaxone in the treatment of acute shigellosis were evaluated in a randomized, placebo-controlled trial (94). Both ampicillin (4 g/d i.v.) and ceftriaxone (1 g/d) reduced the duration of fever, but only the former reduced the duration of culture-positive stools. Neither drug significantly decreased the duration of diarrhea, tenesmus, or abdominal discomfort.

Clinical efficacy of sulbenicillin (α-sulfoxybenzylpenicillin) in the therapy of bronchopulmonary infections was assessed in several studies (95–97). With doses of 4–8 g/d, favorable clinical responses of 90% or greater were observed. Nonetheless, results of such open trials are difficult to evaluate further for a variety of reasons. Inclusion of substantial numbers of patients with exacerbations of chronic bronchopulmonary disease and incomplete bacteriologic data are among the factors which complicate such analyses.

In a trial comparing the combination of ticarcillin (18 g/d) plus tobramycin with ceftazidime (4 g/d) in the treatment of gram-negative osteomyelitis, 'arrest' of the infection was demonstrated in all 9 patients treated with the combination and in 6 of 9 receiving ceftazidime (98). Failures in the latter group could be traced to various mechanical factors. Despite the small number of patients studied, the strengths of this report included documentation of infection by bone biopsy and relatively long follow-up periods. Ticarcillin (300 mg/kg/d) plus tobramycin combinations or piperacillin (450 mg/kg/d) alone appeared to be equally effective in the treatment of children with cystic fibrosis suffering acute exacerbations of pulmonary disease (99). Twenty-six patients in each group were studied; no resistance to piperacillin developed in organisms recovered following treatment with this agent.

The effectiveness of piperacillin relative to that of cefoxitin was examined in several studies representing a variety of clinical situations: prophylaxis for elective intra-abdominal surgery (100), prophylaxis for Cesarian section (101), treatment of obstetric/gynecologic infections (102), and treatment of various microbiologically documented infections (103). In each study, piperacillin was found to be effective in approximately 90% of cases, with no significant differences from results obtained with cefoxitin. In such comparative trials with agents that are generally effective, failure to demonstrate statistically significant differences does not necessarily indicate that such differences do not exist (because of Type II errors). However, as discussed by Silverblatt (104), it is often not worth the trouble or expense to carry out studies with sufficiently large numbers of patients to document small significant differences.

Finally, 4 prospective randomized studies have assessed regimens which include a penicillin in the empirical therapy of febrile neutropenic patients. Kramer et al (105) compared a carbenicillin + cefalotin + gentamicin combination with ceftazidime alone or ceftazidime + vancomycin. No statistically significant differences between the groups, either in overall initial clinical response (57% in the double- and triple-drug arms) or in the response of bacteremic episodes, were detected. However, fewer superinfections were encountered in the vancomycin + ceftazidime group, and fewer deaths due to infection occurred in this group as well. In an EORTC trial, over 700 patients were randomized to receive either azlocillin, ticarcillin or cefotaxime, each in combination with amikacin (106). Although response rates among all patients with documented or possible infections and among those with single gram-negative rod bacteremia were higher for those receiving azlocillin (70% and 66%, respectively) than for those treated with ticarcillin (59% and 47%), these differences were not significant. Considering only episodes of gram-negative bacteremia, multiple logistic regression analysis did, however, demonstrate superiority of the azlocillin-containing regimen. Response was also affected by persistent profound neutropenia and susceptibility of the isolate to the β-lactam employed (all isolates were susceptible to amikacin). A particular strength of this study was the strict definition of favorable response, which required that no change in antibiotics be deemed necessary during the course of therapy. On the other hand, design of the study did not require that amikacin dose be adjusted to achieve specific serum concentrations. Also, both azlocillin and ticarcillin were administered in 6-hourly doses; whether more frequent dosing would have altered these results is a matter of speculation.

Two trials utilized double β-lactam combinations in one study arm. DeJongh et al (107) compared moxalactam (8 g/d)+piperacillin (300 mg/kg/d, administered in 4 doses) with moxalactam+amikacin. For all evaluable episodes, overall response rates (approx. 70%) were equivalent. Although more patients with documented gram-negative infections responded to moxalactam+piperacillin (85%) than to moxalactam+amikacin (54%), the numbers were small and these differences did not reach statistical significance. Skin rashes and hypokalemia occurred equally in both groups, while nephro- and oto-toxicities were seen more frequently in the moxalactam+amikacin arm. Antibiotic resistance emerged in two pathogens recovered from patients treated with the double β-lactams. Moxalactam (2 g every 4 hours)+ticarcillin (4 g every 4 hours) was compared with two regimens containing aztreonam (with vancomycin, and with vancomycin+amikacin) (108). Responses to the aztreonam (approx. 70%) and ticarcillin (approx. 63%) regimens were similar, both in patients with documented infections and overall. Comparable responses were also observed in single gram-negative rod infections; however, gram-positive infections responded more favorably to regimens which included vancomycin.

FUTURE DIRECTIONS

The application of new techniques for the study of penicillin-binding proteins will, no doubt, continue to advance studies on the role of these targets in the action of, and bacterial resistance to, the penicillins. The discovery of γ-lactams and other non-β-lactams which bind to PBPs and inhibit peptidoglycan synthesis is a notable event. Infections due to gram-negative bacteria which possess inducible, chromosomally mediated β-lactamases remain a therapeutic challenge. Recent observations pertaining to characteristics of these enzymes under sequential stages of derepression must be confirmed and extended. New penicillins will be evaluated not only for their capacity to act as inducers of β-lactamases, but also for their ability to act as selectors of derepressed mutants.

Development of new classes of penicillins continues at a basic research level. As new parenteral antibiotics are introduced, efforts to devise enterally absorbable derivatives will also continue. The recent description of a temocillin prodrug illustrates this point. Clinical studies remain the cornerstone on which antibiotic selection strategies are based. In the present highly competitive environment, comparative trials will be undertaken not only to document efficacy of new agents, but also to demonstrate therapeutic equivalence between potentially more cost-effective antimicrobial agents and other, more expensive, regimens in clinical use.

REFERENCES

1. Eliopoulos GM (1987) Penicillins. In: Peterson PK, Verhoef J (Ed), *The Antimicrobial Agents Annual 2*, 153. Elsevier, Amsterdam.
2. Rolinson GN (1986) β-Lactam antibiotics. *J. Antimicrob. Chemother., 17*, 5.
3. Neu HC (1986) β-Lactam antibiotics: structural relationships affecting in vitro activity and pharmacologic properties. *Rev. Infect. Dis., 8, Suppl 3*, S237.
4. White AR, Cooper CE, Griffin KE, Slocombe B (1986) Antibacterial activity of re-solved temocillin epimers. *J. Antimicrob. Chemother., 18*, 335.
5. Basker MJ, Merrikin DJ, Ponsford RJ, Slocombe B, Tasker TCG (1986) BRL 20330, an oral prodrug of temocillin: bioavailability studies in man. *J. Antimicrob. Chemother., 18*, 399.
6. Burton G, Best DJ, Dixon RA, Kenyon RF, Lashford AG (1986) Studies on 6α-sub-stituted penicillins. II. Synthesis and structure-activity relationships of 6β-(2-aryl-2-sulfoacetamido)-6α-methoxy penicillanic acids. *J. Antibiot., 39*, 1419.
7. Ohi N, Aoki B, Shinozaki T, Moro K, Noto T, Nehashi T, Okazaki H, Matsunaga I (1986) Semisynthetic β-lactam antibiotics. I. Synthesis and antibacterial activity of new ureidopenicillin derivatives having catechol moieties. *J. Antibiot., 39*, 230.
8. VanLanduyt HW, Lambert A, Boelaert J, Gordts B (1986) In vitro activity of BRL 36650, a new penicillin. *Antimicrob. Agents Chemother., 29*, 362.
9. Mandell W, Neu HC (1986) Antimicrobial activity and β-lactamase stability of for-amidocillin. *Antimicrob. Agents Chemother., 29*, 769.
10. Hoy JF, Rolston KVI, Ho DH, Alvarez M, Thirolf P, Bodey GP (1986) In vitro activi-ty of BRL-36650, a new semisynthetic penicillin. *Antimicrob. Agents Chemother., 29*, 972.
11. Verbist L (1986) In-vitro activity of BRL-36650, a novel β-lactamase-stable penicillin, against multiply resistant gram-negative organisms. *J. Antimicrob. Chemother., 18*, 351.
12. Malouin F, Bryan LE (1986) Modification of penicillin-binding proteins as mecha-nisms of β-lactam resistance. *Antimicrob. Agents Chemother., 30*, 1.
13. Reynolds PE (1986) From whole organisms to crystallography: the changing face of the target of β-lactam antibiotics. *J. Antimicrob. Chemother., 17*, 129.
14. Handwerger S, Tomasz A (1986) Alterations in kinetic properties of penicillin-binding proteins of penicillin-resistant *Staphylococcus pneumoniae*. *Antimicrob. Agents Chemother., 30*, 57.
15. Hakenbeck R, Ellerbrok H, Briese T, Handwerger S, Tomasz A (1986) Penicillin-binding proteins of penicillin-susceptible and -resistant pneumococci: immunological relatedness of altered proteins and changes in peptides carrying the β-lactam binding site. *Antimicrob. Agents Chemother., 30*, 553.
16. Schryvers AB, Wong SS, Bryan LE (1986) Antigenic relationships among penicillin-binding proteins 1 from members of the families Pasteurellaceae and Enterobacteria-ceae. *Antimicrob. Agents Chemother., 30*, 559.
17. Reynolds PE, Fuller C (1986) Methicillin-resistant strains of *Staphylococcus aureus*: presence of identical additional penicillin-binding protein in all strains examined. *FEMS Microbiol. Lett., 33*, 251.
18. Tonin E, Tomasz A (1986) β-Lactam-specific resistant mutants of *Staphylococcus au-reus*. *Antimicrob. Agents Chemother., 30*, 577.
19. Reynolds PE, Brown DFJ (1985) Penicillin-binding proteins of beta-lactamase-re-

sistant strains of *Staphylococcus aureus*: effect of growth conditions. *FEBS Lett., 192,* 28.

20. Hartman BJ, Tomasz A (1986) Expression of methicillin resistance in heterogeneous strains of *Staphylococcus aureus*. *Antimicrob. Agents Chemother., 29,* 85.

21. Qoronfleh MW, Wilkinson BJ (1986) Effects of growth of methicillin-resistant and -susceptible *Staphylococcus aureus* in the presence of β-lactams on peptidoglycan structure and susceptibility to lytic enzymes. *Antimicrob. Agents Chemother., 29,* 250.

22. Heneine N, Stewart PR (1986) Physiological determination of methicillin resistance in *Staphylococcus aureus*: comparison of clinical and genetically derived isolates. *J. Antimicrob. Chemother., 17,* 705.

23. Blanchard T, Poston SM, Reynolds PJ (1986) Recipient characteristics in the transduction of methicillin resistance in *Staphylococcus epidermidis*. *Antimicrob. Agents Chemother., 29,* 539.

24. Georgopapadakou NH, Dix BA, Mauriz YR (1986) Possible physiological functions of penicillin-binding proteins in *Staphylococcus aureus*. *Antimicrob. Agents Chemother., 29,* 333.

25. Faruki H, Sparling PF (1986) Genetics of resistance in a non-β-lactamase-producing gonococcus with relatively high-level penicillin resistance. *Antimicrob. Agents Chemother., 30,* 856.

26. Dougherty TJ (1986) Genetic analysis and penicillin-binding protein alterations in *Neisseria gonorrhoeae* with chromosomally mediated resistance. *Antimicrob. Agents Chemother., 30,* 649.

27. Boyd DB, Elzey TK, Hatfield LD, Kinnick MD, Morion Jr JM (1986) γ-Lactam analogues of the penems. *Tetrahedron Lett., 27,* 3453.

28. Boyd DB, Foster BJ, Hatfield LD, Hornback WJ, Jones ND, Munroe JE, Swartzendruber JK (1986) γ-Lactam analogues of carbapenems. *Tetrahedron Lett., 27,* 3457.

29. Nozaki Y, Katayama N, Ono H, Tsubotani S, Harada S, Okazaki H, Nakao Y (1987) Binding of a non-β-lactam antibiotic to penicillin-binding proteins. *Nature (London), 325,* 179.

30. Bauernfeind A (1986) Classification of β-lactamases. *Rev. Infect. Dis., 8, Suppl 5,* S470.

31. Bush K, Sykes RB (1986) Methodology for the study of β-lactamases. *Antimicrob. Agents Chemother., 30,* 6.

32. Philippon AM, Paul GC, Thabaut MP, Jacoby GA (1986) Properties of a novel carbenicillin-hydrolyzing β-lactamase (CARB-4) specified by an IncP-2 plasmid from *Pseudomonas aeruginosa*. *Antimicrob. Agents Chemother., 29,* 519.

33. Livermore DM, Jones CS (1986) Characterization of NPS-1, a novel plasmid-mediated β-lactamase, from two *Pseudomonas aeruginosa* isolates. *Antimicrob. Agents Chemother., 29,* 99.

34. Shlaes DM, Medeiros AA, Kron MA, Currie-McCumber C, Papa E, Vartian CV (1986) Novel plasmid-mediated β-lactamase in members of the family Enterobacteriaceae from Ohio. *Antimicrob. Agents Chemother., 30,* 220.

35. Philippon AM, Paul GC, Jacoby GA (1986) New plasmid-mediated oxacillin-hydrolyzing β-lactamase in *Pseudomonas aeruginosa*. *J. Antimicrob. Chemother., 17,* 415.

36. Medeiros A, Levesque R, Jacoby GA (1986) An animal source for the ROB-1 β-lactamase of *Haemophilus influenzae* type b. *Antimicrob. Agents Chemother., 29,* 212.

37. Reid AJ, Amyes SGB (1986) Plasmid penicillin resistance in *Vibrio cholerae*: identification of new β-lactamase SAR-1. *Antimicrob. Agents Chemother., 30,* 245.

38. Livermore DM, Moosdeen F, Lindridge MA, Kho P, Williams JD (1986) Behavior

of TEM-1 β-lactamase as a resistance mechanism to ampicillin, mezlocillin and azlocillin in *Escherichia coli. J. Antimicrob. Chemother., 17*, 139.

39. Nichols WW, Milne LM (1986) Derepressed β-lactamase synthesis in strains of *Pseudomonas aeruginosa* isolated from patients with cystic fibrosis. *J. Antimicrob. Chemother., 17*, 549.

40. Sanders CC, Watanakunakorn C (1986) Emergence of resistance to β-lactams, aminoglycosides, and quinolones during combination therapy for infection due to *Serratia marcescens. J. Infect. Dis., 153*, 617.

41. Curtis NAC, Eisenstadt RL, Rudd C, White AJ (1986) Inducible Type I β-lactamases of gram-negative bacteria and resistance to β-lactam antibiotics. *J. Antimicrob. Chemother., 17*, 51.

42. Sanders CC, Sanders Jr WE (1986) Type I β-lactamases of gram-negative bacteria: interactions with β-lactam antibiotics. *J. Infect. Dis., 154*, 792.

43. Eng RHK, Smith SM, Cherubin CE (1986) In vitro emergence of β-lactam-resistant variants of *Pseudomonas aeruginosa. J. Antimicrob. Chemother., 17*, 717.

44. Gates ML, Sanders CC, Goering RV, Sanders WE (1986) Evidence for multiple forms of Type I chromosomal β-lactamase in *Pseudomonas aeruginosa. Antimicrob. Agents Chemother., 30*, 453.

45. Tuomanen E, Durack DT, Tomasz A (1986) Antibiotic tolerance among clinical isolates of bacteria. *Antimicrob. Agents Chemother., 30*, 521.

46. Tuomanen E (1986) Phenotypic tolerance: the search for β-lactam antibiotics that kill nongrowing bacteria. *Rev. Infect. Dis., 8, Suppl 3*, S279.

47. Sherris JC (1986) Problems in in vitro determination of antibiotic tolerance in clinical isolates. *Antimicrob. Agents Chemother., 30*, 633.

48. Tomasz A, De Vegvar M-L (1986) Construction of a penicillin-tolerant laboratory mutant of *Staphylococcus aureus. Eur. J. Clin. Microbiol., 5*, 710.

49. Yee Y, Farber B, Mates S (1986) Mechanism of penicillin-streptomycin synergy for clinical isolates of viridans streptococci. *J. Infect. Dis., 154*, 531.

50. Miller MH, El-Sokkary MA, Feinstein SA, Lowy FD (1986) Penicillin-induced effects on streptomycin uptake and early bactericidal activity differ in viridans group and enterococcal streptococci. *Antimicrob. Agents Chemother., 30*, 763.

51. Zenilman JM, Miller MH, Mandel LJ (1986) In vitro studies simultaneously examining effect of oxacillin on uptake of radiolabeled streptomycin and on associated lethality in *Staphylococcus aureus. Antimicrob. Agents Chemother., 30*, 877.

52. Henry NK, Wilson WR, Geraci JE (1986) Treatment of streptomycin-susceptible enterococcal experimental endocarditis with combinations of penicillin and low- or high-dose streptomycin. *Antimicrob. Agents Chemother., 30*, 725.

53. Backes RJ, Rouse MS, Henry NK, Geraci JE, Wilson WR (1986) Activity of penicillin combined with an aminoglycoside against group B streptococci in vitro and in experimental endocarditis. *J. Antimicrob. Chemother., 18*, 491.

54. Lyon MD, Smith KR, Saag MS, Cloud GA, Cobbs CG (1986) In vitro activity of piperacillin, ticarcillin, and mezlocillin alone and in combination with aminoglycosides against *Pseudomonas aeruginosa. Antimicrob. Agents Chemother., 30*, 25.

55. Fu KP, Hetzel N, Hung PP, Gregory FJ (1986) Synergistic activity of apalcillin and gentamicin in a combination therapy in experimental *Pseudomonas* bacteremia of neutropenic mice. *J. Antimicrob. Chemother., 17*, 499.

56. Gutmann L, Vincent S, Billot-Klein D, Acar JF, Mrena E, Williamson R (1986) Involvement of penicillin-binding protein 2 with other penicillin-binding proteins in lysis

of *Escherichia coli* by some β-lactam antibiotics alone and in synergistic lytic effect of amdinocillin (mecillinam). *Antimicrob. Agents Chemother., 30*, 906.

57. Kusser W, Ishiguro EE (1986) Lysis of nongrowing *Escherichia coli* by combinations of β-lactam antibiotics and inhibitors of ribosomal function. *Antimicrob. Agents Chemother., 29*, 451.

58. Mackenzie AMR, Chan FTH (1986) Combined action of chloramphenicol and ampicillin on chloramphenicol-resistant *Haemophilus influenzae. Antimicrob. Agents Chemother., 29*, 565.

59. Bamberger DM, Peterson LR, Gerding DN, Moody JA, Fasching CE (1986) Ciprofloxacin, azlocillin, ceftizoxime and amikacin alone and in combination against gram-negative bacilli in an infected chamber model. *J. Antimicrob. Chemother., 18*, 51.

60. Chin NX, Jules K, Neu HC (1986) Synergy of ciprofloxacin and azlocillin in vitro and in a neutropenic mouse model of infection. *Eur. J. Clin. Microbiol., 5*, 23.

61. Bakker-Woudenberg IAJM, Lokerse AF, Vink-Van den Berg JC, Roerdink FH, Michel MF (1986) Effect of liposome-entrapped ampicillin on survival of *Listeria monocytogenes* in murine peritoneal macrophages. *Antimicrob. Agents Chemother., 30*, 295.

62. Van den Broek PJ, Buys LFM, Mattie H, Van Furth R (1986) Effect of penicillin G on *Staphylococcus aureus* phagocytosed by human monocytes. *J. Infect. Dis., 153*, 586.

63. Van den Broek PJ, Buys LFM, Mattie H, Van Furth R (1986) Comparison of the effect of phenoxymethyl penicillin, cloxacillin, and flucloxacillin on *Staphylococcus aureus* phagocytosed by human monocytes. *J. Antimicrob. Chemother., 17*, 767.

64. Hand WL, King-Thompson NL (1986) Contrasts between phagocytic antibiotic uptake and subsequent intracellular bactericidal activity. *Antimicrob. Agents Chemother., 29*, 135.

65. Anderson R, Joone G, Van Rensburg CEJ (1986) An in vitro investigation of the intracellular bioactivity of amoxicillin, clindamycin, and erythromycin for *Staphylococcus aureus. J. Infect. Dis., 153*, 593.

66. Moreillon P, Francioli P, Overholser D, Meylan P, Glauser MP (1986) Mechanisms of successful amoxicillin prophylaxis of experimental endocarditis due to *Streptococcus intermedius. J. Infect. Dis., 154*, 801.

67. Gilsdorf JR, Jesperson JM (1986) Effect of antibiotics on adherence of *Haemophilus influenzae* type b. *Antimicrob. Agents Chemother., 30*, 370.

68. Pascual-Lopez A, Van der Auwera P, Lieppe S, Klastersky J (1986) BRL-36650: in vitro studies and assessment of serum bactericidal activity after single-dose administration in volunteers. *Antimicrob. Agents Chemother., 29*, 757.

69. Saito A, Nakashima M (1986) Pharmacokinetic study of lenampicillin (KBT-1585) in healthy volunteers. *Antimicrob. Agents Chemother., 29*, 948.

70. Akbaraly JP, Sarlangue J, Sautarel M, Heinzel G, Peyraud J, Martin C (1985) Pharmacocinétique de l'apalcilline en pédiatrie. *Pathol. Biol., 33*, 309.

71. Guglielmo BJ, Flaherty JF, Batman R, Barrier SL, Gambertoglio JG (1986) Comparative pharmacokinetics of low- and high-dose ticarcillin. *Antimicrob. Agents Chemother., 30*, 359.

72. Colaizzi PA, Coniglio AA, Poynor WJ, Vishniavsky N, Karnes HT, Polk RE (1986) Comparative pharmacokinetics of two multiple-dose mezlocillin regimens in normal volunteers. *Antimicrob. Agents Chemother., 30*, 675.

73. Colaizzi PA, Polk RE, Poynor WJ, Raffalovich AC, Cefali EA, Beightol LA (1986) Comparative pharmacokinetics of azlocillin and piperacillin in normal adults. *Antimicrob. Agents Chemother., 29*, 938.

74. Van Laethem Y, Klastersky J (1986) Serum bactericidal activity of mezlocillin, ceftazidime, mezlocillin/amikacin against *Klebsiella pneumoniae* and *Pseudomonas aeruginosa. Eur. J. Clin. Microbiol., 5*, 110.

75. Paton DM (1986) Comparative bioavailability and half-lives of cloxacillin and flucloxacillin. *Int. J. Clin. Pharmacol. Res., 6*, 347.

76. Bergan T, Engeset A, Olszewski W, Ostby N, Solberg R (1986) Extravascular penetration of highly protein-bound flucloxacillin. *Antimicrob. Agents Chemother., 30*, 729.

77. Barza M, Peckman C, Baum J (1986) Transscleral iontophoresis of cefazolin, ticarcillin, and gentamicin in the rabbit. *Ophthalmology, 93*, 133.

78. Sonntag MR, Zoppi M, Fritschy D, Maibach R, Stocker F, Sollberger J, Büchli W, Hess T, Hoigné R (1986) Exantheme unter häufig angewandten Antibiotika und antibakteriellen Chemotherapeutika (Penicilline, speziell Aminopenicilline, Cephalosporine und Cotrimoxazol) sowie Allopurinol. *Schweiz. Med. Wochenschr., 116*, 142.

79. DeHaan P, Bruynzeel P, Van Ketel WG (1986) Onset of penicillin rashes: relation between type of penicillin administered and type of immune reactivity. *Allergy, 41*, 75.

80. Wendel Jr GD, Stark BJ, Jamison RB, Molina RD, Sullivan TJ (1985) Penicillin allergy and desensitization in serious infections during pregnancy. *N. Engl. J. Med., 312*, 1229.

81. Anderson JA (1986) Cross-sensitivity to cephalosporins in patients allergic to penicillin. *Pediatr. Infect. Dis., 5*, 557.

82. Hannedouche T, Godin M, Fillastre JP (1986) Vascularites d'hypersensibilité d'origine médicamenteuse. *Ann. Méd. Interne, 137*, 57.

83. Sattler FR, Weitekamp MR, Ballard JO (1986) Potential for bleeding with the new beta-lactam antibiotics. *Ann. Intern. Med., 105*, 924.

84. Fletcher C, Pearson C, Choi SC, Duma RJ, Evans HJ, Qureshi GD (1986) In vitro comparison of antiplatelet effects of β-lactam antibiotics. *J. Lab. Clin. Med., 108*, 217.

85. Al-Hadramy MS, Aman H, Omer A, Khan MA (1986) Benzylpenicillin-induced neutropenia. *J. Antimicrob. Chemother., 17*, 251.

86. Kleinman MS, Presberg JE (1986) Cholestatic hepatitis after dicloxacillin-sodium therapy. *J. Clin. Gastroenterol., 8*, 77.

87. Wright DN, Hale DC, Saxon B, Matsen JM (1986) In vitro inactivation of aminoglycosides by apalcillin. *Antimicrob. Agents Chemother., 29*, 353.

88. Kaye D (1986) Prophylaxis for infective endocarditis: an update. *Ann. Intern. Med., 104*, 419.

89. Markovitz DM, Beutner KR, Maggio RP, Reichman RC (1986) Failure of recommended treatment for secondary syphilis. *J. Am. Med. Assoc., 255*, 1767.

90. Tunér K, Nord CE (1986) Impact on peritonsillar infections and microflora of phenoxymethylpenicillin alone versus phenoxymethylpenicillin in combination with metronidazole. *Infection, 14*, 129.

91. Kim KS, Kaplan EL (1985) Association of penicillin tolerance with failure to eradicate group A streptococci from patients with pharyngitis. *J. Pediatr., 107*, 681.

92. Scheld WM, Sydnor Jr A, Farr B, Gratz JC, Gwaltney Jr JM (1986) Comparison of cyclacillin and amoxicillin for therapy of acute maxillary sinusitis. *Antimicrob. Agents Chemother., 30*, 350.

93. Mattucci KF, Levin WJ, Habib MA (1986) Acute bacterial sinusitis: minocycline *vs* amoxicillin. *Arch. Otolaryngol., 112*, 73.

94. Kabir I, Butler T, Khanam A (1986) Comparative efficacies of single intravenous doses of ceftriaxone and ampicillin for shigellosis in a placebo-controlled trial. *Antimicrob. Agents Chemother., 29*, 645.

95. Ginesu F, Ortu AR, Schena GP, Casali L, Cabiddu R, Ticca MA, Foddai GA, Cardia P, Ligia GP, Torrazza PL, Coghe M, Bande G (1985) Multicentre clinical and bacteriological study of sulbenicillin in patients with bronchopulmonary infection. *Drugs Exp. Clin. Res., 11,* 885.

96. Saccarola L, Crisafi V, Cannizzaro G, Calvo MV, Pesce L, Macaluso S (1985) Results of treatment with sodium sulbenicillin in thirty elderly patients with acute bronchopulmonary infection. *Drugs Exp. Clin. Res., 11,* 895.

97. Macchioni PL, DelDin G, Filippi G, Baricchi R, Bertani A, Portioli I (1985) Clinical assessment of sulbenicillin in acute respiratory tract infection. *Drugs Exp. Clin. Res., 11,* 879.

98. Sheftel TG, Mader JT (1986) Randomized evaluation of ceftazidime or ticarcillin and tobramycin for the treatment of osteomyelitis caused by gram-negative bacilli. *Antimicrob. Agents Chemother., 29,* 112.

99. Jackson MA, Kusmiesz H, Shelton S, Prestidge C, Kramer RI, Nelson JD (1986) Comparison of piperacillin *vs* ticarcillin plus tobramycin in the treatment of acute pulmonary exacerbations of cystic fibrosis. *Pediatr. Infect. Dis., 5,* 440.

100. Baker RJ, Donahue PE, Finegold SM, Johnson WC, Middleton JR, Monafo WW, Wilson SE (1985) A prospective double-blind comparison of piperacillin, cephalothin and cefoxitin in the prevention of postoperative infections in patients undergoing intra-abdominal operations. *Surg. Gynecol. Obstet., 161,* 409.

101. Benigno BB, Ford LC, Lawrence WD, Ledger WJ, Ling FW, McNeeley SG (1986) A double-blind, controlled comparison of piperacillin and cefoxitin in the prevention of postoperative infection in patients undergoing cesarian section. *Surg. Gynecol. Obstet., 162,* 1.

102. Scalambrino S, Regallo M, Spreafico P, Epis A, Landoni F, Zanini A, Rescaldani R, Mangioni C (1986) Piperacillin versus cefoxitin in the treatment of infections in obstetrics ans gynecology. *Curr. Ther. Res., 40,* 49.

103. McCloskey RV (1986) Clinical comparison of piperacillin and cefoxitin in patients with bacteriologically confirmed infections. *Antimicrob. Agents Chemother., 30,* 354.

104. Silverblatt FJ (1987) Clinical trials and statistical rigor – are the benefits necessarily worth the cost? *J. Infect. Dis., 155,* 168.

105. Kramer BS, Ramphal R, Rand KH (1986) Randomized comparison between two ceftazidime-containing regimens and cephalothin-gentamicin-carbenicillin in febrile granulocytopenic cancer patients. *Antimicrob. Agents Chemother., 30,* 64.

106. Klastersky J, Glauser MP, Schimpff SC, Zinner SH, Gaya H, EORTC Antimicrobial Therapy Project Group (1986) Prospective randomized comparison of three antibiotic regimens for empirical therapy of suspected bacteremic infection in febrile granulocytopenic patients. *Antimicrob. Agents Chemother., 29,* 263.

107. DeJongh CA, Joshi JH, Thompson BW, Newman KA, Finley RS, Moody MR, Salvatore PC, Tenney JH, Drusano GL, Schimpff SC (1986) A double beta-lactam combination versus an aminoglycoside-containing regimen as empiric antibiotic therapy for febrile granulocytopenic cancer patients. *Am. J. Med., 80, Suppl 5C,* 101.

108. Jones PG, Rolston KVI, Fainstein V, Elting L, Walters RS, Bodey JP (1986) Aztreonam therapy in neutropenic patients with cancer. *Am. J. Med., 81,* 243.

CHAPTER 15

Quinolones

TOM BERGAN

The quinolones (Fig. 1) currently represent the group of antibacterial agents with the most innovative developments. The current wave of new, third-generation quinolones started with piperazinyl substitution and fluorination of the nalidixic acid nucleus. This resulted in norfloxacin, which has a considerably extended antibacterial spectrum compared with any of the otherwise improved quinolones such as cinolinic acid, pipemidic acid, piromidic acid, oxolinic acid, flumequin, or rosoxacin. The presently better documented fluorinated quinolones are ciprofloxacin, enoxacin, norfloxacin, ofloxacin, pefloxacin and the more recent amifloxacin, the trifluorinated fleroxacin (Ro 23-6240), CI-934, NY-198, AT-3295, AT-3765, E-3432, E-3846, S-25932, pirfloxacin, difloxacin (A-56619), A-56620 and A-60969. The properties of the newer quinolones and their probable therapeutic position are now reasonably well elucidated and will be summarized below.

ACTIVITY

Mechanism of action

The quinolones block bacterial gyrase, which has two functions:
1. Reducing the space needed for the chromosome to make it fit inside the bacterial cell (1). The enterobacterial chromosome is some 500–700 times longer than the length or the diameter of the cell. To reduce space, the gyrase causes supercoiling (supertwisting) of a number of loops (domains) of helical, double-stranded DNA which are each joined together and attached to an RNA backbone.
2. Sealing and nicking of DNA Each DNA domain is synthesized separately, but the gyrase catalyzes covalent bonds between them after the completion of supertwisting. For the genes to be activated, the DNA must first uncoil and the two DNA strands separated before transcription of mRNA. This process starts by opening the covalent bonds at each end of the DNA domain (nicking).

The enzyme (also called topoisomerase II) consists of 4 pieces, two α-monomers (MW = 105,000 daltons) and two β-monomers (MW = 95,000 daltons). The α-subunits are responsible for recognizing a key DNA sequence and for DNA nicking;

Antimicrobial Agents Annual 3
P.K. Peterson and J. Verhoef, editors
© Elsevier Science Publishers BV, 1988

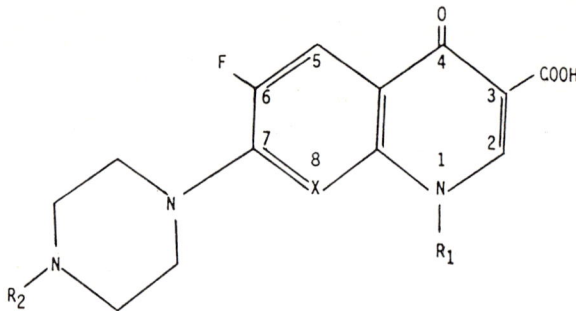

Fig. 1   Structural formula of nucleus of fluorinated quinolones.

	Substituents		
	R_1	R_2	X
Ciprofloxacin	C_3H_5	H	CH
Enoxacin	C_2H_5	H	N
Nalidixic acid	As enoxacin, but without F substitution of C6 and with a CH$_3$ substituent instead of a piperazinyl group at C7		
Norfloxacin	C_2H_5	H	CH
Ofloxacin	C_3H_6O (cyclic from N_1 to X)	CH_3	C
Pefloxacin	C_2H_5	CH_3	CH
Fleroxacin	C_2H_4F	CH_3	CF

the β-subunits cause DNA supercoiling.

    Quinolones block the gyrase activity by attachment to the gyrase α-subunits. Quinolones like ciprofloxacin and ofloxacin appear also to interact with the β-monomers.

    Quinolones cause increases in bacterial cell size; rod-shaped bacteria become filamentous and ultimately burst. Consequently, the quinolones are bactericidal. A post-antibiotic effect is observed with ciprofloxacin against both gram-negative and gram-positive bacteria (N Chin, HC Neu, personal communication, 1986).

    Other gyrase blockers are coumermycin and novobiocin, but these only interact with the β-monomers of the enzyme.

    There is some disagreement about whether uptake of quinolones into bacterial cells occurs by simple, passive diffusion or by an active, energy-consuming process (2, 3). No competition between different quinolones (enoxacin and ciprofloxacin) is apparent and energy-motive mechanisms are apparently not involved. Observations that anaerobic conditions reduce the activity of the quinolones (JT Smith, personal communication, 1986) suggest an active mechanism. Uptake is porin-dependent and intracellular binding forces are weak.

Spectrum of activity

The fluorinated quinolones are highly active against gram-negative bacteria including enterobacteria, *Pseudomonas aeruginosa, Haemophilus, Branhamella* and gonococci (4). The activity is less against gram-positive species, although they are usually within the therapeutic range. Generally, ciprofloxacin has lower minimal inhibitory concentrations (MICs) than the other quinolones. Ciprofloxacin is active against *Chlamydia trachomatis* and some mycoplasmas. *Legionella pneumophila* is susceptible to ciprofloxacin and ofloxacin. The anaerobic bacteria, *Pseudomonas cepacia* and *Pseudomonas maltophilia* are resistant to the quinolones. All fluorinated quinolones are highly active against most pathogens of the urinary and intestinal tracts and against gonococci.

The MICs of the fluorinated quinolones are much lower than those of aminoglycosides, amoxicillin, and third-generation cephalosporins for gram-negative rods, including multiresistant strains. The quinolone activity against gram-positive cocci is comparable to that of aminoglycosides and aminopenicillins, but better than that of cephalosporins. The activity against aerobic organisms is in general comparable with that of imipenem, which is more active than the quinolones against some aerobic species and, moreover, acts against anaerobic bacteria.

The in vitro bactericidal activity of ciprofloxacin, ofloxacin and pefloxacin is unchanged by β-lactam antibiotics, gentamicin and fosfomycin, but is significantly decreased against some strains by chloramphenicol, clindamycin, doxycyclin, erythromycin, fusidic acid and rifampicin (5, 6). The rate of kill is increased by aminoglycosides (6).

However, the therapeutic implications of such in-vitro results are uncertain. A thigh model (in neutropenic mice) infected with staphylococci and streptococci showed that clinical results obtained with ciprofloxacin and either erythromycin or vancomycin were similar. Against anaerobes, ciprofloxacin acted synergistically with cefotaxime, cefoxitin, clindamycin, metronidazole and mezlocillin (7). Antagonism occurred with less than 10% of the strains when ciprofloxacin was combined with clindamycin or cefoxitin. Cytostatic alkylating drugs, antimetabolites and alkaloids did not interfere in vitro. However, fluorouracil and mitomycin C enhanced the bactericidal activity of ciprofloxacin (8). Some synergy was reported for ciprofloxacin + azlocillin against *P. aeruginosa* in a model in vitro simulating the fluctuating concentrations occurring in vivo (9).

These findings in vitro on synergism and antagonism are consistent with observations of bacteridical activity and killing rates in sera of people receiving pefloxacin alone or in combination with other antibacterial agents (10).

Resistance mechanisms

Resistance to quinolones results primarily from structural changes of outer membrane porins or of the gyrase (11). Quinolone resistance emerges only from mutation. The rate of mutations in strains exposed to fluorinated quinolones is unusually low, less than 10^{-12} compared to 10^{-8}–10^{-10} with other earlier quinolones like nalidixic acid (12) or 10^{-6}–10^{-8} for most antibiotics. R-factor-mediated resistance has never been detected for quinolones. Indeed, R-factors produced by genetic engineering are unstable and are lost by the culture progeny (4). Quinolones at subinhibitory concentrations have cured bacteria for extrachromosomal DNA coding, e.g. for pathogenicity factors (13–15). Lack of R-factors and loss of plasmids by cells exposed to subinhibitory concentrations of quinolones are explained by the key function of gyrase in the organization of DNA during replication and transfer of R-factor DNA from a donor to a recipient. When the gyrase is blocked, DNA neosynthesis or transfer cannot occur. Emergence of resistance due to selection of resistant mutants proceeds somewhat more slowly than the more rapid spread of R-factors which may involve whole populations of susceptible strains. Thus, quinolones would appear to have a relatively low risk of resistance development. Selection of mutants under therapeutic conditions has been demonstrated in mice infected intraperitoneally by *Enterobacter cloacae* and given single doses of pefloxacin (16).

However, evidence that the infecting pathogen rarely persists during treatment with quinolones results from a recent analysis of carefully monitored patients who received ciprofloxacin (17). An assessment was made of 1540 evaluable patients (with urinary tract, respiratory tract, intra-abdominal and skin structure infections from whom cultures were taken before, during and after therapy, with testing of the susceptibility of the organisms. Some 1933 causative strains were isolated; of these, only 27 (1.4%) strains developed a low-level resistance against ciprofloxacin during therapy, and treatment failed in only 5 of these cases. The most frequent species were *P. aeruginosa* (more than half of the strains), *Serratia* spp. and *Klebsiella pneumoniae*. The infections actually resolved in 7 of the patients (urinary and respiratory tract infections) and either improvement or an undetermined outcome was noted in the remaining 15 patients.

Although selection of resistant mutants has caused treatment failure with, e.g., ciprofloxacin and norfloxacin (18), the mutants grow more slowly than the wild types and are replaced by the latter susceptible strains within 7–14 days. This has occurred, e.g., with *P. aeruginosa* colonizing the lower respiratory tract of patients with cystic fibrosis (19–22).

CLINICAL PHARMACOLOGY

When the same doses are given, pefloxacin and ofloxacin cause higher serum levels than either ciprofloxacin or norfloxacin (23, 24). The significance of the differences in absolute values, however, is somewhat offset by different intrinsic antibacterial activity of the compounds (MICs and rate of killing) and the consequences of bioactive metabolites produced from certain quinolones (see below). Thus, a crossover study on identical doses showed higher bactericidal serum titers for ciprofloxacin and norfloxacin than for ofloxacin when values were considered in relation to their absolute serum concentrations (23).

Serum concentrations essentially reach steady-state levels after the very first dose of ciprofloxacin and norfloxacin (4, 25, 26). This means that higher initial doses of these drugs are not necessary. For pefloxacin and ofloxacin, on the other hand, higher concentrations are reached during steady state than after the first dose. For these compounds, a larger initial dose might therefore be considered.

Elimination

An update on the pharmacokinetic properties of the quinolones appear in Table 1. The major difference from the status presented in *Annual 2* is that it has now emerged beyond doubt that the serum half-life ($t_{1/2}$) of 6–7 hours originally claimed for ofloxacin is overestimated by a factor of about two. In addition, the ofloxacin $t_{1/2}$ spans over a wider range of differences in healthy volunteers than those of the other quinolones. A review of the literature made in June 1986 showed that a large body of individual serum curves of healthy volunteers ($n = 322$) gave a mean ofloxacin $t_{1/2}$ of 4.5 hours. Comparable values of most other new key quinolones were found: ciprofloxacin about 4 hours; enoxacin 4.8 hours; and norfloxacin 4.6 hours (Table 2) (27).

The comparability of ofloxacin, ciprofloxacin and norfloxacin has also been substantiated directly by several recent studies and by cross-over studies (Table 3 in Ref. 4). The U.S. producer of ofloxacin reported a $t_{1/2}$ of 3.8 hours after one *oral* dose (28). Intravenous doses of 0.025–0.2 g ofloxacin gave $t_{1/2}$ values of 2.7, 2.8, 3.3 and 3.5 hours (29). A terminal, slower phase of elimination of ofloxacin with $t_{1/2}$ of 9–13 hours was observed, but this later phase started only when the serum concentrations had dropped below therapeutic levels. Elimination of the quinolones occurs in principle by 3 major routes: renal, metabolic and transintestinal. The renal route combines glomerular filtration and active tubular secretion; the latter is blocked by probenecid. The amount of renal elimination ranges from 30 to 60% of the dose for ciprofloxacin and norfloxacin from 75 to 95% for ofloxacin.

Metabolites and their relative amounts are shown in Table 3. Ofloxacin normally fails to render detectable metabolites in serum, while the other quinolones do. A substantial portion of pefloxacin is transformed to norfloxacin to the effect that 38% of the dose is excreted in urine as norfloxacin, another 38% as *N*-oxide pefloxacin, and only 24% as the parent compound (39). The antibacterial activity of unchanged pefloxacin as such is slightly lower or similar to that of norfloxacin against some species. Thus, after pefloxacin administration, norfloxacin contributes significantly to its antibacterial activity in both serum and urine.

Transintestinal elimination   The transintestinal route of elimination has been documented only recently, so far only for ciprofloxacin (40). In healthy volunteers, a single intravenous dose of ciprofloxacin resulted in a recovery of about 15% of the dose in feces (approximately one half as the parent compound and the other half as metabolites). Since less than 1% of the drug is eliminated in the bile, the

Table 1   *Pharmacokinetics of major fluorinated quinolones and nalidixic acid*

Drug	Protein binding (%)	Serum C_{max} (mg/l, dose = 500 mg)	Oral bioavailability (%)	$t_{1/2}$ (h)	Excretion (%) urine		Transintestinal (feces) (parent + metabolites)*	Extravascular penetration**
					Parent compound	Metabolites*		
Ciprofloxacin	35	2.0	85	3–4.5	30–60	7	15	117–120
Enoxacin	50	3.5	90	3–6	40–50	NA+	NA	114–130
Nalidixic acid	90	0.3	NA	1.5	5	90	<5	NA
Norfloxacin	15	2.0	70–80++	3–4.5	30–40	20	NA	106
Ofloxacin	10	8.5	90–95	(3–)3.5–5(–7)	70–90	5–10	<5	120
Pefloxacin	25	7.5	83+++	6–14	10	50–60	NA	NA
Fleroxacin	23	7.5	96	9.5	60–70	15	NA	90

*Biliary excretion < 1% for ciprofloxacin, nalidixic acid, and ofloxacin.

**Percentage of blister fluid area under the concentration curve (AUC) relative to serum AUC.

+NA = not available.

++Since intravenous formulation of norfloxacin is missing, the value is an estimate made in analogy with ciprofloxacin, since serum levels, $t_{1/2}$ and amount of dose eliminated in urine are similar for both drugs.

+++Based on AUCs of pefloxacin. Calculation adding up metabolites has given more than 100% bioavailability, but since the same molecule contributes to more than one of the classes (and concentration curves) of metabolites, this approach overestimates the bioavailability.

References: 10, 23–33 (German product manual for enoxacin).

Table 2   *Pharmacokinetics of quinolones in healthy subjects based on review of the literature*

Quinolone	No. of serum curves	Serum $t_{1/2}$* (h)
Ciprofloxacin	695	3.9
Enoxacin	62	4.8
Fleroxacin	90	10.1
Norfloxacin	205	4.6
Ofloxacin	322	4.5
Pefloxacin	53	11.2

*Mean of values of each individual curve. In the case of ofloxacin one of the producers has recently argued that the studies with the shorter $t_{1/2}$ values have had methodologic flaws (short observation period, few samples during elimination) and should be omitted. Some of these studies, however, were submitted for approval of the drug in the Federal Republic of Germany and data were initially reportedly used for recalculations leading to $t_{1/2}$ of 6–7 hours. The 'flaws' must therefore have been surmountable at that time. Repeated requests in the interests of free flow of academic information to have the original serum concentrations of the disputed studies made available for purposes of calculating the $t_{1/2}$ for control purposes, have regrettably failed. Thus, the scientific community cannot assess the alternate $t_{1/2}$ and we are, consequently, bound to accept the published data as they are. It may be presumed that methodologic deviations do not systematically affect only one compound and that with such a large body of information, the number of $t_{1/2}$ which may be within the erroneously low range would be cancelled out by an equal contribution covering the higher range.
**D. Herbold (personal communication, 1987).

substance reaches the lumen of the colon mainly by passage across the intestinal wall, either in intestinal secretions or by other mechanisms.

Reduced renal function   The quinolones are differentiated regarding the consequences of reduced renal function on the rate of elimination (4). Thus for ofloxacin, which is eliminated almost completely by the kidneys, the $t_{1/2}$ starts to increase already as soon as the renal function drops below clearances of about 30 ml/min. The ofloxacin $t_{1/2}$ reaches 40–50 hours at clearances below 10 ml/min (Table 4). For ciprofloxacin and norfloxacin, on the other hand, the $t_{1/2}$ is raised only to 5–10 hours, even in terminal renal failure, and the increase starts only at about a low function, corresponding to a creatinine clearance of about 15 ml/min (4, 41). This difference with a more favorable pattern for ciprofloxacin and norfloxacin occurs because the alternative, non-renal routes of elimination (metabolism and transintestinal elimination) render high capacity reserves (Table 5). Thus, in subjects with renal failure, the alternative pathways of ciprofloxacin and norfloxacin elimination compensate completely for the reduced renal capacity and these routes serve as safety valves in the event of reduced kidney function.

Table 3   *Metabolism of fluorinated quinolones eliminated in urine*

		Ciprofloxacin Oral	Intravenous	Enoxacin	Ofloxacin	Norfloxacin	Pefloxacin
Primary metabolites							
N-Demethylquinolone	H₂N-R			0.3	1.5		20.2 (= norfloxacin)
7-Aminoquinolone (piperazine removed)	HN⟨N-R (M-3)					0.6-0.8 (M-5)	
Oxoquinolone	(M-3)	6.2	5.6	7.5		4.6-6 (M-1)	6.2*
Ethylene diaminoquinolone (open, oxidized ring)	H₂N—NH-R (M-1)	1.4	1.3	0.8		1.1-1.8 (M-2)	
N-Oxide quinolone	CH₃-N⟨N-R (O)				1.2		23.2
Secondary metabolites							
N-Formylquinolone	O=C-N(H)⟨N-R (M-4)	0.1	0.1	0.1		0.25 (M-4)	
N-Acetylquinolone	O=C-N(CH₃)⟨N-R			0.3		0.25 (M-4)	
N-Sulfoquinolone	HO₃S-N⟨N-R (M-2)	3.7	2.6				
N-Acetylethylene diamino-quinolone	CH₃-C(=O)-HN—NH-R						
Glucuronide quinolone					traces	0.2-0.5 (M-3)	traces
Urinary elimination							
Unchanged		45	61.5	44	85-95	20-40	9.3
Total			71		90-95	28-46	60
			56			(0-48 h)	(0-72 h)

*Both as oxo-norfloxacin (5.4%) and oxo-pefloxacin (0.8%).

References: Data on file Bayer AG, F.R.G.; Astra Alab Sweden; W. Christ, personal communication, 1986; Refs 30-38.

R = quinolone ring nucleus, differences as shown in Fig. 1 (R), e.g. for norfloxacin:

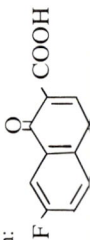

Table 4   *Serum half-life of fluorinated quinolones in renal failure*

Compound	$t_{1/2}$ (h)
Ciprofloxacin	5–10
Enoxacin	± 40
Norfloxacin	5–10
Ofloxacin	40–50
Pefloxacin	11–15

References 4, 32.

The $t_{1/2}$ values of the ciprofloxacin metabolites are only slightly longer in reduced renal function than that of the parent compound, whereby accumulation
to excessive levels should not become a problem (T Bergan, SB Thorsteinsson, R
Solberg, unpublished results).

Liver failure   Liver failure has a similar impact on ciprofloxacin and norflocaxin
$t_{1/2}$ as renal failure, i.e. the $t_{1/2}$ stays below 10 hours (4). Pefloxacin $t_{1/2}$ is considerably
increased from about 11 hours in healthy volunteers to $35 + 19$ hours in patients
with cirrhosis (42).

Table 5   *Percentage of the dose of intravenous ciprofloxacin eliminated by various routes
in patients with renal failure compared with healthy volunteers*

	Normal renal func-tion	Renal failure
Urine		
Parent drug	62.3	21.6
Metabolites	12.2	6.5
Total	74.5	28.1
Feces		
Parent drug	10.1	35.4
Metabolites	7.1	37.5
Total	17.2	65.9
Urine + feces		
Parent drug	72.4	57.0
Metabolites	19.3	37.0
Total	91.7	94.0

R Rohwedder, SB Thorsteinsson, H Scholl, T Bergan, unpublished data.

Table 6   Incidence (%) of side effects of treatment with major quinolones

	Ciprofloxacin		Enoxacin	Norfloxacin	Ofloxacin	Pefloxacin
	Americas	Europe/Japan				
No. patients evaluated	1241[a]	3918[b]	2407[f]	4844[c]	3701[d]	781[e]
Central nervous system	4.4	1.0	1.2	1.5	0.9	1.1
Gastrointestinal	8.1	3.7	3.8	3.9	3.0	4.2
Dermatologic	1.9	0.8	0.7	0.6	0.6	2.4
Urogenital					0.3	0
Other	1.8	0.6	0.4	0.1	0.2	
Musculoskeletal disorders	0.2	0.08	0.04	0.1	0	0.9
Eye	0.2	0.1			0	
Hematologic	0.1	1.3				
Metabolic/nutritional	4.2	7.6				
Cardiovascular	0.5	0.07	0.1			
Incidence adverse reactions*	22.6	15.1	6.2	6.6	4.7	
Patients with adverse reactions	13.4	10.2		3.2	3.8	
Patients withdrawn due to side effects			6.5	1.2	1.4	1.3

[a]G. Arcieri, oral presentation, Second European Symposium of Clinical Microbiology, Brighton, 1985, and Refs 48–52.
[b]Dr P. Schacht, personal communication, 1987.
[c]Ref. 49.
[d]Personal communication, 1986, Hoechst AG, F.R.G. Incidence of adverse reactions in Europeans 2.8% while 2.4% of the patients showed such reactions (50).
[e]Rhône-Poulenc, product manual in French, 1985.
[f]Ref. 51.
*When one and the same patient experienced several types of reactions, each is recorded; therefore the total incidence of reactions is higher than the number of patients with reactions.

Table 7   *Therapeutic efficacy of major quinolones*

Diagnosis	Ciprofloxacin		Enoxacin		Norfloxacin		Ofloxacin		Pefloxacin	
	No.	Effect* (%)	No.	Effect (%)	No.	Effect (%)	No.	Effect (%)	No.	Effect (%)
Urinary tract	1522	94	1025	79	1417	94	1287	85	115	90
Respiratory tract	926	89	2386	75	188	65	269	68	120	73
Bacterial enteritis	111	96	131	85	125	96	143	75	56	68
Ear-nose-throat**	155	90	383	68	777	73	116	85	20	80
Otitis media			131	60	108	80	47	64	12	92
Skin and soft tissues	592	97	350	69			472	84	108	90
Gynecologic	96	94	12	100						
Gonorrhea***	100% (250 mg)		100% (600 mg)		100% (800 mg)		100% (200 mg) 100% (400 mg)		100% (800 mg)	
Intra-abdominal	45	93	145	89						
Bacteremia	56	93							52	87
Osteomyelitis	43	98							70	91
Bone joints	20	77	67	99						
Eye	83	92	19	79	44	71	51	92		
Pneumonia			51	86			59	90		

*Effect refers to bacterial resolution and clinical improvement, except for skin structures and infections treated with enoxacin and pefloxacin where bacterial eradication was not documented in available data.

**Tonsillitis, sinusitis, otitis.

***Expected cure rates for documented doses; based on available literature and personal communication with producers.

References: Ref. 4, German product manual on enoxacin, personal communication from each producer.

Tissue penetration

Since the fluorinated quinolones are small molecular substances with a low serum protein binding, they penetrate readily into tissues. The total concentration in suction skin blisters exceed serum levels by 10–20% (without significant differences) (4). Concentrations are high in prostate tissue and secretion. Ciprofloxacin reaches high concentrations in female genital organs, maxillary sinus mucosa, skin and muscle. Intracellular ciprofloxacin concentrations in leukocytes rise to 5.5 times the extracellular levels after the cells have been kept in physiologic solution for 2 hours (CSF Easmon, personal communication, 1986). Therefore, quinolones enhance phagocytic killing of bacteria (43, 44).

The cerebrospinal fluid (CSF) concentrations of ciprofloxacin and pefloxacin are about 40–60% of the serum concentrations during meningeal irritation and 2–20% when meninges are uninflamed (45; P Schacht, personal communication, 1986). The concentrations of ofloxacin in CSF are 50–60% of the serum levels when there is no distinct meningeal irritation (46). In adult patients with inflamed meninges, a mean CSF concentration of 2.1 mg/l ofloxacin was found 2 hours after oral doses of 200 mg b.i.d. for 2 days and 1.4 mg/l after 12 hours; the corresponding serum levels were 6.8 and 3.1 mg/l (47).

Concentrations in maternal milk remain below detectable levels. Ciprofloxacin and norfloxacin concentrations in bone are therapeutically significant. Low levels have been found in saliva. The levels in sputum have been 75–115% of the serum levels of enoxacin, ofloxacin and pefloxacin, and about 50% for ciprofloxacin (4).

ADVERSE EFFECTS AND DRUG INTERACTIONS

The most frequent complaints during use of quinolones are nausea, upper gastrointestinal discomfort, and dizziness. The reactions are usually mild and rarely necessitate changing to another antibacterial drug. The incidence of side effects appear similar for the various drugs when based on data of the type submitted to government licensing bodies (Table 6).

During the past year, however, the German market has offered a useful feedback complementing the results of early clinical studies monitored by the industrial developers. Reports of side effects to the 'Arzneimittelkommission der deutschen Aerzteschaft' reporting to the 'Bundesgesundheitsamt' (BGA) have indicated that ofloxacin (after some 1.7 million therapeutic courses) has caused several instances of serious central nervous system (CNS) reactions (53). The neurotoxic reactions have ranged from insomnia, dizziness, headache, visual disturbances, and psychomotoric restlessness to more severe psychotic events like hallucinations and disorientation. Although the reactions have been temporary, ofloxacin administration has even necessitated a number of admissions to psychiatric hospitals. The recommended doses of ofloxacin are lower than for other quinolones, although the curative effect of routine doses appears inferior to that of the other quinolones (see below and Table 7).

After about 2.0 million prescriptions, norfloxacin has been associated only with 1 case of transient, mild disorientation, which did not require hospitalization. Since norfloxacin has been on the German market for a longer period of time than other fluorinated congeners, experience is more complete with norfloxacin than with the other fluorinated quinolones. Ciprofloxacin has been on the same market only since February 1987, too short for a comparable feedback to the BGA, but CNS changes appear less insignificant; nearly 20% of the ciprofloxacin reactions involving the CNS include restlessness, tremors and dizziness (48).

The higher rate of CNS side effects, like the higher penetration into CSF (and eye), seen for ofloxacin than with ciprofloxacin and norfloxacin would be related to the higher lipid solubility of ofloxacin.

Use of pefloxacin has been troubled by the discovery of cataract in beagle dogs; this has blocked government approval in Germany and elsewhere, but re-assessment may change this.

Enoxacin produces a high frequency of nausea, which is more prominent during concomitant theophylline therapy because of mutual interaction of the metabolism of enoxacin and theophylline. No such interaction occurs with ofloxacin and the interference is much less with ciprofloxacin, norfloxacin and pefloxacin than with enoxacin (4, 54; Hekster, personal communication, 1986). Pefloxacin has caused aspermia and testicular atrophy (4).

Quinolones accumulate in cartilage from which they disappear only slowly. Blister formation and ulcerations have been observed in cartilage of young experimental animals, mainly in weight-bearing joints. Although it is difficult to extrapolate these changes to man, quinolones are, consequently, now recommended only after completion of adolescence, and not during pregnancy or lactation. However, the fact that nalidixic acid has been given for decades without apparent deleterious effects on joints makes it uncertain whether this phenomenon really represents a major problem.

One phenomenon which has been the focus of attention (55; SB Thorsteinsson, T Bergan, R Rohwedder, H Scholl, unpublished results), is specific quinolone crystals in urine. We have observed ciprofloxacin crystal formation more frequently at high urinary pH (at 7.2 and above). One dose of 1000 mg given orally to 12 healthy volunteers followed by microscopy of freshly voided urine at 37° C showed quinolone crystals in 4 subjects after ciprofloxacin and in 2 cases after norfloxacin, but not after ofloxacin or nalidixic acid. After the urine was allowed to cool down, however, crystals of all the 3 fluorinated drugs appeared. Although the in vivo frequencies are different, the in vitro observations after cooling suggest that all 3 drugs, in principle, have similar potential.

The consequences of formation of quinolone crystals is uncertain at the present time. We have never observed any deleterious effects of crystals (by chemical methods and microscopy to detect hematuria) (54; Thorsteinsson et al, unpublished results). In this connection, it is quite interesting that no crystals could be detected in a patient who developed hematuria consistently when given ciprofloxacin 3 times (56, 57).

The following doses would appear safe from the point of view of crystal formation: ciprofloxacin 500 mg orally or 400 mg intravenously; 800 mg norfloxacin orally; and 1000 mg ofloxacin orally.

Intravenous ciprofloxacin may elicit local skin reactions, but the erythematous reaction is of little concern if the drug is infused into the larger cubital vein rather than into veins on the dorsum of the hand (SB Thorsteinsson, R Rohwedder, T Bergan, unpublished results). The rash develops around the site of the infusion and is accompanied by a local burning sensation. The rash, however, may recede even during the infusion and disappears within minutes after the infusion is stopped.

The absorption of fluorinated quinolones is unaffected or only slightly delayed by food, pirencepine (anti-muscarinic drug) and ranitidine (H2-receptor antagonist), but the total serum concentration (AUC) is unaffected. Antacids based on Mg—OH— and Ag—OH markedly reduce the absorption of both ciprofloxacin and ofloxacin, probably due to chelate formation with the quinolone. *N*-Bamyl-scopolamine bromide, which retards enteric motility, slows down absorption of ciprofloxacin. Metoclopramine, which enhances intestinal motility, causes earlier quinolone peaks, but does not significantly lower serum concentrations (shown for ciprofloxacin and ofloxacin). Pharmacokinetic interaction is not observed with β-lactam antibiotics or aminoglycosides.

Since coffeine is metabolized by the same pathways as theophylline and thus delays elimination of the latter (58), it is relevant to note that caffeine may also be eliminated more slowly by fluorinated quinolones. Enoxacin (800 mg) has a clear-cut effect, but ciprofloxacin (250 mg) and ofloxacin (200 mg) at lower doses have had insignificant consequences (55).

Ecology

The fluorinated quinolones significantly decrease the numbers of fecal enterobacteria, but otherwise leave the microflora virtually unchanged (25, 59–61). Thus, the quinolones have no impact on more than 99.9% of the normal microflora and normalization occurs within 7–14 days. This makes the fluorinated quinolones uniquely ecologically compatible.

CLINICAL USES

Three infectious disease entities have emerged as the major targets of the fluorinated quinolones: urinary tract infections (lower and upper plus acute and uncomplicated infections and prophylaxis in urosurgery), gonorrhea, and bacterial enteritis. This is because the therapeutic results have been consistently satisfactory for these diseases using the recommended drug regimens (Table 7), although slight underdosing may apply to one of the drugs, as suggested by the fact that the dose is clearly lower in relation to activity in vitro than to the other quinolones, and that this correlates with the lower cure rate with this drug (Table 7). Generalized salmonelloses with high fever and severe malaise would favor initial parenteral administration, to be followed by oral administration of a quinolone as soon as the patient shows signs of stable improvement.

In the case of urinary tract infections, comparative studies have shown that both ciprofloxacin (250 mg b.i.d.) and norfloxacin (400 mg b.i.d.) are more effective than other alternatives such as amoxicillin, trimethoprim + sulfamethoxazole, nalidixic acid, or pipemidic acid (49, 62, 63). Ofloxacin (200 or 300 mg b.i.d.) has been as effective as or better than trimethoprim + sulfamethoxazole, nalidixic acid, nitrofurantoin or pipemidic acid (64, 65). In urinary tract infections, the same (statistically) cure rates have been obtained by increasing doses of 250, 500 and 750 mg ciprofloxacin b.i.d. which produced cure rates of 93, 93, and 97% (66). Ofloxacin doses of 200, 300 and 400 mg b.i.d. resulted in a lower cure rate at the usually recommended dose (200 mg b.i.d.) and higher, similar to those of ciprofloxacin and norfloxacin, after the higher doses (93 and 94%) (67). In small studies, single doses of ciprofloxacin (500 mg) and norfloxacin (800 mg) in complicated urinary tract infections have had similar cure rates (68) as had ciprofloxacin (250 mg b.i.d.) versus ofloxacin (400 mg b.i.d.) (69).

Against bacterial enteritis, the fluorinated quinolones appear to hold particular promise. An efficacy rate of 100% has been observed with 400 mg norfloxacin b.i.d. for 3 days against *Salmonella, Shigella, Vibrio cholerae, V. parahaemolyticus, Aeromonas hydrophila, Edwardsiella tarda*, and *Plesiomonas shigelloides* (S Lolekha, personal communication, 1986). The effect was distinctly better than that obtained with either trimethoprim + sulfamethoxazole or a placebo, both in terms of clinical symptoms and signs, and duration of discharge of the infecting strain. Ciprofloxacin b.i.d. for 5 days was effective in 75% of the cases caused by *Salmonella* and in 100% by *Shigella* (60, 70–74).

The quinolones with an intravenous formulation (ciprofloxacin, perfloxacin) are also very suitable for severe systemic infections (75, 76).

In adequate doses, one single dose of any of the fluorinated quinolones has been effective for gonorrhea (ciprofloxacin 250 mg, enoxacin 600 mg, norfloxacin 800 mg, ofloxacin 200–400 mg, pefloxacin 800 mg) (47, 62, 77).

Chancroid has been effectively treated by 500 mg ciprofloxacin twice daily for 13 days (78). The results are less favorable with a single dose of ciprofloxacin (78).

Chlamydia trachomatis and *Ureaplasma urealyticum* may be eradicated by 750 mg ciprofloxacin twice daily for 1 week, but 10–40% of the patients are not cured (79). The same applies to doses of 200 mg b.i.d. for 10 days (L Fransen, D Avonts, J Vidfont, P Piot, personal communication, 1986). Ciprofloxacin, thus emerges as a useful supplement after erythromycin or tetracyclines for non-gonococcal urethritis. A regimen of ofloxacin (100 mg t.i.d. for 14 days) may also cure chlamydial urethritis (80).

The use of fluorinated quinolones in upper and lower respiratory tract infections is fraught with two major problems: (a) minimal inhibitory concentrations of relevant pathogens, in particular gram-positive bacteria such as the pneumococci, are high compared to the levels reached in relevant body fluids; (b) a number of antibiotics including penicillins are already well established as effective in respiratory tract infections.

Ciprofloxacin (200 mg b.i.d. orally) has been found comparable to doxycycline in respiratory tract infections treated in general practice (cure rates of 82% and 79%) (81). Ciprofloxacin (200–400 mg b.i.d.) has been documented in a sufficient number of patients to allow assessment of its effect on different respiratory tract infections (82–86) (Table 8). The cure rates were above 94% for *Haemophilus influenzae, E. coli*, and *Branhamella catarrhalis*, 91% for pneumococci, 82–83% for staphylococci and *K. pneumoniae*, and 45% for *P. aeruginosa*. Ciprofloxacin (750 mg b.i.d. orally) has been as good for chronic bronchopulmonary infections in cystic fibrosis as a combination of azlocillin and tobramycin given intravenously (22, 83). Ciprofloxacin therefore appears to be an acceptable alternative in the treatment of respiratory tract infections.

Common respiratory tract pathogens like pneumococci and staphylococci respond poorly to ofloxacin; depending on the dose, the eradication rates have been 76% and 80% in 53 patients treated for lower respiratory tract infections (chronic bronchitis and similar) (87). The response rates were 93–100% for *Haemophilus*, enterobacteria and *Branhamella*, and 34% for *P. aeruginosa* (87). Ofloxacin (200–300 mg b.i.d.) versus amoxicillin (1 g b.i.d. or t.i.d.) in lower respiratory tract infections showed overall microbiologic eradication rates of 95% and 73% respectively (88). Similar differences occurred in another study with an 'excellent' clinical response in 73% of the patients treated with ofloxacin and 35% with amoxicillin (89). A dose range study of 200, 300 and 400 mg b.i.d. ofloxacin showed respective cure rates of 43, 52 and 80% in upper respiratory tract infections and of 34, 55 and 48% in lower respiratory tract infections (67). Bacteriologic results indicate eradication rates of 85, 89 and 85% in upper respiratory tract infections and 72, 84 and 83% in lower respiratory tract infections. The incidence of patients with side effects increased from 4.1% with doses of 200 mg b.i.d. to 6.4% with 400 mg b.i.d. and the number of patients who dropped out because of side effects increased from 1.6 to 2.0%. For the treatment of infective episodes in bronchiectasis, ofloxacin (200 mg t.i.d.) was distinctly more effective and better tolerated than amoxicillin (1 g t.i.d.) (90). Ten days' treatment of chronic bronchitis with 400 mg ofloxacin bid has seemed comparable to 750–1000 mg (!) ciprofloxacin b.i.d., and 400 mg b.i.d. enoxacin or pefloxacin (91). The side effects were distinctly more apparent with enoxacin than with ciprofloxacin, and developed least with pefloxacin (91). Ofloxacin has improved the condition of patients with cystic fibrosis during treatment, but without eliminating the pathogen (92).

Quinolones have been used to successfully treat chronic osteomyelitis caused by gram-negative species, including *P. aeruginosa* (93–97).

Fluorinated quinolones, in particular ciprofloxacin, have been found effective in curing soft tissue infections caused by a wide range of gram-positive cocci (staphylococci, streptococci), pseudomonas, and enterobacteria (98, 99).

Ciprofloxacin and norfloxacin have been useful both prophylactically and therapeutically in neutropenic patients (100–103).

Table 8   *Clinical results of ciprofloxacin treatment of upper and lower respiratory tract infections*

Diagnosis	No. of patients	Clinical effectiveness				Cure rate (%)
		Excellent	Good	Poor	Unchanged	
Lower respiratory tract						
Acute bronchitis	102	15	74	5	8	87
Chronic bronchitis	163	9	117	21	16	77
Bronchiectasis	102	13	68	16	5	79
Bronchopneumonia	84	12	61	4	7	87
Panbronchiolitis	35	4	23	2	6	77
Subtotal	486	53	343	48	42	82
Upper respiratory tract						
Acute tonsillitis	60	21	34	4	1	92
Acute otitis media	12	9	3	0	0	100
Acute sinusitis	16	7	7	1	1	88
Acute pharyngitis	37	14	20	1	2	92
Chronic sinusitis	15	2	11	0	2	87
Subtotal	140	53	75	6	6	91
Grand total	626	106	418	54	48	84

Ref. 86.

DOSING

In the urinary tract infections, twice-daily doses of 125–250 mg of ciprofloxacin appear therapeutically equivalent to 200–400 mg norfloxacin (Table 9). The doses of 100–200 mg ofloxacin are slightly less effective, but are recommended by the producer, probably because these were used and thus documented in clinical studies employed for governmental approval. This situation was reflected by bacteriologically documented cure rates in urinary tract infections of 94% for both ciprofloxacin and norfloxacin compared with 85% for ofloxacin (2) (Table 2). Because one cannot on a purely clinical basis with certainty differentiate between lower and upper urinary tract involvement, it would seem preferable always to use the higher doses. The cure rates have been lower for enoxacin and pefloxacin. Recommended regimens both of enoxacin and pefloxacin are 400 mg b.i.d.

Cure of gonorrhea can be expected with single oral doses of 250 mg ciprofloxacin, 600 mg enoxacin, 800 mg norfloxacin, 200–400 mg ofloxacin, or 800 mg pefloxacin. Chlamydial urethritis is not cured by single doses, but 1 week of 500 mg ciprofloxacin b.i.d. has cured 91% and 10–14 days' duration seems better (4). Norfloxacin and ciprofloxacin have both effectively cured some cases of prostatitis.

Cure of bacterial enteritis has been impressively documented with ciprofloxa-

Table 9   Dosing of major quinolones (mg per dose × no. doses per 24 h)*

Diagnosis	Ciprofloxacin	Enoxacin	Norfloxacin	Ofloxacin	Pefloxacin
Urinary tract infection					
Uncomplicated, lower	250 × 2	400 × 2	200–400 × 2	100 × 2	400 × 2
Complicated, upper	250–500 × 2	400 × 2	400 × 2	200 × 2	400 × 2
Gonorrhea, single dose	250	600	800	200 or 400	400
Bacterial enteritis	250–500 × 2	(400 × 3)	400 × 2–3	200 × 2	400 × 3
Typhoid fever	250–500 × 2	—	400 × 2–3	(200 × 2)	400 × 3
Shigellosis	250–500 × 2	200 × 3	400 × 2	200 × 2	400 × 2
Reduced renal function*					
15–30 ml/min GFR (ser. creat. 2.5–5 ml/min)	normal	normal × ½	normal	normal × ½	normal?
Under 15 ml/min GFR (ser. creat. > 5 ml/min)	normal × ½	normal × ¼	normal × ½	100 × 1	normal × ½
Soft tissue infections	500 × 2	—	—	(200 × 2)	(400 × 2)
Upper respiratory tract	250–750 × 2	—	—	(200 × 2)	(400 × 2)
Lower respiratory tract	250–750 × 2	—	—	(200 × 3)	(400 × 2)
Otitis, sinusitis	250–500 × 2	—	—	(200 × 3)	(400 × 2)
Septicemia, neutropenia	750 × 2	—	—	—	(400 × 2)
Biliary system	500 × 2	—	—	—	—
Bone system, joints	500 × 2	—	—	—	—

*Based on company recommendations and published literature.
**Monitoring of serum levels of parent compound and metabolites needed.
GFR = glomerular filtration rate; ser. creat. = serum creatinine. Brackets indicate need for further documentation or recommendation not to follow producer's recommendation.

cin, norfloxacin and ofloxacin. The recommended doses given 2–3 times daily for 3–5 days (under guidance of clinical response) appear to be 250–500 mg ciprofloxacin, 400 mg enoxacin, 400 mg norfloxacin, or 200 mg ofloxacin. Systemic infections like salmonelloses will require longer periods of treatment than other causes as directed by patient condition and speed of recovery.

Soft-tissue structure infections appear to be effectively cured by ciprofloxacin. Because of a more modest activity against relevant gram-positive species, ofloxacin is less satisfactory.

The only quinolone which seems to be sufficiently satisfactory that it can be considered as an alternative for respiratory tract infections is ciprofloxacin. Pneumococci are eradicated less well by ofloxacin than ciprofloxacin. However, a penicillin for the treatment of respiratory tract infections and otitis media is still preferred because of the relatively lower activity of quinolones against gram-positive organisms. Ciprofloxacin would be considered as a second- or third-line drug, together with erythromycin, trimethoprim + sulfamethoxazole, and tetracyclines, depending on allergy, symptoms, causative organism, and whether previous treatment has failed.

FUTURE DIRECTIONS AND CONCLUSIONS

The currently most favorable fluorinated quinolones appear to be ciprofloxacin and norfloxacin. At recommended doses, these have comparable therapeutic effects against urinary tract infections, gonorrhea and bacterial gastroenteritis (including shigellosis, systemic salmonellosis, and watery diarrheas). The good effect in gonorrhea, regardless of β-lactamase production, offers a most interesting potential for the quinolones. Ciprofloxacin is useful also against osteomyelitis caused by gram-negative rods. Ciprofloxacin has been more extensively documented in both basic and clinical studies than the other quinolones, has the advantage that an intravenous dosage form is available, and that it has a documented good effect in infections of other than urinary tract infections, gonorrhea and enteritis. The efficacy rates of recommended doses of ofloxacin appear slightly less than for ciprofloxacin and norfloxacin (Table 7), but increasing the ofloxacin doses may significantly reduce the tolerance. In particular, the effects on CNS functions including induction of psychosis and consequent hospitalization in a distinct number of cases has been a problem with ofloxacin, although the reactions are fully reversible. The cure rates of pefloxacin are generally comparable to those of ciprofloxacin and norfloxacin.

Being orally administered broad-spectrum antimicrobial agents, the quinolones have considerable potential for significantly reducing treatment costs. Oral drugs reduce costs, since supplies and equipment for parenteral drugs become unnecessary and health personnel work time is less. Oral dosage forms have less iatrogenic consequences than intravenous ones. Effective drugs reduce the duration of hospitalization. Broad-spectrum compounds make unnecessary the use of multiple drug regimens; polypharmacy has more side effects, may be more costly and may lead to incorrect administration. Patients with multiresistant strains can be more readily treated outside hospitals by an effective oral dosage form. Development of resistance appears to be less of a problem with quinolones than with most other antimicrobial agents and the former are ecologically more favorable since the normal microflora is little affected. Consequently, it would seem advisable, from the point of view of both economy and good antibiotic policy-making, to include one or two of the fluorinated quinolones on the list of approved drugs in health institutions.

REFERENCES

1. Smith JT (1984) Awakening of the slumbering potential of the 4-quinolone antibacterials. *Pharm. J., 20*, 299.
2. Bedard J, Wong S, Brejan LE (1986) Mechanism of transport of enoxacin into *Escherichia coli*. In: *Abstracts, 26th Interscience Conference on Antimicrobial Agents and Chemotherapy, New Orleans, LA, 1986*, No. 945.
3. Diver JM, Piddock LJV, Wise R (1986) Investigations into the uptake of five fluoroquinolones by *E. coli* KL-16. In: *Abstracts, 26th Interscience Conference on Antimicrobial Agents and Chemotherapy, New Orleans, LA, 1986*, No. 946.
4. Bergan T (1986) Quinolones. In: Peterson PK, Verhoef J (Eds), *The Antimicrobial Agents Annual 1*, 164. Elsevier, Amsterdam.
5. Haller I (1986) Influence of several antibiotics on the bactericidal activity of new quinolones against staphylococci and enterococci in vitro. In: *Abstracts, 26th Interscience Conference on Antimicrobial Agents and Chemotherapy, New Orleans, LA, 1986*, No. 346.
6. Smith JT (1986) Should 4-quinolones be used in combination therapy? In: *Abstracts, 26th Interscience Conference on Antimicrobial Agents and Chemotherapy, New Orleans, LA, 1986*, No. 347.
7. Whiting JL, Cheng N, Chow AW (1986) Synergistic combinations of ciprofloxacin and other agents against anaerobic bacteria. In: *Abstracts, 26th Interscience Conference on Antimicrobial Agents and Chemotherapy, New Orleans, LA, 1986*, No. 348.
8. Bauernfeind A (1986) Influence of cytostatics on the antibacterial activity of ciprofloxacin. In: *Abstracts, 26th Interscience Conference on Antimicrobial Agents and Chemotherapy, New Orleans, LA, 1986*, No. 349.
9. Dudley M, Blaser J, Kuepker M, Gilbert D, Zinner S (1986) Synergism between ciprofloxacin and azlocillin *vs Ps. aeruginosa* in an in vitro model: effect of simultaneous *vs* 'staggered' dosing. In: *Abstracts, 26th Interscience Conference on Antimicrobial Agents and Chemotherapy, New Orleans, LA, 1986*, No. 1123.
10. Lieppe S, Van der Auwera P, Vandermies A, Klastersky J (1986) Bactericidal activity and killing rate of serum in volunteers receiving pefloxacin alone or in combination with ceftazidime, piperacillin or mezlocillin against *Pseudomonas aeruginosa*. In: *Abstracts, 26th Interscience Conference on Antimicrobial Agents and Chemotherapy, New Orleans, LA, 1986*, No. 582.
11. Wolfson JS, Hooper DC, Ng EY, Souza KS, McHugh GL, Swartz MN (1986) Studies of mechanisms of action of and resistance to ofloxacin in *Escherichia coli*. In: *Ab-*

stracts, *26th Interscience Conference on Antimicrobial and Chemotherapy, New Orleans, LA, 1986*, No. 950.

12. Smith JT (1986) The mode of action of 4-quinolones and possible mechanism of resistance. *J. Antimicrob. Chemother., 18, Suppl D*, 21.

13. Mehtar S, Blakemore PH, George R, Pitt T (1986) In vivo elimination of plasmids from *Serratia marcescens* by ciprofloxacin. In: *Abstracts, 26th Interscience Conference on Antimicrobial Agents and Chemotherapy, New Orleans, LA, 1986*, No. 952.

14. Weisser J, Wiedemann B (1986) Elimination of plasmids by enoxacin and ofloxacin at near inhibitory concentrations. *J. Antimicrob. Chemother., 18*, 575.

15. Michel-Briand Y, Uccelli V, Laporte JM, Plesiat P (1986) Elimination of plasmids from Enterobacteriaceae by 4-quinolone derivatives. *J. Antimicrob. Chemother., 18*, 667.

16. Vladoianu JR, Bellido F, Lucain C, Regamey P, Pechere JC (1986) Decreased susceptibility to quinolones in *Enterobacter cloacae* associated to (*sic!*) altered OMP F porin. In: *Abstracts, 26th Interscience Conference on Antimicrobial Agents and Chemotherapy, New Orleans, LA, 1986*, No. 948.

17. Schacht P, Hullmann R (1986) Development of resistance during phase II and II clinical trials with ciprofloxacin. In: *Abstracts, Congress on Bacterial and Parasitic Drug Resistance, Bangkok, 1986*, p 109. HN Press, Bangkok.

18. Ogle JW, Reller LB, Vasil ML (1986) Development of resistance in *Pseudomonas aeruginosa* to imipenem, norfloxacin, or ciprofloxacin. In: *Abstracts, 26th Interscience Conference on Antimicrobial Agents and Chemotherapy, New Orleans, LA, 1986*, No. 111.

19. Bender SW, Posselt HG, Wonne R, Stover B, Strehl R, Shah PM, Bauernfeind A (1986) Ciprofloxacin treatment of patients with cystic fibrosis and *Pseudomonas* bronchopneumonia. In: Neu HC, Weuta H (Eds), *Proceedings, Current Clinical Practice Series, 34*, p 272. Excerpta Medica, Amsterdam.

20. Shalit I, Stutman HR, Marks MI (1987) Randomized study of two dosage regimens of ciprofloxacin for treating chronic bronchopulmonary infection in patients with cystic fibrosis. *Am. J. Med., 32, Suppl 4A*, 189.

21. Scully BE, Nakatomi M, Ores C, Davidson S, Neu HC (1987) Ciprofloxin therapy in cystic fibrosis. *Am. J. Med., 82, Suppl 4A*, 196.

22. Bosso JA, Black PG, Matsen JM (1987) Ciprofloxin versus tobramycin plus azlocillin in pulmonary exacerbations in adult patients with cystic fibrosis. *Am. J. Med., 82, Suppl 4A*, 180.

23. Beerman D, Wingender W, Zeiler HJ, Forster D, Graefe KH, Schacht P (1984) Comparative pharmacokinetics of three new quinolone carboxylic acid antibiotics after oral administration in healthy volunteers. *J. Clin. Pharmacol., 24*, 403.

24. Krech T, Naumann P, Copp C, Crea A (1985) Antibacterial in vitro activity of norfloxacin, ciprofloxacin, ofloxacin and pefloxacin. *Chemioterapia, 4(2), Suppl*, 447.

25. Bergan T, Delin C, Johnsen S et al (1986) Pharmacokinetics of ciprofloxacin and effect of repeated dosage on salivary and fecal microflora. *Antimicrob. Agents Chemother., 29*, 298.

26. Wise R, Lister D, McNulty, CAM, Griggs D, Andrews JM (1986) The comparative pharmacokinetics of five quinolones. *J. Antimicrob. Chemother., 18, Suppl D*, 71.

27. Bergan T (1987) Pharmakokinetik von Ciprofloxacin. *Fortschr. Antimikrob. Antineoplast. Chemother., 6*, 447.

28. Flor S, Weintraub H, Beals B, Tack K (1986) Pharmacokinetics of ofloxacin in humans after single dose and during multiple dose administration. In: *Abstracts, 26th*

Interscience Conference on Antimicrobial Agents and Chemotherapy, New Orleans, LA, 1986, No. 483.

29. Lode H, Kirch P, Olschewski H, Sievers G, Hoffken G, Borner K, Verhoef M, Koepper P (1986) Pharmacokinetics of parenteral ofloxacin in volunteers. In: *Abstracts, 26th Interscience Conference on Antimicrobial Agents and Chemotherapy, New Orleans, LA, 1986*, No. 484.

30. Borner K, Hoffken G, Prinzing C, Lode H (1984) Renale Ausscheidung von Ciprofloxacin und einigen Metaboliten nach einmaliger oraler oder intravenöser Applikation von 50 mg. *Fortschr. Antimikrob. Antineoplast. Chemother., 3*, 695.

31. Borner K, Lode H (1986) Biotransformation von ausgewählten Gyrasehemmern. *Infection, 14, Suppl 1*, 54.

32. Dagrosa EE, Verho M, Malerczyk V (1985) Pharmacokinetik von Ofloxacin. *Fortschr. Antimicrob. Antineoplast. Chemother., 5–5*, 819.

33. Montay G, Goueffon Y, Roquet F (1984) Absorption, distribution, metabolic fate and elimination of pefloxacin mesylate in mice, rats, dogs, monkeys and humans. *Antimicrob. Agents Chemother., 25*, 463.

34. Ozaki T, Uchida H, Irikura T (1981) Studies on metabolism of AM-715 (norfloxacin) in humans by high performance liquid chromatography. *Chemotherapy (Tokyo), 29, Suppl 4*, 128.

35. Shimada J, Yamaji T, Ueda Y et al (1983) Mechanism of renal excretion of AM-715, a new quinolonecarboxylic acid derivative, in rabbits, dogs, and humans. *Antimicrob. Agents Chemother., 23*, 1.

36. Sudo K, Hashimoto K, Kurata T et al (1984) Metabolic disposition of DL-8280: the third report metabolism of 14C-DL-8280 in various animal species. *Chemotherapy (Tokyo), 32*, 1203.

37. Swanson BN, Bopparia KK, Vlasses PH et al (1983) Norfloxacin disposition after sequentially increasing oral doses. *Antimicrob. Agents Chemother., 23*, 284.

38. Vree TB, Wijnands WJA, Guelen PJM (1986) Pharmacokinetics, metabolism and renal excretion of quinolones in man. *Pharmaceut. Weekbl. Sci. Ed., 8*, 29.

39. Frydman AM, LeRoux Y, Lefebvre MA, Fourtillan JB, Gaillot J (1986) Pharmacokinetics of pefloxacin after repeated intravenous and oral administration (400 mg bid in young healthy volunteers). *J. Antimicrob. Chemother., 17, Suppl B*, 65.

40. Rohwedder R, Thorsteinsson SB, Bergan T (1986) In: *Abstracts, Congress on Bacterial and Parasitic Drug Resistance, Bangkok, 1986*, p 64, H.N. Press, Bangkok.

41. Webb DB, Roberts DE, Williams JD, Asscher AW (1986) Pharmacokinetics of ciprofloxacin in healthy volunteers and patients with impaired kidney function. *J. Antimicrob. Chemother., 18, Suppl D*, 83.

42. Danan G, Montay G, Cunci R, Erlinger S (1985) Pefloxacin kinetics in cirrhosis. *Clin. Pharmacol. Ther., 38*, 439.

43. Easmon CSF, Crane JP, Blowers A (1986) Effect of ciprofloxacin on intracellular organism: in-vitro and in-vivo studies. *J. Antimicrob. Chemother., 18, Suppl D*, 43.

44. Desnottes JF, Jacotot F, Bruel J, Bassoullet MT, Niel G (1986) Effects of pefloxacin on phagocytosis function of rat macrophages and polymorphonuclear leucocytes. *J. Antimicrob. Chemother., 17, Suppl B*, 53.

45. Dow J, Chazal J, Fryman AM, Janny P, Woehrle R, Djebbar F, Gaillot J (1986) Transfer kinetics of pefloxacin into cerebrospinal fluid after one hour iv infusion of 400 mg in man. *J. Antimicrob. Chemother., 17, Suppl B*, 81.

46. Rietbrock N, Staib AH (1987) Gyrase-Hemmer: unerwünschte zentralnervose Wirkun-

gen. *Dtsch. Med. Wochenschr., 112*, 201.

47. Stahl JP, Croize J, Akbaraly JP, Bru JP, Guyot A, Leduc D, Fourtillan JB, Micoud M (1986) Diffusion of ofloxacin into cerebrospinal fluid of patients with bacterial meningitis. In: *Abstracts, 9th International Congress of Infectious and Parasitic Diseases, Munich, July 20-26, 1986*, No. 716. Futuramed Verlag, Munich.
48. Arcieri G, August R, Becker N et al (1986) Clinical experience with ciprofloxacin in the USA. *Eur. J. Clin. Microbiol., 5*, 220.
49. Bergan T (1986) Norfloxacin: a review of clinical experiences. *J. Am. Med. Assoc. SE Asia, Spec. Suppl, April*, 57.
50. Blomer R, Bruch H, Zahlten RN (1986) Zusammen gefasste Ergebnisse der klinischen Phase II und III: Studien mit Ofloxacin (HOE 280) in Europa. *Infection, 14, Suppl 1*, 102.
51. Ishigami J (1985) Discussion. *Res. Clin. Forums, 7*, 107.
52. Schacht P, Deck K, Arcieri G, Ryoki T (1986) Overview of international clinical studies of ciprofloxacin, with special reference to safety. In: Neu HC, Weuta H (Eds), *Proceedings, 1st International Ciprofloxacin Workshop, Leverkusen, 1985*, p 435. Excerpta Medica, Amsterdam.
53. Arzneimittelkommission der deutschen Arzteschaft (1987) Neue Risikofaktoren zu Ofloxacin (Tarivid). *Dtsch. Aerztebl., 84*, B178.
54. Thorsteinsson SB, Bergan T, Oddsdottir S et al (1986) Crystalluria and ciprofloxacin, influence of urinary pH and hydration. *Chemotherapy (Tokyo) 32*, 404.
55. Luthy R (1986) Discussion. In: Neu HC, Weuta H (Eds), *Proceedings, 1st International Ciprofloxacin Workshop, Leverkusen, 1985*, p 69. Excerpta Medica, Amsterdam.
56. Staib AH, Harder S, Mieke S, Beer C, Stille W (1987) Gyrase inhibitors impair caffeine elimination in man. *Methods Find. Exp. Clin. Pharmacol., 9*, 193.
57. Garlando F, Tanber MG, Joos B, Oelz O, Luthy R (1985) Ciprofloxacin-induced haematuria. *Infection, 13*, 177.
58. Zilly W, Ziegler M, Richter E (1986) Interaktion zwischen Coffein und Theophyllin. *Med. Klin., 81*, 560.
59. Bergan T, Delin C, Johansen S et al (1986) Pharmacokinetics of ciprofloxacin and effect of repeated dosage on salivary and fecal microflora. *Antimicrob. Agents Chemother., 29*, 298.
60. Diridl G, Pichler H, Wolf D (1986) Four weeks' treatment of adult chronic *Salmonella* carriers with ciprofloxacin and its influence on the faecal flora. In: Neu H, Weuta H (Eds), *Proceedings, 1st International Ciprofloxacin Workshop, Leverkusen, 1985*, p 370. Excerpta Medica, Amsteram.
61. Reeves DS (1986) The effect of quinolone antibacterials on the gastrointestinal flora compared with that of other antibacterials. *J. Antimicrob. Chemother., 18, Suppl D*, 89.
62. Neu HC, Weuta H (Eds) (1986) *Proceedings, 1st International Ciprofloxacin Workshop, Leverkusen, 1985*, pp 287, 325. Excerpta Medica, Amsterdam.
63. Norrby R, Rylander M, Sandberg T et al (1987) Coordinated multicentre study of norfloxacin versus trimethoprim-sulfamethoxazole treatment of symptomatic urinary tract infections. *J. Infect. Dis., 155*, 170.
64. Cox CE, Callery SV, Tack KJ (1986) Clinical experience with ofloxacin in urinary tract infection. *Infection, 14, Suppl 4*, S303.
65. Blomer R, Bruch K, Zahlten RN (1986) Zusammengefasste Ergebnisse der klinischen Phase II – und III – Studien mit Ofloxacin (HOE 280) in Europa. *Infection, 14, Suppl 1*, S102.

66. Cox CE (1986) Comparative study of three dosage regimens of ciprofloxacin in the treatment of urinary tract infections. In: Neu HC, Weuta H (Eds), *Proceedings, 1st International Ciprofloxacin Workshop, Leverkusen, 1985*, p 291. Excerpta Medica, Amsterdam.

67. Grassi GG (1986) A multicentre study on clinical efficacy of ofloxacin in respiratory and urinary tract infections. *Infection, 14, Suppl 4*, S300.

68. Naber KG, Bartosik-Wich B (1986) ciprofloxacin versus norfloxacin in the treatment of complicated urinary tract infections: in vitro activity, serum and urine concentrations, safety and therapeutic efficacy. In: Neu HC, Weuta H (Eds), *Proceedings, 1st International Ciprofloxacin Workshop, Leverkusen, 1985*, p 314. Excerpta Medica, Amsterdam.

69. Kromann-Andersen B, Sommer P, Pers C et al (1986) Clinical evaluation of ofloxacin versus ciprofloxacin in complicated urinary tract infections. *Infection, 14, Suppl 4*, S305.

70. Heise-Reinecker E, Rusckmeyer J, Rosenfeld M (1986) Clinical efficacy of ciprofloxacin in *Salmonella* carriers. In: Neu HC, Weuta H (Eds), *Proceedings, 1st International Ciprofloxacin Workshop, Leverkusen, 1985*, p 373. Excerpta Medica, Amsterdam.

71. Limson BM (1986) Efficacy and safety of ciprofloxacin in uncomplicated typhoid fever. In: Neu HC, Weuta H (Eds), *Proceedings, 1st International Ciprofloxacin Workshop, Leverkusen, 1985*, p 362. Excerpta Medica, Amsterdam.

72. Pichler H, Diridl G, Wolf D (1986) Ciprofloxacin versus placebo in the treatment of acute bacterial diarrhoea. In: Neu HC, Weuta H (Eds), *Proceedings, 1st International Ciprofloxacin Workshop, Leverkusen, 1985*, p 357. Excerpta Medica, Amsterdam.

73. Ramirez CA, Bran JL, Mejia CR, Garcia JF (1986) Clinical efficacy of ciprofloxacin in typhoid fever. In: Neu HC, Weuta H (Eds), *Proceedings, 1st International Ciprofloxacin Workshop, Leverkusen, 1985*, p 365. Excerpta Medica, Amsterdam.

74. Schonwald S, Breitenfeld V, Car V, Gmajnicki B (1986) Treatment of acute diarrhoeal syndrome with ciprofloxacin: pilot study. In: Neu HC, Weuta H (Eds), *Proceedings, 1st International Ciprofloxacin Workshop, Leverkusen, 1985*, p 353. Excerpta Medica, Amsterdam.

75. Lauwers S, Vincken W, Naessens A, Pierard D (1986) Efficacy and safety of pefloxacin in the treatment of severe infections in patients hospitalized in intensive care units. *J. Antimicrob. Chemother., 17, Suppl B*, 111.

76. Mehtar S, Drabu YJ, Blakemore PH (1986) Efficacy and safety of ciprofloxacin in severe systemic infections. In: Neu HC, Weuta H (Eds), *Proceedings, 1st International Ciprofloxacin Workshop, Leverkusen, 1985*, p 414. Excerpta Medica, Amsterdam.

77. Ariyarit C, Panikabutra K, Chitwarakon A, Wongba C, Buatiang A (1986) Efficacy of ofloxacin in uncomplicated gonorrhoea at different dose levels: a double-blind dose response study. In: *Abstracts, 9th International Congress on Infectious and Parasitic Diseases, Munich, 1986*, No. 719. Futuramed Verlag, Munich.

78. Plummer FA (1986) Ciprofloxacin in chancroid: dose-finding and comparison with co-trimoxazole. In: Neu HC, Weuta H (Eds), *Proceedings, 1st International Ciprofloxacin Workshop, Leverkusen, 1985*, p 346. Excerpta Medica, Amsterdam.

79. Oriel JD (1986) Ciprofloxacin in the treatment of gonorrhoea and non-gonococcal urethritis. *J. Antimicrob. Chemother., 18, Suppl D*, 129.

80. Saito I (1986) Clinical evaluation of ofloxacin in treatment of non-gonococcal urethritis. In: Ishigami J (Ed), *Proceedings, 14th International Congress of Chemotherapy, Kyoto, 1985*, p 1817. University of Tokyo Press, Tokyo.

81. Bantz PM, Grote J, Peters-Haertel W, Stahmann J, Timm J, Kasten R, Bruck H (1987) Low-dose ciproflaxin in respiratory tract infections: a randomized comparison with doxycycline in general practice. *Am. J. Med. 82, Suppl 4A*, 208.

82. Gleadhill TC, Ferguson WP, Lowry RC (1986) Efficacy and safety of ciprofloxacin in patients with respiratory infections in comparison with amoxycillin. *J. Antimicrob. Chemother., 18, Suppl D*, 133.

83. Rubio TT, Shapiro C (1986) Ciprofloxacin in the treatment of pseudomonas infections in cystic fibrosis. *J. Antimicrob. Chemother., 18, Suppl D*, 147.

84. Davies BI, Maesen FPV, Baur C (1986) Ciprofloxacin in the treatment of acute exacerbations of chronic bronchitis. *Eur. J. Clin. Microbiol., 5*, 226.

85. Ernst JA, Sy ER, Colon-Lucca H, Sandhu N, Rallos T, Lorian V (1986) Ciprofloxacin in the treatment of pneumonia. *Antimicrob. Agents Chemother., 29*, 1088.

86. Mohr CP (1986) Ciprofloxacin-Therapie bei Infektionen der oberen und unteren Luftwege. *Krankenhausarzt, 59*, 667.

87. Kobayashi H (1986) Clinical evaluation of ofloxacin in lower respiratory tract infections. *Infection, 14, Suppl 4*, S279.

88. Devogelaere R, Maes P (1986) Ofloxacin in lower respiratory tract infections – a comparison with amoxicillin. *Infection, 14, Suppl 4*, S283.

89. Lam WK, Chau PY, So SY, Leung YK, Chan JCK, Sham MK (1986) A double-blind randomized study comparing ofloxacin episodes in bronchiectasis. *Infection, 14, Suppl 4*, S290.

90. Lam WK, Chau PY, So SY, Leung YK, Chan JCK, Sham MK (1986) A double-blind randomized study comparing ofloxacin and amoxicillin in treating infective episodes in bronchiectasis. In: *Abstracts, 9th International Congress on Infectious and Parasitic Diseases, Munich, 1986*, No. 714. Futuramed Verlag, Munich.

91. Davies BI, Maesen FPV, Teengs JP, Baur C (1986) Neue orale Chinolon-Verbindungen bei chronischer Bronchitis. *Infection, 14, Suppl 1*, S73.

92. Kurz CC, Marget W, Harms K, Bertele RM (1986) Kreuzstudie über die Wirksamkeit von Ofloxacin und Ciprofloxacin bei oraler Anwendung. *Infection, 14, Suppl 1*, S82.

93. Giamarellou H, Galanakis N, Dendrinos C, Stefanon J, Daphnis E, Daikos GK (1986) Evaluation of ciprofloxacin in the treatment of *Pseudomonas aeruginosa* infections. *Eur. J. Clin. Microbiol., 5*, 232.

94. Follath F, Bindschedler M, Wenk M, Frei R, Stalder H, Reber H (1986) Use of ciprofloxacin in the treatment of *Pseudomonas aeruginosa* infections. *Eur. J. Clin. Microbiol., 5*, 236.

95. Gilbert DN, Tice AD, Marsh PK, Craven PC (1987) Oral ciprofloxacin therapy for chronic contiguous osteomyelitis caused by aerobic gram-negative bacilli. *Am. J. Med., 82, Suppl 4A*, 254.

96. Slama TG, Misinski J, Sklar S (1987) Oral ciprofloxin therapy for osteomyelitis caused by aerobic gram-negative bacilli. *Am. J. Med., 82, Suppl 4A*, 259.

97. Greenberg RN, Tice AD, Marsh PM, Craven PC, Reilly PM, Bollinger M, Weinandt WJ (1987) Randomized trial of ciprofloxacin compared with other antimicrobial therapy in the treatment of osteomyelitis. *Am. J. Med., 82, Suppl 4A*, 266.

98. Fass RJ (1986) Treatment of skin and soft tissue infections with oral ciprofloxacin. *J. Antimicrob. Chemother., 18, Suppl D*, 153.

99. Wood MJ, Logan MN (1986) Ciprofloxacin for soft tissue infections. *J. Antimicrob. Chemother., 18*, Suppl D, 159.

100. Bow EJ, Louie TJ, Rayner E (1985) Norfloxacin versus trimethoprim/sulfamethoxaz-

ole for infection prevention in patients with acute leukemia. In: *Abstracts, 25th Interscience Conference on Antimicrobial Agents and Chemotherapy, Minneapolis, 1985*, No. 150.

101. Karp JE, Hendricksen C, Redden T et al (1985) Double-blind randomized trial of prophylactic norfloxacin on infections in acute leukemia. In: *Abstracts, 25th Interscience Conference on Antibacterial Agents and Chemotherapy, Minneapolis, 1985*, No. 149.

102. Smith GM, Leyland MJ, Farrell ID, Geddes AM (1986) Preliminary evaluation of ciprofloxacin, a new 4-quinolone antibiotic, in the treatment of febrile neutropenic patients. *J. Antimicrob. Chemother., 18, Suppl D*, 165.

103. Wood ME, Newland AC (1986) Intravenous ciprofloxacin in the treatment of infection in immunocompromised patients. *J. Antimicrob. Chemother., 18, Suppl D*, 175.

CHAPTER 16

Rifampin

JOAN E. KAPUSNIK and MERLE A. SANDE

The rifamycins are a group of antibiotics isolated from *Nocardia mediterranei*. Rifampin (rifampicin) is a semisynthetic antibiotic derivative of rifamycin B (3-(4-methylpiperazin-1-yliminomethyl)rifamycin SV). Rifampin is a zwitterion and is soluble in organic solvents and water at acidic pH. It has been extensively used in the treatment of tuberculosis and Hansen's disease (leprosy) and for chemoprophylaxis of meningococcal disease (1, 2). More recently its utility in the treatment of infections caused by other bacterial pathogens has been more widely recognized (3, 4). The debate as to whether or not rifampin should be used in short courses for the treatment of non-tuberculous infections or whether it should be withheld for fear of the inadvertent generation of rifampin-resistant *Mycobacterium tuberculosis* is still alive (5). This Chapter will focus more closely on the place of rifampin in this newer area of antibacterial indications.

ACTIVITY

Rifampin has a unique antimicrobial mechanism of action. It is bactericidal and inhibits DNA-dependent RNA polymerase at its β-subunit, stopping chain initiation. Since this mechanism is unique, bacterial cross-resistance with other classes of antimicrobial agents has not been observed to occur (6). Rifampin is active in vitro against most aerobic gram-positive cocci and bacilli and against aerobic gram-negative organisms, such as *Escherichia coli, Klebsiella* species, *Proteus* species, *Pseudomonas* species, *Haemophilus influenzae, Neisseria* species, and *Brucella* species. Most mycobacteria, *Chlamydia*, rickettsiae, and anaerobic bacteria including some *Bacteroides* species are also susceptible. Certain fungi, including *Candida* species, and viruses have been shown in vitro to be inhibited by high concentrations of rifampin (7–12).

Of interest most recently, however, is the antistaphylococcal activity of rifampin. It is active against both *Staphylococcus aureus* and *Staphylococcus epidermidis*. It is the most active antimicrobial by weight against susceptible strains (7, 13). In one study the minimum inhibitory concentration for 90% (MIC_{90}) of rifampin

Antimicrobial Agents Annual 3
P.K. Peterson and J. Verhoef, editors

for 75 strains of *S. aureus* ranged from 0.004 to 0.03 μg/ml for both methicillin-susceptible and methicillin-resistant isolates (14). Similarly, 90% of methicillin-resistant, coagulase-negative staphylococci (25 strains) were inhibited by 0.02 μg/ml of rifampin (15).

Clinically the major drawback to the use of rifampin for staphylococcal infections has been the rapid emergence of high-level rifampin resistance (16, 17). Unfortunately, staphylococci, as with mycobacteria and other bacteria, quickly become resistant (MIC > 512 μg/ml) to rifampin when it is used alone. In vivo this can be significant, especially under two circumstances: (a) when there is a large bacterial inoculum at the site of infection ($> 10^6$); (b) when rifampin is used as single drug therapy for a prolonged period.

In a given bacterial inoculum the spontaneous mutation rate is 1 in 10^6 colony-forming units that will be found to have high-level rifampin resistance. The mechanism appears to be due to a single amino acid change in the β-subunit of RNA polymerase, which results in a conformational change of this target enzyme. Subsequent binding or attachment of the rifampin molecule at this altered target site occurs much less readily, if at all (18). Thus, in situations with large bacterial populations or with continuous rifampin exposure sensitive organisms are killed, leaving the highly resistant subpopulations to emerge as the dominant phenotype. In a clinical setting rifampin-resistant strains have emerged even when multiple-drug therapy has been used (19, 20).

To combat the problem of bacterial resistance, combination chemotherapy has usually been recommended (21). Finding the ideal companion drug for rifampin has been difficult since most classes of antibiotics, especially β-lactams, produce either an indifferent or antagonistic effect when tested with rifampin in vitro (22). In vitro studies (serum bactericidal titers and time-kill curves) have shown the combination of rifampin and erythromycin, trimethoprim, or clindamycin to have increased bactericidal activity (23). Others as well have shown trimethoprim in combination with rifampin to have increased bactericidal activity against staphylococci as well as other bacteria (24–26). These non-β-lactam antimicrobial agents and other drugs (e.g. ciprofloxacin, teicoplanin) combined with rifampin appear to warrant further in vivo testing.

The observed in vitro antagonism or reduction in antibacterial activity, which has been observed utilizing the classical testing methods (checkerboard or time-kill studies), however, has not been consistent with clinical experience or the experience in animal models of infection. Studies utilizing an animal model of *S. aureus* endocarditis has demonstrated enhanced killing by rifampin (in various dosages) with cloxacillin, compared to animals administered either drug alone, despite in vitro studies suggesting antagonism with the combination (27). Results of a placebo-controlled, double-blinded clinical trial also suggest enhanced efficacy with a combination of rifampin plus a β-lactam or vancomycin in severely ill patients (28).

The explanation for this in vitro/in vivo discrepancy is unclear. The success of this drug in vivo may be partially explained by the exceptional antistaphylococcal activity of rifampin plus its ability to distribute widely to tissues and penetrate into hidden recesses of infection (see 'Clinical Pharmacology' below). Clinically, the addition of the β-lactam antibiotic for the most part is done to effectively kill the minority of rifampin-resistant strains, and thus prevent their emergence into the majority population.

Rifampin has offered benefits in the treatment of infections caused by methicillin-resistant *S. aureus* and *S. epidermidis* where vancomycin is the primary drug used. This observation may be due to differences in pharmacologic properties for these two agents, as they do not penetrate to the same degree to potential sites of infection. Vancomycin penetrates less well into many tissues and body fluids, including the cerebrospinal fluid (CSF). However, combining vancomycin with rifampin has failed in a few instances to prevent the emergence of rifampin-resistant strains for both *S. aureus* and *S. epidermidis* when large numbers of organisms were present in deep-seated infections (29, 30).

In summary, there seem to be two major reasons for the slow clinical acceptance of rifampin for routine treatment of bacterial infections: (a) the antagonistic or indifferent effects in vitro observed from tested combinations, even though these results are not predictive of relative in vivo efficacy; (b) the rapid emergence of high-level rifampin-resistant strains. Rifampin-induced adverse reactions and drug-drug interactions have also played a role in reducing the appeal of this drug (see below).

CLINICAL PHARMACOLOGY

Rifampin possesses unique pharmacokinetic properties. It is highly lipid-soluble, which allows it to penetrate into various tissues and bodily fluids that would be considered 'hidden recesses', including the central nervous system, bone, and abscess cavities. The drug is also concentrated within phagocytic cells, thus facilitating the subsequent killing of sequestered intraleukocytic staphylococci (31–34). In experimental infections of localized or disseminated staphylococcal abscesses and chronic osteomyelitis, rifampin has proven to be a most effective antistaphylococcal drug. Its lipophilic property also increases the ability of the drug to access ocular fluids, respiratory and nasal secretions. This is especially important because it makes rifampin useful for the eradication of susceptible organisms from the nasopharynx (for bacterial 'carrier-states'). Rifampin administration has been shown to eliminate effectively the nasopharyngeal carriage of *Neisseria meningitidis, Haemophilus influenzae*, and group A streptococci in asymptomatic patients (35–38). It has also been used in combination with other agents (trimethoprim + sulfamethoxazole) to eradicate colonization of methicillin-resistant and methicillin-sensitive *S. aureus* (39, 40).

Rifampin is commercially available only in an oral capsule dosage form. An intravenous preparation is available for investigational use from the manufacturer (Merrell Dow Pharmaceuticals Inc., Cincinnati, Ohio, U.S.A.). A 600 mg oral dosage produces a peak serum drug concentration of 7–8 $\mu g/ml$ (approx. 2 h after the dose), and a trough concentration (24 h later) of 1–2 $\mu g/ml$ (41, 42). The drug is widely distributed throughout the body, and penetrates well into most tissues (e.g. lung, liver, kidney) (43, 44). Rifampin crosses the placenta, producing clinically significant concentrations of drug in the fetus and amniotic fluid (45). Rifampin penetrates inflamed meninges and achieves effective concentrations in the CSF for most susceptible organisms after usual oral dosages (46). The CSF concentration may increase 4- to 8-fold in patients with meningitis (47). The protein-binding of rifampin in serum is in the range of 80–90% (48, 49).

Rifampin is mostly metabolized by the liver to desacetyl-rifampin, which also has some antimicrobial activity. This metabolite is rapidly eliminated in the bile, but reabsorption via enterohepatic recirculation does occur. A small percent (16%) of rifampin is excreted unchanged into the urine (50). The elimination half-life of rifampin (parent compound) has been observed to be 1.5–5 hours. The half-life is prolonged in patients with severe liver disease, but is unaffected by renal insufficiency (51, 52).

ADVERSE EFFECTS AND DRUG INTERACTIONS

Mild gastrointestinal symptoms are the most common side effects from rifampin therapy. As common is the discoloration of urine and of other bodily secretions to a red color. This red discoloration has been used as a marker for monitoring the patients' medication compliance. Also reported is the red discoloration of soft contact lenses by rifampin (53).

Some patients have developed a 'flu-like' syndrome, which is thought to be a febrile immunological reaction to the drug. There is some evidence to suggest that this syndrome is dose-related and related to once-weekly (intermittent) dosing (54). This syndrome has been rarely associated with renal failure or hepatorenal syndrome (55). The topic of rifampin-induced renal insufficiency has recently been reviewed and the literature still confirms acute interstitial nephritis as the most common presentation. However, the clinicopathologic spectrum reported for rifampin-induced renal failure includes acute hemoglobinuric renal failure secondary to hemolysis, diffuse intravascular coagulopathy, renal cortical necrosis, proliferative glomerulonephritis, nephrotic syndrome, hypokalemic renal tubular acidosis, and light-chain proteinuria with or without obstructive nephropathy (56, 57). The avoidance of dehydration or contrast dye use during rifampin therapy may reduce the potential for light-chain-induced acute renal failure.

Thrombocytopenia has been observed and is postulated to be due to the effects of anti-rifampin antibodies (58). This side effect also has been more commonly associated with intermittent (twice weekly), high-dose (>900 mg/d) regimens. Patients experiencing this side effect may require dosage reduction and/or be switched to a daily treatment regimen (59). Other hematologic side-effects have also been reported, including leukopenia, hemolysis, and anemia (60–62).

Rifampin has been reported to cause hepatic dysfunction, ranging from fulminant hepatitis with encephalopathy, to uncomplicated jaundice (63). The hepatitis in patients receiving isoniazid + rifampin resembles the clinical picture for isoniazid-induced hepatitis (64). The incidence, however, increases from 1% for isoniazid alone, to 5–8% during combination therapy (65). The effect of rifampin on the metabolism of isoniazid in human volunteers has been investigated. Rifampin was observed to induce hepatic microsomal enzymes, however, it did not increase the urinary appearance of the metabolites of isoniazid. Therefore, it is not possible to predict the effect of rifampin on isoniazid hepatotoxicity (66). The use of rifampin and isoniazid is not contraindicated in individuals (e.g. alcoholics with cirrhosis) who do not have significant pre-existing hepatic disease, which is evident by significant changes in prothrombin time or encephalopathy (67).

Rifampin is a potent hepatic enzyme-inducer, which explains the many reported drug-drug interactions. In fact, rifampin is reported to induce its own metabolism (desacetylation). Rifampin has been shown to increase menstrual irregularities and cause amenorrhea, presumably by inducing the metabolism or reducing the activity of endogenous hormones. Probably via a similar mechanism rifampin therapy is associated with an increase in the rate of unwanted pregnancies in patients taking oral contraceptives (68, 69). Patients should be advised to use an alternative method of birth control during rifampin therapy.

Rifampin has also been observed to antagonize the clinical effects, and increase the metabolism of warfarin, corticosteroids, quinidine, diazepam, digoxin, phenytoin, cyclosporin, verapamil and theophylline (70–78). It may be necessary to increase the dosages of these agents during rifampin therapy. Of great importance is the newly recognized rifampin-cyclosporin interaction in the post-organ-transplantation setting (79–81). In this situation a rifampin-corticosteroid interaction is important as well. Rifampin is a potent inducer of cyclosporin and steroid metabolism and additionally appears to have an immunosuppressive effect shown to be an interference with mechanisms involved in specific transplantation tolerance. Caution should be exercised when using rifampin in transplant recipients and cyclosporin levels should be monitored more closely.

The simultaneous oral administration of para-aminosalicylic acid (PAS) may impair the gastrointestinal absorption of rifampin (82), as does taking rifampin with food (83). When PAS and rifampin are to be used concurrently, as they are commonly for the treatment of tuberculosis, their administration should be separated by an interval of 8–12 hours.

CLINICAL USES

Rifampin is one of the most effective antimicrobial agents for the treatment of the various mycobacterial infections, but is always used in combination with another agent(s) (84, 85). Rifampin is the drug of choice for chemoprophylaxis in household contacts of patients with infections due to *Neisseria meningitidis* and *H. influenzae* meningitis (35, 86–88).

Studies have also confirmed the efficacy of rifampin for the elimination of the staphylococcal nasal carrier-state, which is important for hemodialysis patients, intravenous drug users, or in other persons, such as health-care providers (39, 89). The successful eradication of methicillin-resistant *S. aureus* colonization has been achieved utilizing rifampin in combination with a variety of other antimicrobials (e.g. trimethoprim + sulfamethoxazole, erythromycin, novobiocin, fusidic acid) (40, 90–92).

The effect of single-dose rifampin (600 mg) on the oral microflora has been evaluated in 17 healthy volunteers as a preliminary study to delineate the possible role of rifampin as pre-operative prophylaxis for patients undergoing head and neck surgery (93). Such surgical procedures are associated with a high infection rate. Salivary specimens cultured prior to and after rifampin administration revealed that both aerobic and anaerobic bacterial growth was inhibited by the drug. This result is not surprising since rifampin attains high salivary concentrations. Clinical trials will be necessary to determine the role of rifampin, alone or in combination with another antimicrobial agent, for the prophylaxis of head and neck surgery.

The treatment of patients with recurrent furunculosis (who also are nasal carriers of *S. aureus*) has been studied using 7–10 days therapy with the combination of rifampin + cloxacillin (3). All patients studied had previously failed at least 3 courses of conventional antistaphylococcal therapy. Thirty-one of 32 patients were cured of their recurrent boils and had *S. aureus* eliminated from their nasal secretions. Only 6 of the 31 patients needed 2–3 additional treatment courses.

Rifampin penetrates into phagocytic cells where it remains microbiologically active and kills susceptible organisms that survive in the intracellular environment (e.g. staphylococci). This characteristic has been examined in various animal models of *S. aureus* infection (94–96). Following intraperitoneal inoculation of organisms, animal survival was significantly increased in those that received rifampin, compared to animals given only methicillin or penicillin. Also, abscess formation from a subcutaneous injection of *S. aureus* was significantly reduced in animals receiving rifampin, compared to those receiving β-lactam antimicrobial agents. These observations suggest the importance of rifampin in the therapy of infections that involve large collections of neutrophils and sequestered *S. aureus*. Thus, as an example, rifampin may offer a particular advantage to patients with chronic granulomatous disease, a state where patients are unable to eradicate staphylococcal infections because of 'hidden' intracellular foci (97–99).

The successful treatment of patients with deep-seated staphylococcal infections (e.g. osteomyelitis, endocarditis) depends largely upon sufficient and sustained antimicrobial concentrations at the site of infection. Staphylococcal osteomyelitis is an infection associated with the formation of pus and sequestra. Rifampin concentrations in diseased bone were in one study observed to be above the MIC of the infecting organism for up to 24 hours after a single 40 mg/kg dose (100). Osteomyelitis in an animal model has been shown to be more effectively treated with combination therapy that included rifampin (101–103). Human studies have evaluated the role of rifampin in the treatment of chronic staphylococcal osteomyelitis

(104). Various agents have been used in combination with rifampin. Results revealed a microbiologic cure in 20 of 21 patients (95%); however, 30% of patients did not have a clinical cure. Clinical failures were possibly because of unresolved polymicrobial infection, inflammatory sinus drainage, or the inability to culture the organisms causing persistent infection ('culture-negative' infection).

Cloxacillin and rifampin, alone or in combination, were studied in the treatment of experimental *S. aureus* endocarditis (105). Four of 5 combination drug regimens produced an improved rate of eradication of the organisms from cardiac vegetations. 'Peak' serum samples taken for serum bactericidal titer (SBTs) failed to predict the observed efficacy improvement for the animals receiving rifampin + oxacillin. An anecdotal report of 2 patients with endocarditis caused by methicillin-tolerant *S. aureus* demonstrated cure with the combination of rifampin (20 mg/kg/d) with an aminoglycoside (106). The isolates from these patients were tested in vitro and efficacy with this regimen was predicted.

In experimental models of *S. epidermidis* endocarditis, rifampin was observed to be quite active (107, 108). Cure rates in patients treated for methicillin-resistant *S. epidermidis* prosthetic valve endocarditis were improved significantly by the addition of rifampin to antimicrobial regimens (109).

The treatment of infections in the presence of a foreign body truly tests an antimicrobial agent's ability to eradicate infection, in as much as investigations have demonstrated that phagocytic cell activity is markedly reduced in the presence of a prosthesis or foreign body. Under these conditions polymorphonuclear leukocytes (PMNs) exhibit a significant reduction in their ability to function properly (generate superoxide in response to a particulate or a soluble stimulus) (110). This inability to respond is probably a result of the 'activation' of PMNs by the foreign body. This activated state is sustained with no recovery phase and is followed by degranulation and loss of bactericidal capacity. Under these circumstances rifampin therapy may be especially useful since the drug penetrates well into PMNs and is active within neutrophils that have been 'inactivated' (by the presence of a foreign body) (111).

A clinical trial has examined the potential value of using the combination of rifampin and a β-lactam or vancomycin for the treatment of a wide variety of staphylococcal infections (112). In at least one study the patients that were given the combination regimen had a significantly better outcome. A better clinical outcome was again not consistent with the results of SBTs from these patients. The addition of rifampin to therapy was shown to reduce peak and trough SBTs, compared to the SBTs from patients receiving the standard single-drug, β-lactam treatment. Another report suggests that rifampin + minocycline is useful in the treatment of a variety of severe infections due to multiresistant (methicillin-resistant and aminoglycoside-resistant) *S. aureus* (113).

Meningitis due to *S. aureus* has been reviewed in a small retrospective study of 10 patients (114). Six patients treated with rifampin plus a semisynthetic penicillin regimen were cured, in contrast to 3 of 4 patients who died that were treated with non-rifampin combinations. Further trials with rifampin in combination with other antistaphylococcal antibiotics for the treatment of staphylococcal meningitis are warranted.

DOSING

Adults should receive a dosage of 600 mg and children 10–20 mg/kg daily (not to exceed 600 mg/d) for the treatment of *M. tuberculosis*. This same regimen can be administered on 4 consecutive days for the eradication of the *N. meningitidis* or *H. influenzae* carrier-states. It is generally recommended that rifampin be administered once daily, either 1 hour before or 2 hours after meals. The once-daily dosage interval was designed, however, for the treatment of infections caused by mycobacteria and for eradication of carrier-states. The new role of rifampin in the treatment of bacterial infections may require more frequent dosing. For example, in the treatment of deep-seated staphylococcal infections the authors recommend twice-daily dosing, 300–600 mg dosages every 12 hours for adults. Therapy for pediatric non-tuberculous infections requires a dosage of 15 mg/kg twice daily (115).

Patients who are unable to swallow the commercially available capsules should receive a suspension (1 mg/ml). To prepare this suspension, empty the contents of four 300 mg capsules and mix with 20 ml simple syrup; shake vigorously, then add 100 ml simple syrup for a total volume of 120 ml. Stability studies indicate that this suspension is stable for 6 weeks if refrigerated. Shake the suspension before each dose is administered (116).

FUTURE DIRECTIONS

New, long-acting rifamycin SV derivatives (cyclopentylrifampins) are being investigated for their activity against *M. tuberculosis* (117), as well as for their antistaphylococcal activity (118, 119). Anecdotal reports, and experience in our institution with patients who have deep-seated *S. aureus* infections (endocarditis, osteomyelitis) that are treated with vancomycin alone, have been disappointing (HF Chambers, personal communication). These infections were notable for refractory bacteremia while on antibiotics. The addition of rifampin with or without an aminoglycoside cleared their bacteremia in some cases. Therefore, patients with deep-seated *S. aureus* infections accompanied by persistent bacteremia may benefit from early combination therapy which includes rifampin.

Rifampin has a very broad spectrum of antibacterial, antifungal and antiviral activity. The significance of this broad in vitro activity needs to be tested in vivo in animal models of infection in order to assess its potential clinical usefulness. The role of rifampin in the treatment of other non-tuberculous infections and non-staphylococcal infections is slowly being elucidated. Experimental infections and in humans with brucellosis (120–122), *Legionella* pneumonia (123–125), and listeriosis (126) have been treated successfully using combination therapies that include rifampin.

REFERENCES

1. Long MW, Snider Jr DE, Farer LS (1979) U.S. Public Health Service Cooperative Trial of three rifampin-isoniazid regimens in treatment of pulmonary tuberculosis. *Am. Rev. Respir. Dis., 119*, 879.
2. Sanders WE (1976) Rifampin. *Ann. Intern. Med., 85*, 82.
3. Kapusnik JE, Parenti F, Sande MA (1984) The use of rifampin in staphylococcal infections – a review. *J. Antimicrob. Chemother., 13, Suppl C*, 61.
4. Gruneberg RN, Emmerson AM, Ridgway GL (1984) Rifampicin-containing antibiotic combinations in the treatment of difficult infections. *J. Antimicrob. Chemother., 13, Suppl C*, 49.
5. Gruneberg RN, Emmerson AM, Cremer AWF (1985) Rifampicin for non-tuberculous infections? *Chemotherapy, 31*, 324.
6. Wehrli W, Staehelin M (1971) Actions of rifamycins. *Bacteriol. Rev., 35*, 290.
7. Thornsberry C, Hill BC, Swenson JM, McDougal LK (1983) Rifampin: spectrum of antibacterial activity. *Rev. Infect. Dis., 5, Suppl 3*, S412.
8. Atlas E, Turck M (1968) Laboratory and clinical evaluation of rifampin. *Am. J. Med. Sci., 256*, 247.
9. Kunin CM, Brandt D, Wood H (1969) Bacteriologic studies of rifampin, a new semisynthetic antibiotic. *J. Infect. Dis., 119*, 132.
10. McCabe WR, Lorian V (1968) Comparison of the antibacterial activity of rifampicin and other antibiotics. *Am. J. Med. Sci., 256*, 255.
11. Varaldo PE, Debbia E, Schito GC (1985) In vitro activities of rifapentine and rifampin, alone and in combination with six other antibiotics, against methicillin-susceptible and methicillin-resistant staphylococci of different species. *Antimicrob. Agents Chemother., 27*, 615.
12. Tuazon CU, Shamsuddin D, Miller H (1982) Antibiotic susceptibility and synergy of clinical isolates of *Listeria monocytogenes. Antimicrob. Agents Chemother., 21*, 525.
13. Sabath LD, Garner C, Wilcox C, Finland M (1976) Susceptibility of *Staphylococcus aureus* and *Staphylococcus epidermidis* to 65 antibiotics. *Antimicrob. Agents Chemother., 9*, 962.
14. Traczewski MM, Goldmann DA, Murphy P (1983) In vitro activity of rifampin in combination with oxacillin against *Staphylococcus aureus. Antimicrob. Agents Chemother., 23*, 571.
15. Lowy FD, Chang DS, Lash PR (1983) Synergy of combinations of vancomycin, gentamicin, and rifampin against methicillin-resistant, coagulase-negative staphylococci. *Antimicrob. Agents Chemother., 23*, 932.
16. Acar JF, Goldstein FW, Duval J (1983) Use of rifampin for the treatment of serious staphylococcal and gram-negative infections. *Rev. Infect. Dis., 5, Suppl 3*, S502.
17. Moorman DR, Mandell GL (1981) Characteristics of rifampin-resistant variants obtained from clinical isolates of *Staphylococcus aureus. Antimicrob. Agents Chemother., 20*, 709.
18. Wehrli W (1983) Rifampin: mechanism of action and resistance. *Rev. Infect. Dis., 5, Suppl 3*, S407.

211

19. Chamovitz B, Bryant RE, Gilbert DN, Hartstein AI (1985) Prosthetic valve endocarditis caused by *Staphylococcus epidermidis*. *J. Am. Med. Assoc., 253*, 2867.
20. Eng RHK, Smith SM, Tillem M, Cherubin C (1985) Rifampin resistance: development during therapy of methicillin-resistant *Staphylococcus aureus* infection. *Arch. Intern. Med., 145*, 146.
21. Sande MA (1983) The use of rifampin in the treatment of nontuberculous infections: an overview. *Rev. Infect. Dis., 5, Suppl 3*, S399.
22. Watanakunakorn C, Tisone JC (1982) Antagonism between nafcillin and oxacillin and rifampin against *Staphylococcus aureus*. *Antimicrob. Agents Chemother., 22*, 920.
23. Hackbarth CJ, Chambers HF, Sande MA (1986) Serum bactericidal activity of rifampin in combination with other antimicrobial agents against *Staphylococcus aureus*. *Antimicrob. Agents Chemother., 29*, 611.
24. Farrell W, Wilks M, Drasar FA (1977) The action of trimethoprim and rifampicin in combination against gram-negative rods resistant to gentamicin. *J. Antimicrob. Chemother., 3*, 459.
25. Gruneberg RN, Emmerson AM (1977) The interaction between rifampicin and trimethoprim: an in vitro study. *J. Antimicrob. Chemother., 3*, 453.
26. Arioli V, Berti M, Carniti G, Rossi E (1977) Interaction between rifampicin and trimethoprim in vitro and in experimental infections. *J. Antimicrob. Chemother., 3*, 87.
27. Zinner SH, Lagast H, Klastersky J (1981) Antistaphylococcal activity of rifampin with other antibiotics. *J. Infect. Dis., 144*, 365.
28. Van der Auwera P, Klastersky J, Thys JP et al (1985) Double-blind, placebo-controlled study of oxacillin combined with rifampin in the treatment of staphylococcal infections. *Antimicrob. Agents Chemother., 28*, 467.
29. Simon GL, Smith RH, Sande MA (1983) Emergence of rifampin-resistant strains of *Staphylococcus aureus* during combination therapy with vancomycin and rifampicin: a report of two cases. *Rev. Infect. Dis., 5, Suppl 3*, S507.
30. Karchmer AW, Archer GA, and the Endocarditis Study Group (1984) Methicillin-resistant *Staphylococcus epidermidis* (SE) prosthetic valve (PV) endocarditis (E). In: *Program and Abstracts, 24th Interscience Conference of Antimicrobial Agents and Chemotherapy, Washington, DC, 1984*, p 177. American Society of Microbiology, Washington, DC.
31. Nesthus I, Haneberg B, Glette J, Solberg CO (1985) The influence of antimicrobial agents on macrophage-associated *Staphylococcus aureus*. *Acta Pathol. Microbiol. Immunol. Scand., 93*, 189.
32. Mandell GL (1973) Interaction of intraleukocytic bacteria and antibiotics. *J. Clin. Invest., 52*, 1673.
33. Hand WL, Corwin RW, Steinberg TH, Grossman GD (1984) Uptake of antibiotics by human alveolar macrophages. *Am. Rev. Respir. Dis., 129*, 933.
34. Mandell GL, Vest TK (1972) Killing of intraleukocytic *Staphylococcus aureus* by rifampin: in vitro and in vivo studies. *J. Infect. Dis., 125*, 486.
35. Beaty HN (1983) Rifampin and minocycline in meningococcal disease. *Rev. Infect. Dis., 5, Suppl 3*, S451.
36. Fleming DW, Leibenhaut MH, Albanee D et al (1985) Secondary *Haemophilus influenzae* type b in day-care facilities: risk factors and prevention. *J. Am. Med. Assoc., 254*, 509.
37. Glode MP, Daum RS, Boies EG et al (1985) Effect of rifampin chemoprophylaxis on carriage eradication and new acquisition of *Haemophilus influenzae* type b in contacts. *Pediatrics, 76*, 537.

38. Tanz RR, Shulman ST, Barthel MJ et al (1985) Penicillin plus rifampin eradicates pharyngeal carriage of group A streptococci. *J. Pediatr., 106*, 876.
39. Wheat LJ, Kohler RB, Luft FC, White A (1983) Long-term studies of the effect of rifampin on nasal carriage of coagulase-positive staphylococci. *Rev. Infect. Dis., 5, Suppl 3*, S459.
40. Ellison III RT, Judson FN, Peterson LC et al (1984) Oral rifampin and trimethoprim/ sulfamethoxazole therapy in asymptomatic carriers of methicillin-resistant *Staphylococcus aureus* infections. *West. J. Med., 140*, 735.
41. Radner DB (1973) Toxicologic and pharmacologic aspects of rifampin. *Chest, 64*, 213.
42. Kucer A, Bennett NMcK (1979) Rifampicin (Rifampin). In: Kucer A, Bennett NMcK (Eds), *The Use of Antibiotics: A Comprehensive Review with Clinical Emphasis, 3rd ed.*, p 552. Heinemann Medical Books, London.
43. Kenny MT, Strates B (1981) Metabolism and pharmacokinetics of the antibiotic rifampin. *Drug Metab. Rev., 12*, 159.
44. Sensi P, Maggi N, Furesz S, Maffii G (1967) Chemical modifications and biological properties of rifamycins. *Antimicrob. Agents Chemother., 1967*, 699.
45. Binda G, Domenichini E, Gottardi A et al (1971) Rifampicin, a general review. *Arzneim.-Forsch., 21*, 1907.
46. Barling RWA, Selkon JB (1978) The penetration of antibiotics into cerebrospinal fluid and brain tissue. *J. Antimicrob. Chemother., 4*, 203.
47. D'Oliveira JJG (1972) Cerebrospinal fluid concentrations of rifampin in meningeal tuberculosis. *Am. Rev. Respir. Dis., 106*, 432.
48. Bowman G (1973) Protein binding of rifampicin: a review. *Scand. J. Respir. Dis., Suppl 84*, 40.
49. Bowman G, Ringberger VA (1974) Binding of rifampicin by human plasma proteins. *Eur. J. Clin. Pharmacol., 7*, 369.
50. Nitti V, Virgilio R, Patricolo MR, Iuliano A (1977) A pharmacokinetic study of intravenous rifampicin. *Chemotherapy, 23*, 1.
51. Acocella G, Bonollo L, Gariroldi M et al (1972) Kinetics of rifampicin and isoniazid administered alone and in combination to normal subjects and patients with liver disease. *Gut, 13*, 47.
52. Acocella G (1983) Pharmacokinetics and metabolism of rifampin in humans. *Rev. Infect. Dis., 5, Suppl 3*, S428.
53. Harris J, Jenkins P (1985) Discoloration of soft contact lenses by rifampicin. *Lancet, 2*, 1133.
54. Dickinson JM, Mitchison DA, Lee SK et al (1977) Serum rifampicin concentration related to dose size and to the incidence of the 'flu' syndrome during intermittent rifampicin administration. *J. Antimicrob. Chemother., 3*, 445.
55. Flynn CT, Rainford DJ, Hope E (1974) Acute renal failure and rifampin: danger of unsuspected intermittent dosage. *Br. Med. J., 2*, 482.
56. Soffer O, Nassar VH, Campbell Jr WG, Bourke D (1987) Light chain cast nephropathy and acute renal failure associated with rifampin therapy. *Am. J. Med., 82*, 1052.
57. Cohn JR, Fye DL, Sills JM, Francos GC (1985) Rifampicin-induced renal failure. *Tubercle, 66*, 289.
58. Blajchman MA, Lowry RC, Petit JE, Stradling P (1970) Rifampin-induced immune thrombocytopenia. *Br. Med. J., 3*, 24.
59. Poole G, Stradling P, Worlledge S (1971) Potentially serious side effects of high-dose twice-weekly rifampicin. *Br. Med. J., 3*, 343.

60. Girling DJ (1977) Adverse reactions to rifampicin in antituberculosis regimens. *J. Antimicrob. Chemother., 3*, 115.
61. Stradling P (1973) Side-effects observed during intermittent rifampicin therapy. *Scand. J. Respir. Dis., Suppl 84*, 129.
62. Van Assendelft AHW (1985) Leucopenia in rifampicin chemotherapy. *J. Antimicrob. Chemother., 16*, 407.
63. Grosset J, Leventis S (1983) Adverse effects of rifampin. *Rev. Infect. Dis., 5, Suppl 3*, S440.
64. Gutman L (1978) More adverse reactions to rifampicin. *J. Antimicrob. Chemother., 4*, 283.
65. Pessayre D, Bentata M, Degott C et al (1977) Isoniazid-rifampin fulminant hepatitis. *Gastroenterology, 72*, 284.
66. Timbrell JA, Park BK, Harland SJ (1985) A study of the effects of rifampicin on isoniazid metabolism in human volunteer subjects. *Hum. Toxicol., 4*, 279.
67. Cross FS, Long MW, Banner AS, Snider Jr DE (1980) Rifampin-isoniazid therapy of alcoholic and nonalcoholic tuberculosis patients in a U.S. Public Health Service Cooperative Therapy trial. *Am. Rev. Respir. Dis., 122*, 349.
68. Skolnick JL, Stoler BS, Katz DB, Anderson WH (1976) Rifampin, oral contraceptives, and pregnancy. *J. Am. Med. Assoc., 236*, 1382.
69. Orme MLE, Back DJ, Breckenridge AM (1983) Clinical pharmacokinetics of oral contraceptive steroids. *Clin. Pharmacokinet., 8*, 95.
70. O'Reilly RA (1975) Interaction of chronic daily warfarin therapy and rifampin. *Ann. Intern. Med., 83*, 506.
71. Twum-Barima Y, Carruthers SG (1981) Quinidine-rifampin interaction. *N. Engl. J. Med., 304*, 1466.
72. Powell-Jackson PR, Gray BJ, Heaton RW et al (1983) Adverse effect of rifampicin administration on steroid-dependent asthma. *Am. Rev. Respir. Dis., 128*, 307.
73. Gault H, Longerich L, Dawe M, Fine A (1984) Digoxin-rifampin interaction. *Clin. Pharmacol. Ther., 35*, 750.
74. Kay L, Kampmann JP, Svendsen TL et al (1985) Influence of rifampicin and isoniazid on the kinetics of phenytoin. *Br. J. Clin. Pharmacol., 20*, 323.
75. Powell-Jackson PR, Jamieson AP, Gray BJ et al (1985) Effect of rifampicin administration on theophylline pharmacokinetics in humans. *Am. Rev. Respir. Dis., 131*, 939.
76. Cassidy MJD, Van Zuyl-Smitt R, Pascoe MD et al (1985) Effect of rifampicin on cyclosporin A blood levels in a renal transplant recipient. *Nephron, 41*, 207.
77. Barbarash RA (1985) Verapamil-rifampin interaction. *Drug Intell. Clin. Pharmacol., 19*, 559.
78. Rahn KH, Mooy J, Bohm R, Van der Vet A (1985) Reduction of bioavailability of verapamil by rifampin. *N. Engl. J. Med., 312*, 920.
79. Offerman S, Keller F, Molzahn M (1985) Low cyclosporin A blood levels and acute graft rejection in a renal transplant recipient during rifampin treatment. *Am. J. Nephrol., 5*, 385.
80. Farge D, Charpentier B, Simonneau G et al (1985) Rifampin and acute cellular rejection in renal transplantation. *Néphrologie, 6*, 53.
81. Coward RA, Raftery AT, Brown CB (1985) Cyclosporin and antituberculous therapy. *Lancet, 1*, 1342.
82. Bowman G, Hanngren A, Malmborg A-S et al (1971) Drug interaction: decreased serum concentrations of rifampicin when given with P.A.S. *Lancet, 1*, 800.

83. Polasa K, Krishnaswamy K (1983) Effect of food on bioavailability of rifampicin. *J. Clin. Pharmacol., 23*, 433.

84. Raleigh JW (1972) Rifampin in treatment of advanced pulmonary tuberculosis. *Am. Rev. Respir. Dis., 105*, 397.

85. Bullock VE (1983) Rifampin in the treatment of leprosy. *Rev. Infect. Dis., 5, Suppl 3*, S606.

86. Murphy TV, Chrane DF, McCracken Jr GH, Nelson JD (1983) Rifampin prophylaxis vs. placebo for house-hold contacts of children with *Haemophilus influenzae* type b disease. *Am. J. Dis. Child., 137*, 627.

87. Band JD, Fraser DW, Ajello G (1984) Prevention of *Haemophilus influenzae* type b disease. *J. Am. Med. Assoc., 251*, 2381.

88. Guttler RB, Counts GW, Avent CK, Beatty HN (1971) Effect of rifampin and minocycline on meningococcal carrier rates. *J. Infect. Dis., 124*, 199.

89. Wheat L, Kohler RB, White AL, White A (1981) Effect of rifampin on nasal carriers of coagulase-positive staphylococci. *J. Infect. Dis., 144*, 177.

90. Finley RS, Schimpff SC, Fortner CL, Wiernik PH (1982) Rifampin and cloxacillin in the reduction of staphylococcal colonization. *Clin. Pharmacol., 1*, 370.

91. Ward TT, Winn RE, Harstein AI, Sewell DL (1981) Observations relating to an inter-hospital outbreak of methicillin-resistant *Staphylococcus aureus*: role of antimicrobial therapy in infection control. *Infect. Control, 2*, 453.

92. Walsh TJ, Auger FA, Tatem BA et al (1986) Novobiocin and rifampin in combination against methicillin-resistant *Staphylococcus aureus*: an in-vitro comparison with vancomycin plus rifampin. *J. Antimicrob. Chemother., 17*, 75.

93. Appelbaum PC, Spangler SK, Potter CR, Sattler FR (1986) Reduction of oral flora with rifampin in healthy volunteers. *Antimicrob. Agents Chemother., 29*, 576.

94. Mandell GL (1983) The antimicrobial activity of rifampin: emphasis on the relation to phagocytes. *Rev. Infect. Dis., 5, Suppl 3*, S463.

95. Suter F, Maserati R, Concia E et al (1984) Rifampicin in collections of pus: a kinetic study in human abscesses. *J. Antimicrob. Chemother., 13, Suppl C*, 43.

96. Lobo MC, Mandell GL (1972) Treatment of experimental staphylococcal infection with rifampin. *Antimicrob. Agents Chemother., 2*, 195.

97. Hays NT, Regelmann WE, Quie PG (1983) The use of rifampin in patients with chronic granulomatous disease of childhood: clinical notes. *Rev. Infect. Dis., 5, Suppl 3*, S522.

98. Lorber B (1980) Rifampin in chronic granulomatous disease. *N. Engl. J. Med., 303*, 111.

99. Hoger PH, Vosbeck K, Seger R, Hitzig WH (1985) Uptake, intracellular activity, and influence of rifampin on normal function of polymorphonuclear leukocytes. *Antimicrob. Agents Chemother., 28*, 667.

100. Norden CW (1983) Experimental chronic staphylococcal osteomyelitis in rabbits: treatment with rifampin alone and in combination with other antimicrobial agents. *Rev. Infect. Dis., 5, Suppl 3*, S491.

101. Norden CW (1975) Experimental osteomyelitis. IV. Therapeutic trials with rifampin alone and in combination with gentamicin, sisomicin, and cephalothin. *J. Infect. Dis., 132*, 493.

102. Norden CW (1980) Treatment of experimental staphylococcal osteomyelitis with rifampin and trimethoprim alone and in combination. *Antimicrob. Agents Chemother., 17*, 591.

103. Norden CW, Schaffer M (1983) Treatment of experimental chronic osteomyelitis due to *Staphylococcus aureus* with vancomycin and rifampin. *J. Infect. Dis., 147,* 352.

104. Norden CW, Fierer J, Bryant RE et al (1983) Chronic staphylococcal osteomyelitis: treatment with regimens containing rifampin. *Rev. Infect. Dis., 5, Suppl 3,* S495.

105. Zak O, Scheld WM, Sande MA (1983) Rifampin in experimental *Staphylococcus aureus* endocarditis in rabbits. *Rev. Infect. Dis., 5, Suppl 3,* S481.

106. Suter F, Maserati R, Carnevale G et al (1984) Management of staphylococcal endocarditis in drug addicts: combined therapy with oral rifampicin and aminoglycosides. *J. Antimicrob. Chemother., Suppl 13,* 57.

107. Archer GL, Johnston JL, Vazquez GJ, Haywood III HB (1983) Efficacy of antibiotic combinations including rifampin against methicillin-resistant *Staphylococcus epidermidis*: in vitro and in vivo studies. *Rev. Infect. Dis., 5, Suppl 3,* S522.

108. Kobasa WD, Kaye KL, Shapiro T, Kaye D (1983) Therapy for experimental endocarditis due to *Staphylococcus epidermidis. Rev. Infect. Dis., 5, Suppl 3,* S533.

109. Karchmer AW, Archer GL, Dismukes WE (1983) *Staphylococcus epidermidis* causing prosthetic valve endocarditis: microbiologic and clinical observations as guides to therapy. *Ann. Intern. Med., 98,* 447.

110. Tshefu K, Zimmerli W, Waldvogel FA (1983) Partial efficacy of short term rifampin administration in the prevention of foreign body infection. *Rev. Infect. Dis., 5, Suppl 3,* S475.

111. Zimmerli W, Lew PD, Waldvogel FA (1984) Pathogenesis of foreign body infection: evidence for a local granulocyte defect. *J. Clin. Invest., 73,* 1191.

112. Van der Auwera P, Thys JP, Meunier-Carpentier F, Klastersky J (1984) The combination of oxacillin with rifampin in staphylococcal infections: a review of laboratory and clinical studies of the Institut Jules Bordet. *J. Antimicrob. Chemother., 13, Suppl C,* 31.

113. Clumeck N, Marcelis L, Amiri-Lamraaski MH, Gordts B (1984) Treatment of severe staphylococcal infections with a rifampicin-minocycline association. *J. Antimicrob. Chemother., Suppl 13,* 17.

114. Gordon JJ, Harter DH, Phair JP (1985) Meningitis due to *Staphylococcus aureus. Am. J. Med., 78,* 965.

115. Straneo G, Ferre R, Gattei G et al (1985) Rifampicin in the treatment of paediatric non-tuberculous infections. *J. Clin. Trials, 22,* 135.

116. Package insert (1981) Merrell Dow Pharmaceuticals Inc., Subsidiary of The Dow Chemical Company, Cincinnati, OH.

117. Pan Yu-Xuan, Liu Su-Mei, Li Wei-Wen (1985) Laboratory studies on antituberculous activity of cyclopentylrifampicin. II. A long-acting antituberculotic cyclopentylrifampicin. *Chin. J. Antibiot., 10,* 305.

118. Easmon CSF, Crane JP (1984) Comparative uptake of rifampicin and rifapentine (DL473) by human neutrophils. *J. Antimicrob. Chemother., 13,* 585.

119. Varaldo PE, Debbia E, Schito GC (1985) In vitro activities of rifapentine and rifampin, alone and in combination with six other antibiotics, against methicillin-susceptible staphylococci of different species. *Antimicrob. Agents Chemother., 27,* 615.

120. Ariza J, Gudiol F, Pallares R et al (1985) Comparative trial of rifampin-doxycycline versus tetracycline-streptomycin in the therapy of human brucellosis. *Antimicrob. Agents Chemother., 28,* 548.

121. Montanari M, Gandini T, Torre D, Dietz A (1985) Treatment of brucellosis: clinical experience with an association of rifampicin and doxycycline. *Minerva Med., 76,* 1407.

122. Salata RA, Ravdin JI (1985) *Brucella species.* In: Mandell GL, Douglass Jr RG, Bennett JE (Eds), *Principles and Practice of Infectious Diseases, 2nd ed.,* p 1283. Wiley Medical Publications, New York.

123. Parry MF, Stampleman L, Hutchinson JH et al (1985) Waterborne *Legionella bozemanii* and nosocomial pneumonia in immunosuppressed patients. *Ann. Intern. Med., 103,* 205.

124. Pasculle AW, Dowling JN, Frola FN et al (1985) Antimicrobial therapy of experimental *Legionella micdadei* pneumonia in guinea pigs. *Antimicrob. Agents Chemother., 28,* 730.

125. Saito A, Sawatari K, Fukuda Y et al (1985) Susceptibility of *Legionella* pneumonia in guinea pigs. *Antimicrob. Agents Chemother., 28,* 15.

126. Hawkins AE, Bortolussi R, Issekutz AC (1984) In vitro and in vivo activity of various antibiotics against *Listeria monocytogenes* type 4b. *Clin. Invest. Med., 7,* 335.

CHAPTER 17

Tetracyclines

DAVID N. WILLIAMS

The tetracycline antibiotics were the first 'broad spectrum' antibiotics and were, initially, effective against a wide range of gram-positive and gram-negative organisms. As a group, the tetracyclines are now less generally used, in large part due to the development of antimicrobial resistance and the appearance of newer and more effective agents in the chemotherapeutic armamentarium. Currently, tetracyclines are used predominantly outside the hospital where they account for up to 39% of antibiotic prescriptions in the United Kingdom (1), while in the United States, a recent survey of outpatient drug use from selected retail pharmacies ranked tetracycline as twentieth overall, and fourth in antibiotics (2). Since the appearance of *Annual 2* (3), the role of tetracyclines in combination with other antibiotics in the treatment of infections due to certain intracellular bacteria has been further evaluated, as has the increasing importance of this family of drugs in the treatment of Lyme disease.

The basic structure consists of a hydroxynaphthacene nucleus, containing, as the name implies, 4 fused benzene rings. Substitution on the rings accounts for the number and diversity of tetracyclines. The first tetracyclines – chlortetracycline and oxytetracycline – were the result of an intensive screening of soil organisms for antimicrobial properties. Chlortetracycline was isolated from *Streptomyces aureofaciens* in 1947, and oxytetracycline from *Streptomyces rimosus* in 1950. The parent compound, tetracycline, was produced by the catalytic dehalogenation of chlortetracycline in 1953. The semisynthetic congeners, doxycycline and minocycline, were discovered in 1966 and 1972, respectively.

ACTIVITY

Mechanism of action

The penetration of the gram-negative bacterial cell wall by tetracyclines is, as is the case for most antibiotics, more difficult than that of gram-positive organisms. It probably occurs as a result of both passive diffusion and an active transport

Antimicrobial Agents Annual 3
P.K. Peterson and J. Verhoef, editors
© Elsevier Science Publishers BV, 1988

system. Once within the bacterial cell, the primary mechanism of antibacterial action is inhibition of protein synthesis by binding to the 30S ribosomal subunit, so as to block the binding of aminoacyl *t*RNA to the acceptor site of the *m*RNA ribosome complex. This prevents the addition of new amino acids to the growing peptide chain. For a more detailed description the reader is referred to the review by Chopra et al (4). Tetracyclines are bacteriostatic drugs, and as such should not be used for the treatment of infections in granulocytopenic (WBC $< 500/mm^3$) patients, or those with infective endocarditis.

Spectrum of activity

Tetracycline is felt to be the most representative congener, and therefore routine sensitivities are determined using the standard 30 μg antimicrobial disc. Differences in antimicrobial activity between the congeners do exist, but as a generaliza-

Table 1   *Susceptibility of selected micro-organisms to tetracycline, minocycline and doxycycline*,***

Organism	Tetracycline	Minocycline	Doxycycline
Gram-positive bacteria			
Staphylococcus aureus	100.00	3.1–6.3	25.00
Streptococcus pyogenes	3.10	0.80	0.80
Streptococcus pneumoniae	0.80	0.20	0.20
Gram-negative bacteria			
Neisseria gonorrhoeae	1.60	1.60	1.60
Haemophilus influenzae	6.30	3.10	3.10
Brucella spp.	2.00	2.00	1.00
Pasteurella multocida	0.40	0.40	0.40
Anaerobes			
Bacteroides fragilis	32.00	8.00	8.00
Clostridium perfringens	64.00	32.00	8.00
Other			
Mycoplasma pneumoniae	1.60	1.60	1.60
Legionella pneumophila		4.00	4.00
Chlamydia trachomatis	0.12	0.06	
Nocardia asteroides	32.00	4.00	32.00
Mycobacterium marinum	20.00	10.00	10.00

*Adapted from various sources (Refs 5–14). Organisms should be considered susceptible if the MICs are 4 μg/ml or less.
**Expressed as the antimicrobial concentration (μg/ml) required to inhibit 90% of isolates (MIC_{90}).

tion, doxycycline and minocycline are the most active. The superior activity of minocycline against *Staphylococcus aureus* and *Nocardia asteroides* and of doxycycline against *Bacteroides fragilis* deserve emphasis, but the clinical relevance is questionable. Increasing microbial resistance, particularly true of many of the gram-positive organisms, has led to a decline in the utility of tetracyclines. Resistance was initially noted with strains of *S. aureus*, but later resistance, the prevalence of which depended in part on geographic location, was seen in *Streptococcus pneumoniae* and β-hemolytic streptococci. Tetracyclines retain activity against community isolates of aerobic gram-negative organisms, such as *Escherichia coli* and *Klebsiella*, but isolates of *Pseudomonas aeruginosa* and *Proteus mirabilis* are resistant. Resistance has been described in about 5% of isolates of *Haemophilus influenzae*, and to an increasing extent for *Neisseria gonorrhoeae*, but again the prevalence varies from place to place. Tetracyclines are active against a number of other micro-organisms, including *Chlamydia, Mycoplasma*, rickettsiae, and spirochetal organisms, which has important clinical implications. They are also active, to some degree, against mycobacterial, fungal and protozoal organisms (Table 1) (5–14).

Resistance mechanisms

Resistance to tetracyclines is primarily plasmid(R-factor)-mediated, most of which is inducible, i.e. bacteria express their resistance following exposure to subinhibitory concentrations of the drug. Resistant bacterial isolates accumulate less drug than their sensitive parent strains (4). There has been a great deal of interest of late in the use of tetracycline in animal husbandry (as animal food additives for growth promotion and prophylaxis) and particularly its relationship to resistance in gram-negative organisms (15). Recently there have been reports (16) of isolates of *Neisseria gonorrhoeae* which are highly resistant (MICs of 16–64 μg/ml) to tetracycline. The mechanism of resistance has been shown to be due to the acquisition of the resistance determinant *tet*M, a transposon-borne determinant found initially in the genus *Streptococcus*, and more recently in *Mycoplasma hominis, Ureaplasma urealyticum*, and *Gardnerella vaginalis* (17).

CLINICAL PHARMACOLOGY

There are 10 tetracyclines in clinical use, although not all are available in all countries: chlortetracycline, oxytetracycline, tetracycline, demeclocycline, methacycline, clomocycline, lymecycline, rolitetracycline, doxycycline and minocycline. For the most part, the discussion will focus on tetracycline (as the standard or parent drug), doxycycline and minocycline.

Tetracycline has a half-life of 10 hours, compared with 15 hours for minocycline and 18 hours for doxycycline. Tetracycline is traditionally dosed 4 times a day, while doxycycline and minocycline are usually given on a once- and twice-a-day basis, respectively. The reported degree of protein binding varies, depending on the methods used: tetracycline is about 60% protein-bound, while doxycycline and minocycline are 80–90% protein-bound.

Following oral administration, drug absorption occurs primarily in the stomach and proximal small intestine, the degree of absorption varying from almost 100% for doxycycline and minocycline to 80% for tetracycline. The well-known impairment of tetracycline absorption with concomitant milk and antacid ingestion appears to be least with doxycycline. Following oral administration of 500 mg of tetracycline, peak serum levels of about 3–4 μg/ml occur at approximately 1–3 hours, falling to about 2 μg/ml at 8 hours. Peak serum levels following a 200 mg dose of oral doxycycline or minocycline are around 2.5 μg/ml at 2 hours. Peak (30 min after drug administration) serum level following a 500 mg intravenous dose of tetracycline is around 8 μg/ml and 4 μg/ml following a 200 mg intravenous dose of doxycycline or minocycline. The intravenous formulations are usually given slowly over a period of an hour because of local thrombophlebitis, while intramuscular administration of these drugs is not recommended because of local irritation. Doxycycline is the most favored, and best tolerated, intravenous formulation.

Following oral absorption there is an active enterohepatic circulation, resulting in biliary levels that are at least 5- to 10-fold higher than the corresponding serum levels. The tetracyclines, especially minocycline and doxycycline, are lipophilic and are thus highly diffusible, resulting in penetration of 'difficult tissues' such as the brain, eye and prostate. Cerebrospinal fluid levels are about 20% of serum levels. Doxycycline has been shown to diffuse into the inflamed and non-inflamed prostate in therapeutic concentrations (18). Minocycline is able to penetrate respiratory secretions, hence its former role in the treatment of the meningococcal carrier state. Tetracyclines also penetrate into the sebum and are excreted in perspiration, properties which attest to their usefulness in the treatment of acne. Problems arise as a result of their ability to cross the placental barrier, which is of importance because of the avidity with which they bind to calcium, interfering with dental and bone growth in the unborn child. They are also excreted in breast milk.

All tetracyclines are excreted, in varying degrees, in urine and feces. Urinary excretion depends on the glomerular filtration rate with recovery rates of 60% for tetracycline, 35% for doxycycline and 10% for minocycline (19). With the exception of doxycycline, the tetracyclines should be avoided in renal insufficiency. Doxycycline appears to have 'an alternate route' of excretion in renal failure in that it diffuses into the intestinal lumen, and in this alkaline milieu cationic chelation occurs (doxycycline binds with calcium or magnesium in the gut lumen). The chelated doxycycline cannot be reabsorbed and thus the main route of excretion is fecal (20).

ADVERSE EFFECTS AND DRUG INTERACTIONS

Adverse effects

Hypersensitivity True hypersensitivity is rare, resulting in various rashes and even anaphylaxis. Because of cross-sensitivity, such manifestations would preclude use of all members of the tetracycline family. Treatment of spirochetal infections frequently results in a Jarisch-Herxheimer reaction.

Photosensitivity This classically occurs with demeclocycline, but is of importance and concern with other tetracyclines, most notably doxycycline because of its use in the prophylaxis of traveler's diarrhea. It is now thought that the photosensitivity is a toxic rather than an allergic reaction, and is presumably related to drug accumulation in the skin.

Hyperpigmentation There are reports of increased skin pigmentation and pigment accumulation in the thyroid with chronic use of tetracyclines. The black thyroid gland of minocycline therapy is innocuous, and appears to be due to lipofuscins (21).

Dental and bone effects Tetracyclines achieved some notoriety many years ago because of unwanted dental staining. The color varies from a grey-brown to yellow. It is most likely to occur between the fourth and sixth month of intrauterine life and in the neonate before first dentition. However, the threat of interference with dental and, to a lesser degree, bone growth persists through to the age of 8 years. Many authorities urge avoidance of tetracyclines until the age of 12 years. Dental staining seems to be dose-dependent, and to some degree drug-dependent. It is least likely with doxycycline because of less avid chelation. Thus, in pediatric practice, while doxycycline might be appropriately recommended in the treatment of an episode of Rocky Mountain spotted fever or other rickettsial or spirochetal infection, repeated courses of any tetracycline must be avoided.

Gastrointestinal effects Tetracyclines may cause diarrhea as a result of a dose-related chemical effect, often in those congeners that are less well absorbed. Diarrhea may also occur as a result of staphylococcal superinfection, or the more contemporary problem of antibiotic-associated colitis due to colonization with *Clostridium difficile*. Tetracyclines are very acidic in solution (doxycycline has a pH of 3.0) and there are increasing reports of esophageal ulceration occurring, particularly in elderly patients with pre-existing gastroesophageal disease. Thus, patients should be encouraged to take tetracycline (and especially doxycycline) with liberal amounts of fluid and at least an hour or so before retiring.

Genital and oral mucosa *Candida* overgrowth may be a problem. Glossitis and cheilosis probably represent sensitivity reactions.

Hepatic toxicity Liver changes, manifest histologically as microvesicular fatty change, have been described most typically in pregnant women with pre-existing renal insufficiency receiving more than 2 g/d of intravenous tetracycline. A high mortality resulted.

Renal toxicity Renal failure is predisposed to by the tetracycline-induced reduction of protein synthesis, resulting in increased azotemia from amino acid catabolism. In addition, a number of specific problems are seen. Thus, demeclocycline can cause renal tubular damage and use of this may be made in the treatment of resistant edema associated with inappropriate antidiuretic hormone secretion. Another phenomenon, no longer seen, is the Fanconi syndrome of renal tubular acidosis, which was associated with use of outdated tetracycline which degraded to the epianhydro form.

Neurotoxicity Giddiness, vertigo and ataxia are seen exclusively with minocycline and seem to occur primarily in females (22). Raised intracranial pressure can be seen at all ages, and is most typically seen in infants.

Bleeding diathesis A bleeding diathesis can occur as a result of interference with endogenous vitamin K production.

Drug interactions

Reduced absorption Reduced absorption of oral tetracyclines can occur due to interaction with food and divalent metals, e.g. calcium, magnesium and aluminum (important constituents of antacids) as well as with iron preparations. Tetracyclines chelate divalent metals and the resulting compound cannot be absorbed.

Hepatic metabolism A number of drugs, particularly the antiepileptic drugs carbamazepine, diphenylhydantoin and barbiturates, induce hepatic metabolism of tetracyclines and thus reduce their serum half-life. This has been best described with doxycycline.

Augmentation of nephrotoxicity The anesthetic agent, methoxyflurane, can cause nephrotoxicity when administered with tetracycline. Renal problems may occur when tetracyclines are administered concomitantly with diuretics.

Interaction with other antibiotics Tetracyclines are bacteriostatic agents and antagonism may result from the concomitant administration of a bactericidal antibiotic. This issue is controversial and is based on the observations of Lepper and Dowling in the early 1950s, when concurrent use of penicillin and tetracycline in the treatment of pneumococcal meningitis resulted in a poorer outcome than when penicillin was used alone (23).

CLINICAL USES

Tetracycline administration should be avoided in children (under the age of 12 years), in pregnant women, and in those with liver and kidney disease (doxycycline is the exception). Although tetracyclines were the first broad-spectrum antibiotics, they can no longer be used as initial therapy for most unknown acute infections. Rather, they should be used in specific situations, and this discussion focuses on a few of the many indications.

Spirochetal infections

Tetracycline is the drug of choice in adults for the treatment of the cutaneous manifestation of Lyme disease (erythema chronicum migrans). Administration of oral tetracycline 250 mg 4 times a day for 10 days has been shown not only to reduce the duration of the rash, but also to prevent the important sequelae of arthritis, meningitis and carditis. Arthritic sequelae have been successfully treated with oral penicillin or with oral tetracycline (30 mg/kg body weight per day for 4 weeks) (24). More refractory cases of arthritis and those with meningitis should be treated with parenteral penicillin (25). Tetracycline has also been used in the treatment of relapsing fever (due to *Borrelia recurrentis*) as well as an alternative drug in the treatment of syphilis. Recent data have shown the efficacy of doxycycline in both the treatment (26) and prophylaxis of leptospirosis.

Genital infections

Chlamydia trachomatis is an important pathogen in a number of genital infections, including urethritis, pelvic inflammatory disease and epididymitis. Increasingly, there is concern that patients with urethritis may harbor both *Neisseria gonorrhoeae* and *Chlamydia trachomatis* concomitantly, and there is, further, the added concern regarding resistance. This has prompted the recommendation that periodic testing for antimicrobial sensitivity of a sample of *N. gonorrhoeae* isolates and all isolates associated with treatment failure should be an integral part of gonorrhea control programs (27). Thus, currently, treatment for uncomplicated genital gonococcal infection consists of a penicillin or a cephalosporin, followed by a 7-day course of oral tetracycline hydrochloride (500 mg q.i.d.) or doxycycline (100 mg b.i.d.). Similarly, the importance of appropriate treatment of pelvic inflammatory disease has been emphasized because of the high rate of infertility following inadequate treatment of this syndrome. *N. gonorrhoeae, E. coli* and other aerobic gram-negative coliforms, *Bacteroides fragilis*, and *Chlamydia* may all play a role. For that reason a tetracycline is now invariably included as part of any therapeutic regimen for pelvic inflammatory disease. Because so many of the common sexually transmitted infections (*C. trachomatis, Ureaplasma urealyticum, N. gonorrhoeae*, syphilis, lymphogranuloma venereum, granuloma inguinale, and chancroid) are for the most part susceptible to tetracycline, this family of drugs has great utility in this setting.

Urinary tract infections

The designation of microbial sensitivity or resistance is based on the concept of easily achievable *serum* concentrations of a given drug. Thus, urinary infections may be cured despite apparent resistance in vitro because of the enormously higher *urinary* drug concentrations. Moreover, the tetracyclines are more active in an acid pH and this, together with the increased concern for *Chlamydia* infection, ensures a role for these drugs in urinary infections. For example, the dysuria-frequency syndrome, which clinically presents rather insidiously, with pyuria and a negative urine culture, is often due to *Chlamydia*. While in *acute* prostatitis virtually all antibiotics penetrate the inflamed prostate, the treatment of chronic prostatitis is a formidable challenge. Recent work has emphasized the etiologic role of *Chlamydia*, and pharmacologic data indicate that doxycycline is one of only a handful of drugs that penetrate the non-inflamed prostate (18).

Respiratory infections

Tetracyclines are still widely used in the treatment of various respiratory problems, especially the treatment of acute exacerbations of chronic bronchitis. The drugs may be used episodically or continuously during the winter months. Patients with atypical pneumonia, where *Mycoplasma pneumoniae, Chlamydia psittaci, Coxiella burnetii, Francisella tularensis* and *Legionella pneumophila* are all etiologic considerations, should be considered for tetracycline therapy, alone or in combination. It should be emphasized, however, that tetracyclines should not be used to treat acute pharyngitis or pneumonia, because of the increasing prevalence of resistant isolates of β-hemolytic streptococci, *Streptococcus pneumoniae* and *Haemophilus influenzae*.

Gastrointestinal infections

Tetracyclines have been shown to be useful both in the treatment and prophylaxis of cholera. One of the commonest uses of tetracycline nowadays is prophylaxis of traveler's diarrhea. Suitable candidates for such prophylaxis include those visiting high-risk areas on business, patients with some underlying health problem that might increase their susceptibility to infection (achlorhydria, gastric resection, and acid therapy), or elderly people who may be particularly vulnerable to dehydration. Prophylaxis (with doxycycline 100 mg daily) should not exceed 3 weeks (28).

Combination therapy

Tetracycline retains an important role in the treatment of a diverse list of organisms in combination with other drugs. Its utility in the treatment of difficult cases of amebiasis and drug-resistant *Plasmodium falciparum* is discussed elsewhere in this volume. Tetracycline remains an important drug in the treatment of melioidosis (due to *Pseudomonas pseudomallei*) when it is used for a prolonged period (3 months or more), usually combined with chloramphenicol or trimethoprim + sulfamethoxazole for the first month of therapy. Severe infections with *Yersinia pestis* and *Brucella* species are probably best treated with a combination of tetracycline and streptomycin. A recent comparative trial of a 30-day course of the combination of doxycycline and rifampicin versus tetracycline and streptomycin, for the treatment of brucellosis (due to *Brucella melitensis*), found the rifampin + doxycycline combination to be less effective in preventing relapses (38.8% *vs* 7.1% with the tetracycline + streptomycin combination) (29). Finally, in the treatment of *Mycobacterium fortuitum* and *M. chelonei* infections, doxycycline + amikacin is a useful combination, while minocycline alone, for 8–16 weeks, is appropriate initial therapy for *M. marinum* infection.

DOSING

For reasons previously cited, no pediatric doses are given. Usual adult doses are as follows:

a. Tetracycline 250–500 mg, orally, 4 times per day. Available in 250 and 500 mg capsules.

b. Doxycycline 100 mg once or twice per day (50 and 100 mg capsules). Doxycycline hyclate is the favored intravenous formulation, and may be given in a dose of 100 mg once or twice per day.

c. Minocycline 100 mg twice a day (50 and 100 mg capsules).

REFERENCES

1. Hamilton-Miller JMT (1984) Use and abuse of antibiotics. *Br. J. Clin. Pharmacol., 18*, 469.
2. Baum C, Kennedy DL, Forbes MF, Jones JK (1982) Drug use and expenditures in 1982. *J. Am. Med. Assoc., 253*, 382.
3. Williams DN (1987) Tetracyclines. In: Peterson PK, Verhoef J (Eds), *The Antimicrobial Agents Annual 2*, p 194. Elsevier, Amsterdam.
4. Chopra I, Howe TGB, Linton AH, Linton B, Richmond MH, Speller DCE (1981) The tetracyclines: prospects at the beginning of the 1980's. *J. Antimicrob. Chemother., 8*, 5.
5. Neu HC (1978) A symposium on the tetracyclines: a major appraisal. *Bull. NY Acad. Med., 54*, 141.

6. Steigbigel NH, Reed CW, Finland M (1968) Susceptibility of common pathogenic bacteria to seven tetracycline antibiotics in vitro. *Am. J. Med. Sci., 255*, 179.
7. Hall WH, Opfer BJ (1984) Influence of inoculum size on comparative susceptibility of penicillinase-positive and -negative *Neisseria gonorrhoeae* to 31 antimicrobial agents. *Antimicrob. Agents Chemother., 26*, 192.
8. Farrell ID, Hinchcliffe PM, Robinson L (1976) Sensitivity of *Brucella* spp. to tetracycline and its analogues. *J. Clin. Pathol., 29*, 1097.
9. Rosenthal SL, Freundlich LF (1976) In vitro antibiotic sensitivity of *Pasteurella multocida. Health Lab. Sci., 13*, 246.
10. Sutter VL, Finegold SM (1976) Susceptibility of anaerobic bacteria to 23 antimicrobial agents. *Antimicrob. Agents Chemother., 10*, 736.
11. Edelstein PH, Meyer RD (1980) Susceptibility of *Legionella pneumophila* to twenty antimicrobial agents. *Antimicrob. Agents Chemother., 18*, 403.
12. Oriel JD, Ridgway GL (1983) Comparison of tetracycline and minocycline in the treatment of non-gonococcal urethritis. *Br. J. Vener. Dis., 59*, 245.
13. Gutmann L, Goldstein FW, Kitzis MD, Hautefort B, Darmon C, Acar JR (1983) Susceptibility of *Nocardia asteroides* to 46 antibiotics, including 22 β-lactams. *Antimicrob. Agents Chemother., 23*, 248.
14. Sanders WJ, Wolinsky E (1980) In vitro susceptibility of *Mycobacterium marinum* to eight antimicrobial agents. *Antimicrob. Agents Chemother., 18*, 529.
15. Holmberg SD, Osterholm MT, Senger KA, Cohen ML (1984) Drug-resistant *Salmonella* from animals fed antimicrobials. *N. Engl. J. Med., 311*, 617.
16. Centers for Disease Control (1986) Plasmid-mediated tetracycline-resistant *Neisseria gonorrhoeae* – Georgia, Massachusetts, Oregon. *Morbid. Mortal. Weekly Rep., 35*, 304.
17. Morse SA, Johnson SR, Biddle JW, Roberts MC (1986) High-level tetracycline resistance in *Neisseria gonorrhoeae* is the result of acquisition of streptococcal tetM determinant. *Antimicrob. Agents Chemother., 30*, 664.
18. Ristuccia AM, Cunha BA (1982) Current concepts in antimicrobial therapy of prostatitis. *Urology, 20*, 338.
19. Fabre J, Milek E, Kalfopoulos P et al (1971) The kinetics of tetracycline in man: excretion, penetration in normal inflammatory tissues, behavior in renal insufficiency and hemodialysis. *Schweiz. Med. Wochenschr., 101*, 625.
20. Whelton A, Schach von Wittenau M, Twomey TM, Walker WG, Bianchine JR (1974) Doxycycline pharmacokinetics in the absence of renal function. *Kidney Int., 5*, 365.
21. Gordon G, Sparano BM, Kramer AW, Kelly RG, Iatropoulos MJ (1984) Thyroid gland pigmentation and minocycline therapy. *Am. J. Pathol., 117*, 98.
22. Williams DN, Laghlin LW, Lee Y-H (1974) Minocycline: possible vestibular side effects. *Lancet, 2*, 744.
23. Lepper MH, Dowling JF (1951) Treatment of pneumococcal meningitis with penicillin compared with aureomycin. *Arch. Intern. Med., 188*, 489.
24. Culp RW, Eichenfield AH, Davidson RS, Drummon DS, Christofersen MR, Goldsmith DP (1987) Lyme arthritis in children. *J. Bone Jt Surg., 69*, 96.
25. Steere AC, Green J, Schoen RT, Taylor E, Hutchison GJ, Rahn DW, Malawista SW (1985) Successful parenteral penicillin therapy of established Lyme arthritis. *N. Engl. J. Med., 312*, 869.
26. McLain JBL, Ballou WP, Harrison SM, Steinweg DL (1984) Doxycycline therapy for leptospirosis. *Ann. Intern. Med., 100*, 696.

27. Centers for Disease Control (1985) Treatment guidelines. *Sex. Transm. Dis., 34*, 75S.
28. Dupont HL, Ericsson DC, Johnson PC (1985) Chemotherapy and chemoprophylaxis of traveler's diarrhea. *Ann. Intern. Med., 102*, 260.
29. Ariza J, Gudiol F, Pallares R, Rufi G, Fernandez-Viladrich P (1985) Comparative trial of rifampin-doxycycline versus tetracycline-streptomycin in the therapy of human brucellosis. *Antimicrob. Agents Chemother., 28*, 548.

CHAPTER 18

Sulfonamides and trimethoprim

WALTER T. HUGHES

Trimethoprim, sulfonamides and the combination of these drugs are especially useful in the treatment of infections of the urinary tract. Trimethoprim + sulfamethoxazole has gained prominence in the short-course treatment and prophylaxis of lower urinary tract infection. Experimental evidence suggests that trimethoprim alone, or in combination with sulfamethoxazole, in concentrations well below the minimum inhibitory concentration (MIC) can reduce the synthesis, expression and adhesive properties of Type 1 fimbriae of *Escherichia coli*. Such an effect might prevent adherence of *E. coli* to host cells, thereby aborting colonization and infection.

STRUCTURE, DERIVATION

Sulfisoxazole (sulfafurazole; 3,4-dimethyl-5-sulfanilamidoisoxazole), sulfamethoxazole (5-methyl-3-sulfanilamido-isoxazole) and trimethoprim (2,4-diamino-5-[3,4,5-trimethoxybenzyl]pyrimidine) are the compounds currently in greatest usage.

ACTIVITY

An interesting and important recent observation has been made on the subliminal activity of trimethoprim + sulfamethoxazole on certain gram-negative bacilli. While the therapeutic effects of antibiotics have traditionally been attributed to either the killing or the inhibition of growth of the microbe, Schifferli et al (1) have provided evidence for an additional strategy. Using concentrations of trimethoprim and sulfamethoxazole that do not inhibit bacterial growth, these investigators showed that *E. coli* grown in concentrations of trimethoprim + sulfamethoxazole which were 1/32 the MIC for each drug, together induced a marked reduction in fimbrial synthesis, expression and hemagglutinating activity. Neither

Antimicrobial Agents Annual 3
P.K. Peterson and J. Verhoef, editors
© Elsevier Science Publishers BV, 1988

agent alone in these concentrations produced an effect. However, fimbrial subunit synthesis was inhibited in bacteria grown in one-half the MIC of trimethoprim alone. Since pathogenic bacteria must adhere to the host cell surfaces to establish colonization and subsequently infection, this interference with bacterial adhesive mechanisms before infection occurs may provide a prophylactic approach to some diseases and might account in part for the effectiveness of trimethoprim + sulfamethoxazole as a prophylactic agent in urinary tract infections.

CLINICAL PHARMACOLOGY

Most reports of pharmacokinetics have been directed to normal individuals, those with renal impairment and patients with acute infections. An additional important group of patients has recently been studied at the University of Chile (2). The pharmacokinetics of trimethoprim + sulfamethoxazole was examined in 7 malnourished (marasmic) infants being treated for urinary tract infections. Comparison of the values in these patients was made with 10 infants who were nutritionally normal. It was discovered that the elimination half-life of sulfamethoxazole in the malnourished infants was prolonged (0.6 *vs* 4.9 h) in the normal infants. Also, a greater area under the curve (573 *vs* 328 μg/ml/h) was observed in the malnourished group. This disparity was explained by the differences in body fluid distribution between the two groups.

Consideration is sometimes given to the use of sulfonamides in the treatment of central nervous system infections. Useful information has been generated from a study of the pharmacokinetics of trimethoprim and sulfamethoxazole in the cerebrospinal fluid and serum (3). After a single infusion of 5 mg of trimethoprim and 25 mg of sulfamethoxazole per kilogram over a 2-hour period, peak concentrations in the spinal fluid were 1.0 and 13.8 μg/ml, respectively. A loading dose of the drug combination, based on 10–12 mg trimethoprim and a maintenance dose of 8.0 mg/kg every 8 hours should yield a steady-state peak concentration of at least 5 μg/ml trimethoprim and 160 μg/ml of sulfamethoxazole in the serum. The study found that the spinal fluid penetration was 18% for trimethoprim and 12% for sulfamethoxazole. Another study showed that the administration of tetroxoprim and sulfadiazine orally resulted in spinal fluid concentrations above the MIC for most susceptible bacteria (4). It should be noted that both these studies were done in patients without meningitis or meningeal inflammation. Generally, in most studies drugs administered during active meningitis achieve higher concentrations in spinal fluid than occurs with non-inflamed meninges.

It has been well-established that patients with acquired immunodeficiency syndrome (AIDS) have a high incidence of exaggerated adverse effects of trimethoprim + sulfamethoxazole *(The Antimicrobial Agents Annual 1)*. A recent study of the pharmacokinetics of the usual high doses of the drug used to treat *Pneumocystis carinii* pneumonia may shed some light on these problems as well as provide data on dosage in these individuals (5). Of 7 patients with AIDS and *P. carinii* pneumonia treated with daily doses of 20 mg/kg trimethoprim and 100 mg/kg sulfamethoxazole, mean plasma drug levels at $1\frac{1}{2}$ hours post-dose were 8.7 μg/ml on days 2–4 of treatment and 9.4 μg/ml on days 8–10 of treatment. For the same two periods mean sulfamethoxazole levels of 274 and 343 μg/ml, respectively, were obtained. This established ratios of trimethoprim + sulfamethoxazole of 1:32 and 1:36, respectively. Other studies in non-AIDS patients report lower levels of sulfamethoxazole and a ratio of about 1:20 when using the same dosage of drugs. In the 7 patients studied here all required a change in therapy because of side effects. This study suggests that high serum levels of sulfamethoxazole might account for some of the adverse reactions and that AIDS patients may retain higher concentrations of the drug than non-AIDS patients receiving the same dosages.

ADVERSE EFFECTS

Stevens-Johnson syndrome has been associated with sulfonamide administration, but the frequency of its occurrence is rare. An unusual variant was investigated in a 78-year-old man who experienced a generalized bullous erythema multiforme with simultaneous involvement of the esophagus following administration of trimethoprim + sulfamethoxazole (6). Specific immunoglobulin G, but not E, antibodies to both drugs were detected. Trimethoprim, but not sulfamethoxazole, transformed sensitized lymphocytes. The studies suggested that the adverse reactions of the skin and esophagus were immune-mediated. Another disturbing recent report is the association of erythema multiforme and the topical use of sulfacetamide in an 8 year-old boy with conjunctivitis (7).

At many medical centers trimethoprim + sulfamethoxazole is used prophylactically in patients with leukemia. The drugs may be given over relatively long periods of time and the possibility of bone marrow suppression exists. A placebo-controlled study in children with acute lymphocytic leukemia at the University of Minnesota randomized patients to 6-month periods of a placebo or trimethoprim + sulfamethoxazole (8). During the administration of the drug combination significant reductions were noted in the average white blood cell count, neutrophil count, lymphocyte count and platelet count compared with values obtained during the comparable placebo period. However, no clinical evidence of these abnormalities was apparent. In fact, the infections were significantly fewer in the drug-treated than the placebo-managed group.

Several years ago Asmar et al (9) reported a remarkably high rate of neutropenia and thrombocytopenia in children with otitis media or urinary tract infections treated with trimethoprim + sulfamethoxazole. For example, neutropenia (<1500 neutrophils/mm^3) developed in 34% of the children receiving trimethoprim + sulfamethoxazole but in only 5% receiving amoxicillin. Recently, Feldman et al (10) conducted a similar study in which 90 children with otitis media were randomized to receive trimethoprim + sulfamethoxazole or amoxicillin and the patients were carefully studied for subsequent hematologic abnormalities. Neutropenia devel-

231

oped at least once in 28 (57%) of the 49 children given trimethoprim + sulfamethoxazole and in 22 (54%) of the 41 who received amoxicillin. These changes were transient and appeared to have no effect on the course of the infection or welfare of the patients. In neither the study of Asmar et al nor that of Feldman et al were the etiologic agents identified. It seems reasonable to expect that some were of viral etiology, which might have accounted for some decrease in white blood cell counts.

Some of the adverse hematologic reactions encountered in the treatment of *P. carinii* pneumonitis resemble those of folic acid deficiency. In some areas it has become a practice to routinely administer folinic acid during trimethoprim + sulfamethoxazole therapy. This has raised the question of whether folinic acid might block the antimicrobial activity of the drug combination. A recent study in rats by D'Antonio et al (11) shows that the administration of folinic acid does not impair the capacity of trimethoprim + sulfamethoxazole to prevent or treat the infection.

Acute recurrent pancreatitis has recently been reported to be temporally associated with two courses of trimethoprim + sulfamethoxazole (12). While drug-induced pancreatitis has been described with sulfonamides alone, this case represents the first report of this complication with the drug combination. The mechanism is not known.

CLINICAL USES

Urinary tract infection

Within recent years efforts have been made to reduce the course of antibiotic treatment for bacteriuria and lower urinary tract infection. Several studies have yielded promising results. In a clinical trial 40 elderly patients with bacteriuria served to evaluate the effect of one-day treatment with trimethoprim (13). All patients given the drug obtained sterile urine, while all patients receiving the placebo remained bacteriuric. However, of the 20 patients initially cured with trimethoprim 14 (70%) had recurrent bacteriuria after 6 weeks.

A single-dose of trimethoprim + sulfamethoxazole was compared with a 10-day course of therapy of the drug combination in 203 women with lower urinary tract infections. Of the 11 women given a single dose 87% were cured and of the 92 treated for 10 days 89% were cured 1 week after therapy. No difference in recurrence rates was found between the two groups 6 months after the therapy (14).

In a randomized comparison of single-dose, 3-day and 10-day courses of trimethoprim + sulfamethoxazole in 279 women with uncomplicated urinary tract infection comparable results were obtained with the 3 regimens 2 and 6 weeks after treatment (15). However, adverse reactions were significantly greater in patients treated with the 10-day course (28%) than in those treated with the single-dose (5%) or 3-day course (9%). Single-dose therapy with trimethoprim + sulfamethoxazole was compared with single doses of amoxicillin and cyclacillin in the management of 38 women with acute cystitis. Trimethoprim + sulfamethoxazole was superior to the other two drugs (16). In a multicenter study of 370 patients treated with either trimethoprim + sulfamethoxazole or norfloxacin the percentage of patients with bacteriologic eradication was 97% for the norfloxacin group and 90% for the trimethoprim + sulfamethoxazole group (17).

A major problem in the management of urinary tract infections is the high rate of recurrence after seemingly adequate antibiotic treatment. The prophylactic administration of trimethoprim + sulfamethoxazole was evaluated in 72 children with recurrent urinary tract infections, vesicoureteral reflux or both (18). A relatively low dose of 2 mg trimethoprim and 10 mg sulfamethoxazole per kilogram daily or for 3 days per week was given orally. A significant reduction in infections was noted when compared with the previous year. With daily prophylaxis the infection rate was 5.4 cases per 1000 patient-months compared with 285.4 cases in the year before prophylaxis; side effects occurred in 11% of patients. When the prophylaxis was limited to 3 days per week the infection rate was 15.7 cases per 1000 patient-months compared to 313.6 cases during the year before prophylaxis; side effects were noted in 3% of these patients.

Trimethoprim alone has also been found to be effective prophylactically. Although Macrodantin (nitrofurantoin) was more effective in preventing bacteremia, it was associated with more side effects than trimethoprim (19).

Respiratory tract infections

Two studies have compared trimethoprim alone with trimethoprim + sulfamethoxazole in the treatment of lower respiratory tract infections of bacterial, or presumed bacterial, etiology (20, 21). Favorable responses occurred in both studies with either drug regimen in 80% or greater of patients treated.

Patients with AIDS have exaggerated reactions to trimethoprim + sulfamethoxazole. Of 34 AIDS patients treated with the drug combination for *P. carinii* pneumonitis 22 (65%) developed adverse reactions (22). These reactions included leukopenia in 20, hepatotoxicity in 12, fever in 8, rash in 6 and 'immediate' reactions in 2 patients. While some of these reactions were not clearly documented as drug-related, it is reasonable to conclude that the AIDS patient is at greater risk for such reactions.

Central nervous system infections

Trimethoprim + sulfamethoxazole has been evaluated for the prevention of bacterial infections following ventriculostomy or shunting procedures. Of those undergoing shunting procedures there was a higher infection rate in the placebo group (14 of 60 patients) than in the drug-treated group (4 of 62 patients). There were no differences in the infection rates between similarly treated groups of 52 ventriculostomy patients (23).

Two reports (24, 25) describe successful treatment of *Listeria* monocytogenes meningitis with trimethoprim + sulfamethoxazole. In a review of previously published cases with bacteremia or meningitis caused by *L. monocytogenes* all 7 cases were considered cured following treatment with this combination (24).

Infections in patients with underlying disease

In recent studies the prophylactic use of trimethoprim + sulfamethoxazole has resulted in the reduction of infectious episodes in patients with chronic granulomatous disease (26) and acute lymphocytic leukemia (27, 28). These confirm the findings in earlier studies.

The administration of trimethoprim + sulfamethoxazole alone with metronidazole was compared with the administration of metronidazole alone or a double placebo for effects on the course of Crohn's disease. No differences in the groups were apparent after 4 weeks of treatment (29).

The clinical course of Wegener's granulomatosis improved in 11 of 12 patients treated with antimicrobial agents, primarily trimethoprim + sulfamethoxazole (30). The explanation for this response has not been elucidated.

Ascending cholangitis is a frequent complication of congenital hepatic fibrosis and infection accounts for about half of the deaths with this disease. Sanchez et al (31) successfully treated 2 patients with hepatic fibrosis and cholangitis using prolonged courses of trimethoprim + sulfamethoxazole. This report helps substantiate the claims in two earlier studies on the successful use of this drug combination (32, 33).

Other infections

A group of 72 adults with typhoid fever responded favorably and without complications or adverse effects to either trimethoprim + sulfamethopyrazine or trimethoprim + sulfamethoxazole (34). The authors conclude that either of these drug combinations is safe and effective.

A prospective blinded study of 135 men with genital lesions caused by *Haemophilus ducreyi* (chancroid) revealed that trimethoprim + sulfamoxole given for 5 days was totally effective in achieving a cure, whereas only 78% were cured with a single dose of the combination (35).

DOSING

No recent changes have been made on approved dosages and routes of administration (see *Antimicrobial Agents Annual 1*).

FUTURE DIRECTIONS

Two particular adverse reactions to trimethoprim + sulfamethoxazole require more basic investigation as to the mechanism responsible for their occurrence: these include the exaggerated reactions in patients with AIDS and the erythema multiforme bulbosa (Stevens-Johnson syndrome) which may occur in presumably normal individuals. The expanding use of this drug combination for antimicrobial prophylaxis in cancer patients, organ transplant recipients, and certain immunodeficiency disorders seems generally warranted if cases are carefully chosen and carefully followed. More precise details on doses and intervals of administration are needed.

REFERENCES

1. Schifferli DM, Abraham SN, Beachey EH (1986) Influence of trimethoprim and sulfamethoxazole on the synthesis, expression and function of type 1 fimbriae of *Escherichia coli. J. Infect. Dis. 154*, 490.
2. Bravo IG, Bravo ME, Plate G et al (1984) The pharmacokinetics of cotrimazole sulphonamide in malnourished (marasmic) infants. *Pediatr. Pharmacol., 4*, 167.
3. Dudley MN, Levitz RE, Quitiliani R et al (1984) Pharmacokinetics of trimethoprim and sulfamethoxazole in serum and cerebrospinal fluid of adult patients with normal meninges. *Antimicrob. Agents Chemother., 26*, 811.
4. Albert F, Bishop-Frendling GB, Vergin H (1984) Diffusion of tetroxoprim/sulphadiazine into the cerebrospinal fluid of neurosurgical patients. *Fortschr. Med., 102*, 1064.
5. Bowden FJ, Harmon PJ, Lucas CR (1986) Serum trimethoprim and sulphamethoxazole levels in AIDS. *Lancet, 1*, 853.
6. Heer M, Altorfer J, Burger HR, Walti M (1985) Bullous esophageal lesions due to cotrimoxazole: an immune-mediated process? *Gastroenterology, 88*, 1954.
7. Genvert GI, Cohen EJ, Donnenfeld ED, Blecher MH (1985) Erythema multiforme after use of topical sulfacetamide. *Am. J. Ophthalmol., 99*, 465.
8. Woods WG, Daigle AE, Hutchinson RJ (1984) Myelosuppression associated with cotrimoxazole as a prophylactic antibiotic in the maintenance phase of childhood acute lymphocytic leukemia. *J. Pediatr., 105*, 639.
9. Asmar BI, Maqbool S, Dajani AS (1981) Hematological abnormalities after oral trimethoprim-sulfamethoxazole therapy in children. *Am. J. Dis. Child., 135*, 1100.
10. Feldman S, Doolittle M, Lott L et al (1985) Similar hematologic changes in children receiving trimethoprim-sulfamethoxazole or amoxicillin for otitis media. *J. Pediatr., 106*, 995.
11. D'Antonio RG, Johnson DB, Winn RE et al (1986) Effect of folinic acid on the capacity of trimethoprim-sulfamethoxazole to prevent and treat *Pneumocystis carinii* pneumonia in rats. *Antimicrob. Agents Chemother., 29*, 327.
12. Antonow DR (1986) Acute pancreatitis associated with trimethoprim-sulfamethoxazole. *Ann. Intern. Med., 104*, 363.
13. Renneberg J, Paerregaard A (1984) Single-day treatment with trimethoprim for asymptomatic bacteriuria in the elderly patient. *J. Urol., 132*, 934.

14. Prentice RD, Wu LR, Gehlbach SH et al (1985) Treatment of lower urinary tract infections with single-dose trimethoprim-sulfamethoxazole. *J. Fam. Pract., 20,* 551.

15. Gossius G, Vorland L (1984) A randomized comparison of high-dose versus three-day and ten-day therapy with trimethoprim-sulfamethoxazole for acute cystitis in women. *Scand. J. Infect. Dis., 16,* 373.

16. Hooton TM, Remning K, Stamm WE (1985) Single-dose therapy for cystitis in women: a comparison of trimethoprim-sulfamethoxazole, amoxicillin and cyclacillin. *J. Am. Med. Assoc., 253,* 387.

17. Sabbaj J, Hoagland VL, Shih WJ (1985) Multiclinic comparative study of norfloxacin and trimethoprim-sulfamethoxazole for the treatment of urinary tract infections. *Antimicrob. Agents Chemother., 27,* 297.

18. Labbe J (1984) Comparison of 2 methods for co-trimoxazole prophylaxis of urinary tract infection in children. *Can. Med. Assoc. J., 131,* 1229.

19. Brumfitt W, Smith GW, Hamilton-Miller JMT, Gargan RA (1985) A clinical comparison between macrodantin and trimethoprim for prophylaxis in women with recurrent urinary tract infections. *J. Antimicrob. Agents Chemother., 16,* 111.

20. Haataja M, Hanninen P, Platin LH et al (1985) Trimethoprim or cotrimoxazole in pneumonia. *Curr. Ther. Res. Clin. Exp., 37,* 191.

21. Brumfitt W, Hamilton-Miller JMT, Havard CW, Tansley H (1985) Trimethoprim alone compared to co-trimoxazole in lower respiratory infections: pharmacokinetics and clinical effectiveness. *Scand. J. Infect. Dis., 17,* 99.

22. Small GB, Harris CA, Friedland GH, Klein RS (1985) The treatment of *Pneumocystis carinii* pneumonia in the acquired immunodeficiency syndrome. *Arch. Intern. Med., 145,* 837.

23. Blomstedt GC (1985) Results of trimethoprim-sulfamethoxazole prophylaxis in ventriculostomy and shunting procedures: a double-blind randomized trial. *J. Neurosurg., 62,* 694.

24. Spitzer PG, Hammer SM, Karchmer AW (1986) Treatment of *Listeria monocytogenes* infection with trimethoprim-sulfamethoxazole: case report and review of the literature. *Rev. Infect. Dis., 8,* 427.

25. Armstrong RW, Slater B (1986) *Listeria monocytogenes* meningitis treated with trimethoprim-sulfamethoxazole. *Pediatr. Infect. Dis., 5,* 712.

26. Kremens B, Seger RA, Von Voss H, Wahn V (1985) Chronic granulomatous disease: improved prognosis with early diagnosis and specific therapy: report of five cases. *Monatsschr. Kinderheilkd., 133,* 284.

27. Goorin AM, Hershey BJ, Levin MJ et al (1985) Use of trimethoprim-sulfamethoxazole to prevent bacterial infections in children with acute lymphoblastic leukemia. *Pediatr. Infect. Dis., 4,* 265.

28. Kovatch AL, Wald ER, Albo VC et al (1985) Oral trimethoprim/sulfamethoxazole for prevention of bacterial infection during the induction phase of cancer chemotherapy. *Pediatrics, 76,* 754.

29. Ambrose NS, Allan RH, Keighley MRB et al (1985) Antibiotic therapy for treatment in relapse of intestinal Crohn's disease: a prospective randomized study. *Dis. Colon Rectum, 28,* 81.

30. DeResnee RA, McDonald TJ, Weiland LH (1985) Wegener's granulomatosis: observations on treatment with antimicrobial agents. *Mayo Clin. Proc., 60,* 27.

31. Sanchez C, Gonzalez E, Garau J (1986) Trimethoprim-sulfamethoxazole treatment of cholangitis complicating congenital hepatic fibrosis. *Pediatr. Infect. Dis., 5,* 360.

32. Kocoshis SA, Riely CA, Burrel M et al (1980) Cholangitis in a child due to biliary tract abnormalities. *Dig. Dis. Sci., 25,* 59.
33. Rogers CA, Isenberg JN, Leonard AS et al (1976) Ascending cholangitis diagnosed by percutaneous hepatic aspiration. *J. Pediatr., 88,* 83.
34. Schiraldi O, Sforza E, Piaia F (1985) Effect of a new sulfatrimethoprim combination (trimethoprim-sulfamethopyrazine) in typhoid fever: a double-blind study on 72 adult patients. *Chemotherapy (Basel), 31,* 68.
35. Dylewski J, Nsanze H, D'Costa L et al (1985) Trimethoprim + sulphamoxole in the treatment of chancroid: comparison of two single dose treatment regimens with a five day regimen. *J. Antimicrob. Chemother., 16,* 103.

CHAPTER 19

Vancomycin and teicoplanin

KENT B. CROSSLEY

In 1986, studies of vancomycin were published which continue to broaden our understanding of the activity, pharmacokinetic behavior and clinical efficacy of this agent. Substantial information about teicoplanin was also reported within the past year. The structure of the teicoplanin complex is shown in Figure 1 (1). Teicoplanin has now been extensively evaluated in European clinical trials, the results of which are just being published. Studies in the United States are currently underway.

A number of related glycopeptide antibiotics are in early stages of clinical and laboratory evaluation at the present time.

ACTIVITY

Mechanism of action

Vancomycin and teicoplanin act by inhibiting synthesis of cell wall peptidoglycan by forming bonds with the D-Ala-D-Ala terminal of muramyl pentapeptides. The affinity constant of teicoplanin for D-Ala-D-Ala-agarose is 4–5 times that of vancomycin.

Spectrum of activity

Studies published in 1986 confirm the excellent activity of both vancomycin and teicoplanin against gram-positive cocci. A number of comparative studies, in vitro evaluations of combination therapy and in vivo experiments have been reported.

Del Bene et al (2) examined a heterogeneous collection of isolates of *Staphylococcus aureus*, *S. epidermidis* and *S. haemolyticus* to determine the activity of a variety of antimicrobial agents. Methicillin-resistant and methicillin-susceptible isolates of *S. aureus* were susceptible to similar low concentrations of teicoplanin and vancomycin. Methicillin-resistant isolates of *S. haemolyticus* were substantial-

Antimicrobial Agents Annual 3
P.K. Peterson and J. Verhoef, editors
© Elsevier Science Publishers BV, 1988

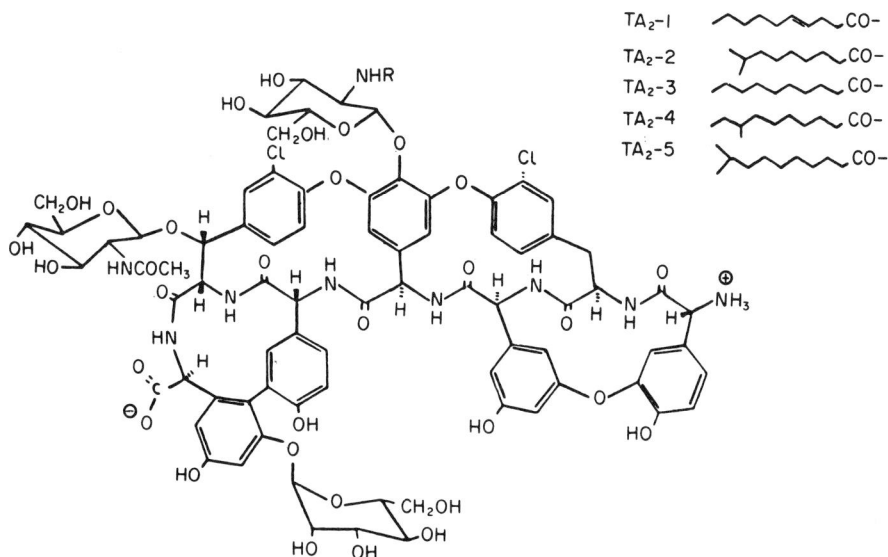

Fig. 1   Structure of teicoplanin complex. TA_2-1 to TA_2-5 are the components of the complex, each characterized by a specific fatty acid moiety (R). Reproduced from Parenti (1) by courtesy of The Journal of Hospital Infection.

ly less susceptible to teicoplanin than vancomycin. With 20 strains, the 90% minimum inhibitory concentration (MIC_{90}) for teicoplanin was 16 μg/ml and 2 μg/ml with vancomycin. In contrast, against methicillin-susceptible coagulase-negative staphylococci, teicoplanin was slightly more active than vancomycin (2).

Moorhouse et al (3) confirmed the excellent activity of teicoplanin against methicillin-resistant *S. aureus*. Brumfitt and Hamilton-Miller (4) reported activity of teicoplanin and vancomycin against 38 isolates of coagulase-negative staphylococci isolated from patients with peritonitis associated with continuous ambulatory peritoneal dialysis. The two drugs were virtually identical in activity against these organisms. A report from the University of Virginia Medical Center examined antibiotic susceptibility of 50 strains of coagulase-negative staphylococci isolated from patients with hospital-acquired bacteremia. Teicoplanin was slightly more active against both *S. epidermidis* isolates (37 strains) and other coagulase-negative staphylococci (13 strains) (5).

Against streptococci, additional evidence has accumulated to suggest that the glycopeptide antibiotics are less active than some other agents. Meylan et al (6) found that the majority of a group of 24 strains of viridans streptococci were not effectively killed by vancomycin. The authors suggested that examination of reduction in colony counts over time was a more accurate measure of susceptibility than the minimum bactericidal concentration (MBC). Shanson and Tadayon (7) confirmed that teicoplanin has greater inhibitory activity than vancomycin against

extra references

streptococci but reported that both drugs were not bactericidal at concentrations less than 16 μg/ml. Teicoplanin plus gentamicin and vancomycin plus gentamicin were synergistic against all 16 tested strains of penicillin-tolerant viridans streptococci or enterococci.

A number of other antibiotics in combination with vancomycin or teicoplanin were examined in reports published in 1986. Ho and Klempner (8) found that vancomycin and clindamycin usually were indifferent or antagonistic against isolates of *S. aureus*. In another study (9), the serum bactericidal activity of vancomycin and teicoplanin (as well as nafcillin) was markedly reduced when rifampin was also present. However, Debbia et al (10), using similar techniques, showed indifference or an additive effect when teicoplanin was combined with rifampin. A third study which examined only vancomycin in combination with rifampin using a checkerboard technique showed indifference (11).

Several reports of experimental infection were published during the past year. Traub demonstrated that although vancomycin was not very active against *Clostridium perfringens* type A in vitro, the drug was as effective as penicillin G or imipenem against this organism in a murine model (12). Arioli et al (13) investigated the activity of teicoplanin alone or with rifampin or gentamicin in the treatment of experimental streptococcal or staphylococcal endocarditis. Rather small numbers of animals were examined, but the authors reported that teicoplanin was more active than vancomycin and that either of these drugs, in combination with rifampin or gentamicin, was significantly more active than single drug therapy.

Barry et al (14) evaluated the activity of teicoplanin and vancomycin and recommended modification of the current zone size standards for disk susceptibility testing. The authors recommended that ≤ 10 mm be interpreted as resistance with both drugs and zones of ≥ 14 mm (teicoplanin) or ≥ 15 mm (vancomycin) be defined as susceptible. Several recent papers have described isolates of *Neisseria gonorrhoeae* which are susceptible to vancomycin (15). This is of considerable importance because the media generally used for isolation of *N. gonorrhoeae* contain vancomycin.

Barr et al (16) examined the effect of various antibiotics on the transfer of a plasmid specifying tetracycline resistance in *S. aureus*. β-Lactam antibiotics dramatically increased the rate of transfer when present in subinhibitory concentrations. Vancomycin and teicoplanin had no effect on the rate of plasmid transfer.

CLINICAL PHARMACOLOGY

Although analysis of teicoplanin serum concentrations has been primarily by means of a microbiologic assay, an enzyme receptor assay has been described (17). Results of the two techniques correlate closely. Vancomycin serum levels are measured by a number of different procedures; refinements and simplifications in the liquid-chromatographic determination procedure were reported in 1986 (18).

Additional information about the pharmacokinetics of vancomycin in infants was published last year. Naqvi et al (19) found that infants less than 41 weeks post-conception had significantly lower vancomycin clearance rates and greater beta-half-lives than infants 3–6 months of age. Spivey (20) reported a marked prolongation of vancomycin beta-half-life in children receiving indomethacin for treatment of patent ductus arteriosus (20). Schaible et al (21) also examined vancomycin kinetics in infants and found relationships similar to those noted by Naqvi et al (19).

A recent pharmacokinetic study compares individualized dosing using a one-compartment model with use of the nomograms published by Moellering and Matzke. The authors of this study found that individualized dosing resulted in more accurate predictions of vancomycin serum concentration than the nomograms (22). Several extensive reviews of vancomycin pharmacokinetics were published in the clinical pharmacy literature in 1986 (23–25).

Use of vancomycin in a few specific clinical situations has been further defined. Harford et al (26) demonstrated that intravenous administration of a single 1 gram dose of vancomycin yielded end-of-dwell dialysate levels above 3 μg/ml for 7 days in each of 5 patients with peritoneal dialysis-associated peritonitis. Matzke et al (27) reported the effect of hemofiltration on vancomycin kinetics in 5 patients. The drug was removed by hemofiltration; the rate of flow was a significant determinant of vancomycin clearance. Brater et al (28) describe the serum clearance of vancomycin in 10 patients with thermal injury; vancomycin clearance correlated closely with creatinine clearance.

Only a few studies of teicoplanin kinetics appeared in 1986. Lagast et al (29) reported the half-life of teicoplanin to be 32.2 hours. Wise et al (30) reported a very similar half-life and noted that the drug rapidly penetrated non-inflamed peritoneal fluid and chemically induced blister fluid. These authors found that by 96 hours, approximately half of the dose of the drug was recovered in urine.

ADVERSE EFFECTS AND DRUG INTERACTIONS

The now well-recognized association between rapid vancomycin administration and flushing and hypotension ('red man's syndrome' or 'red neck syndrome') may also occur following the slow infusion of this drug (31). The mechanism of this reaction is reviewed in another study (32).

Two case-reports further document the occurrence of neutropenia in patients receiving vancomycin (33, 34). Evidence that tobramycin nephrotoxicity is enhanced by the administration of vancomycin was reported from studies in male rats (35). Appel et al (36) have comprehensively reviewed information about nephrotoxicity with this drug. They suggest that the risk of renal toxicity is limited.

McElrath et al (37) described a patient with methicillin-resistant *S. aureus* endocarditis who was treated with vancomycin and developed rash and fever. The patient was subsequently treated with teicoplanin, and fever and rash again developed. This report suggests that significant cross-reactions between these two agents may be of potential concern.

241

CLINICAL USES

Several studies which extend our understanding of the use of vancomycin in the treatment of intracranial infection were published in 1986. Levy et al (38) measured vancomycin levels in fluid from a brain abscess and found concentrations which approach those present in serum. Osborn et al (39) and Pau et al (40) describe use of vancomycin in the treatment of ventricular shunt infections; both authors suggest doses of 4–5 mg administered within the ventricle every 24–72 hours.

Vancomycin and bacitracin were compared for treatment of *Clostridium difficile*-induced diarrhea. Bacitracin, 25 000 units 4 times each day, was as effective as 500 mg of vancomycin 4 times each day in this randomized, double-blind, prospective study (41).

Two reports have described treatment of ocular infection with vancomycin using either a solution prepared in saline or phosphate-buffered artificial tears or intravitreal administration (42, 43). Both techniques were effective and associated with a minimum of toxicity.

The effect of vancomycin versus placebo when combined with gentamicin and ticarcillin for empiric therapy of granulocytopenic patients with fever was examined by Karp et al (44). These authors found that gram-positive infection was significantly less frequent when vancomycin rather than placebo was used. Winston et al (45) compared norfloxacin with vancomycin/polymyxin for use in antimicrobial decontamination of the bowel in granulocytopenic patients. These authors found that norfloxacin was better tolerated and more efficacious than vancomycin/polymyxin.

An increasing number of studies of the clinical use of teicoplanin were published in 1986. The drug was examined for use in dental prophylaxis and found to be efficacious in a small study (46). Williams et al (47) described the use of this drug in treating 94 patients with gram-positive infection. The drug was efficacious and side effects were limited to high-tone hearing loss (1 patient), rash (2 patients), and drug fever (1 patient). Glupczynski et al (48) reported a similar series of 47 patients. These authors observed no significant adverse effects and concluded that the drug was efficacious and well tolerated.

One report, published in early 1987, perhaps inappropriately questioned the efficacy of teicoplanin. The study compared teicoplanin and flucloxacillin in the treatment of severe staphylococcal infection; teicoplanin was significantly less effective. However, the doses of teicoplanin used are substantially less than those currently recommended (49).

REFERENCES

1. Parenti F (1986) Structure and mechanism of action of teicoplanin. *J. Hosp. Infect., 7, Suppl A*, 79.
2. Del Bene VE, John Jr JF, Twitty JA, Lewis JW (1986) Anti-staphylococcal activity

of teicoplanin, vancomycin, and other antimicrobial agents: the significance of methicillin resistance. *J. Infect. Dis., 154,* 349.

3. Moorhouse EC, Mulvihill TE, Jones L, Mooney D, Falkiner FR, Keane CT (1985) The in-vitro activity of some antimicrobial agents against methicillin-resistant *Staphylococcus aureus. J. Antimicrob. Chemother., 15,* 291.

4. Brumfitt W, Hamilton-Miller JMT (1986) Activity of teicoplanin against coagulase-negative staphylococci isolated from patients undergoing continuous peritoneal dialysis. *Eur. J. Clin. Microbiol., 5,* 48.

5. Ponce de Leon S, Guenthner SH, Wenzel RP (1986) Microbiologic studies of coagulase-negative staphylococci isolated from patients with nosocomial bacteraemias. *J. Hosp. Infect., 7,* 121.

6. Meylan PR, Francioli P, Glauser MP (1986) Discrepancies between MBC and actual killing of viridans group streptococci by cell-wall-active antibiotics. *Antimicrob. Agents Chemother., 29,* 418.

7. Shanson DC, Tadayon M (1986) Activity of teicoplanin compared with vancomycin alone, and combined with gentamicin, against penicillin tolerant viridans streptococci and enterococci causing endocarditis. *J. Hosp. Infect., 7, Suppl A,* 65.

8. Ho JL, Klempner MS (1986) In vitro evaluation of clindamycin in combination with oxacillin, rifampin, or vancomycin against *Staphylococcus aureus. Diagn. Microbiol. Infect. Dis., 4,* 133.

9. Hackbarth CJ, Chambers HF, Sande MA (1986) Serum bactericidal activity of rifampin in combination with other antimicrobial agents against *Staphylococcus aureus. Antimicrob. Agents Chemother., 29,* 611.

10. Debbia E, Pesce A, Schito GC (1986) In vitro interactions between teicoplanin and other antibiotics against enterococci and staphylococci. *J. Hosp. Infect., 7, Suppl A,* 73.

11. Walsh TJ, Auger F, Tatem BA, Hansen SL, Standiford HC (1986) Novobiocin and rifampicin in combination against methicillin-resistant *Staphylococcus aureus:* an in-vitro comparison with vancomycin plus rifampicin. *J. Antimicrob. Chemother., 17,* 75.

12. Traub WH (1986) *Clostridium perfringens* type A: comparison of in vitro and in vivo activity of twelve antimicrobial drugs. *Chemotherapy (Basel), 32,* 59.

13. Arioli V, Berti M, Candiani G (1986) Activity of teicoplanin in localized experimental infections in rats. *J. Hosp. Infect., 7, Suppl A,* 91.

14. Barry AL, Thornsberry C, Jones RN (1986) Evaluation of teicoplanin and vancomycin disk susceptibility tests. *J. Clin. Microbiol., 23,* 100.

15. Koelbl JA, Catlin BW (1986) Vancomycin hypersusceptibility in *Neisseria gonorrhoeae* isolated from patients involves diverse mutations. *Antimicrob. Agents Chemother., 29,* 687.

16. Barr V, Barr K, Millar MR, Lacey RW (1986) Beta-lactam antibiotics increase the frequency of plasmid transfer in *Staphylococcus aureus. J. Antimicrob. Chemother., 17,* 409.

17. Cavenaghi L, Corti A, Cassani G (1986) Comparison of the solid phase enzyme receptor assay (SPERA) and the microbiological assay for teicoplanin. *J. Hosp. Infect., 7, Suppl A,* 85.

18. Rosenthal AF, Sarfati I, A'Zary E (1986) Simplified liquid-chromatographic determination of vancomycin. *Clin. Chem., 32,* 1016.

19. Naqvi SH, Keenan WJ, Reichley, Fortune KP (1986) Vancomycin pharmacokinetics in small, seriously ill infants. *Am. J. Dis. Child., 140,* 107.

20. Spivey JM (1986) Vancomycin pharmacokinetics in neonates. *Am. J. Dis. of Child.,* *140*, 859.

21. Schaible DH, Rocci Jr ML, Alpert GA, Campos JM, Paul MH, Polin RA, Plotkin SA (1986) Vancomycin pharmacokinetics in infants: relationships to indices of maturation. *Pediatr. Infect. Dis., 5*, 304.

22. Rybak MJ, Boike SC (1986) Individualized adjustment of vancomycin dosage: comparison with two dosage nomograms. *Drug Intell. Clin. Pharm., 20*, 64.

23. Rybak MJ, Boike SC (1986) Monitoring vancomycin therapy. *Drug Intell. Clin. Pharm., 20*, 757.

24. Cheung RPF, DiPiro JT (1986) Vancomycin: an update. *Pharmacotherapy, 6*, 153.

25. Matzke GR, Zhanel GG, Guay DRP (1986) Clinical pharmacokinetics of vancomycin. *Clin. Pharmacokinet., 11*, 257.

26. Harford AM, Sica DA, Tartaglione T, Polk RE, Dalton HP, Poynor W (1986) Vancomycin pharmacokinetics in continuous ambulatory peritoneal dialysis patients with peritonitis. *Nephron, 43*, 217.

27. Matzke GR, O'Connell MB, Collins AJ, Keshaviah PR (1986) Disposition of vancomycin during hemofiltration. *Clin. Pharmacol. Ther., 40*, 425.

28. Brater DC, Bawdon RE, Anderson SA, Purdue GF, Hunt JL (1986) Vancomycin elimination in patients with burn injury. *Clin. Pharmacol. Ther., 39*, 631.

29. Lagast H, Dodion P, Klastersky J (1986) Comparison of pharmacokinetics and bactericidal activity of teicoplanin and vancomycin. *J. Antimicrob. Chemother., 18*, 513.

30. Wise R, Donovan A, McNulty AM, Waldron R, Andrews JM (1986) Teicoplanin, its pharmacokinetics, blister and peritoneal fluid penetration. *J. Hosp. Infect., 7, Suppl A*, 47.

31. Davis RL, Smith AL (1986) The 'red man's syndrome' and slow infusion of vancomycin. *Ann. Intern. Med., 104*, 285.

32. Southorn PA, Plevak DJ, Wright AJ, Wilson WR (1986) Adverse effects of vancomycin administered in the perioperative period. *Mayo Clin. Proc., 61*, 721.

33. Koo KB, Bachand RL, Chow AW (1986) Vancomycin-induced neutropenia. *Drug Intell. Clin. Pharm., 20*, 780.

34. Henry K, Steinberg I, Crossley KB (1986) Vancomycin-induced neutropenia during treatment of osteomyelitis in an outpatient. *Drug Intell. Clin. Pharm., 20*, 783.

35. Wood CA, Kohlhepp SJ, Kohnen PW, Houghton DC, Gilbert DN (1986) Vancomycin enhancement of experimental tobramycin nephrotoxicity. *Antimicrob. Agents Chemother., 30*, 20.

36. Appel GB, Given DB, Levine LR, Cooper GL (1986) Vancomycin and the kidney. *Am. J. Kidney Dis., 8*, 75.

37. McElrath MJ, Goldberg D, Neu HC (1986) Allergic crossreactivity of teicoplanin and vancomycin. *Lancet, 1*, 47.

38. Levy RM, Gutin PH, Baskin DS, Pons VG (1986) Vancomycin penetration of a brain abscess: case report and review of the literature. *Neurosurgery, 18*, 632.

39. Osborn JS, Sharp S, Hanson EJ, MacGee E, Brewer JH (1986) *Staphylococcus epidermidis* ventriculitis treated with vancomycin and rifampin. *Neurosurgery, 19*, 824.

40. Pau AK, Smego Jr RA, Fisher MA (1986) Intraventricular vancomycin: observations of tolerance and pharmacokinetics in two infants with ventricular shunt infections. *Pediatr. Infect. Dis., 5*, 93.

41. Dudley MN, McLaughlin JC, Carrington G, Frick J, Nightingale CH, Quintiliani R (1986) Oral bacitracin *vs* vancomycin therapy for *Clostridium difficile*-induced diar-

rhea: a randomized double-blind trial. *Arch. Intern. Med., 146*, 1101.

42. Fleischer AB, Hoover DL, Khan JA, Parisi JT, Burns RP (1986) Topical vancomycin formulation for methicillin-resistant *Staphylococcus epidermidis* blepharoconjunctivitis. *Am. J. Ophthalmol., 101*, 283.

43. Smith MA, Sorenson JA, Lowy FD, Shakin JL, Harrison W, Jakobiec FA (1986) Treatment of experimental methicillin-resistant *Staphylococcus epidermidis* endophthalmitis with intravitreal vancomycin. *Ophthalmology, 93*, 1328.

44. Karp JE, Dick JD, Angelopulos C, Charache P, Green L, Burke PJ, Saral R (1986) Empiric use of vancomycin during prolonged treatment-induced granulocytopenia. *Am. J. Med., 81*, 237.

45. Winston DJ, Ho WG, Nakao SL, Gale RP, Champlin RE (1986) Norfloxacin versus vancomycin/polymyxin for prevention of infections in granulocytopenic patients. *Am. J. Med., 80*, 884.

46. Maskell JP, Carter JLB, Boyd RB, Williams RJ (1986) Teicoplanin as a prophylactic antibiotic for dental bacteraemia. *J. Antimicrob. Chemother., 17*, 651.

47. Williams AH, Gruneberg RN, Webster A, Ridgway GL (1986) Teicoplanin in the treatment of infection caused by gram-positive organisms. *J. Hosp. Infect., 7, Suppl A*, 101.

48. Glupczynski Y, Lagast H, Van der Auwera P, Thys JP, Crokaert F, Yourassowsky E, Meunier-Carpentier F, Klastersky J, Kains JP, Serruys-Schoutens E (1986) Clinical evaluation of teicoplanin for therapy of severe infections caused by gram-positive bacteria. *Antimicrob. Agents Chemother., 29*, 52.

49. Calain P, Krause K-H, Vaudaux P, Auckenthaler R, Lew D, Waldvogel F, Hirschel B (1987) Early termination of a prospective, randomized trial comparing teicoplanin and flucloxacillin for treating severe staphylococcal infections. *J. Infect. Dis., 155*, 187.

Flucytosine

CAROL A. KAUFFMAN

Flucytosine (5-fluorocytosine; 5-FC) is a useful antifungal agent for treating infections due to *Candida* and *Cryptococcus*. Flucytosine is almost always used in combination with amphotericin B. Relatively few new data on flucytosine have appeared in the literature in recent years. However, new methods for measuring serum concentrations of flucytosine have been published and several articles dealing with its usefulness in treating cryptococcal meningitis will appear in press in 1987.

ACTIVITY

Flucytosine is active in vitro against most strains of *Cryptococcus neoformans*. The genus *Candida* shows greater variation in susceptibility than *Cryptococcus*, but most strains of *Candida albicans* are susceptible. In addition, some of the dematiaceous fungi that cause chromomycosis are susceptible to flucytosine. Flucytosine exerts its antifungal effect in both yeasts and dematiaceous fungi by conversion to 5-fluorouracil (5-FU) and subsequent inhibition of DNA synthesis (by formation of 5-fluorodeoxyuridine monophosphate, an inhibitor of thymidylate synthetase) and interference with RNA-protein synthetic pathways by incorporation of 5-fluorouridine triphosphate into fungal RNA (1, 2).

Resistance develops quickly when the drug is used alone to treat infection. Recent data suggest that the mechanism of resistance is primarily by decreased UMP pyrophosphorylase activity (3), but previous studies showed that decreased cytosine deaminase activity or decreased flucytosine uptake by the fungal cell also lead to resistance.

CLINICAL PHARMACOLOGY

Flucytosine is well-absorbed orally, exhibits little protein binding, and distributes

Antimicrobial Agents Annual 3
P.K. Peterson and J. Verhoef, editors
© Elsevier Science Publishers BV, 1988

into most body fluids quite well. This makes the drug useful in rather sequestered sites, such as the eye, the nervous system, and joints. The drug achieves excellent levels in peritoneal dialysis fluid in patients on continuous ambulatory peritoneal dialysis. It is excreted almost entirely in the urine as unmetabolized drug; thus, renal failure, commonly seen with administration of amphotericin B therapy, leads to accumulation of flucytosine in the serum.

ADVERSE EFFECTS AND DRUG INTERACTIONS

The major toxic effect of flucytosine is bone marrow depression. This suppression is reversible, is dose-related, occurring when serum drug levels exceed 100 μg/ml, and is most commonly seen during the period of amphotericin-B-induced renal insufficiency when the two drugs are used concomitantly (4, 5). The bone marrow toxicity is presumed due to conversion of the drug to 5-FU (6).

Other side effects of flucytosine include hepatotoxicity, which is uncommonly seen and may be dose-related, and gastrointestinal toxicity, which occurs in about 6–10% of cases and may rarely result in a severe ulcerative enterocolitis (7).

CLINICAL USES

Flucytosine is rarely used as a single agent, the one exception being the short-term treatment of urinary tract candidiasis (8). The drug is almost always combined with amphotericin B therapy for several reasons: combined therapy decreases the emergence of resistance to flucytosine, frequently leads to synergistic antifungal activity, and allows reduction in the daily amphotericin B dosage while still effectively treating the fungal infection, thus decreasing the nephrotoxicity of amphotericin B.

A definite indication for flucytosine use is treatment of cryptococcal meningitis. The results of a cooperative study published in 1979 established the benefits of combined amphotericin B + flucytosine therapy for 6 weeks in this disease (9). Recent data show that 4 weeks of combined therapy with amphotericin B + flucytosine is as efficacious as 6 weeks in certain patient groups (10).

Flucytosine is useful adjunctive therapy in the treatment of serious infections due to *Candida*. While no prospective study has been published comparing the efficacy of combined amphotericin B + flucytosine therapy versus amphotericin B alone in candidiasis, as has been shown with cryptococcosis, several recent studies do document the usefulness of flucytosine in candidiasis. Smego et al (11) and Salaki et al (12) reviewed the use of flucytosine in addition to amphotericin B in treating *Candida* meningitis. Both groups concluded that both amphotericin B and flucytosine should be used in an attempt to provide maximal therapy for this serious infection. Several recent studies point out the increase in candidiasis in premature infants in neonatal intensive care units (13). The use of combined amphotericin B + flucytosine is advocated in this group of patients (14, 15).

In fact, if the organism is sensitive to flucytosine, this drug should always be used to treat severe local *Candida* infections as well as disseminated candidiasis.

Flucytosine is the treatment of choice in many patients with chromomycosis, admittedly an uncommon infection in the United States. In some patients with aspergillosis, flucytosine may be useful adjunctive therapy. Although some early studies commented on the use of flucytosine alone to treat aspergillosis, there is little support for this mode of therapy. Used with amphotericin B, flucytosine may promote killing of *Aspergillus* (16), although a recent study in vitro could not confirm this synergistic action (17).

DOSING

Flucytosine is administered orally at a dose of 150 mg/kg/d. In the face of renal insufficiency, especially when concomitant amphotericin B is given, the dose must be reduced to avoid bone marrow toxicity. Suggested dosing is given in Table 1. Although this gives one an idea of the appropriate dose to use, it is strongly recommended that serum flucytosine levels be measured to be certain to keep the level below 100 μg/ml (4). Levels should be measured weekly to avoid accumulation of drug and subsequent toxicity.

The microbiologic assay for measuring serum flucytosine concentrations, as well as methods for sensitivity testing for flucytosine, have been reviewed recently by a Working Group of the British Society for Mycopathology (18). The methods are very clearly spelled out for incorporation into any hospital laboratory. The drug can also be measured by high-pressure liquid chromatography (19). The newest assay utilizes the observation that flucytosine falsely increases serum creatinine levels when the Kodak 'Ektachem' analyzer is used (20). The drug does not interfere with other automated systems for determining serum creatinine. Thus, one can use the Ektachem system and another system for measuring serum creatinine, and the difference in the results is a measure of serum flucytosine concentration (21).

Table 1   *Flucytosine dosing in renal insufficiency*

Creatinine clearance (ml/min)	Dosage (mg/kg)	Interval (h)
> 40	35	6
20–40	35	12
10–20	35	24
< 10	35	> 24

FUTURE DIRECTIONS

Little can be expected in terms of new developments with this antifungal agent. Indications for its use and methods of dosing will probably not change.

REFERENCES

1. Waldorf AR, Polack A (1983) Mechanisms of action of 5-fluorocytosine. *Antimicrob. Agents Chemother., 23,* 79.
2. Polak A (1983) Mode of action of 5-fluorocytosine and 5-fluorouracil in dematiaceous fungi. *Sabouraudia, 21,* 15.
3. Whelan WL, Kerridge D (1984) Decreased activity of UMP pyrophosphorylase associated with resistance to 5-fluorocytosine in *Candida albicans. Antimicrob. Agents Chemother., 26,* 570.
4. Kauffman CA, Frame PT (1977) Bone marrow toxicity associated with 5-fluorocytosine therapy. *Antimicrob. Agents Chemother., 11,* 244.
5. NIAID Mycoses Study Group (1987) Toxicity of amphotericin B plus flucytosine in 194 patients with cryptococcal meningitis. *Am. J. Med., 83,* 236.
6. Diasio RB, Lakings DE, Bennett JE (1978) Evidence for conversion of 5-fluorocytosine to 5-fluorouracil in humans: possible factor in 5-fluorocytosine clinical toxicity. *Antimicrob. Agents Chemother., 14,* 903.
7. White CA, Traube J (1982) Ulcerating enteritis associated with flucytosine therapy. *Gastroenterology, 83,* 1127.
8. Fisher JF, Chew WH, Shadomy S, Duma RJ, Mayhall CG, House WC (1982) Urinary tract infections due to *Candida albicans. Rev. Infect. Dis., 4,* 1107.
9. Bennett JE, Dismukes WE, Duma RJ, Medoff G, Sande MA, Gallis H, Leonard J, Fields BT, Bradshaw M, Haywood H, McGee ZA, Cate TR, Cobbs CG, Warner JF, Alling DW (1979) A comparison of amphotericin B alone and combined with flucytosine in the treatment of cryptococcal meningitis. *N. Engl. J. Med., 301,* 126.
10. NIAID Mycoses Study Group (1987) Treatment of cryptococcal meningitis with combination amphotericin B and flucytosine: results of a prospective randomized clinical trial. *N. Engl. J. Med., 317,* 334.
11. Smego RA, Perfect JR, Durack DT (1984) Combined therapy with amphotericin B and flucytosine for *Candida* meningitis. *Rev. Infect. Dis., 6,* 791.
12. Salaki JS, Louria DB, Chmel H (1984) Fungal and yeast infections of the central nervous system. *Medicine, 63,* 108.
13. Baley JE, Kliegman RM, Fanaroff AA (1984) Disseminated fungal infections in very low-birth-weight infants: clinical manifestations and epidemiology. *Pediatrics, 73,* 144.
14. Baley JE, Kliegman RM, Fanaroff AA (1984) Disseminated fungal infections in very low-birth-weight infants: therapeutic toxicity. *Pediatrics, 73,* 153.
15. Johnson DE, Thompson TR, Green TP, Ferrieri P (1984) Systemic candidiasis in very low-birth-weight infants (< 1500 grams). *Pediatrics, 73,* 138.
16. Kitahara M, Seth VK, Medoff G, Kobayashi GS (1976) Activity of amphotericin B, 5-fluorocytosine, and rifampin against six clinical isolates of *Aspergillus. Antimicrob. Agents Chemother., 9,* 915.

17. Hughes CE, Harris C, Moody JA, Peterson LR, Gerding DN (1984) In vitro activities of amphotericin B in combination with four antifungal agents and rifampin against *Aspergillus* species. *Antimicrob. Agents Chemother., 25, 560.*

18. Speller CE, Cartwright RY, Evans EGV, Hay RJ, Mackenzie DWR, Milne LJR, Odd FC, Warnock DW (1984) Laboratory methods for flucytosine (5-fluorocytosine): Report of a Working Group of the British Society for Mycopathology. *J. Antimicrob. Chemother., 14, 1.*

19. Schwertschlag U, Nakata LM, Gal J (1984) Improved procedure for determination of flucytosine in human blood plasma by high-pressure liquid chromatography. *Antimicrob. Agents Chemother., 26, 303.*

20. Mitchell RT, Marshall LH, Lefkowitz LB, Stratton CW (1985) Falsely elevated serum creatinine level secondary to the presence of 5-fluorocytosine. *Am. J. Clin. Pathol., 84, 251.*

21. Washburn RG, Klym DM, Kroll MH, Bennett JE (1986) Rapid enzymatic method for measurement of serum flucytosine levels. *J. Antimicrob. Chemother., 17, 673.*

CHAPTER 21

The azoles: miconazole, ketoconazole, itraconazole

ELIZABETH ELSTER WACK and JOHN N. GALGIANI

Major developments in the past year include the investigation of a new orally active triazole, itraconazole. This agent shows promise in a wide range of superficial and deep mycoses. At present, there is no evidence of serious toxicity associated with its use (1). Further comparative clinical studies are underway.

Imidazole derivatives for topical use continue to be developed and tested, particularly for vaginal candidiasis (2). These will not be discussed in detail as there are no clear clinical preferences at this point.

Difficulties remain with in vitro susceptibility testing, but efforts to find a reliable method for predicting sensitivity and clinical response to the antifungal agents continue.

ACTIVITY

In vitro testing of itraconazole has demonstrated a wide range of antifungal activity including activity against the yeasts, dimorphic fungi, and molds. Of particular interest is apparent in vitro activity against *Aspergillus* species. Although such results are very difficult to interpret, they are more encouraging than similar studies with other imidazoles. Thus, they point to the need for further studies in experimental infections and selected patients (3).

Susceptibility tests

Two studies examined the effects of various media on in-vitro susceptibility testing. Doern examined 62 different clinical yeast isolates for susceptibility to amphotericin B, 5-fluorocytosine, ketoconazole, and miconazole using 6 different media in a macrobroth dilution procedure. He concluded that broth dilution susceptibility is best performed with an incubation of 48 hours and that actual

Antimicrobial Agents Annual 3
P.K. Peterson and J. Verhoef, editors
© Elsevier Science Publishers BV, 1988

minimum inhibitory concentrations (MICs) are highly influenced by the medium used (4).

Radetsky et al (5) tested 84 clinical isolates of various *Candida* species for susceptibility to the same 4 antifungal agents using two different media in both agar and microtiter broth dilution systems. He found the microtiter system using RPMI 1640 medium to be the most reliable method. Using a murine model of systemic candidiasis and clinical information from several patients, he was able to corroborate the significance of derived MIC cutoff points.

Mechanism of action

The mechanism of action of the imidazoles has been fully discussed in *Annuals 1 and 2*. Itraconazole appears to interfere with the biosynthesis of cell-membrane ergosterol which is a similar mechanism of action to that of the older azoles (6, 7).

CLINICAL PHARMACOLOGY

The clinical pharmacology of the older imidazoles was discussed in *Annual 1 and 2*. Itraconazole is lipophilic and absorbed after oral administration. Using a bioassay, average itraconazole levels were measured in 10 patients receiving 200 mg/d. Levels were reported as 0.88 and 0.91 µg/ml at 4 and 6 hours after an oral dose 1 week into therapy. After 6 weeks, the levels were 4.1 and 3.8 µg/ml for 4 and 6 hours, respectively. Levels for patients receiving higher doses were correspondingly higher. However, it should be noted that there are several unresolved discrepancies among results obtained by different laboratories and different assay methods. Until these differences have been clarified, the precise serum levels achieved will remain uncertain (8).

ADVERSE EFFECTS AND DRUG INTERACTIONS

One of the major advantages of itraconazole may be its relative freedom from side effects. So far only mild reversible elevations in liver enzymes have been reported. It does not appear to cause the gastrointestinal side effects which have been associated with ketoconazole. However, it is possible that the lessened toxicity is simply a function of dose since the frequency of untoward reactions with ketoconazole increased markedly with higher doses and the experience with itraconazole doses above 400 mg/d is very limited (1).

Two studies this year have carefully documented side effects which have primarily been associated with the older imidazoles. Lavrijsen et al (9) investigated the induction of the hepatic drug-metabolizing enzyme system in rats by miconazole and ketoconazole. Daily doses of 160 mg/kg of ketoconazole produced clearly toxic effects in rats. In contrast, no such increase was observed with itraconazole administered in comparable doses. Induction was dose- and time-dependent. In another study, Ishikawa et al (10) demonstrated platelet dysfunction by inhibition of platelet cyclo-oxygenase in rabbits given intravenous miconazole in doses therapeutic for human subjects. The effect lasted for approximately 24 hours and was reversible.

Inhibition of steroidogenesis

Investigation of the inhibitory effects of imidazole derivatives on steroidogenesis continues. This side effect of imidazoles, especially of ketoconazole, has been turned to therapeutic advantage. Clinical trials of the endocrine uses for ketoconazole are being pursued. Feldman has published an excellent review of this subject with up-to-date references (11). Itraconazole has been found to have no effect on androgen or cortisol metabolism at doses up to 100 mg.

CLINICAL USES

Treatment of superficial fungal infections

Keratomycosis A recent uncontrolled study of miconazole and ketoconazole for the treatment of fungal keratosis suggested that these drugs were useful for empiric therapy of advanced disease. Twenty patients were treated with hourly topical miconazole (along with daily subconjunctival injections with 5 mg for 5 days) and oral ketoconazole 200 mg/d. Healing was seen in 13 of the 20 cases, although vision was often not improved and follow-up was short (12).

Dermatophytoses There is currently little evidence to recommend one imidazole over another in the treatment of dermatophyte infections. Preliminary results of clinical studies suggest that itraconazole is safe and effective for the treatment of dermatomycosis, but comparative studies showing improvement over older therapies have not been done (1).

Vaginal candida As with dermatophytosis, there is little evidence to recommend one imidazole over another in the topical treatment of vaginal candidiasis, although efforts to optimize oral therapy continue. Van der Meijden published a double-blinded, randomized, study of 42 patients and found no difference between 5 days of oral ketoconazole (200 mg/d) and single-dose vaginal miconazole (1200 mg). One week after the start of therapy the mycologic cure rate was 87% in the ketoconazole group and 95% in the miconazole group. There was no long-term follow-up. Oral itraconazole has also been found to be effective therapy for vaginal candidiasis but comparative studies have not been done (14).

Treatment of deep mycosis

Coccidioidomycosis   In an effort to determine the optimal dose of ketoconazole for the treatment of coccidioidomycosis, 112 patients with chronic pulmonary, skeletal or soft tissue infection were treated with 400 or 800 mg/d of the drug. There was no difference in outcome between the two groups. Patients who failed initial therapy were retreated with higher doses of ketoconazole. There were then additional responders, but relapses were more frequent in these patients. Drug intolerance was also a significant problem at higher doses, with gastrointestinal symptoms predominating (15).

Paracoccidioidomycosis and histoplasmosis   There have been encouraging reports of responses to itraconazole in patients with paracoccidioidomycosis and histo-plasmosis. In one study from Argentina, 25 patients with paracoccidioidomycosis were treated with 50 mg/d for approximately 6 months. All patients were cured or showed marked improvement. In the same study, 17 patients with histoplasmo-sis were treated with 100 mg/d until clinical cure was established; then the dose was changed to 50 mg until the completion of 6 months of therapy. Twelve patients were cured, 4 improved, and 1 patient discontinued treatment after 2 months and died (16). In another study from Columbia, 13 patients with paracoc-cidioidomycosis were treated for 6 months with 100 mg/d of itraconazole. Eleven showed major and 2 showed minor improvements (17).

Other systemic infections   Ketoconazole appears to produce some clinical improvement in patients with sporotrichosis. Unfortunately, doses greater than 400 mg/d are necessary and relapse is a significant problem (18). Itraconazole appears to be active in lymphocutaneous sporotrichosis, although the number of patients treated is small and follow-up short (19, 20).

A recent letter reports good results treating disseminated cryptococcosis in 3 patients with acquired immunodeficiency syndrome with 200 mg/d of itraconaz-ole. It must be continued as suppressive therapy, however, after clinical improvement (21).

Prophylaxis in the immunocompromised host

The controversy over the use of imidazoles for fungal prophylaxis in the immuno-compromised host continues. Cauwenbergh (22) published a review of the litera-ture and compilation of 27 published reports. He noted that over 60% of patients became colonized with yeasts during placebo prophylaxis, 30% develop mycosis (from thrush to sepsis) and approximately 5% had autopsy-proven mycosis. Treat-ment with 200 mg of ketoconazole was slightly superior to placebo. With a dose of 600 mg, however, the number of infections was drastically reduced and no pa-tients had autopsy-proven mycosis. Several problems evolved with this therapy. First, there appeared to be a tendency toward infection with *Torulopsis glabrata* and *Aspergillus* species. Secondly, fluctuating blood levels suggested erratic absorption of the drug. The third problem involved the significance of colonization versus infection and the appropriate dosing for the degree of protection sought.

A preliminary non-randomized study (23) of 97 patients comparing ketoconazole with itraconazole prophylaxis in granulocytopenic patients has found itraconazole to be superior to ketoconazole. The incidence of fatal fungal infections was significantly higher among patients receiving ketoconazole 200 mg twice daily than among those receiving the same doses of itraconazole. This trend was especially evident with fatal infections due to *Aspergillus* species.

FUTURE DIRECTIONS

The future will probably see standardization of susceptibility testing of antifungal agents making in vitro studies more reliable. Further clinical trials of itraconazole will delineate the indications for this drug. Meanwhile, the development of newer azole derivatives with even fewer side effects and more benefits will continue.

REFERENCES

1. Cauwenbergh G, De Doncker P, Stoops K, De Dier A, Goyvaerts H, Schuermans V (1987) Itraconazole in the treatment of human mycoses: review of three years of clinical experience. *Rev. Infect. Dis., 9, Suppl 1*, S146.
2. Clissold SP, Heel RC (1986) Tioconazole: a review of its antimicrobial activity and therapeutic use in superficial mycoses. *Drugs, 31*, 29.
3. Van Cutsem J, Van Gerven F, Janssen PAJ (1987) Activity of orally, topically, and parenterally administered itraconazole in the treatment of superficial and deep mycoses: animal models. *Rev. Infect. Dis., 9, Suppl 1*, S15.
4. Doern GV, Tubert TA, Chapin K, Rinaldi MG (1986) Effect of medium composition on results of macrobroth dilution antifungal susceptibility testing of yeasts. *J. Clin. Microbiol., 24*, 507.
5. Radetsky M, Wheeler RC, Roe MH, Todd JK (1986) Microtiter broth dilution method for yeast susceptibility testing with validation by clinical outcome. *J. Clin. Microbiol., 24*, 600.
6. Van den Bossche H, Willemsens G, Marichal P, Cools W, Lauwers W (1984) The molecular basis for the antifungal activities of *N*-substituted azole derivatives: focus on R 51211. In: Trinci APJ, Ryley JF (Eds), *Mode of Action of Antifungal Agents*, p 321. Cambridge University Press, Cambridge.
7. Van den Bossche H (1985) Biochemical targets for antifungal azole derivative: hypothesis of the mode of action. *Curr. Topics Med. Mycol., 1*, 313.
8. Shadomy S, Espinel-Ingroff A, Dismukes WE (1987) Itraconazole serum levels in patients with histoplasmosis and blastomycosis. In: *Abstracts, Annual Meeting of the American Association of Microbiologists, 1987*.
9. Lavrijsen K, Van Houdt J, Thijs D, Meuldermans W, Heykants J (1986) Induction potential of antifungals containing an imidazole or triazole moiety. *Biochem. Pharmacol., 35*, 1867.

10. Ishikawa S, Manabe S, Wada O (1986) Miconazole inhibition of platelet aggregation by inhibiting cyclooxygenase. *Biochem. Pharmacol., 35,* 1787.
11. Feldman D (1986) Ketoconazole and other imidazole derivatives as inhibitors of steroidogenesis. *Endocr. Rev., 7,* 409.
12. Fitzsimons R, Peters AL (1986) Miconazole and ketoconazole as a satisfactory first-line treatment for keratomycosis. *Am. J. Ophthalmol., 101,* 605.
13. Van der Meijden WI, Van der Hoek JCS, Staal HJM, Van Joost T, Stolz E (1986) Double-blind comparison of 200-mg ketoconazole oral tablets and 1200-mg miconazole vaginal capsule in the treatment of vaginal candidosis. *Eur. J. Obstet. Gynec. Reprod. Biol., 22,* 133.
14. Sanz Sanz F, Del Palacio Hernanz A (1987) Randomized comparative trial of three regimens of itraconazole for treatment of vaginal mycoses. *Rev. Infect. Dis., 9, Suppl 1,* S139.
15. Galgiani JN, Stevens DA, Graybill JR, Dismukes WE, Cloud GA (1987) Ketoconazole therapy of progressive coccidioidomycosis: comparison of 400 and 800 mg doses and observations at higher doses. Submitted for publication.
16. Negroni R, Palmieri O, Koren F, Tiraboschi IN, Galimberti RL (1987) Oral treatment of paracoccidioidomycosis and histoplasmosis with itraconazole in humans. *Rev. Infect. Dis., 9, Suppl 1,* S47.
17. Restrepo A, Gomez I, Robledo J, Patino MM, Cano LE (1987) Itraconazole in the treatment of paracoccidioidomycosis: a preliminary report. *Rev. Infect. Dis., 9, Suppl 1,* S51.
18. Calhoun DL, Galgiani JN, Stevens DA, Waskin H, Bonner JR, White MP, Mulholand JH, Rumans LW (1986) Ketoconazole treatment of *Sporothrix schenckii* arthritis and other infections. In: *Abstracts, Interscience Conference of Antimicrobial Agents and Chemotherapy, New Orleans, 1986,* Abstract No. 780. American Society for Microbiology, Washington, DC.
19. Borelli D (1987) A clinical trial of itraconazole in the treatment of deep mycoses and leishmaniasis. *Rev. Infect. Dis., 9, Suppl 1,* S57.
20. Lavalle P, Suchii P, De Ovando F, Reynoso S (1987) Itraconazole for deep mycoses: preliminary experience in Mexico. *Rev. Infect. Dis., 9, Suppl 1,* S64.
21. Viviani MA, Tortatano AM, Giani PC, Arici C, Goglio A, Crocchiolo P, Almaviva M (1987) Itraconazole for cryptococcal infection in the acquired immunodeficiency syndrome (Letter to Editor). *Ann. Intern. Med., 106,* 166.
22. Cauwenbergh G (1986) Prophylaxis of mycotic infections in immunocompromised patients: a review of 27 reports and publications. *Drugs Exp. Clin. Res., 12,* 419.
23. Trico G, Joosten E, Boogaerts MA, Van de Pitte J, Cauwenbergh G (1987) Ketoconazole vs. itraconazole for antifungal prophylaxis in patients with severe granulocytopenia: preliminary results of two nonrandomized studies. *Rev. Infect. Dis., 9, Suppl 1,* S94.

CHAPTER 22

The polyene macrolide antifungal drugs

ANNE MARIE ANGELES and ALAN M. SUGAR

The antifungal spectrum of the polyenes has not changed since the appearance of *Annual 1* and indications for their use have remained relatively stable (1). However, as reviewed in Chapter 21 of this volume, increasing experience with ketoconazole has confirmed the place of oral therapy for many systemic mycoses previously treatable only with parenteral amphotericin B. It is also very clear that seriously ill patients, often with underlying immunosuppression, still require amphotericin B for adequate therapy of fungal infection. As in the previous two volumes of this series, our purpose is to review critically the information that has been published about the polyene antifungals since the completion of the chapter for *Annual 2*. In keeping with the relative importance of amphotericin B as the polyene of greatest usefulness, most of the literature over the past 12 months has been devoted to this drug.

ACTIVITY

Susceptibility testing

As discussed previously, the definitive in vitro antifungal susceptibility test has yet to be proposed. In an attempt to reduce some of the variability, Doern et al (2) analyzed the susceptibility of 62 yeast isolates in 6 different media with 4 antifungal agents (including amphotericin B). Using a macrobroth dilution method, they found that data obtained from 48-hour incubations were more reproducible than those obtained at 24 hours. The actual minimum inhibitory concentrations (MICs) were influenced by the test media used, i.e. amphotericin B MICs obtained using buffered yeast nitrogen broth were 8–16-fold higher than those found using other media. Casein-yeast-glucose broth gave the most reproducible results for all agents. However, correlation of absolute MIC data with clinical response has yet to be shown. Therefore, one is left without sufficient guidelines for interpretation of these test results.

Antimicrobial Agents Annual 3
P.K. Peterson and J. Verhoef, editors
© Elsevier Science Publishers BV, 1988

In an attempt to correlate in vitro MICs with in vivo response to antifungal agents, Radetsky et al (3) describe 7 patients who were treated with a single antifungal agent. The outcome of therapy was known for all patients. The isolates obtained from these patients were then evaluated in a murine model of systemic candidiasis. MICs of 4 antifungal agents were determined in 2 different media (RPMI-1640 and casamino acid media) using both macrodilution and microtiter methods. Discordance between the 2 techniques was noted in 9.3% of assays for imidazole susceptibility when casamino acid medium was used. Disagreement of susceptibility results by microtiter dilution with different media was noted in 55% of isolates exposed to 5-fluorocytosine and 38% of isolates exposed to amphotericin B. There was a 96% concordance for imidazoles. Susceptibility cut-offs were based on the distribution of MICs and the outcome of treated infections in the patients from whom the isolate was obtained. This study offers some promise that in vitro methods might be useful predictors of clinical outcome.

Mechanism of action

The basic mechanism of activity of the polyene antifungal agents is ascribed to the sterol binding capacity of the drugs. In an interesting series of experiments, Shimokawa et al (4) found that *Candida albicans* mutants which had high MICs to amphotericin B grew slower and did not form hyphae when compared with parental strains that were susceptible to amphotericin B. Analysis of sterol composition by gas chromatography and mass spectrometry revealed that the amount of ergosterol was decreased with concomitant increase in 14-methylsterols, ergosterol precursors. The authors postulate that these mutants manifest a defect in the 14-demethylation of the sterol ring, but the association between altered sterol composition and defective morphogenesis and its role in virulence need further clarification. This study confirms the importance of cell membrane ergosterol to sensitivity to amphotericin B.

As discussed in *Annual 2* (5), Brajtburg and colleagues have shown that low-density lipoproteins (LDL) and high-density lipoproteins (HDL) inhibited the toxic effects of amphotericin B and nystatin against red blood cells (RBCs) (6). They have extended these observations to other smaller polyenes (less than 7 double bonds), such as etruscomycin, filipin, and fungichromin (7). RBCs and *C. albicans* were incubated with LDL or HDL and the polyenes and the leakage of intracellular potassium from damaged cells was measured. The study indicated that the lipoproteins abrogated the effects of the polyenes on RBCs. They also found that these small polyenes caused more disruption of erythrocytes than they did to viable *C. albicans* blastospores as compared with the larger polyenes, such as amphotericin B, nystatin and candicidin. These larger polyenes were more disruptive to the fungus than to the erythrocytes, suggesting that the larger polyenes may be more clinically useful. The basis for the preferential effects on fungal rather than mammalian cells seems to be that the smaller polyenes preferentially bind to cholesterol and the larger bind to ergosterol. Since the primary sterol in mammalian cell membranes is cholesterol and ergosterol represents the major sterol in cell membranes of fungi, these data suggest that of the available polyenes, amphotericin B remains the sole clinically useful polyene for systemic administration.

In continuing studies designed to elucidate the role of oxidative metabolites produced by incubation of *C. albicans* with amphotericin B in causing cell damage, Sokol-Anderson et al (8) investigated the role of oxygen in mediating some of the effects seen with polyenes. *C. albicans* protoplasts were exposed to amphotericin B under hypoxic conditions. Amphotericin-B-mediated lysis of protoplasts was reduced by 80% in the absence of oxygen. Furthermore, under these conditions, leakage of intracellular potassium from the protoplasts was not observed. In the presence of oxygen, however, both lysis of cells and loss of intracellular potassium occurred. Exogenous catalase and/or superoxide dismutase protected protoplasts from lysis caused by amphotericin B, supporting the theory that endogenous catalase might play a role in fungal cell resistance to amphotericin B and that hydrogen peroxide is involved in amphotericin-B-induced cellular damage. Because of the differential effect of amphotericin B on lysis and permeability (hypoxia allows loss of intracellular potassium, while the presence of oxygen permits both ion leakage and cell lysis), these data suggest that there are at least two mechanisms of oxidative damage modulated by amphotericin B.

In other related studies, using a mouse model of listeriosis, AKR mice were pretreated with amphotericin B, then infected with *Listeria monocytogenes*, and demonstrated longer survival, while C57BL/6 mice had a shorter survival. The explanation for increased resistance to listeriosis of AKR mice following administration of amphotericin B is postulated to be the result of immune stimulation or a direct effect of the drug on host immune cells, such as macrophages. To evaluate this theory, the authors examined in vitro survival of murine spleen and RBCs from both mouse strains. AKR and C57BL/6 cells were preincubated with amphotericin B, then infected with *Listeria*, under aerobic conditions; cells from both strains demonstrated a resistance to disruption when infected (AKR > C57BL/6). Under hypoxic conditions, the AKR and C57BL/6 cells had no greater resistance to disruption, whether or not the cells were preincubated with amphotericin B. These data suggest that oxidative damage plays a role in amphotericin-B-induced activity. AKR mice have higher cellular levels of catalase than the other mouse strain, suggesting that catalase was protecting AKR cells, important in the immune response to *Listeria* from oxidative damage due to amphotericin B (9). The specific mechanisms of oxidative damage were not determined and the role of adjunctive use of oxidizing agents with amphotericin B to modulate immune function warrants further investigation.

Chemiluminescence (an indirect measurement of respiratory burst activity) was shown to be reversibly decreased when mouse spleen cells were incubated with amphotericin B or ketoconazole (10), suggesting that these agents may decrease immune cell activity. The clinical significance of these observations is unclear. However, other literature suggests that amphotericin B can cause immune enhancement in other systems (see *Annual 2*).

CLINICAL PHARMACOLOGY

No new data were presented over the past year regarding the pharmacology of systemically administered amphotericin B. However, since problems with fungal keratitis and endophthalmitis continue to be an increasingly recognized problem, interest persists in improving our understanding of the pharmacokinetic parameters of topical or intraocular amphotericin B. Using a rabbit model, O'Day et al (11) studied the pharmacokinetics and corneal penetration of topically applied polyene antibiotics. Carbon-14-labelled natamycin and amphotericin B were dissolved in distilled water and applied to rabbit eyes in a 20 μl drop to normal and debrided corneas and concentrations in the aqueous humor were determined at different time intervals following administration. As we would expect, both drugs had poor penetration into the cornea when the epithelium was intact, but small amounts of drug appeared when the corneal epithelium was debrided. Concentrations of the drugs in the corneas were comparable: amphotericin B at 5 minutes (0.05 μg/ml), at 30 minutes (0.46 μg/ml) and at 1 hour (0.16 μg/ml). Physical factors such as blinking were thought to at least partially explain these results. However, drug concentrations were measured by liquid scintillation counts, and the presence of biologically active drug was not determined. Furthermore, binding of amphotericin B to other parts of the eye which might act as a depot were not considered.

Intravitreal administration of amphotericin B and vitrectomy are also used in the treatment of fungal endophthalmitis. To assess the potential for increased toxicity of amphotericin B in the absence of the vitreous humor, Baldinger et al (12) performed experiments in rabbits (each animal's paired eye served as a control, receiving the appropriate manipulation, vitrectomy versus non-vitrectomy). Histologic examination of retina was done after injection of 5, 10, 50 and 250 μg of amphotericin B. They found that at 50 and 250 μg of amphotericin B, extensive retinal necrosis was seen whether or not vitreous humor was present. At the lower doses, even though segmental microscopic necrosis was seen with or without vitrectomy, these eyes appeared grossly normal, and scotopic electroretinography, which assesses retinal function, was unaffected. Therefore, vitrectomy does not appear to increase the degree of amphotericin B toxicity to the retina at doses employed clinically (5–10 μg). Since these studies were performed in rabbits, the implications for intravitreal amphotericin B therapy of human infections are not clear.

Liposomal encapsulation of amphotericin B

The incorporation of amphotericin B into lipid vesicles (liposomes) represents an effort to decrease toxicity and increase efficacy. The pharmacokinetics in animals was reviewed in *Annuals 1 and 2* (1, 5). A clinical study designed to evaluate efficacy of liposomal amphotericin B in a select population has been reported (13). In patients with underlying hematologic malignancies with hepatosplenic fungal infections (7 with *Candida*, 1 with *Aspergillus*) who failed conventional therapy with amphotericin B, all responded to the liposomal formulation. No data are given regarding dose, toxicity or distribution of the drug to allow better understanding of the mechanisms of effect of this liposomal amphotericin B preparation. However, X-ray manifestations of space-occupying lesions were provided and resolution of these hepatosplenic defects concomitant with administration of liposomal amphotericin B was demonstrated. Further studies with this approach are clearly indicated.

Additional animal data with liposomal amphotericin B in the treatment of visceral leishmaniasis showed improved (2-fold) activity of liposomal amphotericin B as compared with systemic amphotericin B (15). Toxicity was difficult to evaluate in this animal model, but the demonstration of efficacy suggests potential for trials against kala-azar in human subjects (14).

Maher et al (15) have attempted to define more precisely the pharmacokinetics of intraperitoneally administered amphotericin B. Since amphotericin B is prepared as a colloidal suspension with sodium deoxycholate, the effects of the polyene or the dispersant on the pharmacology of amphotericin B was studied in a rabbit model. Amphotericin B was shown to increase ultrafiltration without affecting urea clearance. In contrast, deoxycholate changed urea clearance inconsistently and decreased ultrafiltration at low doses (1 mg/kg). At high doses (10 mg/kg), deoxycholate caused peritoneal irritation and increased urea clearance without changing ultrafiltration. These adverse effects of sodium deoxycholate suggest that amphotericin B as currently formulated will affect both ultrafiltration and urea clearance in patients undergoing peritoneal dialysis. This implies that the commercially available preparation of amphotericin B increases solute transport and decreases the efficiency of fluid removal primarily because of the deoxycholate component of the preparation. Therefore, powdered amphotericin B dissolved directly into the dialysate without an irritating solvent might have fewer effects on these parameters and be the preferred method of administration. However, since amphotericin B is insoluble in water, the actual concentration of drug present in the dialysate may be quite variable. The clinical applicability of these data is limited by the lack of an appropriate alternative solvent.

ADVERSE EFFECTS AND DRUG INTERACTIONS

The multiple side effects of amphotericin B and other polyenes are well known and many methods have been proposed to minimize or eliminate these toxic manifestations (reviewed in *Annual 1*). The successful use of dantrolene (a skeletal muscle relaxant) for amphotericin-B-induced rigors was reported (16). Three patients received dantrolene following the development of rigors after 1 dose of amphotericin B. The rigors were unresponsive to diphenhydramine hydrochloride, morphine sulfate, meperidine and/or lorazepam. In contrast to the use of meperidine (17), there was no increase in nausea and vomiting with dantrolene. The use of this drug to treat amphotericin-B-induced rigors requires more study.

Although the use of neutrophil transfusions has been almost completely abandoned in the routine care of febrile immunocompromised patients, the interaction between amphotericin B and neutrophils has created interest in the past (see *Annual 1* or *2*) and some literature continues to address this issue. A letter to the editor describes a case of acute pulmonary decompensation 30 min after infusion of amphotericin B in a granulocytopenic patient who did not receive granulocyte transfusions (18). Administration of amphotericin B 4 days later yielded an identical decompensation which resolved when amphotericin B was stopped. The mechanism for this toxicity is unclear, although the patient did receive platelet and red cell transfusions which contain leukocytes and might predispose to pulmonary leukostasis. Continued aggressive evaluation of pulmonary complications in granulocytopenic patients is needed to further our understanding of the interaction between leukocytes and amphotericin B.

CLINICAL USES

Indications for the use of amphotericin B remain virtually the same as those over the past several years. However, increasing experience with the imidazoles suggests that some fungal infections can be treated with these oral agents. In general, non-immunosuppressed patients with blastomycosis, coccidioidomycosis or histoplasmosis can be treated with imidazoles (ketoconazole) (see Chapter 21). Patients with immunodeficiencies or neutropenia do not seem to respond well to oral therapy and amphotericin B remains the drug of choice in treating serious infections caused by dimorphic or opportunistic fungi. Furthermore, *Aspergillus* infections and zygomycoses remain untouched by available imidazole therapy.

Amphotericin B as an adjunct to cytotoxic therapy

In vivo animal experiments have continued to suggest that amphotericin B may have a role in potentiating the effects of chemotherapeutic agents. In mice, a dose of amphotericin B of 0.5 mg/mouse followed by lomustine increased cytotoxicity to lymphocytic leukemia cells 20-fold when compared with lomustine alone (19). The role of amphotericin B in this clinical setting needs to be studied further.

Antiviral activity of amphotericin B methyl ester

In an interesting experiment, Schaffner et al (20) demonstrated in vitro activity of amphotericin methyl ester against human immunodeficiency virus (HIV), the etiologic agent of the acquired immunodeficiency syndrome (AIDS) (20). However, since amphotericin methyl ester has been shown to be neurotoxic, the clinical utility of this observation is questionable.

DOSING

Systemic fungal infections require the use of systemic fungal therapy. Optimal total doses, duration of therapy and mode of therapy remain empirically derived,
although general guidelines have already been discussed in *Annuals 1 and 2*. Some
investigators have been able to show benefit from combining local and systemic
therapy.

Polsky et al (21) retrospectively evaluated 23 patients with cryptococcal meningitis. Ten were treated with intraventricular amphotericin B, administered via
a subcutaneous reservoir, plus intravenous amphotericin. The other 13 were treated with intravenous therapy alone. Efficacy was evaluated in the 13 patients treated for a first episode of meningitis. Six patients who were treated with combination
therapy were evaluable: 1/6 died during therapy, 6/6 had sterilization of cerebrospinal fluid (CSF) with concomitant decline in titer of cryptococcal antigen.
Seven patients who received intravenous amphotericin B alone were evaluable,
but they fared poorly: 6/7 died, and only 3/7 had CSF sterilization. This suggests
benefit of combination therapy, but additional prospective evaluation is needed
before advocating its routine use, especially considering the well-known problems
with intraventricular reservoirs.

Coccidioidal meningitis requires administration of amphotericin B into the
CSF. Typically, doses of 0.5 mg 3 times a week are instilled into the lumbar space
or into the ventricular space either by direct percutaneous puncture or via a reservoir. In a modification of this approach, high-dose (1.0–1.5 mg 3 times a week)
intrathecal amphotericin B plus intravenous amphotericin B was used to treat patients with coccidioidal meningitis (22). Over a 12-year period, 11 patients were
treated: 8/11 reverted to normal CSF (including complement-fixation titers) during therapy. Of these 8 patients, 3/8 relapsed, 2/8 required continuous therapy because of immunosuppression, and the remaining 3 had normal CSF with no evidence of residual infection, 30–66 months after antifungal therapy was
discontinued. The amphotericin B was administered by lumbar hyperbaric injection in 6 patients and by the intracisternal route in 5 patients. Serious toxicity with
permanent residual neurologic deficits was noted in 5 patients treated via the lumbar route. Intracisternal amphotericin B had more numerous but transient side
effects. These data show a dose-related survival and suggest that a minimal intrathecal dose totalling 40 mg of amphotericin B be administered in 6 months.
However, further clinical experience is needed before routine use of high-dose intrathecal administration can be advocated.

Naegleria fowleri is known to be sensitive to amphotericin B both in vitro and
in vivo in mice but has not been effective clinically in man. In an effort to explain
this discrepancy, Ferrante (23) postulates that, given the assumption that the
mechanism of action of amphotericin B is on the plasma membrane, when the
ameba membrane is disrupted by high doses of amphotericin B, cytopathogenic
substances could be released from the amebae causing additional tissue damage.
He suggests that using low doses of amphotericin B which would inhibit the phag-

ocytic properties of the ameba, rather than full therapeutic doses which disrupt the organism, may be one approach to prevent the harmful processes of phagocytosis and toxin release. Obviously a clinical trial would be needed to further evaluate this theory.

FUTURE DIRECTIONS

Amphotericin B continues to be the mainstay for most systemic infections. Liposomal-encapsulated amphotericin B continues to be available only for patients failing conventional therapy, and, while preliminary clinical studies have shown efficacy, further clinical studies with this preparation need to be done. More important is the need to define a standardized, commercially feasible liposomal system that can be manufactured in sufficient quantities, with a long shelf-life for large-scale clinical trials. If this can be done, and preliminary data are supported, liposomal amphotericin B could represent a major advance in decreasing the toxicity of the current preparation of the drug.

REFERENCES

1. Sugar AM (1986) The polyene macrolide antifungal drugs. In: Peterson PK, Verhoef J (Eds), *The Antimicrobial Agents Annual 1*, p 229. Elsevier, Amsterdam.
2. Doern GV, Tubert TA, Chapin K, Rinaldi MG (1986) Effect of media composition on results of macrobroth dilution antifungal susceptibility testing of yeasts. *J. Clin. Microbiol., 24,* 507.
3. Radetsky M, Wheeler RC, Roe MH, Todd JK (1986) Microtiter broth dilution method for yeast susceptibility testing with validation by clinical outcome. *J. Clin. Microbiol., 24,* 600.
4. Shimokawa O, Kato Y, Nakayama H (1986) Accumulation of 14-methyl sterols and defective hyphal growth in *Candida albicans. J. Med. Vet. Mycol., 24,* 327.
5. Sugar AM (1987) The polyene macrolide antifungal drugs. In: Peterson PK, Verhoef J (Eds), *The Animicrobial Agents Annual 2*, p 228. Elsevier, Amsterdam.
6. Brajtburg J, Elberg S, Bolard J, Kobayashi GS et al (1984) Interaction of plasma lipoproteins with amphotericin B. *J. Infect. Dis., 149,* 986.
7. Brajtburg J, Elberg S, Kobayashi GS, Medoff G (1986) Effects of serum lipoproteins on damage to erythrocytes and *Candida albicans* cells by polyene antibiotics. *J. Infect. Dis., 153,* 623.
8. Sokol-Anderson ML, Brajtburg J, Medoff G (1986) Amphotericin B induced oxidative damage and killing of *Candida albicans. J. Infect. Dis., 154,* 76.
9. Brajtburg J, Elberg S, Kobayashin GS, Medoff G (1986) Toxicity and induction of resistance to *Listeria monocytogenes* infection by amphotericin B in inbred strains of mice. *Infect. Immun., 54,* 303.
10. Abruzzo GK, Giltinan DM, Capizzi TP, Fromtling RA (1986) Influence of six antifungal agents on the chemiluminescence response of mouse spleen cells. *Antimicrob. Agents Chemother., 29,* 602.

11. O'Day DM, Head WS, Robinson RD, Clanton JA (1986) Corneal penetration of topical amphotericin B and natamycin. *Curr. Eye Res., 5,* 877.

12. Baldinger J, Doft BH, Burns SA, Johnson B (1986) Retinal toxicity of amphotericin B in vitrectomised versus non-vitrectomised eyes. *Br. J. Ophthalmol., 70,* 657.

13. Shirkhoda A, Lopez-Berestein G, Holbert JM, Luna MA (1986) Hepatosplenic fungal infection: CT and pathologic evaluation after treatment with liposomal amphotericin B. *Radiology, 159,* 349.

14. Berman JD, Hanson WL, Chapman WL, Alving CR, Lopez-Berestein G (1986) Anti-leishmanial activity of liposome-encapsulated amphotericin B in hamsters and monkeys. *Antimicrob. Agents Chemother., 30,* 847.

15. Maher JF, Hirszel P, Chakrabarti E, Bennett RB (1986) Contrasting effects of amphotericin B and the solvent sodium desoxycholate on peritoneal transport. *Nephron, 43,* 38.

16. Gross MH, Fulkerson WJ, Moore JO (1986) Prevention of amphotericin B induced rigors by dantrolene. *Arch. Intern. Med., 146,* 1587.

17. Burks C, Aisner J, Fortner CL et al (1980) Meperidine for the treatment of shaking chills and fever. *J. Am. Med. Assoc., 140,* 483.

18. Haber RH, Oddone EZ, Gurbel PA, Stead WW (1986) Acute pulmonary decompensation due to amphotericin B in the absence of granulocyte transfusions. *N. Engl. J. Med., 315,* 836.

19. Valeriote F, Dieckman J, Chabot G (1986) Schedule-dependent potentiation of lomustine cytotoxicity by amphotericin B in mice. *J. Natl. Cancer Inst., 76,* 521.

20. Schaffner CP, Plescia OJ, Pontani D et al (1986) Anti-viral activity of amphotericin B methyl ester: inhibition of HTLV III replication in cell culture. *Biochem. Pharmacol., 35,* 4110.

21. Polsky B, Depman MR, Gold JW et al (1986) Intraventricular therapy of cryptococcal meningitis via a subcutaneous reservoir. *Am. J. Med., 81,* 24.

22. Labadie EL, Hamilton RH (1986) Survival improvement in coccidioidal meningitis by high-dose intrathecal amphotericin B. *Arch. Intern. Med., 146,* 2013.

23. Ferrante A (1986) Amphotericin B doses for primary amoebic meningoencephalitis. *Lancet, 2,* 35.

CHAPTER 23

Albendazole, mebendazole and levamisole

G.B.A. OKELO

An important development in the field of parasitic diseases during the last few years has been the successful use of albendazole in the treatment of inoperable hydatid disease (1–3). Since the writing of *Annual 1*, results of several clinical studies with albendazole and mebendazole have been published (4–9). Although levamisole is still being studied for its immunomodulatory capacities, results are conflicting, and often disappointing. The reader is also referred to *Annual 1*.

Albendazole

Albendazole is a new benzimidazole derivative. The benzimidazoles belong to a class of chemical substances which have potent anthelmintic activity. The molecular formula of albendazole is $C_{12}H_{15}N_3O_2S$ and its molecular weight is 265 daltons (10); its structural formula is shown in Figure 1.

ACTIVITY

Mechanism of action

Albendazole interferes with the normal metabolism of the parasite. It selectively blocks glucose uptake by intestinal helminths and their tissue-dwelling larvae (10). This inhibition of glucose uptake leads to depletion of glycogen storage with-

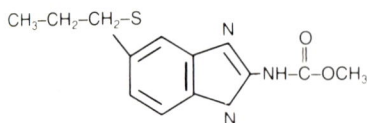

Fig. 1 Structure of albendazole.

Antimicrobial Agents Annual 3
P.K. Peterson and J. Verhoef, editors
© Elsevier Science Publishers BV, 1988

in the parasite which then results in reduced formation of adenosine triphosphate (ATP). ATP is essential for reproduction and survival of the parasite, and the parasite eventually dies (10).

Spectrum of activity

The spectrum of activity of albendazole includes *Nematoda, Cestoda* and *Echinococcus* infections in man. Thus, albendazole is active against *Ascaris*, hookworms, *Taenia solium* and *T. saginata, Trichuris trichiura, Strongyloides stercoralis, Hymenolepis nana, H. diminuta* (11) and *Echinococcus granulosus* (2, 3, 12). It is also effective against pre-intestinal stages of *Necator americanus* (11). Since the use of albendazole is still limited, it is not yet known whether resistant parasites have emerged.

CLINICAL PHARMACOLOGY

Since no new data have been published on the clinical pharmacology of albendazole, the reader is referred to *Annual 1*.

ADVERSE EFFECTS

Albendazole appears to be a safe drug. Only minor and infrequent side-effects occur, e.g. dryness of the mouth, mild epigastric discomfort, nausea, weakness and diarrhea. These side-effects have not been proved to be related definitely to the drug since intestinal helminthiasis itself may be associated with these same symptoms. Two cases of slight, transient neutropenia and 2 patients out of many hundreds of cases studied showed transient elevation of the enzymes SGOT and SGPT (11, 13).

CLINICAL USES

Albendazole has been successfully used in the treatment of infections caused by *Ascaris lumbricoides, Ancylostoma duodenale, Necator americanus, Trichuris trichuria, Enterobius vermicularis, Strongyloides stercoralis, Taenia solium, T. saginata, Hymenolepis nana* and *H. diminuta*.

Albendazole in the treatment of intestinal helminthiasis in children

In 116 children between 2 and 15 years of age entered in a clinical trial of albendazole, examination of their stools revealed ova of one or more intestinal helminths. The drug was administered as a single 400-mg dose (20 ml of 2% suspension) to all the patients except those with *Hymenolepis nana* infection who received treatment for 3 consecutive days. The stools were re-examined on days 7 and 14 post-treatment, and after 3 months for *Taenia* infections. Patients were considered cured if all parasitological examinations of the feces were negative after treatment. After a single oral dose, albendazole was highly effective in ascariasis (91.9%), ancylostomiasis caused by *Ancylostoma duodenale* (87.2%), and *H. nana* infection (71.4%). The drug was well tolerated, and no abnormalities were observed in hematological or blood chemistry values. Since the drug is safe and effective as a single-dose treatment of common helmintic infections, it should be considered for mass therapy in the community (5).

Ovicidal effects of albendazole in human ascariasis, ancylostomiasis and trichuriasis

Albendazole, a broad-spectrum anthelmintic, was administered as a 400 mg single-dose to 20 patients harboring *Ascaris*, hookworms (4 cases each of *Ancylostoma duodenale* and *Necator americanus*) and trichuriasis (10 cases). Feces were obtained before treatment and during the following 5 days. Coprocultures were made for 90 days for *Ascaris* and *Trichuris* eggs; hookworm eggs were cultured by the Harada-Mori technique for at least 8 days. Albendazole was ovicidal against all 4 genera of nematodes (6).

As mentioned above, albendazole has also been shown to be of great value in the treatment of patients with human hydatid disease (2, 12).

In a recent study radiological evidence of remission was seen in 15 of 22 patients with cysts caused by *Echinococcus granulosus*, treated with albendazole (10 mg/kg/d). In 5 patients the cysts virtually disappeared (12).

DOSING

Intestinal helminths

For adults and children over 2 years of age, 2 tablets (or 400 mg) or 20 ml of suspension is usually adequate as a single dose against intestinal helminths (11, 13). If a cure is not achieved, the same dose can be repeated after 3 weeks. Alternatively, a dose of 400 mg/d for 3 days may be more efficacious (10). No purgation or fasting is necessary. The drug should not be used in pregnancy or in epileptic patients.

Human hydatid disease

Patients with hydatid disease should be given 10 mg/kg body weight in 2 daily doses for 8–12 weeks. Larger doses, e.g. 15–20 mg/kg body weight, may be necessary, especially for hepatic hydatids (2, 12). Pulmonary hydatids tend to respond faster. In patients with hydatid disease who require surgery, albendazole should be given both pre- and postoperatively to avoid recurrence of infection. There is evidence now from work done in Kenya in 1986 that the effective dose is 20 mg/kg body weight twice daily for 8 weeks or longer (13).

FUTURE DIRECTIONS

Albendazole should be investigated for its possible value in other infections, e.g. filarial infections, schistosomiasis, and infections due to *Dracunculus medinensis.*

Mebendazole

Mebendazole (5-benzoyl-2-methoxycarbonylamino-benzimidazole) is a benzimidazole derivative with potent broad-spectrum anthelmintic activity. Its structural formula is shown in Figure 2.

ACTIVITY

Mechanism of action

Mebendazole inhibits glucose uptake by the parasite: this action is irreversible. The parasite is then immobilized, eventually dies and is expelled from the gut. The drug can also inhibit the development of larvae of hookworms and eggs of *Trichuris* to the next stages of development. The drug also acts on the myotubular apparatus of the parasite's cells causing disruption and autolysis of the cells. It enters the cell by diffusion.

Spectrum of activity

The spectrum of activity of mebendazole is broad. It is effective against *Ascaris lumbricoides* (15), hookworms (16,17), capillariasis (18), *Enterobius vermicularis, Trichuris trichiura,* all the cestodes (11), *Strongyloides stercoralis* (11), and hydatid disease (2). In preliminary studies it has also been shown to be effective against filariasis (19), but more studies are needed before mebendazole can be recommended for use in this condition.

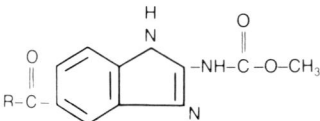

Fig. 2   Structure of mebendazole.

CLINICAL PHARMACOLOGY

After its oral administration, very little of mebendazole is absorbed from the gut, and only 10% is excreted via the kidney in the form of a decarboxylated metabolite. However, when the drug is given in very large doses such as 4–8 g/d along with a fatty meal, its absorption is improved and therapeutic levels of 100 ng/ml are achieved against hydatid disease (2).

The serum half-life of the drug is about 6 hours (2, 20).

ADVERSE EFFECTS

In clinical use in man little toxicity of mebendazole has been noted. Occasional diarrhea and abdominal pain may occur. Bone marrow depression is very rare. During the use of this drug in hydatidosis there may be a release of massive amounts of parasitic antigens into the circulation and this may result in immune complex nephritis from deposition in the kidneys (2).

CLINICAL USES

Mebendazole is used in the treatment of all human nematode infections. No purgation is necessary. Mebendazole is also useful in infections caused by cestodes and intestinal capillariasis (18). However, in a study carried out in Ghana, mebendazole was no more effective in treating onchocerciasis than placebo. In this well-designed study the follow-up was 12 months (7). Van Hoegaerden and Flocard (9) reported successful treatment of 4 patients with loiasis. They concluded that mebendazole is more effective than diethylcarbamazine citrate. Mebendazole may be effective in human hydatid disease provided that it is given concomitantly with fat to improve its absorption so as to achieve a serum drug level of above 100 ng/ml (2). In this situation it should be given for a minimum of 4–8 weeks or longer.

DOSING

In the administration of the drug the oral route is used. No parenteral form is available. In treating cestodes and nematodes a dose of 100 mg twice daily for 3–4 days is usually effective (16); a repeat course 3 weeks later is usually not required. In a study from Indonesia a single dose of mebendazole (500 mg) was effective in treating soil-transmitted nematodes (21).

In *Capillaria philippinensis* a dose of 200 mg twice or thrice daily for a minimum of 3 weeks is effective (18).

In human hydatid disease the dosage must be adjusted so as to achieve a blood level of the drug above 100 ng/ml and again the drug must be given concomitantly with a fatty meal to enhance its absorption. The duration of treatment in hydatidosis is 8 weeks or longer (2).

FUTURE DIRECTIONS

Future studies of mebendazole will include more precise definition of the pharmacokinetics in hydatidosis using radioimmunoassay or high-performance liquid chromatography assays. A more soluble form of the drug and a parenteral formulation are needed.

Levamisole

Levamisole is the levo-isomer of tetramisole, a synthetic anthelmintic which was first described by Thienpont et al in 1966 (22). Its structural formula is given in Figure 3.

ACTIVITY

Levamisole acts by stimulating transmission at a ganglionic site which produces muscular paralysis of the parasite. In high concentrations it also acts by inhibiting fumarate reductase (23) which is essential for the metabolism of the parasite. These two actions contribute to the anthelmintic activity of the drug. Another interesting mode of action of levamisole is its effect on the immune system. It appears to enhance cell-mediated immunity by stimulation of precursor T-lymphocytes to mature T-cells (24). So far, resistant parasites have not been demonstrated.

CLINICAL PHARMACOLOGY

Levamisole is rapidly absorbed from the gastrointestinal tract with peak levels of about 0.5 ng/ml being reached in 2–4 hours after an oral dose of 150 mg in adults. Levamisole is subjected to a high first-pass metabolism, resulting in less than 5% of the oral dose appearing unchanged in the urine.

The half-life of elimination is about 4 hours (25, 26).

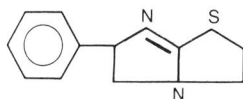

Fig. 3 Structure of levamisole.

ADVERSE EFFECTS

Levamisole is relatively safe with a low incidence of side-effects, especially when used in single doses or other short-course treatment regimens. Some of the side-effects reported on prolonged use include nausea and vomiting, and very rarely reversible agranulocytosis (27).

CLINICAL USES

Levamisole is useful in the treatment of ascariasis, *Ancylostoma duodenale* infection, strongyloidiasis and trichuriasis. Levamisole has been used as adjunctive therapy of malignancies (24, 28, 29) and also in the treatment of rheumatic diseases (27, 30, 31), immunodeficiencies (32), and idiopathic nephrotic syndrome (33).

DOSING

Levamisole is administered orally. A single oral dose of 150 mg is usually effective in nematode infections. No purgation is necessary.

FUTURE DIRECTIONS

The immunostimulant activity of levamisole will need further investigation in the future with a view to its increased usage in malignancies, systemic acne, immunodeficiency states such as acquired immune deficiency syndrome (AIDS), and rheumatic diseases. Its possible carcinogenicity also needs to be looked into in the future. The role of the immunostimulant activity of levamisole needs evaluation in patients with diffuse cutaneous leishmaniasis who are usually immunosuppressed.

REFERENCES

1. Morris DL (1983) Chemotherapy of hydatid disease. *J. Antimicrob. Chemother., 11,* 494.
2. Okelo GBA (1984) *Studies on Human Hydatid Disease in Kenya.* Thesis, University of Nairobi.
3. Saimot AG, Cremieux AC, Hay JM et al (1983) Albendazole as a potential treatment for human hydatidosis. *Lancet, 2,* 652.
4. Morris DL, Dykes PW, Marriner S et al (1985) Albendazole: objective evidence of response in human hydatid disease. *J. Am. Med. Assoc., 253,* 2053.
5. Prasad R, Mathur PP, Taneja VK, Jagota SC (1985) Albendazole in the treatment of intestinal helminthiasis in children. *Clin. Ther., 7,* 164.

6. Maisonneuve H, Rossignol JF, Addo A et al (1985) Ovicidal effects of albendazole in human ascariasis, ancylostomiasis and trichuriasis. *Ann. Trop. Med. Parasitol., 79,* 79.
7. Taylor HR, Awadzi K, George T et al (1985) Fluorescein angiographic studies of mebendazole treatment for onchocerciasis. *Trop. Med. Parasitol., 36,* 7.
8. Bekhti A (1985) Serum concentrations of mebendazole in patients with hydatid disease. *Int. J. Clin. Pharmacol. Ther. Toxicol., 23,* 635.
9. Van Hoegaerden M, Flocard F (1985) Mebendazole treatment of loiasis. *Lancet, 1,* 1278.
10. Smith, Kline and French Laboratories Ltd (1982) *Zentel (Albendazole S.K. & F.): A Significant Advance in the Chemotherapy of Helminthiasis.* Smith, Kline and French Laboratories Ltd., Welwyn Gardens City, Hertfordshire AL7 1EY, U.K.
11. Firth M (Ed) (1983) *Albendazole in Helminthiasis.* International Congress and Symposium Series No. 61, Royal Society of Medicine, London.
12. Morris DL, Dykes PW, Dickson B et al (1983) Albendazole in hydatid disease. *Br. Med. J., 286,* 103.
13. Okelo GBA (1986) Hydatid disease research and control in Turkana. III. Albendazole in the treatment of inoperable hydatid disease in Kenya: a report on 12 cases. *Trans. R. Soc. Trop. Med. Hyg., 80,* 193.
14. Garcia E (1981) Report on the double-blind trial to evaluate albendazole in intestinal helminthiasis. Unpublished document on file, Medical Department, Janssen Pharmaceutica.
15. Chavaria (1974) Unpublished document on file, Medical Department, Janssen Pharmaceutica.
16. Cartwright-Taylor L, Okelo GBA, Pamba HO (1982) Mebendazole: a preliminary study comparing its efficacy against hookworm with pyrantel pamoate (Combantrin) and bephenium hydroxynaphthoate (Alcopar) in patients at Kenyatta National Hospital. *East Afr. Med. J., 59,* 214.
17. Vakil et al (1974) Unpublished document on file, Medical Department, Janssen Pharmaceutica.
18. Singson CN, Banzon TC, Cross JH (1975) Mebendazole in the treatment of intestinal capillariasis. *Am. J. Trop. Med. Hyg., 24,* 932.
19. Fierlafijn E, Vanparijs OF, Raeymaekers AHM et al (1973) Mebendazole in enterobiasis: a placebo-controlled trial in a paediatric community. *Trop. Geogr. Med., 25,* 242.
20. Dawson M, Braithwaite PA, Roberts MS, Watson TR (1985) The pharmacokinetics and bioavailability of a tracer dose of (^{3}H)-mebendazole in man. *Br. J. Clin. Pharmacol., 19,* 79.
21. Abadi K (1985) Single dose mebendazole therapy for soil-transmitted nematodes. *Am. J. Trop. Med. Hyg., 34,* 129.
22. Thienpont D, Vanparijs OF, Raeymaekers AHM et al (1966) Tetramisole (R 8299), a new potent broad spectrum anthelmintic. *Nature (London), 209,* 1084.
23. Van den Bossche H (1972) Biochemical effects of tetramisole. In: *Comparative Biochemistry of Parasites,* p 117, Academic Press, New York-London.
24. Chirigos MA (Ed) (1978) Immune modulation and control of neoplasia by adjuvant therapy. *Prog. Cancer Res. Ther., 7.*
25. Adams JG (1978) Pharmacokinetics of levamisole. *J. Rheumatol., 5, Suppl 4,* 137.
26. Graziani G, De Martin GL (1977) Pharmacokinetic studies on levamisole: on the

pharmacokinetics and relative bioavailability of levamisole in man. *Drug Exp. Clin. Res., 2,* 235.

27. Mielants H, Veys EM (1978) A study of the haematological side effects of levamisole in rheumatoid arthritis with recommendations. *J. Rheumatol., 5,* 77.

28. Niimoto M, Hattori T, Ito I (1984) Levamisole in postoperative adjuvant immunochemotherapy for gastric cancer: a randomized controlled study of the MIC + Tegafur regimen with or without levamisole. *J. Cancer Immunol. Immunother., 18,* 13.

29. Robustelli-Della-Cuna G, Pavesi L, Knerich R (1984) Radio-chemo-immunotherapy (CCNU plus levamisole) for the treatment of metastatic brain tumours: a pilot study. *J. Neurol. Oncol., 2,* 237.

30. Huskisson EC, Adams JG (1980) An overview of the current status of levamisole in the treatment of rheumatic diseases. *Drugs, 19,* 100.

31. Halberg B, Bentzon MW, Crohn O (1984) Double-blind trial of levamisole, penicillamine and azothioprine in rheumatoid arthritis: clinical, biochemical, radiological and scintigraphic studies. *Dan. Med. Bull., 31,* 403.

32. Lawrence DR, Bennett PN (1980) *Clinical Pharmacology, 5th ed.* Churchill-Livingstone, Edinburgh.

33. Niaudet P, Drachman R, Gagnadoux MF, Brou'er M (1984) Treatment of idiopathic nephrotic syndrome with levamisole. *Acta Paediatr. Scand., 73,* 637.

CHAPTER 24

Drug treatment of amebiasis

SHARON L. REED and DAVID A. KATZENSTEIN

Infection with *Entamoeba histolytica* is an important cause of morbidity and mortality in the Third World and a major public health concern in developed countries, where the prevalence approaches 30% in homosexual populations (1, 2). Amebic infection causes a broad spectrum of disease. The majority of patients are asymptomatic, but amebae may invade the colon of others or even reach the bloodstream to cause distant abscesses, particularly of the liver. Recent studies of the epidemiology and pathogenesis of amebiasis suggest that this variability of clinical symptoms may be related to differences in the pathogenic potential of different strains of *Entamoeba*.

It had been widely held that any isolate of *E. histolytica* was potentially invasive and should be eradicated. Several lines of evidence, however, suggest that strains may differ in virulence. Pioneering epidemiological studies by Sargeaunt in several continents (3–5) have led to the identification of distinct isoenzyme patterns (zymodemes) which differentiate strains of *E. histolytica* isolated from asymptomatic patients from those that cause invasive disease (colitis or amebic liver abscess). Further analysis of these clinical isolates in our laboratory revealed that only the pathogenic strains were resistant to complement-mediated lysis, a characteristic that permits them to survive hematogenous dissemination from the bowel (6). Only non-pathogenic zymodemes of *E. histolytica* have been isolated from homosexual patients in London and the United States and their presence has not been associated with any gastrointestinal symptoms (7, 8). Futhermore, Nanda and colleagues found that all asymptomatic cyst passers spontaneously eradicated the parasite within 1–18 months (9). These findings have led to a growing controversy in the management of the most common clinical syndrome of amebic infection, asymptomatic cyst passing. It has been argued that treatment may not be indicated for homosexual men in non-endemic areas (7). Conversely, it has been reported that a strain of *E. histolytica* converted from a non-pathogenic to a pathogenic zymodeme in vitro. Although this event has never been demonstrated in the human host, the possibility is unsettling (10). The controversy over the correct therapy of asymptomatic patients is far from settled and will require more long-term follow-up studies.

Antimicrobial Agents Annual 3
P.K. Peterson and J. Verhoef, editors
© Elsevier Science Publishers BV, 1988

Drugs used in the treatment of amebiasis have traditionally been classified according to their primary site(s) of activity (Table 1). Luminal amebicides are compounds which are poorly absorbed from the gastrointestinal tract and therefore achieve high local levels in the colon. Their antiamebic activity is limited to cysts within the lumen and trophozoites which are close to the intestinal mucosa. Tissue amebicides are drugs which achieve high concentrations in the blood and tissues by virtue of rapid absorption or parenteral administration. These drugs are effective against trophozoites within tissue, but do not eradicate amebas from the stool. The development of nitroimidazole compounds, especially metronidazole, has been a major advance in the treatment of invasive amebic disease. These compounds are the first amebicidal drugs which appear to be effective at all sites.

Metronidazole has been widely accepted as the preferred drug for the treatment of amebic dysentery and amebic liver abscess. Newer nitroimidazole compounds — tinidazole, ornidazole, and nimorazole — are as effective, but have not yet been shown to offer significant advantages over metronidazole. One important characteristic of the nitroimidazoles is their clinical efficacy in single-dose or abbreviated regimens in severe invasive disease (11) (Table 2). This is particularly important in endemic areas with limited access to hospitalization. Although this short-course therapy is clinically effective and convenient, it does not eradicate the cysts of *E. histolytica* from the stool (12).

Reported relapses after metronidazole therapy alone may be due to the failure to eradicate all amebae from the bowel (13). Studies have shown that more than 40% of asymptomatic cyst passers may continue to harbor cysts in their stool after

Table 1 *Drugs used in the treatment of amebiasis*

Drug	Activity in lumen	Intestinal wall	Liver
Diiodohydroxyquin (Diodoquin)	+ + +	+	−
Diloxanide furoate (Furamide)	+ + +	+ +	−
Paromomycin (Humatin)	+ + +	+ +	−
Tetracycline and oxytetracycline	+ +	+ +	+
Chloroquine	+	+	+ +
Dehydroemetine and emetine	−	+ + +	+ + +
Metronidazole and tinidazole	+ + +	+ + +	+ + +

+ + + = effective as a single agent, most patients will be cured by parasitologic and/or clinical criteria; + + indicates that a drug is effective, but should not be used alone; + indicates minimal activity; − = no activity.

Table 2 *Abbreviated courses of nitroimidazoles in the treatment of amebiasis**

Drug	Dose	Duration
Amebic liver abscess		
Metronidazole	2.4 g	once
Ornidazole	2.0 g	once
Tinidazole	2.0 g	once
Amebic dysentery		
Metronidazole	800 mg	b.i.d. × 5 d
Tinidazole	2 g	q.i.d. × 3 d
Secnidazole	2 g	once

*These regimens are clinically effective; however, the parasitologic cure rate (eradication of cysts from the stool) is often low.

5–10 days of metronidazole or tinidazole treatment (14, 15). Luminal agents alone have been used to treat asymptomatic cyst passers and added to metronidazole therapy of colitis or liver abscesses to ensure sterilization of the bowel.

RECOMMENDATIONS FOR TREATMENT

Asymptomatic cyst passers

The necessity of treating all asymptomatic patients with cysts of *E. histolytica* in the stool is debatable. If undertaken, treatment is best accomplished with one of the luminal amebicides, diloxanide furoate, diiodohydroxyquin, or paromomycin. These drugs are generally less toxic and less expensive than metronidazole and are specifically effective in the lumen of the large intestine. Parasitologic cure is obtained in about 90% of patients treated with any of these agents. Diloxanide furoate is considered the drug of choice, primarily because a relatively short course is effective and toxicity is extremely rare (16).

Intestinal amebiasis and liver abscess

Patients should be treated with metronidazole, 750 mg 3 times per day for 10 days (Table 3). In patients who are too sick to take medicines by mouth, parenteral metronidazole, 500 mg every 6 hours is very effective (17). Dehydroemetine (1 mg/kg/d) or chloroquine (600 mg base daily for 2 days then 300 mg base daily for 2–3 weeks) can be added for patients who are seriously ill or after relapse, but there is no evidence that combined therapy is more effective. Treatment with a luminal agent, diloxanide furoate or diiodohydroxyquin, should follow initial therapy to ensure eradication of *E. histolytica* from the stool.

Table 3 *Effective regimens in amebiasis*

Drug	Adult dose	Pediatric dose	Side-effects and toxicity
Asymptomatic cyst passers			
Diloxanide furoate (Furamide)*	500 mg t.i.d. × 10 d	20 mg/kg/d in 3 doses	Excessive flatulence is common, but no other toxic effects have been noted
Diiodohydroxyquin (Diodoquin)	650 mg t.i.d. × 20 d	30–40 mg/kg/d in 3 doses	Absorption of free iodine may result in dermatitis, goiter, or abnormal thyroid function tests; contraindicated in patients with hepatic failure or history of iodine allergy
Paromomycin (Humatin)	500 mg t.i.d. × 7 d	25–30 mg/kg/d in 3 doses	Rarely, systemic absorption has caused vestibular and nephrotoxicity; diarrhea at high doses
*Invasive amebiasis***			
Metronidazole (Flagyl)	750 mg t.i.d. × 10 d	50 mg/kg/d in 3 doses	Disulfiram (Antabuse) reactions if alcohol is consumed; gastrointestinal side effects (nausea, vomiting, epigastric pain, diarrhea) occur rarely; contraindicated in pregnant or lactating women because of theoretical teratogenic risk
and/or			
Dehydroemetine*	1 mg/kg/d i.m. as a single daily dose, not to exceed 90 mg/d		Cardiac toxicity is less than that of emetine, but patients should be monitored with daily ECGs; treatment should be halted if QT prolongation, arrhythmias, hypotension, or anginal pain occurs; gastrointestinal toxicity includes nausea, vomiting and diarrhea
and/or			
Chloroquine (base) (Atabrine)	600 mg × 2 d, then 300 mg qd × 20 d	10 mg/kg/ d × 20 d	Contraindicated in patients with psoriasis, porphyria, or those with retinal disease

* Available in the United States only as an investigational drug through the Center for Disease Control.
** A luminal agent should be added to each regimen in doses used for asymptomatic cyst passers.

The majority of patients treated medically for invasive amebiasis are afebrile and pain-free within 72 hours. The addition of a second drug, dehydroemetine 1 mg/kg/d or chloroquine 300 mg/d (18), or therapeutic aspiration should be considered for patients who do not respond. Amebic abscesses should be aspirated to rule out a pyogenic abscess, when the diagnosis is uncertain, as an adjunct to medical therapy when pain and fever persist beyond 3–5 days, and to minimize the risk that a large left lobe abscess will rupture into the pericardium (19). If an amebic liver abscess extends into the peritoneum, pleural space or pericardium, aspiration or surgical drainage is essential.

FUTURE DIRECTIONS

Although resistance to the highly effective 5-nitroimidazoles has never been demonstrated, their use has been limited by potential teratogenicity (20) and relative inability to eradicate cysts. The search for amebicidal agents that are free of mutagenic effects and more efficient luminal agents should be greatly aided by axenic culture systems and animal models of hepatic and intestinal infection (reviewed in Ref. 21). Experimental amebicidal compounds developed in the past few years include caerulomycin, an antibiotic obtained from *Streptomyces caeruleus* (22), novel tetrahydroquinolones (23), extracts from the plant, *Berberis aristata* (24), and new imidazole-derivatives (25). Future clinical studies should also answer the question about the need to treat asymptomatic cyst carriers with luminal agents.

REFERENCES

1. Quinn T, Stamm WE, Goodell SE et al (1983) The polymicrobial origin of intestinal infections in homosexual men. *N. Eng. J. Med., 309,* 576.
2. Keystone JS, Keystone DL, Proctor LM (1980) Intestinal parasitic infections in homosexual men: prevalence, symptoms and factors in transmission. *Can. Med. Assoc. J., 123,* 512.
3. Sargeaunt PG, Williams JE, Green JD (1978) The differentiation of invasive and non-invasive *E. histolytica* by isoenzyme electrophoresis. *Trans. R. Soc. Trop. Med. Hyg., 72,* 519.
4. Sargeaunt PG, Jackson TFHG, Simjee A (1982) Biochemical heterogeneity of *Entamoeba* isolates, especially those from liver abscess. *Lancet, 1,* 1386.
5. Sargeaunt PG, Williams JE, Jackson TFHG et al (1982) A zymodeme study of *Entamoeba histolytica* in a group of South African schoolchildren. *Trans. R. Soc. Trop. Med. Hyg., 76,* 401.
6. Reed SL, Curd JG, Gigli I et al (1986) Activation of complement by pathogenic and nonpathogenic *Entamoeba histolytica. J. Immunol., 136,* 2265.
7. Allason-Jones E, Mindel A, Sargeaunt P et al (1986) *Entamoeba histolytica* as a commensal intestinal parasite in homosexual men. *N. Engl. J. Med., 315,* 353.
8. Mathews HM, Moss DM, Healy GR et al (1986) Isoenzyme analysis of *Entamoeba histolytica* isolated from homosexual men. *J. Infect. Dis., 153,* 793.

9. Nanda R, Anand BS, Baveja U (1984) *Entamoeba histolytica* cyst passers: clinical features and outcome in untreated subjects. *Lancet, 2,* 301.

10. Mirelman D, Bracha R, Wexler A et al (1986) Changes in isoenzyme patterns of a cloned culture of nonpathogenic *Entamoeba histolytica* during axenization. *Infect. Immun., 54,* 827.

11. Lasserre R, Jaroonvesama N, Kurathong S et al (1983) Single day drug treatment of amebic liver abscess. *Am. J. Trop. Med. Hyg., 32,* 723.

12. Powell SJ, Elsden-Dew R (1972) Some new nitroimidazole derivatives: clinical trials in amebic liver abscess. *Am. J. Trop. Med. Hyg., 21,* 518.

13. Gregory P (1976) A refractory case of hepatic amoebiasis. *Gastroenterology, 70,* 585.

14. Pehrson P, Bengtsson E (1984) Treatment of non-invasive amoebiasis: a comparison between tinidazole and metronidazole. *Ann. Trop. Med. Parasitol., 78,* 505.

15. Spellman R, Ayala SC, Desanchez CE (1976) Double-blind test of metronidazole and tinidazole in the treatment of asymptomatic *Entamoeba histolytica* and *Entamoeba hartmanni* carriers. *Am. J. Trop. Med. Hyg., 25,* 549.

16. Wolfe MS (1973) Nondysenteric intestinal amebiasis treatment with diloxanide furoate. *J. Am. Med. Assoc., 224,* 1601.

17. Nair KG, Kothari N, Sheth UK (1974) Intravenous metronidazole in amoebic liver abscess. *Lancet, 1,* 1238.

18. Katzenstein DA, Rickerson V, Braude AI (1982) New concepts of amebic liver abscess. *Medicine, 61,* 237.

19. Adams EB, MacLeod IN (1977) Invasive amebiasis. II. Amebic liver abscess and its complications. *Medicine, 56,* 325.

20. Roe FJ (1977) Metronidazole: review of uses and toxicity. *J. Antimicrob. Chemother., 3,* 205.

21. Neal RA (1983) Experimental amoebiasis and the development of anti-amoebic compounds. *Parasitology, 86,* 175.

22. Chatterjee DK, Raether W, Iyer N et al (1984) Caerulomycin, an antifungal antibiotic with marked in vitro and in vivo activity against *Entamoeba histolytica. Z. Parasitenkd., 70,* 569.

23. Slighter RG, Yarinsky A, Drobeck HP et al (1980) Activity of quinfamide against natural infections of *Entamoeba criceti* in hamsters: a new potent agent for intestinal amoebiasis. *Parasitology, 81,* 157.

24. Subbaiah TV, Amin AH (1967) Effect of berberine sulphate on *Entamoeba histolytica. Nature (London), 215,* 527.

25. Ray DK, Shrivastava VB, Tendulkar JS et al (1983) Comparative studies on the amoebicidal activity of known 5-nitroimidazole derivatives and CG 10213-Go in golden hamsters, *Mesocricetus auratus,* infected in the liver or caecum or both with trophozoites of *Entamoeba histolytica. Ann. Trop. Med. Parasitol., 77,* 287.

CHAPTER 25

Diethylcarbamazine and ivermectin

BRUCE M. GREENE

Diethylcarbamazine

Diethylcarbamazine (DEC) is widely used as an antifilarial drug in both man and animals (1). Both its mechanism of action and the mechanism of complications and side effects associated with its use are poorly understood.

DEC is 1-diethylcarbamyl-4-methylpiperazine. It is manufactured as the dihydrogen citrate salt of DEC, which is a highly water-soluble and heat-stable white powder.

ACTIVITY

DEC is predominantly a microfilaricidal agent. The mechanism of this effect is unknown, but it is presumed to facilitate in some way the immune mechanisms of the host in most cases, perhaps by unmasking microfilarial antigens.

Spiro et al (2) examined the effect of DEC on intracellular transport and processing of chondroitin sulfate proteoglycan in melanoma cells. Using a combination of biochemical, immunochemical, and morphologic studies, they concluded that DEC inhibits vesicular transport of molecules from the endoplasmic reticulum to the Golgi apparatus, and from the Golgi apparatus to the plasma membrane. DEC thus appears to have a unique pharmacologic effect, as had been suggested in previous studies (3).

CLINICAL PHARMACOLOGY

DEC is well absorbed after oral administration, and reaches a peak after 1–3 hours. A single dose of 6 mg/kg produces a peak level of approximately 3 μg/ml. Following a dose of 200 mg, the half-life was estimated to be 8 hours, and after 800 mg, 12 hours (1). Based on animal studies, the drug appears to be rapidly and

Antimicrobial Agents Annual 3
P.K. Peterson and J. Verhoef, editors
© Elsevier Science Publishers BV, 1988

widely disseminated throughout the major organs. DEC is excreted from the kidneys and the gastrointestinal and biliary tracts.

ADVERSE EFFECTS AND DRUG INTERACTIONS

In normal subjects, DEC is extremely safe. In animal studies, no true teratogenicity has been documented, and the drug is considered safe for human use during pregnancy.

Persons infected with filariae, however, demonstrate a variety of adverse effects following treatment with DEC. Best described are the signs and symptoms seen in *Onchocerca volvulus* infected persons, in whom treatment with DEC frequently leads to pruritus, lymph node swelling and tenderness, rash, fever and arthralgias (4, 5). Dizziness is common, and in some subjects is associated with orthostatic hypotension. DEC administration also leads to ocular complications including punctate keratitis, anterior uveitis, chorioretinitis and optic neuritis (4). The proportion of subjects who experience one or more of these side effects is quite variable, but in general relates to the intensity of infection. Persons with lymphatic filariaisis and *Loa loa* infection may have systemic symptoms similar to those seen with *O. volvulus* infection, but the magnitude is usually less. In addition, pain and tenderness over the sites where adult worms dwell may also be seen. Sutanto et al (6) studied adverse reactions following a single dose of DEC (5 mg/kg) in *Brugia malayi*-infected persons in Indonesia. Fever, anorexia and headache were most commonly observed (in 14, 12, and 12 of 15 subjects, respectively), followed by arthralgia (5/15), myalgia (5/15), nausea/vomiting (4/15), and lymph node pain (3/15). Two persons developed postural hypotension and 1 respiratory distress. Thus, reactions to DEC in *B. malayi* infection are common and are frequently temporarily debilitating. These adverse effects are thought to result in part from massive killing of microfilariae, and perhaps, except in *O. volvulus* infection, adult worms. It appears that a multitude of inflammatory mediators are triggered during this reaction. It is possible that, through enhancement of complement activation, modulation of leukotriene metabolism or other effects, DEC contributes directly to the exaggerated inflammatory response associated with treatment of some infected individuals.

CLINICAL USES

DEC continues to be used widely for treatment of human filarial infections. Two recent reports provide additional support to the value of DEC therapy in lymphatic filariasis (7, 8). Its usage in treatment of *O. volvulus* infection is severely limited by the adverse effects mentioned above. Noteworthy is the emergence of ivermectin as a possible alternative to DEC for treatment of onchocerciasis (see below).

DOSING

DEC is administered orally, at a dosage of 4–6 mg/kg/d. In persons with heavy *O. volvulus* infection, pretreatment with steroids is recommended, as well as the administration of a 25–50 mg test dose. A test dose is also advisable in *Loa loa* infection. In addition, higher doses and more prolonged therapy than usual may be required to kill *Loa loa*, *Brugia malayi* and *Wuchereria bancrofti* adults. Duration of therapy for most filarial infections is 14–21 days, although optimal dosage and duration have yet to be established in a scientifically valid way. Retreatment may be necessary, especially for a cidal effect against adult worms (9).

FUTURE DIRECTIONS

Ongoing research into the mechanism of action of DEC, using both in vitro and in vivo animal systems should define more precisely how DEC exerts its enhancing or facilitating effect on microfilarial killing. In the field, efforts are underway to define the role of DEC in control of lymphatic filariasis. Alternatives to DEC, especially ivermectin, may play an increasing role in the treatment of human onchocerciasis and possibly other human filarial infections.

Ivermectin

Ivermectin (10), a semisynthetic macrocyclic lactone, is a newly developed drug which shows promise in treatment of human infection with *Onchocerca volvulus*. In animals, the drug also shows activity against a wide variety of nematodes and against arthropods (11).

Ivermectin is a synthetic derivative of avermectin B1a, a naturally occurring substance produced by *Streptomyces avermitilis*. It is a stable compound, produced by selective hydrogenation to yield 22,23-dihydroavermectin B1.

ACTIVITY

In human *O. volvulus* infection, ivermectin is a microfilaricidal agent, and causes a prompt and profound decrease in skin microfilaria counts (12–17). The suppression of microfilariae in the skin lasts for approximately 6–12 months or longer, depending upon the intensity of infection and whether the individual is continually exposed to infected blackflies. In addition, ivermectin has an effect on the adult female worm which leads to failure of egress of microfilariae from the uterus (13). The duration of this effect is unknown, but probably is less than 1 year. In addition to its microfilaricidal effect, ivermectin may have an effect on developing infective larvae (18).

In parallel with the reduction in skin microfilaria counts, there is a decrease in microfilariae in the ocular tissues. Importantly, this occurs without major ocular complications, in contrast to what is commonly seen following DEC therapy. Initial trials are underway to examine ivermectin therapy of lymphatic filariasis.

The mode of action of ivermectin is not clearly established, but it is believed that its behavior as an agonist for gamma-aminobutyric acid (GABA) accounts for its antinematodal effect. Ivermectin has been shown both to potentiate release of GABA and to increase the binding of GABA to its receptor (19–21). Another potentially important effect is inhibition of chitin synthesis (22).

CLINICAL PHARMACOLOGY

Ivermectin is rapidly absorbed after oral administration, and in animal studies has been shown to reach peak plasma levels in approximately 4–6 hours. It is excreted as intact drug, 99% in the feces and less than 1% in urine, with a half-life in man of approximately 12 hours. The avermectins are lipophilic, and tissue distribution reflects this characteristic. However, based on animal studies, ivermectin appears to penetrate into brain tissue very poorly or not at all. This may explain its relative lack of toxicity despite the presence of GABA-mediated neurotransmission in the central nervous system (CNS) of vertebrates.

ADVERSE EFFECTS AND DRUG INTERACTION

As detailed below, the striking finding with the use of ivermectin has been the relative lack of complications when used to treat human *O. volvulus* infection. This contrasts with the frequent occurrence of major side effects and complications associated with the use of DEC when used in the same setting (14–17). Two recently reported studies (16, 17) reconfirm the previously reported superior performance of ivermectin over DEC in treatment of onchocerciasis.

Of greatest concern is the potential for CNS complications. However, none has been documented in man despite treatment of more than 10,000 subjects. Nevertheless, because dogs (specifically collies) have shown unexplained neurotoxicity including coma and death (23), concern that this type of complication may be seen in humans is justified. With regard to other potential toxicity, minor ST-T wave changes on electrocardiograms taken 2 days after therapy have been found (13). The significance of this finding is unclear. Postural hypotension has been observed rarely; this effect is also seen with DEC therapy. Animal studies have revealed no teratogenic effects except at doses toxic or nearly toxic to the mother. Because of possible secretion into breast milk, there is potential for toxicity for nursing infants.

No definite drug interactions have been established. However, because ivermectin appears to modulate benzodiazepam receptors (24), caution is warranted regarding this potential interaction. In addition, because of observed hypotension in some recipients, fluid balance and concurrent antihypertensive therapy must be carefully considered.

CLINICAL USES

Ivermectin is currently undergoing large-scale testing for treatment of human *O. volvulus* infection. The principal effect which has been documented in trials to date is reduction in microfilariae in the skin and in the eye. Few data on the long-term effects of ivermectin on disease are available at present, but preliminary results are quite promising in this regard.

A total of 4 trials have now been reported in which ivermectin (single dose 200 μg/kg) was compared, in a double-blind study, directly to DEC (1300 mg over 8 days) (14–17). All of these studies showed less severe and less frequent systemic reactions with ivermectin than with DEC. Qualitatively, the mild reaction seen in some ivermectin recipients was similar to that seen with DEC with fever, rash and lymph node pain or swelling being the dominant manifestations. The requirement for analgesics and antipruritic agents was greater in the DEC group than in the ivermectin group (14).

The ocular reaction seen thus far with ivermectin therapy has been minimal (25). In contrast to the finding with DEC, the number of punctate opacities seen in ivermectin recipients following therapy did not increase significantly. In addition, significant mobilization of microfilariae into the cornea was not seen in the ivermectin groups as it was in DEC recipients. Limbitis was seen more commonly in the DEC groups than with ivermectin and anterior uveitis was not seen in ivermectin recipients. No significant changes in the posterior segment were detected by clinical examination or by fluorescein angiography. However, ivermectin has not yet been adequately tested in subjects with a similar type and magnitude of pre-existing chorioretinal damage as in the subjects who showed posterior segment changes following DEC therapy. Thus, it is important that ivermectin be tested in such subjects before it can be firmly concluded that it is completely without toxicity for the posterior segment of the eye.

DOSING

Ivermectin is administered orally, on an empty stomach, in a single dose. The optimal dosage remains to be determined, but will probably be approximately 150 μg/kg.

FUTURE DIRECTIONS

The precise mechanism of the microfilaricidal effect of ivermectin and of its effect on adult filariae, and whether ivermectin has activity against other human filariae are presently under investigation. If safety and efficacy studies in larger numbers of onchocerciasis patients confirm initial findings, ivermectin will be used in mass treatment trials as a possible means of disease control. In this regard, preliminary results suggest that ivermectin may prove efficacious in preventing transmission of infection from person to person (26).

REFERENCES

1. Hawking F (1979) Diethylcarbamazine and new compounds for the treatment of filariasis. *Adv. Pharmacol. Chemother., 16,* 129.
2. Spiro RC, Parsons WG, Perry SK, Caulfield JP, Hein A, Reisfeld RA, Harper JR, Austen KF, Stevens RL (1986) Inhibition of post-translational modification and surface expression of a melanoma-associated chondroitin sulfate proteoglycan by diethylcargamazine or ammonium chloride. *J. Biol. Chem., 261,* 5121.
3. Stevens RL, Parsons WG, Austen KR, Hein A, Caulfield JP (1985) Novel inhibition of proteoglycan synthesis and exocytosis by diethylcarbamazine in the swarm rat chondrocyte. *J. Biol. Chem., 260,* 5777.
4. Tayor HR, Greene BM, Langham ME (1980) Controlled clinical trial of oral and topical diethylcarbamazine in treatment of onchocerciasis. *Lancet, 1,* 943.
5. Greene BM, Taylor HR, Brown EJ, Humphrey RL, Lawley TJ (1983) Ocular and systemic complications of diethylcarbamazine therapy of onchocerciasis: association with circulating immune complexes. *J. Infect. Dis., 147,* 453.
6. Sutanto I, Boreham PFL, Munawar M, Purnomo, Partono F (1985) Adverse reactions to a single dose of diethylcarbamazine in patients with *Brugia malayi* infection in Riau Province, west Indonesia. *Southeast Asian J. Trop. Med. Public Health, 16,* 395.
7. Partono F, Purnomo (1985) Combined low dosage and short term standard dose treatment with diethylcarbamazine to control Timorian filariasis. *Acta Trop., 42,* 365.
8. Kimura E, Penaia L, Spears GFS (1985) The efficacy of annual single-dose treatment with diethylcarbamazine citrate against diurnally subperiodic bancroftian filariasis in Samoa. *Bull. WHO, 63,* 1097.
9. Ottesen EA (1985) Efficacy of diethylcarbamazine in eradicating infection with lymphatic-dwelling filariae in humans. *Rev. Infect. Dis., 7,* 341.
10. Campbell WC, Fisher MH, Stapley EO, Albers-Schonberg G, Jacob TA (1983) Ivermectin: a potent new antiparasitic agent. *Science, 221,* 823.
11. Campbell WC, Benz GW (1984) Ivermectin: a review of efficacy and safety. *J. Vet. Pharmacol. Ther., 7,* 1.
12. Aziz MA, Diallo S, Diop IM, Lariviere M, Porta M (1982) Efficacy and tolerance of ivermectin in human onchocerciasis. *Lancet, 2,* 171.
13. Awadzi K, Dadzie KY, Schulz-Key H, Haddock DRW, Gilles HM, Aziz MA (1985) The chemotherapy of onchocerciasis. X. An assessment of four single-dose treatment regimes of MK-933 (Ivermectin) in human onchocerciasis. *Ann. Trop. Med. Parasitol., 79,* 63.

14. Greene BM, Taylor HR, Cupp EW, Murphy RP, White AT, Aziz MA, Schulz-Key H, D'Anna SA, Newland HS, Goldschmidt LP, Auer C, Hanson AP, Freeman SW, Reber EW, Williams PN (1985) Comparison of ivermectin and diethylcarbamazine in the treatment of onchocerciasis. *N. Engl. J. Med., 313,* 133.

15. Lariviere M, Vingtain P, Aziz M, Beauvais B, Weimann D, Derouin F, Ginoux J, Schulz-Key H, Gaxotte P, Basset D, Sarfati C (1985) Double-blind study of ivermectin and diethylcarbamazine in African onchocerciasis patients with ocular involvement. *Lancet, 2,* 174.

16. Diallo S, Aziz MA, Lariviere M, Diallo JS, Diop-Mar I, N'Dir O, Badiane S, Py D, Schulz-Key H, Gaxotte P, Victorius A (1986) A double-blind comparison of the efficacy and safety of ivermectin and diethylcarbamazine in a placebo controlled study of Senegalese patients with onchocerciasis. *Trans. R. Soc. Trop. Med. Hyg., 80,* 927.

17. Awadzi K, Dadzie KY, Schulz-Key H, Gilles HM, Fulford AJ, Aziz MA (1986) The chemotherapy of onchocerciasis. XI. A double blind comparative study of ivermectin, diethylcarbamazine and placebo in human onchocerciasis in northern Ghana. *Ann. Trop. Med. Parasitol., 80,* 433.

18. Court JP, Bianco AE, Townson S, Ham PJ, Friedheim E (1985) Study on the activity of antiparasitic agents against *Onchocerca lienalis* third stage larvae in vitro. *Trop. Med. Parasitol., 36,* 117.

19. Fritz LC, Wang CC, Gorio A (1979) Avermectin B_1a irreversibly blocks postsynaptic potentials at the lobster neuromuscular junction by reducing muscle membrane resistance. *Proc. Natl. Acad. Sci., 76,* 2062.

20. Wang CC, Pong SS (1982) Actions of avermectin B_1a on GABA nerves. In: Sheppard JR, Anderson VE, Eaton JW (Eds), *Membranes and Genetic Disease,* p 373. Alan R. Liss, New York.

21. Terada M, Ishu AI, Kino H, Sano M (1984) *Angiostrongylus cantonensis*: paralysis due to avermectin B_1a and ivermectin. *Exp. Parasitol., 57,* 149.

22. Calcott PH, Fatig RO (1984) Inhibition of chitin metabolism by avermectin in susceptible organisms. *J. Antibiot., 37,* 253.

23. Pulliam JD, Seward RL, Henry RT, Steinberg SA (1985) Investigating ivermectin toxicity in collies. *Vet. Med., June,* 33.

24. Matsumoto K, Kasuya M, Fukuda H (1986) DIDS, an anion transport blocker, modulates ivermectin-induced enhancement of benzodiazepine receptor binding in rat brain. *Gen. Pharmacol., 17,* 519.

25. Taylor HR, Murphy RP, Newland HS, White AT, D'Anna SA, Keyvan-Larijani E, Aziz MA, Cupp EW, Greene BM (1986) Treatment of onchocerciasis: comparison of the ocular effects of ivermectin and diethylcarbamazine. *Arch. Ophthalmol., 104,* 863.

26. Cupp EW, Bernardo MJ, Kiszewski AE, Collins RC, Taylor HR, Aziz MA, Greene BM (1986) The effects of ivermectin on transmission of *Onchocerca volvulus. Science, 231,* 740.

CHAPTER 26

Drugs used in the treatment and prevention of malaria

PHUC NGUYEN-DINH and CARLOS C. CAMPBELL

Both favorable and unfavorable developments have marked the past year in the field of antimalarial chemotherapy. On the negative side, chloroquine-resistant *Plasmodium falciparum* has continued to expand further westward on the African continent, and earlier reports on the potential value of proguanil in preventing multidrug-resistant *P. falciparum* malaria have not been substantiated. On the positive side, promising observations have been made on the reversal in vitro of chloroquine resistance in *P. falciparum*, and simple methods for the parenteral administration of chloroquine and quinine have been shown to be safe and efficient, thus enhancing the potential for the effective use of these compounds in malaria-endemic areas.

Chloroquine and 4-aminoquinolines

Chloroquine (7-chloro-4-[4'-(diethylamino)-1'-methylbutylamino]quinoline) is the most widely used antimalarial drug worldwide, because of its low cost, relative safety and rapidity of action. Chloroquine is the drug of choice for the prevention and treatment of malaria due to *P. vivax, P. ovale* and *P. malariae*. Against these 3 species chloroquine exhibits a schizonticidal effect (destruction of the asexual parasite blood stages, which are responsible for the symptoms of malaria) as well as a gametocytocidal effect (destruction of the sexual blood stages, which are responsible for the transmission of the disease). However, in the case of *P. falciparum*, the causal agent of severe malaria, chloroquine is inactive against the mature gametocytes, and strains of *P. falciparum* resistant to the schizonticidal effect of chloroquine have been noted in an increasing number of areas of the world. Of particular concern is the accelerating westward spread in Africa of chloroquine-resistant *P. falciparum*, which has been recently documented as far west as Benin (1) and Nigeria (2, 3). To date, for unknown reasons, no chloroquine resistance has been yet documented in Central America west of the Panama Canal or on the island of Hispaniola (Haiti and the Dominican Republic).

Several hypotheses have been proposed for the mode of action of chloroquine

Antimicrobial Agents Annual 3
P.K. Peterson and J. Verhoef, editors
© Elsevier Science Publishers BV, 1988

and for parasite resistance to this drug (4, 5). While the mechanisms responsible remain yet to be identified, recent findings will prove useful in orienting future investigations. Parasite response to chloroquine has been found to be influenced by host cell factors; *P. falciparum* isolates tested in erythrocytes containing sickle hemoglobin appeared to be less sensitive to chloroquine in vitro than the same parasites grown in normal erythrocytes (6). Verapamil, a calcium channel blocker, has been found in vitro to reverse drug resistance in two chloroquine-resistant *P. falciparum* isolates (7). An understanding of the biologic mechanisms responsible for these findings might provide useful information on how chloroquine acts and how parasites develop resistance to this drug. In addition, the confirmation in vivo of the potential of verapamil and related compounds for reversing chloroquine resistance would have obvious applications in re-establishing the therapeutic and prophylactic value of chloroquine and other 4-aminoquinolines.

Although chloroquine is most often administered orally, in many endemic areas, especially Africa, parenteral chloroquine is frequently used for treating patients severely ill with *P. falciparum* malaria. However, various authorities (8) have discouraged the parenteral administration of chloroquine because of its association, albeit with an unknown frequency, with hypotension and sudden death. These side effects are probably due to the high, transient peak concentrations found after rapid distribution of the drug following its parenteral administration. That the parenteral administration of chloroquine can be safe, provided that certain guidelines are adopted, has been demonstrated in recent studies. In 15 adult patients in Sri Lanka (9) and in 50 adult patients in Zambia (10), no severe side effects were observed when chloroquine was administered parenterally as slow intravenous perfusion or as small, frequent intramuscular or subcutaneous doses. Intramuscular and subcutaneous administration resulted in satisfactory plasma profiles, with peak concentrations reached at 30–60 minutes following initiation of treatment. Predicted acceptable regimens consist of 2.5 mg of chloroquine base/kg every 4 hours, or 3.5 mg base/kg every 6 hours, for a total of 25 mg/kg. (Oral administration should be substituted as soon as the patient's clinical status permits.) These results were obtained in adults and remain to be verified in children, before parenteral chloroquine, in these recommended regimens, can be adopted in the treatment of severe *P. falciparum* malaria.

Amodiaquine (7-chloro-4-(3'-diethylaminomethyl-4'-hydroxyanilino)-quinoline) has been advocated in areas with chloroquine resistance, because of its marginally greater activity on chloroquine-resistant *P. falciparum*. However, the use of amodiaquine is now limited because of its recently observed association with neutropenia and agranulocytosis. In particular, this drug is no longer recommended for use in malaria chemoprophylaxis (11).

Primaquine and 8-aminoquinolines

Primaquine (8-[4'-amino-1'-methylbutylamino]-6-methoxyquinoline) presents a unique spectrum of antimalarial activity, being both a gametocytocidal compound active on the mature gametocytes of *P. falciparum* and a tissue schizonticidal compound (destroying pre-erythrocytic liver stages and hypnozoites, or dormant liver stages). Primaquine is the drug of choice for eliminating *P. falciparum* gametocytes (thus preventing further transmission of the disease), and for destroying the hypnozoites found in *P. vivax* and *P. ovale* (thus preventing the relapses that occur with these two *Plasmodium* species). Recently, a technique has been developed for evaluating in vitro the effects on liver stage parasites of primaquine and other antimalarial compounds, using parasites of the rodent malaria parasite *P. yoelii* cultured in hepatocytes of the rodent *Thamnomys gazellae* (12).

Pyrimethamine

Pyrimethamine (2,4-diamino-5[*p*-chlorophenyl]-6-ethylpyrimidine) is of limited efficacy when used alone because pyrimethamine resistance is widespread. The principal use of pyrimethamine is found in fixed combinations containing this dihydrofolate reductase (DHFR) inhibitor and sulfa-type compounds, resulting in a synergistic sequential block on the metabolic pathway of folate synthesis.

Recent studies have confirmed that pyrimethamine resistance in *P. falciparum* is associated with an altered dihydrofolate reductase, which has decreased affinity for both pyrimethamine and dihydrofolate (13). In the two pyrimethamine-resistant *P. falciparum* isolates used in these studies, no evidence was found of gene amplification or overproduction of dihydrofolate reductase, which had been earlier reported as alternative potential mechanisms for pyrimethamine resistance.

Proguanil and biguanides

Proguanil (1-[p-chlorophenyl]-5-isopropylbiguanide), another DHFR inhibitor, has been recommended for prevention of malaria by some malariologists because it acts as a causal prophylactic (by eliminating the primary liver stages of the parasites) and is well tolerated. Additional interest in proguanil has been raised during the past few years because of preliminary reports that it was effective, when combined with 4-aminoquinolines, in preventing malaria in areas of multidrug-resistant *P. falciparum*. Recent evidence, however, indicates that it is not the case. In Papua New Guinea, 19 of 120 non-immune adult individuals developed *P. falciparum* malaria during or following prophylaxis with proguanil, 200 mg daily, and chloroquine, 300 mg base weekly (14). Five of the patients developed malaria while taking the proguanil + chloroquine prophylaxis.

Chlorproguanil, a long-acting analog of proguanil, was shown to be equally inefficacious in protecting semi-immune children in areas with chloroquine-resistant *P. falciparum* malaria (15, 16). One hundred children in Burundi and 78 children in Kenya, taking chlorproguanil alone at the dosages recommended for prophylaxis (20 mg weekly), and 100 children in Burundi receiving chlorproguanil combined with chloroquine, did not have a lower malarial attack rate than appropriate control groups receiving either placebo or chloroquine alone. However, the dosage regimen adopted might not have resulted in the drug levels required for eliminating parasites resistant to DHFR inhibitors, especially in view of the fact that the calculated half-life (25 hours) of chlorproguanil (17) is shorter than previously estimated. Whether a higher dosage of chlorproguanil might not have provided better results still remains to be established (16, 17).

Combination of pyrimethamine and sulfa-type compounds

These drug combinations include Fansidar* (pyrimethamine + sulfadoxine), Maloprim (pyrimethamine + dapsone) and Metakelfin (pyrimethamine + sulfalene). They constitute alternative drug formulations that have proven very useful for prevention and treatment of malaria in areas with chloroquine-resistant *P. falciparum*. In the case of Metakelfin, recent in vivo studies in Tanzania, in 336 school children, have shown this drug combination to be markedly more active than chloroquine (18). Because of the side effects observed with Fansidar and Maloprim, Metakelfin should receive more attention in terms of its efficacy and potential for side effects.

Problems associated with the pyrimethamine and sulfa-type drug combinations include the following: concurrent resistance in some *P. falciparum* strains to both chloroquine and these compounds (19); side effects such as agranulocytosis due to pyrimethamine + dapsone (20); or liver function abnormalities, hepatitis and fatal hepatic necrosis associated with sulfadoxine + pyrimethamine (21). The observation of severe cutaneous reactions consisting of erythema multiforme, Stevens-Johnson syndrome or toxic dermal epidermolysis in travelers taking Fansidar for prophylaxis has resulted in recommendations that limit the prophylactic use of this drug (11). Such prophylaxis should be restricted to long-term travelers to areas with highest risk of acquiring malaria due to chloroquine-resistant *P. falciparum*, for whom no other drug regimen would be appropriate. Short-term travelers to areas with chloroquine resistance are advised only to carry Fansidar as a supply to be used for treatment, in case of suspected malarial episodes, under conditions where there is no reliable access to malaria diagnosis and therapy.

Quinine and quinidine

Quinine (-6-methoxy-α-[5-vinylquinuclidin-2-yl]-4-quinolinemethanol), an alkaloid derived from the cinchona bark, is assuming increasing importance. Quinine is effective against multidrug-resistant *P. falciparum*, has a rapid schizonticidal activity, and can be administered by intravenous drip. Thus, it is the drug of choice

---

* Use of trade names is for identification purposes only and does not imply endorsement by the Public Health Service or by the U.S. Department of Health and Human Services.

for treating severe *P. falciparum* malaria, especially in areas of chloroquine resistance. The main drawbacks of quinine reside in its short duration of action (approximate half-life: 10 hours), multiple side effects, and reportedly low curative effect when not combined with another antimalarial drug such as a tetracycline or sulfadoxine + pyrimethamine.

Recently published reports of studies conducted in 1983 in an area of Thailand with a high level of multidrug-resistant *P. falciparum* indicated that quinine, given for 7 days at a dose of 600 mg every 8 hours, combined with a 7-day course of tetracycline, 500 mg 8-hourly, had a high curative effect (92%) in 36 adults (22). More recent, unpublished reports from Thailand of infections unresponsive to this regimen have yet to be confirmed. Some indications exist, however, mainly from in vitro studies, that the efficacy of quinine may be diminishing in several areas of the world. Extensive in vitro monitoring in Thailand showed that between 1982 and 1984 the quinine susceptibility of *P. falciparum* decreased, with a parallel but less marked decrease in susceptibility to mefloquine (23). Additional reports have described in Zaire a decrease of in vitro quinine sensitivity between 1983 and 1985 (24), and decreased in vitro susceptibility to quinine was described in occasional isolates from Benin (1), Senegal (25) and Gabon (26). These findings remain to be evaluated by systematic investigations combining testings of quinine susceptibility in *P. falciparum*.

Such investigations will prove particularly useful in Africa, where quinine will play an increasingly important role because of the expansion of chloroquine resistance. Since in Africa most of the population will have developed some degree of immunity to malaria, specific questions to be adressed will include: the minimum effective dose of quinine for a clinical and/or parasitologic cure; and the role of additional antimalarial drugs, such as tetracycline, in curing *P. falciparum* infections treated with quinine.

While slow intravenous infusion has been the recommended method for administering quinine to patients with severe *P. falciparum* malaria, facilities for intravenous perfusion are not available in most peripheral health posts in malaria-endemic areas. A recent study in 8 adult patients in Thailand showed that intramuscular quinine, administered as a loading dose of 20 mg/kg followed by 10 mg/kg doses at 8-hour intervals, allowed the rapid achievement of inhibitory plasma concentrations of the drug, with a mean interval to peak concentration varying between 4 and 8 hours (median: 5 hours) (27). The plasma concentration profiles and the fever and parasite clearance times were similar to those observed following intravenous quinine infusion. Minor cinchonism (transient deafness and tinnitus) was the only side effect reported. The confirmation of these results in a larger number of patients, including children, would represent a major advance in the logistics of treatment of severe malaria in rural endemic areas.

Quinidine, the dextrorotary isomer of quinine, is equally or more active than quinine against *P. falciparum*. Quinidine is readily available in most hospitals in areas not endemic for malaria and can prove life-saving when quinine is not immediately obtainable for treating severe malaria (28). Not surprisingly, quinidine has been shown to share with quinine a disadvantage not found in other antimalarial drugs such as chloroquine, amodiaquine, mefloquine and halofantrine. Both quinine and quinidine cause hypoglycemia, by stimulation of insulin release (29). This side effect deserves attention, since hypoglycemia can be a serious complication of severe malaria in itself, especially in pregnant women and, as recently demonstrated (30), in children.

Antibiotics

The tetracyclines are among the antibiotics with the best-demonstrated antiplasmodial activity, and will play an important role in the prevention and treatment of malaria due to multidrug-resistant *P. falciparum*. Tetracyclines are considered an important adjunct to quinine in the successful treatment of multidrug-resistant *P. falciparum* (22). For malaria prophylaxis in areas with multidrug resistance, the tetracyclines (especially doxycycline) represent a valuable alternative regimen for persons for whom sulfa-type compounds are contraindicated. The main disadvantage of tetracyclines lies in their side effects; in particular, the sustained use of these drugs for prophylaxis is not recommended for pregnant women and children less than 8 years of age (11).

Mefloquine

Mefloquine (DL-erythro-α-[2-piperid-2-yl]-2,8-bis[trifluoromethyl]-4-quinoline-methanol; WR-142490) is a newly introduced antimalarial drug, structurally related to quinine, with a long duration of action (half life: 14 days) and with demonstrated activity against multidrug-resistant *P. falciparum*. Ultrastructural studies with *P. falciparum* and the rodent malaria parasite *P. berghei* demonstrated the effect of mefloquine to be observable at the level of the parasite food vacuole, as a swelling of the vacuole with loss of pigment (31). Although the drug has been used only on a limited basis, increasing evidence now shows that resistance to mefloquine in *P. falciparum* does occur. In Thailand, a decrease of in vitro sensitivity to quinine of *P. falciparum* field isolates was accompanied by a parallel, but lesser, decrease in the response in vitro to mefloquine (23). In addition, the demonstration that cross-resistance exists not only between mefloquine and quinine, but also between mefloquine and halofantrin and enpiroline, two newer drugs in trial phase, severely limits the potential value of the two latter compounds.

Because of the fear of selecting for mefloquine-resistant parasites, a triple combination of mefloquine + sulfadoxine + pyrimethamine (MSP) has been introduced. This combination is active against multidrug-resistant parasites (22) and does not result in deleterious interactions between the 3 compounds or in enzymatic induction by either compound, at least not in healthy volunteers (32). Nonetheless, the advisability of this combination remains open to question. No information is available to indicate that it will delay the appearance of mefloquine resistance in *P. falciparum*, especially in view of the very different half lives of mefloquine (14 days) and of sulfadoxine + pyrimethamine (90 and 100–200 hours, respectively). In addition, the severe side effects associated with sulfadoxine + pyrimethamine represents a strong disincentive to the use of this triple combination in malaria chemoprophylaxis.

Antimalarial drugs in trial phase

Qinghaosu (artemisinine), a sesquiterpene lactone derived from the Chinese herb *Artemisia annua* L., and the arylaminoalcohols, halofantrine (WR-171 669) and enpiroline (WR-180 409), constitute the major antimalarial drugs currently being investigated. These compounds are characterized by their rapid action and their effectiveness on multidrug-resistant parasites. Resistance to these compounds, however, is a major potential limitation. Resistant mutants to qinghaosu can be induced in vitro, and studies in Southeast Asia indicate that a level of cross-resistance does occur between halofantrine and enpiroline and other aminoalcohols such as quinine and mefloquine.

Table 1   *Malaria chemoprophylactic regimens*

Regimen A: For travel of *any duration* to areas of risk where chloroquine-resistant *P. falciparum* has *not* been reported or where only low-level or focal chloroquine-resistance has been reported: once-weekly use of chloroquine *alone*

Regimen B: For *short-term* travel (3 weeks or less) to areas of risk where chloroquine-resistant *P. falciparum* is endemic: once-weekly use of chloroquine *alone*. In addition, travelers to these areas (except those with histories of sulfonamide intolerance) should carry a treatment dose of Fansidar, which should be taken promptly in the event of a febrile illness during their travel, *when professional medical care is not readily available.* Such presumptive self-treatment is only a temporary measure and prompt medical care is imperative.
Doxycycline *alone* taken daily is an alternative to the regimen described above for short-term travel to areas of risk where there is chloroquine-resistant *P. falciparum*. It is particularly appropriate for those individuals with a history of sulfonamide intolerance

Regimen C: For *prolonged* travel (greater than 3 weeks) in areas where chloroquine-resistant *P. falciparum* is endemic: the use of once-weekly prophylaxis with chloroquine and Fansidar may be indicated. This regimen should be considered for: travelers to areas where the transmission of chloroquine-resistant *P. falciparum* is most intense (such as East and Central Africa, Papua New Guinea, Irian Jaya, Solomon Islands, Vanuatu); travelers to areas where there is limited availability of medical care; and travelers who are elderly, immunocompromised, or who have other significant underlying medical conditions. The potential benefit of the routine prophylactic use of Fandisar for these travelers must be weighted against the risk of a possible serious or fatal adverse reaction. *If weekly use of Fansidar is prescribed, the traveler should be cautioned about the possible side effects*

CLINICAL USES

Tables 1–3 summarize current CDC recommendations regarding the prevention and treatment of malaria using the principal antimalarial drugs currently available.

FUTURE DIRECTIONS

Drug resistance and undesirable side effects restrict noticeably the utility of currently available antimalarial drugs. Only a limited number of new compounds has become available, with a spectrum of resistance and side effects not yet ascertained under actual field conditions. In response to these limitations, various useful approaches can be adopted. Continued research into the mechanisms of drug resistance and their reversal, and detailed pharmocokinetic studies for safer and simpler modes of administration, will help to maximize the usefulness of currently available compounds. Such investigations, together with a rational use of the drugs available and a further search for newer products, should represent the principal elements of malaria chemotherapy practice and research in the foreseeable future.

Table 2   *Drugs used in the prophylaxis of malaria*

Drug	Adult dose	Pediatric dose
Choroquine phosphate (Aralen)	300 mg base (500 mg salt) orally, once per week	5 mg/kg base (8.3 mg/kg salt) orally, once per week, up to maximum adult dose of 300 mg base
Pyrimethamine- +sulfadoxine (Fansidar)	1 tablet (25 mg pyrimethamine and 500 mg sulfadoxine) orally, once per week	2–11 months: 1/8 tablet per week 1–3 years: 1/4 tablet per week 4–8 years: 1/2 tablet per week 9–14 years: 3/4 tablet per week > 14 years: 1 tablet per week
Doxycycline	100 mg orally, once per week	> 8 years: 2 mg/kg of body weight orally per day, up to adult dose of 100 mg/d (contraindicated in children under 8 years of age)
Primaquine	15 mg base (26.3 mg salt) orally, once per day for 14 days, *or* 45 mg base (79 mg salt) orally, once per week for 8 weeks	0.3 mg/kg base (0.5 mg/kg salt) orally once/day for 14 days *or* 0.9 mg/kg base (1.5 mg/kg salt) orally, once per week for 8 weeks

Table 3   Drugs of choice for the treatment of malaria*

Clinical setting	Drug(s) of choice	Pediatric dosage	Adult dosage
Uncomplicated attacks of all species of malaria, **except** P. falciparum acquired in areas of chloroquine resistance	Chloroquine phosphate (Aralen)	10 mg/kg base (up to maximum of 600 mg base), then 5 mg/kg base 6 h later, then 5 mg/kg/d base for 2 days	600 mg base, then 300 mg base 6 h later, then 300 mg base per day for 2 days
Uncomplicated attacks of P. falciparum acquired in areas of chloroquine resistance	quinine sulfate	25 mg/kg/d in 3 divided doses for 3 days (up to 650 mg per dose)	650 mg every 8 h for 3 days
	plus pyrimethamine-+sulfadoxine (Fansidar)**	6–11 mth: 1/4 tablet 1–3 yr: 1/2 tablet 4–8 yr: 1 tablet 9–14 yr: 2 tablets >14 yr: 3 tablets in a single dose	3 tablets in a single dose
	or quinine sulfate plus tetracycline***	same as above 5 mg/kg 4 times daily for 7 days (up to 250 mg per dose)	same as above 250 mg 4 times daily for 7 days
Severe illness, or when oral therapy cannot be administered for any reason	quinine dihydrochloride (intravenous)[+]	25 mg/kg/d (up to 1800 mg/d); give one third over 2–4 hours; then repeat every 8 hours until oral therapy can be commenced	600 mg in 300 ml normal saline over 2–4 hours; repeat in 6–8 hours (maximum 1800 mg/d)
After treatment of P. vivax or P. ovale to prevent relapses	primaquine phosphate[++]	0.3 mg/kg/d base for 14 days (maximum 15 mg/d), or 0.9 mg base once weekly for 8 weeks (maximum 45 mg/w)	15 mg/d base for 14 days, or 45 mg base once weekly for 8 weeks

* Consult experts, including Centers for Disease Control, Atlanta, GA, regarding alternative regimens.

** Fansidar should not be given to persons with known allergy to sulfonamides.

*** The FDA considers tetracycline investigational when used in malaria. Physicians must weigh the benefit of therapy against the possibility of known side effects in children under 8 years of age.

[+]In the USA, quinine dihydrochloride is available from the Centers for Disease Control, Atlanta, GA.

[++]Primaquine may cause severe hemolysis in G6PD-deficient individuals.

REFERENCES

1. Le Bras J, Hatin I, Bouree P, Coco-Cianci O, Garin J-P, Rey M, Charmot G, Roue R (1986) Chloroquine-resistant falciparum malaria in Benin. *Lancet, 2,* 1043.
2. Centers for Disease Control (1987) Chloroquine-resistant *Plasmodium falciparum* malaria in West Africa. *Morb. Mortal. Weekly Rep., 36,* 13.
3. Salako LA, Fadeke Aderounmu A (1987) In vitro chloroquine and mefloquine-resistant *Plasmodium falciparum* in Nigeria. *Lancet, 1,* 572.
4. Krogstad DJ, Schlesinger PH (1987) The basis of antimalarial action: non-weak base effects of chloroquine on acid vesicle pH. *Am. J. Trop. Med. Hyg., 36,* 213.
5. Geary TG, Jensen JB, Ginsburg H (1986) Uptake of (^{3}H)chloroquine by drug-sensitive and -resistant strains of the human malaria parasite *Plasmodium falciparum*. *Biochem. Pharmacol., 35,* 3085.
6. Nguyen-Dinh P, Parvin RM (1986) Haemoglobin S and in vitro chloroquine susceptibility of *Plasmodium falciparum*. *Lancet, 2,* 1278.
7. Martin SK, Oduola AMJ, Milhous WK (1987) Reversal of chloroquine resistance in *Plasmodium falciparum* by verapamil. *Science, 235,* 899.
8. World Health Organization (1984) Advances in malaria chemotherapy: report of a WHO Scientific Group. *WHO Techn. Rep. Ser., 711,* 92.
9. Phillips RE, Warrell DA, Edwards G, Galagedera Y, Theakston RDG, Abeysekera DTD, Dissanayaka P (1986) Divided dose intramuscular regimen and single dose subcutaneous regimen for chloroquine: plasma concentrations and toxicity in patients with malaria. *Br. Med. J., 293,* 13.
10. White NJ, Watt G, Bergqvist Y, Njelesani EK (1987) Parenteral chloroquine for treating falciparum malaria. *J. Infect. Dis., 155,* 192.
11. Centers for Disease Control (1986) *Health Information for International Travel 1986.* Centers for Disease Control, Atlanta, GA.
12. Millet P, Landau I, Baccam D, Miltgen F, Peters W (1985) La culture des schizontes exo-érythrocytaires des *Plasmodium* de rongeurs dans des hépatocytes: un nouveau modèle expérimental pour la chimiothérapie du paludisme. *CR Acad. Sci. Paris, 301,* 403.
13. Walter RD (1986) Altered dihydrofolate reductase in pyrimethamine-resistant *Plasmodium falciparum*. *Mol. Biochem. Parasitol., 19,* 61.
14. Henderson A, Simon JW, Melia W (1986) Failure of malaria chemoprophylaxis with a proguanil-chloroquine combination in Papua New Guinea. *Trans. R. Soc. Trop. Med. Hyg., 80,* 838.
15. Coosemans MH, Barutwanayo M, Onori E, Otoul C, Gryseels B, Wery M (1987) Double-blind study to assess the efficacy of chlorproguanil given alone or in combination with chloroquine for malaria chemoprophylaxis in an area with *Plasmodium falciparum* resistance to chloroquine, pyrimethamine and cycloguanil. *Trans. R. Soc. Trop. Med. Hyg., 81,* 151.
16. Watkins WM, Brandling-Bennett AD, Oloo AJ, Howells RE, Gilles HM, Koech DK (1987) Inadequacy of chlorproguanil 20 mg per week as chemoprophylaxis for falciparum malaria in Kenya. *Lancet, 1,* 125.
17. O'Neil AB, Law B, Haworth SJ, Tuersley LV (1987) Chlorproguanil chemoprophylaxis for falciparum malaria in Kenya. *Lancet, 1,* 572.
18. Kihamia CM, Minjas JN, Ramji BD, Masau BF, Masana L, Donno L (1986) Chloroquine-resistant *Plasmodium falciparum* in Dar es Salaam, Tanzania, and comparative

therapeutic results with Metakelfin. *Curr. Ther. Res., 40,* 141.

19. Miller KD, Lobel HO, Pappaioanou M, Patchen LC, Churchill FC (1986) Failures of combined chloroquine and Fansidar prophylaxis in American travelers to East Africa. *J. Infect. Dis., 154,* 689.

20. Hutchinson DBA, Whiteman PD, Farquhar JA (1986) Agranulocytosis associated with Maloprim: review of cases. *Hum. Toxicol., 5,* 221.

21. Zitelli BJ, Alexander J, Taylor S, Miller KD, Howrie DL, Kuritzki JN, Perez TH, Van Thiel DH (1987) Fatal hepatic necrosis due to pyrimethamine-sulfadoxine (Fansidar). *Ann. Intern. Med., 106,* 393.

22. Meek SR, Doberstyn EB, Gauzere BA, Thanapanich C, Nordlander E, Phuphaisan S (1986) Treatment of falciparum malaria with quinine and tetracycline or combined mefloquine/sulfadoxine/pyrimethamine on the Thai-Kampuchean border. *Am. J. Trop. Med. Hyg., 35,* 246.

23. Suebsaeng L, Wernsdorfer WH, Rooney W (1986) Sensitivity to quinine and mefloquine of *Plasmodium falciparum* in Thailand. *Bull. WHO, 64,* 759.

24. Wery M, Ngimbi NP, Hendrix L, Mpungu MT, Shunguza, Delacollette C (1986) Evolution de la sensibilité de *P. falciparum* à la chloroquine, à la quinine et à la mefloquine entre 1983 et 1985 au Zaïre. *Ann. Soc. Belge Méd. Trop., 66,* 309.

25. Brandicourt O, Druilhe P, Diouf F, Brasseur P, Turk P, Danis M (1986) Decreased sensitivity to chloroquine and quinine of some *Plasmodium falciparum* strains from Senegal in September 1984. *Am. J. Trop. Med. Hyg., 35,* 717.

26. Simon F, Le Bras J, Charmot G, Girard PM, Faucher C, Pichon F, Clair B (1986) Severe chloroquine-resistant falciparum malaria in Gabon with decreased sensitivity to quinine. *Trans. R. Soc. Trop. Med. Hyg., 80,* 996.

27. Wattanagoon Y, Phillips RE, Warrell DA, Silamut K, Looareesuwan S, Nagachinta B, Back DJ (1986) Intramuscular loading dose of quinine for falciparum malaria: pharmacokinetics and toxicity. *Br. Med. J., 293,* 11.

28. Rudnitski G, Miller KD, Padua T, Stull TL (1987) Continuous-infusion quinidine gluconate for treating children with severe *Plasmodium falciparum* malaria. *J. Infect. Dis., 155,* 1040.

29. Phillips RE, Looareesuwan S, White NJ, Chanthavanich P, Karbwang J, Supanaranond W, Turner RC, Warrell DA (1986) Hypoglycemia and antimalarial drugs: quinidine and release of insulin. *Br. Med. J., 292,* 1319.

30. White NJ, Miller KD, Marsh K, Berry CD, Turner RC, Williamson DH, Brown J (1987) Hypoglycemia in African children with severe malaria. *Lancet, 1,* 708.

31. Jacobs GH, Aikawa M, Milhous WK, Rabbege JR (1987) An ultrastructural study of the effects of mefloquine on malaria parasites. *Am. J. Trop. Med. Hyg., 36,* 9.

32. Schwartz DE, Weidekamm E, Mimica I, Heizmann P, Portmann R (1987) Multiple-dose pharmacokinetics of the antimalarial drug Fansimef (pyrimethamine + sulfadoxine + mefloquine) in healthy subjects. *Chemotherapy, 33,* 1.

CHAPTER 27

Pentamidine

JOAN E. KAPUSNIK and JOHN MILLS

STRUCTURE, DERIVATION

The initial discovery and subsequent studies of the chemotherapeutic properties of diamidine compounds (see Table 1), such as pentamidine, were a direct outgrowth of a lengthy search for agents which would disrupt glucose metabolism in trypanosomes (1). Following the introduction of the trypanocidal agents suramin and tryparsamide, in 1919, no other effective trypanocides were developed until 1937 when King et al demonstrated activity of the aliphatic diguanidines towards trypanosomes (2). In the 1930s additional amidine compounds, as well as guanidines, isothioureas and amines with alkyl and alkylene chains were found to have trypanocidal activity both in vitro and in vivo. The structural features, which are thought to influence the chemotherapeutic activity of these compounds are inert, central carbon chains and polar terminal groups (2). Aromatic diamidines exhibit antibacterial, antiprotozoal, antifungal and antitumor activity, although the mechanisms of action are generally not understood (1, 3).

Pentamidine isethionate is an aromatic diamidine derivative with the chemical name, 4:4'-diamidinodiphenoxypentane di-(β-hydroxyethane sulfonate). The drug has a pKa of 11.4, and thus is fully ionized at physiologic pH. Uptake, intracellular distribution and the lethal action of pentamidine may all be dependent upon the affinity of the drug for an uncharacterized anionic receptor (3).

Acquired resistance of pathogenic trypanosomes for this drug is likely to involve at least two alterations in the parasite: (a) a change in the metabolism of the parasite occurs whereby drug-sensitive enzyme reactions are modified, bypassed or eliminated; and (b) a modification in the surface protein structure of the parasite, which is important for uptake of drug. Little evidence exists at present supporting this first proposed mechanism of resistance. However, indirect evidence supports the latter. Some postulate that the development of resistance involves physical change in cellular structure (i.e. the anionic receptor), which would result in reduced drug uptake (4). For both drug-susceptible and drug-resistant strains of trypanosomes, the antiparasitic activity of ionized trypanocidal drugs is pH-dependent with activity increased with increasing pH.

Antimicrobial Agents Annual 3
P.K. Peterson and J. Verhoef, editors
© Elsevier Science Publishers BV, 1988

The pentamidine preparation most commonly used in the United States and Europe is parenteral pentamidine isethionate (Pentam 300 or Lomidine). Drug dosages that are recommended, or that are utilized in studies, are given as milligrams of pentamidine isethionate (1.74 mg of this pentamidine salt contains 1.0 mg of pentamidine base). Another salt form is available outside of the United States, pentamidine mesylate, but has been associated with greater toxicity than the isethionate preparation (see 'Adverse Reactions' below).

ACTIVITY

Pentamidine is active in vitro against most strains of *Trypanosoma brucei gambiense*, some strains of *T. brucei rhodesiense*, but is not active against *T. cruzi* (Chagas' disease). The drug is also active against most strains of *Leishmania*, including *L. donovani*, *L. tropica*, and *L. braziliensis*. Most information on the mechanism of the antiprotozoal action of pentamidine has been derived from studies with trypanosomes. The specific mechanism of action of pentamidine on *Pneumocystis carinii* is not known. Pentamidine has been shown to bind to nucleic acids and thus interferes with the incorporation of nucleotides into RNA and DNA. Pentamidine, in addition, may inhibit thymidinylate synthetase and oxidative phosphorylation, which also would result in the inhibition of phospholipid, DNA, RNA, and protein biosynthesis. Ultrastructural studies with trypanosomes reveal mitochondrial enlargement and fragmentation and also condensation of the kinetoplast DNA in the presence of pentamidine (3, 5, 6). As described above, different species of trypanosomes vary in their susceptibility to pentamidine. These differences are thought to be related to the relative importance of aerobic versus anaerobic glycolysis for the various species. In vivo observations confirm this finding, an example being the clinical cures for infections caused by *T. brucei rhodesiense* and *T. congolense*, compared to drug failures in infections caused by *T. cruzi*.

Pentamidine has been shown to exert antiparasitic effects in vitro on *Leishmania* similar to those seen with trypanosomes (7).

In animals with cutaneous *L. tropica major* infections, pentamidine was shown to reduce skin ornithine decarboxylase activity and polyamine levels, while both of these values remained unchanged in the skin of uninfected animals given pentamidine. Thus, serially monitoring polyamine levels and decarboxylase activity in affected skin may be done in patients to assess treatment efficacy (8).

Although pentamidine has been widely used for treatment of human tropical parasitic diseases, it was rarely used in the developed countries of the temperate zones. Subsequent to the discovery in 1958 of its activity against *P. carinii* and the recognition of this organism as an important cause of pneumonia in immunosuppressed patients — including those with acquired immunodeficiency syndrome (AIDS) — there has been a marked increase in the use of the drug and a greater interest in its pharmacology and therapeutic potential (9, 10).

Pentamidine exerts a lethal effect on *P. carinii*, as assessed by dye exclusion studies (11). Pentamidine-treated *P. carinii* cysts show morphologic changes, including

Table 1   *Representative diamidine compounds*

Stilbamidine	Pentamidine (isethionate salt)*
Hydroxystilbamidine*	Propamidine
Oxystilbamidine	Phenamidine

* Compounds being used clinically

the disappearance of nuclei, nuclear substances, and intracystic bodies (12). Lethal concentrations of pentamidine appear to cause only modest inhibitions of glucose metabolism, amino acid transport, protein synthesis, and RNA synthesis (13).

In vitro studies show that pentamidine inhibits growth of *P. carinii*, which was defined as an increase in the observed numbers of cyst forms over time. This effect was observed at drug concentrations (0.3–9.0 μg/ml) achievable in humans (14).

The aromatic diamidines also are active in vitro against many pathogenic fungi, and have been used in the treatment of blastomycosis, actinomycosis, histoplasmosis, cryptococcosis, and chromoblastomycosis (15). The efficacy in vivo of pentamidine for the treatment of these fungal infections is presently not supported by clinical data. Hydroxystilbamidine, however, is often used as a second-line agent in the treatment of blastomycosis.

CLINICAL PHARMACOLOGY

Pentamidine isethionate is poorly absorbed when taken orally, and thus is recommended only for parenteral use (intravenous or intramuscular).* After administration the drug appears to quickly distribute and bind to tissues with only minimal amounts of drug found in plasma after dosing. Seven patients given a single daily intramuscular injection of 4 mg/kg for 10–12 days had an average steady-state plasma drug concentration of 0.3–0.5 μg/ml (5). This concentration is at least 10 times lower than might be expected if the drug were distributed equally throughout the body. Pentamidine is slowly excreted into the urine and can be detected there for up to 6–8 weeks following cessation of therapy. The disposition of pentamidine appears to be much like that of amphotericin B, in that after administration it quickly distributes and binds to tissues/membranes, then over time is slowly re-released into the systemic circulation (16).

A single-dose pharmacokinetic study in patients with AIDS has confirmed previous pentamidine disposition data (17). Twelve patients received either an intramuscular or intravenous 4 mg/kg dose. The mean peak concentrations in plasma were 209 and 612 ng/ml, respectively. The drug concentrations were low, but consistent with the very large apparent volume of distribution, which was 140 liters after intramuscular and 924 liters after intravenous administration. The renal

---

*Because of severe local reactions which may occur after i.m. administration, most centers use i.v. administration whenever possible.

clearance of pentamidine was observed to be $\leq 5\%$ of total plasma clearance for the single-dose with the serum beta-elimination half-life being approximately 6.5–9.5 hours.

Patients with mild azotemia (as defined solely by an elevated blood urea nitrogen (BUN)) had average steady-state pentamidine plasma concentrations which were higher than in patients with normal renal function (18). In one patient, as the BUN rose from 28 to 102 mg/100 ml, average plasma drug concentration increased from 0.3 to 1.4 μg/ml. Five patients in another study with creatinine clearances of 35–75 ml/min showed no significant difference in plasma clearance or elimination half-life compared to patients with normal renal function (17).

At present, there are not enough data from which one can derive recommendations for pentamidine dosage adjustments in patients with renal insufficiency. Until data from ongoing pharmacokinetic studies are available, we recommend that the daily maintenance dosage of pentamidine be decreased by approximately 50% in patients with severe renal disease (creatinine clearance of approx. 20 ml/min or less). These patients should, however, receive up to three 4 mg/kg daily doses first, as loading doses, before their daily maintenance dose is reduced. This loading dose again is an estimate, since the volume of distribution for pentamidine is very large and a target serum drug concentration has not been described.

Pentamidine disposition studies in animals show that only a small percentage of drug is excreted via the feces, with most being eliminated as the active parent compound in the urine. Pentamidine also has been found to accumulate preferentially in the kidneys and liver of animals, and to a lesser extent in lung tissue (see Table 2) (18, 19). Pentamidine has not been effective in the treatment of human trypanosomal central nervous system infections, and thus is not thought to cross the blood-brain barrier to a significant degree. Currently there are no reported measurements of drug concentrations in cerebrospinal fluid.

ADVERSE REACTIONS

The clinical use of pentamidine has been limited because it must be administered parenterally, and because of the high incidence of drug-related adverse reactions (see Table 3). In a study of 404 patients (without AIDS) with suspected or confirmed *P. carinii* pneumonia (PCP), almost 50% of patients receiving pentamidine

Table 2 *Average concentrations of pentamidine in various organs (µg/g)*

Dose (animal)	Kidney	Liver	Spleen	Lung	Brain	Ref. no
10 mg/kg i.p. (mice)	52	28	11	5	ND*	18
4 mg/kg i.m. (rats)	10.2	8	–	0.8	–	19
20 mg/kg i.m. (rats)	24	55	–	3.2	–	19

* ND = measurement taken, but not detectable.

Table 3 *Adverse reactions in patients treated with pentamidine*

	No. (%) of patients with indicated reactions		
Ref. no.	47	20	49
Patient category	Pediatric	All	AIDS
(total no. patients)	(n = 15)	(n = 189)	(n = 32)
Nephrotoxicity	9 (60)	95 (24)	21 (66)
Abnormal liver enzymes	12 (80)	39 (10)	21 (66)
Leukopenia	2 (13)	17 (4)	13 (41)*
Hypocalcemia	10 (67)	5 (1)	4 (13)
Injection site reactions	10 (67)	74 (18)	0
Hypoglycemia	6 (40)	25 (6)	6 (19)
Immediate reactions	0	39 (10)	19 (59)
Thrombocytopenia	2 (13)	0	4 (13)
Rash	3 (20)	6 (2)	1 (3)
% patients with major and/or minor reactions**	14	47	100
Total number of adverse reactions***	67	189	10

* Includes patients receiving 'bad batch' (see 'Adverse Reactions').
** Some patients experienced multiple reactions.
*** Not all adverse reactions are listed above.

experienced adverse effects directly attributable to pentamidine therapy (20). Of particular importance in this study was the high frequency of renal toxicity, which ranged from reversible azotemia to severe renal dysfunction that contributed to death. In other reports the degree of pentamidine-induced renal insufficiency has varied from azotemia with urine sediment changes, to acute tubular necrosis (21–25). Patients receiving concomitant nephrotoxic agents may be at increased risk of pentamidine-induced nephrotoxicity, as well as patients that are not optimally hydrated during therapy (20, 26, 27). A case of severe pentamidine-induced myoglobinuria and renal failure has also been reported (28).

Pentamidine can also cause either hypoglycemia or hyperglycemia (20, 23, 24, 29, 30). Pancreatic islet cell toxicity from pentamidine may be manifest by an initial hyperglycemia, which may last for minutes, followed by a phase of hypoglycemia lasting for hours, and lastly by a persistent phase of hyperglycemia that may eventually result in insulin-dependent diabetes (30, 31). Studies have shown the hypoglycemic phase to be associated with inappropriately high concentrations of circulating insulin. This evidence supports the hypothesis that pentamidine causes acute pancreatic islet cell inflammation or necrosis and subsequent release of insulin (32, 33). No effect was observed in a single patient treated with pentamidine for a malignant insulinoma (34). Reversal of acute pentamidine-induced hypoglycemia reportedly has been achieved with oral diazoxide therapy (35), although this treatment is not routinely recommended. Pentamidine isethionate is thought to be less pancreatotoxic than the mesylate salt (36). Recently, two AIDS patients were reported to have had fatal acute pancreatitis when treated with pentamidine isethionate for PCP (37).

Pentamidine inhibits platelet aggregation and coagulation in vitro at concentrations greater than 1 $\mu g/ml$ (38). The clinical relevance of this finding is not clear but may impact on patients with severe renal insufficiency. Thrombocytopenia, including thrombocytopenic purpura, has been observed during pentamidine therapy (10, 20, 23). This particular complication has been associated with the combination of both pentamidine and trimethoprim + sulfamethoxazole (39). Pentamidine-induced neutropenia has also been reported (23, 40). In 1984 there was a dramatic increase in the number of reported cases of pentamidine-induced neutropenia. The Center for Disease Control later ascribed this 'epidemic' to be related to a specific batch of pentamidine isethionate (41).

Previously it was recommended that pentamidine be administered only intramuscularly in order to avoid the immediate cardiovascular toxic reactions from intravenous administration (26). Studies in animals suggest that the drug has a direct vasodilatory action on peripheral small arteries and arterioles, believed to be independent of any central nervous system mechanism (42). However, epinephrine and atropine have been administered to patients experiencing pentamidine-induced hypotension without reversal of the syncopal episode (1). In a review of 74 patients receiving pentamidine by intramuscular and intravenous routes, hypotension only occurred in the intramuscular group (43). No hypotension was observed in any of the patients given an intravenous infusion, perhaps because of the slow infusion rate of ≥ 60 minutes. However, hypotension (including postural hypotension) has occurred after intravenous pentamidine administration in our experience and others (44; C.B. Wofsy, personal communication).

Other infusion-related adverse effects include patients who experienced rash at the infusion site (43). The rash did not recur in these patients when they were premedicated with antihistamines. A fatal Herxheimer-like reaction also has been reported in a patient (being treated for PCP) 11 hours after pentamidine administration (45). The patient experienced fever, tachycardia, and hypotension; all bacterial and fungal cultures were negative. At autopsy *P. carinii* was present only in the lung tissue.

It is recommended that pentamidine be administered intravenously. The infusion rate should be slow, over at least 1 hour, thus avoiding the infusion-related side effects and potential complications associated with daily intramuscular injections (e.g. pain and sterile abscesses). Should the patient develop hypotension, fever, or chills during the intravenous infusion, administration time may be increased to 120 minutes (46).

The incidence of pentamidine-induced major and minor adverse reactions, from retrospective and prospective studies, appears to be higher in AIDS patients, compared to other patient populations (see Table 3) (20, 47, 48). The explanation for this consistent observation is not clear. Monitoring more closely for drug-induced adverse reactions is therefore indicated for this group of patients. Guidelines for monitoring pentamidine therapy in AIDS patients have been published (49). The frequency of screening for potential side effects and toxicities is based upon their prevalence and severity.

CLINICAL USES

Pentamidine is currently used for the treatment of both leishmaniasis and trypanosomiasis. Although pentavalent antimonal compounds are considered the most effective drugs for all forms of leishmaniasis, some difficult cases may require the concurrent administration of pentamidine or amphotericin B (50).

Pentamidine (3–5 mg/kg/d for 7–10 d) is also highly effective in the treatment of early cases (before central nervous system involvement) of Gambian and Rhodesian trypanosomiases. It has been widely used for prophylaxis against *Trypanosoma gambiense*, as a single 3–5 mg/kg dose, which is generally considered protective for 3–6 months (51).

The aromatic diamidines were first tested in 1958 by Ivady and Paldy for the treatment of PCP, which was a common complication of cancer or immunosuppressive therapy (9). Pentamidine isethionate, as employed in the treatment of PCP has been recently reviewed (52). Most drug use occurs in 2 classifications of patients: (a) premature or debilitated infants up to 6 months of age; and (b) older children or adults with congenital or acquired immunodeficiencies, including AIDS. Before the introduction of pentamidine, mortality from PCP in these patients was between 50–100%; higher mortality rates were seen in the United States than in Europe, and they were higher in immunosuppressed adults than in children (53–55). From 1958 to 1962 Ivady and co-workers treated 212 such patients in Europe, and reduced their fatality rate from 50 to 3.5% (56). In the United States the efficacy of pentamidine in the treatment of PCP was well documented by Walzer et al (20) in 1974. Sixty-nine of 163 patients (42%) with confirmed PCP recovered when treated with pentamidine. The recovery rate for those treated 9 or more days was 63%. Early diagnosis of infection and institution of therapy were important determinants of a good outcome, as previously emphasized (20, 57).

Hughes et al (47) studied a group of 50 pediatric patients with PCP and compared intramuscular pentamidine therapy (4 mg/kg/d) with oral trimethoprim+sulfamethoxazole (20 and 100 mg/kg/d). This study showed a 58% initial response rate with pentamidine, which increased to 75% when patients who did not respond within 4 days were crossed over to trimethoprim+sulfamethoxazole (TMP+SMX). The initial response rate for TMP+SMX treated patients was 65%, which increased to 77% when the failures were crossed over to pentamidine. The response rate for each drug regimen was equivalent. None of the patients from either group had recurrences. Fourteen of 15 patients treated with pentamidine had adverse reactions, compared with only 1 of 17 patients receiving TMP+SMX. Thus, it was concluded in this patient population that TMP+SMX is as efficacious as pentamidine in the treatment of PCP, and has the added advantages of lesser toxicity and an oral dosage route. A more recent study in the pediat-

305

ric population with PCP has confirmed these results (58).

A retrospective review of 38 patients with AIDS treated for PCP reported these patients to have a higher incidence of adverse reactions from TMP + SMX therapy than from pentamidine (P < 0.005) (23). The appearance of drug-induced toxicity from TMP + SMX was earlier than toxicity associated with pentamidine (7.5 vs 9.5 days into therapy). Subsequently, a prospective, randomized trial was done at the same institution in AIDS patients treated for PCP with TMP + SMX versus pentamidine (48). In 40 patients with first episode PCP there was no significant difference for TMP + SMX and pentamidine regimens when comparing the time to clinical improvement and pulmonary function tests. Minor adverse drug reactions occurred in all patients. Major adverse reactions that necessitated a cross-over to the alternate drug therapy occurred in 50% of patients initially treated with TMP + SMX and 55% of patients initially treated with pentamidine. This study and another (59) have concluded that in the AIDS population either drug regimen is toxic and neither is superior (59). TMP + SMX is still considered as the standard of therapy because its potential toxicities are for the most part less severe and reversible relative to those of pentamidine.

A single clinical trial utilizing aerosolized pentamidine has been published (see 'Future Directions' below).

DOSING

Pentamidine should only be administered by deep intramuscular injection or slow intravenous infusion. The intravenous route is strongly preferred because of lesser toxicity (see 'Adverse Reactions'). For intramuscular injection the contents of each vial (Pentam 300) should be diluted with 3.0 ml of Sterile Water for Injection, USP. The unused portion should be discarded, as long-term stability of this concentrated solution has not yet been confirmed. For intravenous infusion pentamidine may be reconstituted either with Sterile Water for Injection or with 5% dextrose solution. Further dilution for intravenous administration was previously done only using 5% dextrose. However, pentamidine 2 mg/ml appears to be stable for 48 hours in either 5% dextrose or 0.9% sodium chloride when stored at 24° C (60).

The optimal pentamidine treatment regimens for visceral and cutaneous leishmaniasis have not been established. Pentamidine isethionate 4 mg/kg, 3 times weekly for 5–25 weeks, has been recommended for patients with visceral leishmaniasis and 4 mg/kg once weekly until resolution is complete for localized cutaneous leishmaniasis (61). Experts also differ as to the optimal pentamidine dose and duration of therapy for the treatment of African trypanosomiasis. Pentamidine isethionate 4–7 mg/kg/d is recommended for 7–10 days. The higher daily dosage may be associated with increased risk of adverse effects. Longer therapy is sometimes necessary if initial treatment fails.

The recommended adult and pediatric dosage of pentamidine isethionate for the treatment of PCP is 4 mg/kg/d, given as a single daily dose for 12–14 days.

A longer duration of therapy (21 days) has generally been employed in AIDS patients with PCP. Two-week treatment regimens are associated with a high incidence of residual organisms in lung tissue, even in patients who have responded clinically to therapy. This observation may help explain the high relapse or recurrence rate of PCP in AIDS patients (62). Post-treatment suppressive doses have ranged from once weekly to once monthly. Studies are presently underway that are evaluating these regimens.

FUTURE DIRECTIONS

There was initial enthusiasm for the use of pentamidine in the treatment of human babesiosis due to *Babesia microti*, a self-limiting disease (63). However, the drug did not always eradicate the organism and is now seldom used. Efficacy in humans should be more thoroughly investigated in view of pentamidine's effectiveness in animal babesiosis.

Studies in animals have looked at combination therapy of pentamidine and TMP + SMX in the treatment of PCP. These data suggest that such drug therapy is possibly less effective than either regimen alone. This combination therapy question needs still to be resolved in humans. Therapy with pentamidine plus TMP + SMX might allow for a dosage reduction of these otherwise toxic drugs, and thus reduce overall morbidity.

Studies are currently underway that will more carefully define the pharmacokinetic disposition of pentamidine after intravenous infusions in patients with renal insufficiency. This is especially important, as patients experiencing pentamidine-induced renal toxicity may need pentamidine therapy to be continued, and a proper dosage adjustment is necessary.

Further investigations concerning the various mechanisms of action of pentamidine and modes of acquired resistance would be helpful in order to better utilize this agent.

Pentamidine should be continued to be evaluated as post-treatment suppressive therapy in AIDS patients with PCP who cannot tolerate TMP + SMX. Preliminary results have been reported where 7 patients received 4 mg/kg monthly with 2 of 7 (28.5%) patients having a recurrence of PCP, compared to 5 of 10 (50%) in an untreated control group (65). Pentamidine should also be studied for prophylaxis of PCP in patients with AIDS-related condition (ARC) and in AIDS patients who have not yet had PCP.

The development of a less toxic pentamidine analog should be pursued, especially because of the increased cases of PCP in AIDS patients and because toxicity remains the limiting factor in therapy for most patients. Investigators are looking at innovative methods of administration which will hopefully reduce systemic toxicities. Pentamidine has been incorporated into liposomes and administered directly to the lung via aerosolization in healthy animals (66). Also, aerosolized pentamidine isethionate has been administered to AIDS patients with PCP (67). Results are encouraging as extrapulmonary drug tissue concentrations were found to be negligible after aerosol delivery. Aerosolized pentamidine appears to be an effective therapy for PCP in rats (68) and in a preliminary open trial in human subjects (69). Treatment consisted of inhalations of pentamidine aerosol once daily for 21 days. 600 mg of pentamidine isethionate was dissolved in 6 ml sterile water and placed in the Respigard II® nebulizer system. The pentamidine particle size delivered was 1.42 ± 1.88 μm (mass median aerodynamic diameter). Each inhalation session was approximately 20 minutes, with the total doses delivered being about 300 mg. 13 of 15 (87%) patients were treated successfully. No systemic adverse effects were observed in any patient during therapy, with serum pentamidine concentrations being less than 10 ng/ml in 12 of 14 patients. The only adverse reaction was coughing, which was severe in patients who were cigarette smokers. In view of this efficacy rate, along with the reduced incidence of toxicity, a blinded randomized trial of aerosolized pentamidine versus intravenous trimethoprim + sulfamethoxazole has begun (A.B. Montgomery, personal communication). Also, post-treatment suppressive therapy with aerosolized pentamidine is being studied.

REFERENCES

1. Schoenbach EB, Greenspan EM (1948) The pharmacology, mode of action and therapeutic potentialities of stilbamidine, pentamidine, propamidine and other aromatic diamidines – a review. *Medicine, 27,* 327.
2. Lourie EM, Yorke W (1939) Studies in chemotherapy. XXI. The trypanocidal action of certain aromatic diamidines. *Ann. Trop. Med. Parasitol., 33,* 289.
3. Williamson J (1979) Effects of trypanocides on the fine structure of target organisms. *Pharmacol. Ther., 7,* 445.
4. Williamson J (1959) Drug resistance in trypanosomes: effects of inhibitors pH and oxidation-reduction potential on normal and resistant *Trypanosoma rhodesiense. Br. J. Pharmacol., 14,* 443.
5. LymphoMed, Inc. (1984) Pentam 300^R-sterile pentamidine isethionate: package insert prescribing information. Melrose Park, IL.
6. Kaplan HG, Myers CE (1977) Complex inhibition of thymidinylate synthetase by aromatic diamidines: evidence for both rapid, freely reversible and slowly progressive, nonequilibrium inhibition. *J. Pharmacol. Exp. Ther., 201,* 554.
7. Croft SL, Brazil RP (1982) Effect of pentamidine isethionate on the ultrastructure and morphology of *Leishmania mexicana amazonesis* in vitro. *Ann. Trop. Med. Parasitol., 76,* 37.
8. Bachrach U, Abu-Elheiga L, Schnur LF (1983) *Leishmania tropica major:* effect of paramomycin and pentamidine on polyamine levels in the skin of normal and infected mice. *Exp. Parasitol., 55,* 280.
9. Ivady G, Paldy L (1957) A new form of treatment for interstitial plasma cell pneumonia in premature infants with pentavalent antimony and aromatic diamidines. *Monatsschr. Kinderheilkd., 106,* 10.
10. Levy MA, Senior RM, Sneider RE (1974) Severe thrombocytopenia purpura complicating pentamidine therapy for *Pneumocystis carinii* pneumonia. *Cancer, 34,* 441.

11. Pesanti EL (1980) In vitro effects of antiprotozoan drugs and immune serum on *Pneumocystis carinii*. *J. Infect Dis., 141*, 775.
12. Pesanti EL, Cox C (1981) Metabolic and synthetic activities of *Pneumocystis carinii* in vitro. *Infect. Immun., 34*, 908.
13. Mori T, Izumi A, Watanabe K, Ikemoto H (1979) Microscopic studies on the effect of pentamidine on *Pneumocystis carinii*. *Jpn. J. Med., 18*, 64.
14. Pifer LL, Pifer DD, Woods DR (1983) Biological profile and response to antipneumocystis agents of *Pneumocystis carinii* in cell culture. *Antimicrob. Agents Chemother., 24*, 674.
15. Christison IB, Conant NF (1953) Antifungal activity of some aromatic diamidines. *J. Lab. Clin. Med., 42*, 638.
16. Bernard EM, Donnelly HJ, Maher MP, Armstrong D (1985) Use of a new bioassay to study pentamidine pharmacokinetics. *J. Infect. Dis., 152*, 750.
17. Conte Jr JE, Upton RA, Phelps RT et al (1986) Use of a specific and sensitive assay to determine pentamidine pharmacokinetics in patients with AIDS. *J. Infect. Dis., 154*, 923.
18. Waalkes TP, Denham C, De Vita VT (1970) Pentamidine: clinical pharmacologic correlations in man and mice. *Clin. Pharmacol. Ther., 11*, 505.
19. Waldman RH, Pearce DE, Martin RA (1973) Pentamidine isethionate levels in lungs, liver, and kidneys of rats after aerosol or intramuscular administration. *Am. Rev. Respir. Dis., 108*, 1004.
20. Walzer PD, Perl DP, Krogstad DJ et al (1974) *Pneumocystis carinii* pneumonia in the United States: epidemiologic, diagnostic and clinical features. *Ann. Intern. Med., 80*, 83.
21. Wang JJ, Freeman AI, Gaeta JF, Sinks LF (1970) Unusual complications of pentamidine in the treatment of *Pneumocystis carinii* pneumonia. *J. Pediatr., 77*, 311.
22. Misikova Z, Kovacs L, Foltinova A (1979) Nephrotoxicity of pentamidine in treatment of pneumonia in 2 children with acute lymphoblastic leukemia. *Cesk. Pediatr., 34*, 715.
23. Gordin FM, Simon GL, Wofsy CB, Mills J (1984) Adverse reactions to trimethoprim-sulfamethoxazole in patients with acquired immunodeficiency syndrome. *Ann. Intern. Med., 100*, 495.
24. Murdoch JK, Keystone JS (1983) Pentamidine and hypogylcemia. *Ann. Intern. Med., 99*, 879.
25. Emmer M, De Vita VT (1968) *Pneumocystis carinii* pneumonia and pentamidine isethionate toxicity. *Ann. Intern. Med., 69*, 637.
26. Waalkes TP, Makulu DR (1976) Pharmacologic aspects of pentamidine. *Natl Cancer Inst. Monogr., 43*, 171.
27. Stehr-Green JK, Helmick CG (1985) Pentamidine and renal toxicity. *N. Engl. J. Med., 313*, 694.
28. Sensakovie JW, Suarez M, Perez G et al (1985) Pentamidine treatment of *Pneumocystis carinii* pneumonia in the acquired immunodeficiency syndrome. *Arch. Intern. Med., 145*, 2247.
29. Western KA, Perera DR, Schultz MG (1970) Pentamidine isethionate in the treatment of *Pneumocystis carinii* pneumonia. *Ann. Intern. Med., 73*, 695.
30. Bouchard P, Sai P, Reach G et al (1982) Diabetes mellitus following pentamidine-induced hypoglycemia in humans. *Diabetes, 31*, 40.
31. Ganda OP (1984) Pentamidine and hypoglycemia. *Ann. Intern. Med., 100*, 464.

32. Sai P, Boillet D, Boitard CL et al (1983) Pentamidine, a new diabetogenic drug in laboratory rodents. *Diabetologia, 25,* 418.

33. Murphey SA, Josephs AS (1981) Acute pancreatitis associated with pentamidine therapy. *Arch. Intern. Med., 141,* 56.

34. Osei K, Falko JM, Nelson KP (1984) Diabetogenic effect of pentamidine: in vitro and in vivo studies in a patient with malignant insulinoma. *Am. J. Med., 77,* 41.

35. Fitzgerald DB, Young IS (1984) Reversal of pentamidine-induced hypoglycemia with oral diazoxide. *J. Trop. Med. Hyg., 87,* 15.

36. Belehu A, Naafs B (1982) Diabetes mellitus associated with pentamidine mesylate. *Lancet, 1,* 1463.

37. Salmeron S, Pettipretz P, Katlama C et al (1986) Pentamidine and pancreatitis. *Ann. Intern. Med., 105,* 140.

38. Kempin SJ, Jackson CW, Edwards CC (1977) In vitro inhibition of platelet function and coagulation by pentamidine isethionate. *Antimicrob. Agents Chemother., 12,* 451.

39. Milder JE, Walzer PD, Powell Jr RD (1979) Treatment of *Pneumocystis carinii* pneumonia with trimethoprim-sulfamethoxazole and pentamidine: efficacy and toxicity. *South. Med. J., 72,* 1626.

40. Polsky B, Dryjanski J, Whimbey E et al (1984) Severe neutropenia during pentamidine treatment of *Pneumocystis carinii* pneumonia in patients with acquired immunodeficiency syndrome — New York. *J. Am. Med. Assoc., 251,* 1253.

41. Anonymous (1984) Severe neutropenia during pentamidine treatment of *Pneumocystis carinii* pneumonia in patients with acquired immunodeficiency syndrome. *Morbid. Mortal. Wkly Rep., 33,* 65.

42. Bielenberg GW, Krieglstein J (1984) On the hypotensive effect of aromatic amidines and imidazolines. *Arzneim-Forsch./Drug Res., 34,* 958.

43. Navin TR, Fontaine RE (1984) Intravenous versus intramuscular administration of pentamidine. *N. Engl. J. Med., 311,* 1701.

44. Helmick CG, Green JK (1985) Pentamidine-associated hypotension and route of administration. *Ann. Intern. Med., 103,* 480.

45. Stark FR, Crast F, Clemmer T, Ramirez R (1976) Fatal Herxheimer reaction after pentamidine in *Pneumocystis* pneumonia. *Lancet, 1,* 1193.

46. Oliff L (1987) Comments: pentamidine monitoring. *Drug Intell. Clin. Pharm., 21,* 467.

47. Hughes WT, Feldman S, Chaudhary S et al (1978) Comparison of pentamidine isethionate and trimethoprim-sulfamethoxazole in the treatment of *Pneumocystis carinii* pneumonia. *J. Pediatr., 92,* 285.

48. Wharton M, Coleman DL, Fitz G et al (1986) Trimethoprim-sulfamethoxazole or pentamidine for *Pneumocystis carinii* pneumonia in the acquired immunodeficiency syndrome. *Ann. Intern. Med., 105,* 37.

49. Andersen R, Boedicker M, Ma M, Goldstein EJC (1986) Adverse reactions associated with pentamidine isethionate in AIDS patients: recommendations for monitoring therapy. *Drug Intell. Clin. Pharm., 20,* 862.

50. Marsden PD (1979) Current concepts in parasitology. *N. Engl. J. Med., 300,* 350.

51. Apted FIC (1980) Present status of chemotherapy and chemoprophylaxis of human trypanosomiasis in the eastern hemisphere. *Pharmacol. Ther., 11,* 391.

52. Goa KL, Campoli-Richards DM (1987) Pentamidine isethionate: a review of its antiprotozoal activity, pharmacokinetic properties and therapeutic use in *Pneumocystis carinii* pneumonia. *Drugs, 33,* 242.

53. Nelson WE (1979) The respiratory system. In: Nelson WE (Ed), *Textbook of Pediat-*

rics, 11th ed., p 1215. Saunders, Philadelphia.

54. Johnson JF, Rehder TL, Moore GF (1981) *Pneumocystis carinii* pneumonia: review with a case study. *Drug. Intell. Clin. Pharm., 15*, 732.

55. Drake S, Lampasona V, Nicks HL, Schwartzman SW (1985) Pentamidine isethionate in the treatment of *Pneumocystis carinii* pneumonia. *Clin. Pharmacol., 4*, 507.

56. Ivady G, Paldy L, Koltay M et al (1967) *Pneumocystis carinii* pneumonia. *Lancet, 1*, 616.

57. Fortuny IE, Tempero KF, Amsden TW (1970) *Pneumocystis carinii* pneumonia diagnosed from sputum and successfully treated with pentamidine. *Cancer, 26*, 911.

58. Siegel SE, Wolff LJ, Baehner RL, Hammond D (1984) Treatment of *Pneumocystis carinii* pneumonia. *Am. J. Dis. Child., 138*, 1054.

59. Small CB, Harris CA, Friedland GH, Klein RS (1985) The treatment of *Pneumocystis carinii* pneumonia in the acquired immunodeficiency syndrome. *Arch. Intern. Med., 145*, 837.

60. De NC, Alam AS, Kapoor JN (1986) Stability of pentamidine isethionate in 5% dextrose and 0.9% sodium chloride injections. *Am. J. Hosp. Pharm., 43*, 1486.

61. Pearson RD, Hewlett EL (1985) Pentamidine for the treatment of *Pneumocystis carinii* pneumonia and other protozoal diseases. *Ann. Intern. Med., 103*, 782.

62. DeLorenzo LJ, Maguire GP, Wormser GP et al (1985) Persistence of *Pneumocystis carinii* pneumonia in the acquired immunodeficiency syndrome. *Chest, 88*, 79.

63. Francioloi PB, Keithly JS, Jones TC et al (1981) Response of babesiosis to pentamidine therapy. *Ann. Intern. Med., 94*, 326.

64. Kluge RM, Spaulding DM, Spain DJ (1978) Combination of pentamidine and trimethoprim-sulfamethoxazole in the therapy of *Pneumocystis carinii* pneumonia in rats. *Antimicrob. Agents Chemother., 13*, 975.

65. Karaffa C, Rehm S, Calabrese L (1986) Efficacy of monthly pentamidine infusions in preventing recurrent *Pneumocystis carinii* pneumonia in the AIDS patient. In: *Program and Abstracts, 26th Interscience Conference on Antimicrobial Agents and Chemotherapy, New Orleans, 1986*, p 224. American Society for Microbiology, Washington, DC.

66. Debs RJ, Straubinger RM, Brunette EN et al (1987) Selective enhancement of pentamidine uptake in the lung by aerosolization and delivery in liposomes. *Am. Rev. Respir. Dis., 135*, 731.

67. Montgomery AB, Debs RJ, Luce JM et al (1987) Concentration of pentamidine in bronchoalveolar lavage fluid after aerosol and intravenous administration (Abstract). *Am. Rev. Respir. Dis., 135*, A167.

68. Debs RJ, Blumenfeld W, Brunette EN et al (1987) Successful treatment with aerosolized pentamidine of *Pneumocystis carinii* pneumonia in rats. *Antimicrob. Agents Chemother., 31*, 37.

69. Montgomery AB, Debs RJ, Luce JM et al (1987) Aerosolized pentamidine as sole therapy for *Pneumocystis carinii* pneumonia in patients with acquired immunodeficiency syndrome. *Lancet, 2*, 480.

CHAPTER 28

Praziquantel

V. KUMAR, S. GEERTS and J.R.A. BRANDT

Since the publication of *Annual 2*, unfortunately little new information has appeared on praziquantel. The discussion in this Chapter continues to represent a current perspective regarding this agent. Since the previous account of praziquantel therapy (1), most reports on its use have been directed towards the chemotherapeutic management of schistosomiasis, despite the fact that the drug has a wide spectrum of activity and has become the drug of choice against other major trematode and cestode infections of man.

Schistosomiasis

Various dose regimens of praziquantel (1×50, 3×20, 1×40, 2×35, 3×25 or 2×20 mg/kg given in one day) were evaluated for the treatment of schistosomiasis japonica in single- and double-blind, stratified, randomized studies. The side-effects of the treatment were highest (70%) in the 1×50 mg/kg group. Although a single dose is more convenient, administration of the drug in divided doses is recommended and the 2×20 mg/kg schedule is deemed suitable for large-scale field treatment (2).

Schistosomiasis japonica patients with hepatomegaly and/or splenomegaly were treated with 3×20 mg/kg or 1×50 mg/kg single-day praziquantel and compared with an untreated group. One year after treatment, 55% of the treated patients showed marked decrease in hepatosplenomegaly compared with the untreated group of whom 13% improved spontaneously; however, 35% of the cases had increased hepatosplenomegaly (3).

Fifteen patients with hepatosplenic schistosomiasis due to *Schistosoma mansoni* received praziquantel in a single oral dose (30 mg/kg); 14 of these patients exhibited hepatosplenomegaly. Ten patients, including 3 concurrently infected with *S. haematobium*, ceased to pass live eggs while in the others there was a 95% reduction in output of live eggs. Although transient side-effects during treatment were observed in some patients, Bassily et al (4) concluded that praziquantel is the

Antimicrobial Agents Annual 3
P.K. Peterson and J. Verhoef, editors
©Elsevier Science Publishers BV, 1988

treatment of choice for advanced cases of hepatosplenic schistosomiasis and concurrent *S. haematobium* infection. At 40 mg/kg per day for 3 consecutive days this drug cured 8 of 11 patients, showing schistosomal colonic polyposis. In 7 of the cured patients, 3–6 months later, there was a decrease in the size and number of polyps (5).

Praziquantel is apparently more effective in killing late than early developmental stages of *S. mansoni*. In mice it was shown that 3-day-old blood flukes (lung forms) were less responsive to the drug than infections of longer duration (6).

In Maniema (Zaïre) praziquantel treatment (40 mg/kg, single dose) of 90 patients heavily infected with *S. mansoni* provoked an unusually high incidence of transient yet unexplained side-effects. Within 30 minutes of administration of the drug, symptoms of intense abdominal discomfort and hemorrhagic diarrhea were observed in more than half the patients. The frequency of occurrence of these symptoms was correlated with the intensity of infection (7).

In 6 schoolchildren infected with *S. haematobium* the urinary egg output decreased from a mean of 310 eggs to 1 egg per 10 ml, 20 days after treatment with praziquantel. Simultaneously proteinuria, erythrocyturia and leukocyturia were reduced over a period of 2 months. The vesicular polyps had disappeared 1 month after treatment (8). Mott et al (9), however, found that infected individuals with clinical signs of hematuria and proteinuria had lower cure rates (15.4%) than patients without these symptoms, where a cure rate of 96% was obtained.

In laboratory animals infected with *S. mansoni* it has been demonstrated that treatment with praziquantel, besides affecting the parasites, also halted or partly reversed liver fibrosis (10, 11). Furthermore, although the drug has no suppressive effect in vitro on human lymphocyte proliferation (12), it does produce a significant increase in the blastogenic response of peripheral blood mononuclear cells to soluble adult worm antigen (13).

In general, praziquantel is less toxic than other currently used drugs against schistosomiasis such as niridazole, metrifonate and oxamniquine, though a limit to its use in mass chemotherapy is its cost, which is more than 10 times that of metrifonate (14).

Clonorchiasis and opisthorchiasis

The safety of praziquantel and its efficacy against important trematode infections due to *Clonorchis/Opisthorchis* and *Paragonimus* may soon warrant its establishment as a drug of choice for these diseases as well (15).

In a double-blind, placebo-controlled study on the efficacy of praziquantel in *Clonorchis/Opisthorchis* infection in 37 immigrants, mainly from Laos, a one-day treatment at 3×25 mg/kg showed a cumulative cure rate of 96% 60 days after treatment and this appeared to be independent of the intensity of infection. In the placebo control group, the cure rate was 8% during a follow-up period of 60 days. Following treatment acute symptoms developed in 26–27% of the patients as against 6–7% in the placebo control. Most of these symptoms (dizziness, head-ache, nausea, vomiting, pruritic rash, drowsiness) were transient, although in 1 case the pruritic skin rash lasted for several days. The drug had no effect on con-current intestinal nematode infections 30–60 days after treatment and equally a concurrent *Hymenolepis nana* infection was not cured with this treatment schedule (16).

Paragonimiasis

In Lower Mundani, Cameroon, 35 human cases were detected who were excreting eggs of *Paragonimus* species in sputum. They were treated with praziquantel 75 mg/kg per day, administered at 4- to 6-hourly intervals, for 3 days. At 3 months follow-up examination, 97.1% of the patients had been cured (17). Eight docu-mented cases of paragonimiasis in refugee patients from Southeast Asia were treated with this drug at 3×25 mg/kg daily for 2 consecutive days. Six of these were cured parasitologically at 3 months and the seventh at 4 months as judged by ova-negative sputa and stools. Concomitant use of antihistaminic and/or anti-emetic agents is advocated to avert the side-effects of treatment (18).

Fascioliasis

A female patient severely infected with *Fasciola hepatica* was successfully cured parasitologically with praziquantel at 75 mg/kg given in 3 divided doses over a 1-day period. Four days after treatment the levels of hepatic enzymes (SGOT, SGPT, alkaline phosphatase) had begun to decrease (19).

Adult cestode infections

Previous reports on the activity of praziquantel against *Taenia saginata* were con-firmed by Zwierz and Machnicka (20); a single dose of 10 mg/kg eliminated usual-ly, but not always, adult *T. saginata*. One patient of 61 carriers (dosed with 12–20 mg/kg) remained positive after a dose of 12 mg/kg.

Equally for *Hymenolepis nana* two doses of 25 mg/kg administered at an inter-val of 10 days seem to be necessary to obtain a complete cure (21–23).

Metacestode infections

Several studies have been published confirming the efficacy of praziquantel in hu-man cysticercosis. Treatment is particularly effective against cutaneous or paren-chymal (brain) cysticerci (24–27), but ineffective against intraocular cysts (28). Evidence has become available, however, that the commonly used long-term treatment (i.e. 25 mg/kg for 3 or 4 days and 50 mg/kg for 15 days in cutaneous and cerebral cysticercosis respectively) can be shortened and that the same effect can be obtained even using a lower dosage. Pun and Wong (29) obtained a complete cure in a patient with subcutaneous and neurocysticercosis receiving a total dosage of 300 mg/d for 3 days followed by 600 mg/d for a further 3 days. At this dose, which corresponds to 5–10 mg/kg daily for 6 days, fewer side-effects were present, so that steroid coverage was not needed. Zhu et al (30) obtained good results with a total amount of 120 mg/kg divided over 4–6 days in 42 patients who were followed for 1–3 years. In about 60% of the cases, however, 2 or 3 of these treatment courses were necessary to get rid of most of the cysticerci and the neuropsychiatric symptoms. Xu et al (31) used similar doses (120–180 mg/kg divided over 2–6 days) in 200 patients with subcutaneous or cerebral cysticercosis and obtained 83.5% marked and 14.5% moderate improvement (follow-up 1–3 years). They observed that better results were obtained when higher single doses were given, even if the total dosage remained the same.

Cysticerci in the spinal column or in the ventricular cavities did not respond to praziquantel treatment (25, 32). The drug was also less effective in cysticercotic arachnoiditis since remission was observed in only 47% of the patients (25).

In conclusion, the optimal doses and duration of praziquantel therapy are not yet known. For this purpose more information is needed about the amount of praziquantel that penetrates into the brain and the cerebrospinal fluid (CSF) and the level necessary to kill the cysts. Spina-Franca et al (33) observed that about 1/7 of the amount of praziquantel present in the serum penetrated into the CSF, although there were large individual variations.

There is still controversy about the simultaneous use of steroids during praziquantel treatment. Whereas some authors (25, 34) do not always consider them necessary, the majority find them absolutely indispensable to avoid side-effects (35), although they disagree about the dose and duration of the steroid treatment.

Since praziquantel does not seem to be effective against dead or calcified cysts, only patients with active forms of cysticercosis should be selected for praziquantel treatment. Evaluation of the effects of treatment (and a decision about a second treatment course) should not be made earlier than 3 months since this could give rise to misleading interpretation of CT scans: the cavities produced by the cysticerci and the inflammatory reaction around the parasites may still be present even if the therapy has been effective (25).

REFERENCES

1. Brandt JRA, Kumar V, Geerts S (1986) Praziquantel. In: Peterson PK, Verhoef J (Eds), *The Antimicrobial Agents, Annual 1*, p 287. Elsevier, Amsterdam.
2. Nosenas JS, Santos Jr AT, Blas BL et al (1984) Experiences with praziquantel against

Schistosoma japonicum infection in the Philippines. *Southeast Asian J. Trop. Med. Public Health, 15,* 489.

3. Hayashi M, Matsuda H, Tormis LC et al (1984) Clinical study on hepatosplenomegalic schistosomiasis japonica on Leyte Island: follow-up study 4 years after treatment with praziquantel. *Southeast Asian J. Trop. Med. Public Health, 15,* 498.

4. Bassily S, Farid Z, Dunn M et al (1985) Praziquantel for treatment of schistosomiasis in patients with advanced hepatosplenomegaly. *Ann. Trop. Med. Parasitol., 79,* 629.

5. El-Masry NA, Bassily FS, Trabolsi B, Trek Jr M (1985) Treatment of bilharzial colonic polyposis with praziquantel. *J. Infect. Dis., 152,* 1360.

6. Xiao S, Catto BA, Webster Jr LT (1985) Effect of praziquantel on different developmental stages of *Schistosoma mansoni* in vitro and in vivo. *J. Infect. Dis., 151,* 1130.

7. Polderman AM, Gryseels B, Gerold JL et al (1984) Side effects of praziquantel in the treatment of *Schistosoma mansoni* in Maniema, Zaïre. *Trans. R. Soc. Trop. Med. Hyg., 78,* 752.

8. Doehring E, Reider F, Schmidt-Ehry G, Ehrich JHH (1985) Reduction of pathological findings in urine and bladder lesions in infection with *Schistosoma haematobium. J. Infect. Dis., 152,* 807.

9. Mott KE, Dixon H, Osei-Tutu E et al (1985) Effect of praziquantel on hematuria and proteinuria in urinary schistosomiasis. *Am. J. Trop. Med. Hyg., 34,* 119.

10. Morcos SH, Khayval MT, Mansour MM et al (1985) Reversal of hepatic fibrosis after praziquantel therapy of murine schistosomiasis. *Am. J. Trop. Med. Hyg., 34,* 314.

11. El-Hawy AM, Masoud A, El-Badrawy N et al (1985) Hepatic histochemistry and electron microscopy of hamsters infected with *Schistosoma mansoni* and treated with praziquantel. *J. Egyptian Soc. Parasitol., 1,* 249.

12. Odum N, Theander TG, Bygbjerg IC (1984) Effect of praziquantel on human lymphocyte proliferation in vitro. *Eur. J. Clin. Pharmacol., 27,* 311.

13. Ellner JJ, Tweardy DJ, Osman GS et al (1985) Increased blastogenic response to worm antigen and loss of adherent suppressor cell activity after treatment for human infection with *Schistosoma mansoni. J. Infect. Dis., 151,* 320.

14. Conlon CP, Ellis C (1985) Praziquantel. *J. Antimicrob. Chemother., 15,* 1.

15. Hsu CCS, Kron MA (1985) Clonorchiasis and praziquantel. *Arch. Intern. Med., 145,* 1002.

16. Jong EC, Wasserheit JN, Johnson RJ et al (1985) Praziquantel for the treatment of *Clonorchis/Opisthorchis* infections: report of a double-blind placebo-controlled trial. *J. Infect. Dis., 152,* 637.

17. Sam-Abbanyi A (1985) Paragonimose pulmonaire endémique au Lower Mundani (arrondissement de Fontem au Sud-Ouest Cameroun). *Bull. Soc. Pathol. Exot. Fil., 78,* 334.

18. Johnson RJ, Jong EC, Dunning SB et al (1985) Paragonimiasis: diagnosis and the use of praziquantel in treatment. *J. Infect. Dis., 7,* 200.

19. Schiappacasse RH, Mohammadi D, Christie AJ (1985) Successful treatment of severe infection with *Fasciola hepatica* with praziquantel. *J. Infect. Dis., 152,* 1339.

20. Zwierz C, Machnicka B (1985) Praziquantel in the treatment of *Taenia saginata* and *Hymenolepis nana* infections in humans. In: *Proceedings, II International Symposium on Taeniasis/Cysticercosis & Hydatidosis/Echinococcosis, Česke Budějovice, 1985,* p. 43.

21. Campos R, Bressan MCRV, Evangelista MGBF (1984) Activity of praziquantel against *Hymenolepis nana,* at different development stages, in experimentally infected

mice. *Rev. Inst. Med. Trop. São Paulo, 26,* 344.

22. Campos R, Baillot Moreira AA, Silva Pinto PL et al (1984) Tentativa de controle da himenolepiase devide *Hymenolepis nana* por meio do praziquantel, em coletivade semifechada. *Rev. Saude Publica, 18,* 491.

23. Castro MLM, Rezende GL (1985) Estudo da eficacia terapeutica do praziquantel e das alteracões morfologicas dos ovos de *Hypmenolepis nana* apos sua administração em dois esquemas posologicos. *Rev. Inst. Med. Trop. São Paulo, 27,* 40.

24. Baranski MC (1984) Treatment of dermal cysticercosis with praziquantel: a new cestocidal agent. *Rev. Inst. Med. Trop. São Paulo, 26,* 259.

25. Sotelo J, Torres B, Rubio-Donnadieu F et al (1985) Praziquantel in the treatment of neurocysticercosis: long-term follow-up. *Neurology, 35,* 752.

26. Nash TE, Neva FA (1984) Recent advances in the diagnosis and treatment of cerebral cysticercosis. *N. Engl. J. Med., 311,* 1492.

27. Gomez JG, Sanchez E, Pardo P (1984) Treatment of cysticercosis with praziquantel. *Arch. Neurol., 41,* 1022.

28. Kestelyn P, Taelman H (1985) Effects of praziquantel on intraocular cysticercosis: a case report. *Br. J. Ophthalmol., 69,* 788.

29. Pun KK, Wong WT (1984) Successful treatment of neurocysticercosis with low-dose praziquantel. *Trop. Geogr. Med., 36,* 303.

30. Zhu D, Xu W, Qian Y et al (1985) Treatment and follow-up of 50 cases of cerebral cysticercosis with praziquantel (Abstract). *J. Parasitol. Parasit. Dis., 3,* 50.

31. Xu ZB, Chen WK, Zhong HL et al (1985) Praziquantel in treatment of cysticercosis cellulosae: report of 200 cases. *Chin. Med. J., 98,* 489.

32. Carydakis C, Baulac M, Laplane D et al (1984) Cysticerose spinale pure: note sur la liquide céphalo-rachidien. *Rév. Neurol., 140,* 590.

33. Spina-Franca A, Machado LR, Nobrega JPS et al (1985) Praziquantel in the cerebrospinal fluid in neurocysticercosis. *Arq. Neuro-Psiquiatr., 43,* 243.

34. Robles Castillo MCC (1981) Tratamiento médico de la cisticercosis cerebral. *Salua Publica Mexico, 23,* 443.

35. Ciferri F (1984) Praziquantel for cysticercosis of the brain (Letter to Editor). *N. Engl. J. Med., 311,* 733.

CHAPTER 29

Drugs used in the treatment of schistosomiasis

PAUL L. GIGASE and PAUL DEMEDTS

Recent progress in the field of chemotherapy of schistosomiasis has been practically restricted to the further evaluation of the three drugs developed in the seventies, included in the full WHO model list of essential drugs: metrifonate, oxamniquine and praziquantel. Treatment of infected individuals and of heavily infected communities is now deemed advisable, even if the global effects of schistosomiasis on health are still insufficiently known. In recent years non-invasive ultrasonography techniques have been instrumental in confirming the frequency of potentially dangerous organ lesions in urinary and, to a lesser degree, in hepato-intestinal schistosomiasis. It has furthermore been shown both in clinical and in experimental studies that advanced lesions as ureteric obstruction or liver fibrosis are more often reversible after treatment than was previously thought possible (1, 2). The availability of the afore-mentioned drugs has shifted emphasis in schistosomiasis control from snail control to mass chemotherapy which aims essentially at preventing serious disease and at reducing morbidity and, to a lesser extent, transmission (3). Schistosomes, like most other parasitic helminths, do not multiply in their human host and the mere reduction of parasite loads by suppressive therapy can therefore avoid more serious ill effects.

The results of treatment in schistosomiasis are difficult to evaluate due to the limited sensitivity of parasitologic examinations of stools or urine and to the late reversal of serologic reactions. The rectal snip examination is an alternative parasitologic technique, more sensitive, but invasive and not quantitative. The results of the rectal snip examination are sometimes discrepant from those obtained by the more usual methods (4). The determination of schistosomal antigens in blood or urine will certainly become a more appropriate diagnostic tool in the near future.

Metrifonate

Metrifonate (Bilharcil, trichlorfone, trichlorphone) has been used since 1962. It is an organophosphorous ester which is metabolically transformed to dichlorvos (dichlorovinyl dimethyl phosphate), a cholinesterase inhibitor, temporarily para-

Antimicrobial Agents Annual 3
P.K. Peterson and J. Verhoef, editors
© Elsevier Science Publishers BV, 1988

lysing adult schistosomes, although the precise mode of action remains unknown. Metrifonate is administered orally and is rapidly absorbed, metabolized and excreted. The drug is active on both *Schistosoma haematobium* and *S. mansoni* when localized in the urinary tract, but does not impair egg excretion of these parasites in the stools (5). Metrifonate is microfilaricidal but is not a major improvement on diethylcarbamazine. It is effective against hookworms (6). In areas where *S. haematobium* is prevalent, either associated with hookworms or not, anemia, growth and hepatosplenomegaly were favorably influenced by mass treatment of schoolchildren with metrifonate (7–10). As a rule, treatment has more effect on egg output than on cure rates. The recommended mode of administration is 7.5 mg/kg in 2 or 3 doses at fortnightly intervals. After single administration of 10 mg/kg, reductions for up to 3 years in egg excretion in areas of continuous transmission have been observed (11–13).

Side effects of metrifonate are usually mild and limited to transient abdominal pain. No further reports on congenital malformations in children born to mothers who had received metrifonate in pregnancy have been reported after a single possible case (14). No serious toxicity which could clearly be related to cholinesterase inhibition has been observed in more than 20 years of experience with this drug.

The results of therapy even with 3 doses of metrifonate are inferior to those of a single dose of praziquantel. The main advantage of metrifonate in mass treatment schemes is its low cost, although the cost/effectiveness relation is not necessarily better than that of praziquantel (15). Also, the necessity of 3 dosages leads to poor compliance (16). Metrifonate still has a place for indiscriminate suppressive mass treatment in highly endemic areas, especially when hookworms are simultaneously present. It has no indication, however, in the curative treatment of individual cases, e.g. in imported urinary schistosomiasis.

Oxamniquine

The tetrahydroquinoline methanol, oxamniquine (Vansil, Mansil) is active only against *S. mansoni*. Results of trials on *S. haematobium*, *S. intercalatum* and *S. matthei* have been poor and no reports of treatment of Eastern schistosomiasis are available. No clinical activity against other parasitic helminths has been reported. Treatment with oxamniquine kills the male worms and exerts an irreversible dose-dependent effect on the reproductive functions of adult female worms, leaving them unable to reproduce when reunited with males. The mechanisms of action remain largely unknown, but it seems that the drug exerts its schistosomicidal action at least partly by inhibition of nucleic acid synthesis (17). Oxamniquine is experimentally effective on schistosomules of *S. mansoni* which display maximal resistance at 48–96 hours after infection, being more susceptible to the drug both earlier and later (18, 19). In other animal experiments (20) oxamniquine became effective only 5–6 weeks after infection.

Recent reports have revealed a higher incidence of toxicity in man than was initially expected. Some of the side effects are related to the schistosomicidal function, e.g. fever within 3 days after treatment, transient eosinophilia and proteinuria. Clinical and radiologic signs of lung involvement are found in more than 25% of treated patients in Brazil (21) and evidence has been obtained by bronchoalveolar washings of an eosinophilic pneumonia due to the shift of worms to the lungs during treatment (22). Direct toxic reactions are headaches, amnesia, disorientation, confusion and fainting, which have been observed in 2–5% of infections in Kenya even after 1 dose of 15 mg/kg (23, 24). Drowsiness and dizziness are reported in roughly half of treated patients in Brazil while amnesia, behavioral disturbances and seizures are observed in about 5% (25). Stokvis (26) observed patients in the Netherlands with generalized seizures, 2 of them Asian, and considers these complications to be more frequent than has been reported previously.

The therapeutic results of oxamniquine in mansonian schistosomiasis are comparable to those of praziquantel and the now discarded oltipraz. Regression of hepatomegaly and splenomegaly with return to the level of non-infected people has been documented in Brazil 8 years after mass treatment (27). Treatment with oxamniquine of serious cases of schistosomal polyposis in Egypt yielded less satisfactory results than after praziquantel or niridazole therapy (28).

Data on the optimal dosage of oxamniquine are conflicting. The susceptibility of local strains has been incriminated in the varying responses to the drug, but the intensity of infections and the methodologies of evaluation have not always been comparable. In America and West Africa single doses of 15 mg/kg are advocated, with the recommendation that higher doses, of 20 mg/kg, divided or not, should be used in children, known to be less responsive. In East and Central Africa doses of 30, 40 or even 60 mg/kg in 1, 2 or 3 consecutive days are said to be required. In a careful dose-finding trial in Ethiopia, however, a dose of 30 mg/kg was considered optimal for mass treatment (29).

Resistance to oxamniquine can be induced experimentally and parasite strains more or less resistant to treatment have been isolated from human subjects (30). Such strains remain susceptible to praziquantel.

Praziquantel

Praziquantel (Biltricide) has been used since 1976. It is produced in the People's Republic of China under the name of 'pyquiton'. It is a heterocyclic pyrazinoisoquinoline. Its mechanisms of action are still elusive. Interactions with the nucleic acid of the schistosomes, adenosine triphosphate and carbohydrate metabolism have been observed in vitro but do not explain the rapid schistosomicidal effect. *S. mansoni* worms become rapidly dislodged from the portal vessels and show intensive vacuolization of their tegument followed by attachment of leukocytes. Tegumental damage is dose-dependent and more pronounced in male than in female worms. It is also, like the rapid musculature contraction, Ca^{2+}-dependent (31). Egg production in females is inhibited at very low concentration while mass hatching of mature ova followed by immediate death of the miracidia is incited both in vitro and in vivo. Contact of adult male worms with praziquantel in vitro results in increased exposure of parasite antigens, which may enhance the suscepti-bility of the worm to immune mechanisms (32).

No mutagenic, carcinogenic, teratogenic or embryotoxic activity has been ob-served. Immunomodulatory effects of praziquantel have been intensively exam-ined (33). Reductions in size of hepatic granulomas and of delayed footpath swell-ing after injection of soluble antigen were observed in infected mice (34), confirming previous work on granuloma formation in the lung of uninfected mice (35). The implications for protective mechanisms affecting reinfection after pre-vious treatment have been studied in human subjects (36) with the conclusion that nearly all parameters of cell-mediated immunity to schistosomes remain high for at least 2 years after treatment.

The differential responsiveness when hepatosplenic involvement is present has also been evaluated (37). The blastogenic response to soluble adult worm antigen was in fact found to be enhanced 9 months after treatment with praziquantel (38). Trials in mice to attenuate granulomatous responses by combining praziquantel and indomethacin (39) have not demonstrated improvement of inflammatory re-sponses and liver damage contraindicates the combined use of these drugs. In mice treated at different times after infection with *S. mansoni* or *S. bovis* and perfused afterwards for the presence of living worms, praziquantel became effective only from the 5th week on (20), although effects in vitro on developmental stages are different (40, 41).

The spectrum of activity includes all species of human schistosomes, most of the adult cestodes and trematodes of man and some of their larval forms. The efficacy of praziquantel on *S. mekongi* has been questioned on the basis of the presence of living eggs in rectal snips 1 year after treatment with the drug (42). With the same technique, failure of treatment was observed in 7 of 9 patients in-fected with different species of schistosomes and followed in France during 6 years (4). On the other hand, numerous recent studies confirm the efficacy of praziquan-tel including favorable long-term effects on serious complications of the disease such as colonic polyposis (43), cerebral schistosomiasis japonicum with seizures (44), organic urinary tract abnormalities caused by *S. haematobium* (45) and their clinical consequences (46, 47), and chronic salmonellosis associated with *S. man-soni* (48). Trials comparing praziquantel and placebo are instrumental in specify-ing some ill-known repercussions of schistosomiasis on health as shown by the improvement of scores of physical activity of *S. haematobium*-infected schoolchil-dren after treatment (49). Side effects are reported in 50–80% of treated people but are usually benign and related, like other drugs, either to its schistosomicidal activity or to drug toxicity itself in the form of headaches and rashes. Even in ad-vanced cases of hepatosplenomegalic mansonian schistosomiasis, benign side ef-fects occurred in only 50% of treated patients (50). The most serious side effects are severe colicky pain and bloody stools, first mentioned from Zaire, but reported also from the Philippines (51) where a history of occult blood in the stools before therapy and severity of liver involvement were found to be risk factors (52). Such effects could be potentially harmful in people with bleeding tendencies. Hitherto, no mention has been made of the consequences of the cysticercicidal effect, e.g. when concomitant cysticercosis of the central nervous system is present. Praziquantel has no effect on the plasma concentration of contraceptive steroids in women (53).

Recent data reveal a trend towards the use of lower dosages and administration in one dose. In a dose-finding trial against *S. japonicum* infections Chen et al (54) found that neither cure rates nor side effects were significantly different with doses of 30–60 mg/kg and recommend the lower dosages of 30–40 mg/kg for treatment. Kardaman (55) found a slight but non-significant improvement in cure rates when a dose of 40 mg/kg was given divided in 2 doses in one day but he also observed more side effects. Compared with oxamniquine no significant differences in activity are observed between the drugs if they are given in adequate dosages, e.g. 15 mg/kg for oxamniquine and 40 mg/kg for praziquantel (56–58).

FUTURE DIRECTIONS

No further reports have been published on oltipraz (RPM-35972), which has apparently been withdrawn. The reason is its vascular toxicity causing occasional gangrene of the fingertips, not unexpected since recent studies had drawn attention to pain under the fingertips and blurred vision after administration of the drug (59, 60). Recent reports had also stressed the necessity of administration together with fatty food (61). Hycanthone, another promising drug, has been abandoned due to its hepatotoxicity and presumed mutagenic effects. Experimental work on its peculiar properties is still continuing (62, 63).

Amoscanate and its analogs have the advantage of an enlarged anthelminthic spectrum but appear unduly toxic and have no future unless less toxic derivatives are synthetized. Nitrothiamidazole (niridazole, Ambilhar) is still used locally on a large scale, although clearly inferior to present-day drugs in therapeutic efficiency, easiness of administration, frequency and seriousness of side effects.

All things considered, praziquantel emerges as the main drug in the field of schistosomiasis. Metrifonate can compete only in mass treatment of urinary schistosomiasis thanks to its lower cost and perhaps also to its effects on hookworms in areas where both infections are prevalent. Oxamniquine could compete only where *S. mansoni* is concerned, but has no definite advantages and its side effects on the nervous system have perhaps been initially underrated. Emergence of drug resistance (64), although not mentioned hitherto for praziquantel, is an incentive to further research. Synergism between praziquantel and oxamniquine has been described, implying a possibility of lower drug dosages and minimal side effects (65) but has apparently not been further studied. Cost of the drugs remains a major problem, now that mass treatment is considered to be the most realistic way of control for the time being (3).

REFERENCES

1. Naude JH (1984) The natural history of ureteric bilharzia. *Br. J. Urol., 56*, 599.
2. Andrade ZA, Grimaud JA (1986) Evolution of the schistosomal hepatic lesions in mice after curative chemotherapy. *Am. J. Pathol., 124*, 59.
3. WHO Expert Committee (1985) The control of schistosomiasis. *WHO Techn. Rep. Ser., 728*, 110.
4. Chidiac C, Beaucaire G, Mouton Y, Caillaux M, Fourrier A (1986) Echecs du praziquantel dans le traitement des bilharzioses: intérêt de la biopsie de muqueuse rectale et du suivi prolongé. *Méd. Mal. Infect., 5bis*, 380.
5. Doehring E, Poggensee U, Feldmeier H (1986) The effect of metrifonate in mixed *Schistosoma haematobium* and *Schistosoma mansoni* infections in humans. *Am. J. Trop. Med. Hyg., 35*, 323.
6. Kurz KM, Stephenson LS, Latham MC, Kinoti SN (1986) The effectiveness of metrifonate in reducing hookworm infection in Kenyan school children. *Am. J. Trop. Med. Hyg., 35*, 571.
7. Abdel-Salam E, Peters PAS, Abdel Meguid AE, Abdel Meguid AAE, Mahmoud AAF (1986) Discrepancies in outcome of a control program for schistosomiasis haematobia in Fayoum governorate, Egypt. *Am. J. Trop. Med. Hyg., 35*, 786.
8. Stephenson LS, Latham MC, Kinoti SN, Oduori ML (1985) Regression of splenomegaly and hepatomegaly in children treated for *Schistosoma haematobium* infection. *Am. J. Trop. Med. Hyg., 34*, 119.
9. Stephenson LS, Latham MC, Kurz KM, Kinoti SN, Oduori ML, Crompton DW (1985) Relationships of *Schistosoma haematobium*, hookworm and malarial infections and metrifonate treatment to hemoglobin level in Kenyan school children. *Am. J. Trop. Med. Hyg., 34*, 519.
10. Stephenson LS, Latham MC, Kurz KM, Kinoti SN, Oduori ML, Crompton DWT (1985) Relationships of *Schistosoma haematobium*, hookworm and malarial infections and metrifonate treatment to growth of Kenyan school children. *Am. J. Trop. Med. Hyg., 34*, 1109.
11. El-Kholy A, Boutros S, Tamara F, Warren KS, Mahmoud AAF (1984) The effect of a single dose of metrifonate on *Schistosoma mansoni* infection in Egyptian school children. *Am. J. Trop. Med. Hyg., 33*, 1170.
12. Tswana SA, Mason PR (1985) Eighteen month follow-up on the treatment of urinary schistosomiasis with a single dose of metrifonate. *Am. J. Trop. Med. Hyg., 34*, 746.
13. Sellin B, Simonkovich E, Sellin E, Rey JL, Mouchet F (1984) Evolution sur 3 années consécutives de la schistosomiase urinaire après traitement au métrifonate dans un village de savane sèche de Haute-Volta. *Méd. Trop., 44*, 357.
14. Monson MH, Alexander K (1984) Metrifonate in pregnancy. *Trans. R. Soc. Trop. Med. Hyg., 78*, 565.
15. Korte R, Schmidt-Ehry B, Kielmann AA, Brinkman UK (1986) Cost and effectiveness of different approaches to schistosomiasis control in Africa. *Trop. Med. Parasitol., 37*, 149.
16. Sellin B, Rey JL, Simonkovich E, Sellin E, Mouchet F (1986) Essai de lutte par chimiothérapie contre *Schistosoma haematobium* en zone irriguée Sahélienne au Niger. *Méd. Trop., 46*, 21.
17. Pica-Mattocia L, Cioli D (1985) Studies on the mode of action of oxamniquine and related schistosomicidal drugs. *Am. J. Trop. Med. Hyg., 34*, 112.

18. Bickle QD, Andrews BJ (1985) Resistance following drug attenuation (Ro 11–3128 or oxamniquine) of early *Schistosoma mansoni* infections in mice. *Parasitology, 90,* 325.

19. Mastin AJ, Wilson RA, Bickle QD (1985) Induction of resistance to *Schistosoma mansoni* in mice by chemotherapy: migration of schistosomula in primary and challenge infections. *Parasitology, 90,* 519.

20. Sabah AA, Fletcher C, Webbe G, Doenhoff MJ (1986) *Schistosoma mansoni*: chemotherapy of infections of different ages. *Exp. Parasitol., 61,* 294.

21. Pedroso ERP, Lambertucci JR, Rocha MOC (1985) Alteraçoes clinico-radiologicas pulmonares pos tratamento na esquistossomose mansoni aguda e cronica. *Rev. Soc. Bras. Med. Trop., 18,* 23.

22. Davidson BL, El-Kassimi F, Uz-Zaman A, Pillai DK (1986) The 'lung shift' in treated schistosomiasis: bronchoalveolar lavage evidence of eosinophilic pneumonia. *Chest, 89,* 455.

23. Chunge CN, Kimani RG, Gachihi G, Mkoji G, Kamau T, Rashid JR (1985) Serious side effects of oxamniquine during the treatment of *Schistosoma mansoni* in Kenya. *East Afr. Med. J., 62,* 3.

24 Okela GB (1985) Serious side effects of oxamniquine during the treatment of *Schistosoma mansoni* in Kenya. *East Afr. Med. J., 62,* 433.

25. De Carvalho SA, Shikanai-Yasuda MA, Amato Neto V, Shiroma M, Luccas FJC (1985) Neurotoxicidade do oxamniquine no tratamento da infeccao humana pelo *Schistosoma mansoni. Rev. Inst. Med. Trop. Sao Paulo, 27,* 111.

26. Stokvis H, Bauer AGC, Stuiver PC, Malcolm D, Overbosch D (1986) Seizures associated with oxamniquine therapy. *Am. J. Trop. Med. Hyg., 35,* 330.

27. Sleigh AC, Hoff R, Mott KE, Maguire JH, Da França Silva JT (1986) Manson's schistosomiasis in Brazil: 11 year evaluation of successful disease control with oxamniquine. *Lancet, 1,* 635.

28. El-Masry NA, Farid Z, Bassily S (1986) Oxamniquine therapy for schistosomal polyposis: a 1–2 year follow-up study. *J. Trop. Med. Hyg., 89,* 19.

29. Ayele T (1986) Preliminary clinical trial of oral oxamniquine in the treatment of *Schistosoma mansoni* in children in Ethiopia. *East Afr. Med. J., 63,* 291.

30. Dias LC de S, Olivier E (1985) Stability of *Schistosoma mansoni* progeny to antischistosomal drugs. *Rev. Inst. Med. Trop. Sao Paulo, 27,* 186.

31. Xiao SH, Guo HF, Dai ZQ, Zhang RQ (1985) Effect of calcium, magnesium and temperature on praziquantel induced tegument damage of male *Schistosoma japonicum. Acta Pharmacol. Sin., 6,* 59.

32. Harnett W, Kusel JR (1986) Increased exposure of parasite antigens at the surface of adult male *Schistosoma mansoni* exposed to praziquantel in vitro. *Parasitology, 93,* 401.

33. Tawfik AF, Colley DG (1986) Effects of anti-schistosomal chemotherapy on immune responses, protection and immunity. III. An effective regimen of praziquantel does not alter immune capabilities of normal mice. *Am. J. Trop. Med. Hyg., 35,* 118.

34. Botros SS, El-Badrawy N, Metwally AA, Khayyal MT (1986) Study of some immunopharmacological properties of praziquantel in experimental schistosomiasis mansoni. *Ann. Trop. Med. Parasitol., 80,* 189.

35. Botros SS, Metwally AA, Khayyal MT (1984) The immunological aspects of praziquantel in unsensitized mice with experimentally induced schistosome pulmonary granuloma. *Trans. R. Soc. Trop. Med. Hyg., 78,* 569.

36. Colley DG, Barsoum IS, Dahawi SS, Gamil F, Habib M, El-Alamy M (1987) Immune responses and immunoregulation in relation to human schistosomiasis in Egypt. III. Immunity and longitudinal studies of in vitro responsiveness after treatment. *Trans. R. Soc. Trop. Med. Hyg., 80,* 592.
37. Colley DG, Garcia AA, Lambertucci JR, Para JC, Katz N, Rocha RS, Gazzinelli G (1986) Immune responses during human schistosomiasis. XII. Differential responsiveness in patients with hepatosplenic disease. *Am. J. Trop. Med. Hyg., 35,* 793.
38. Ellner JJ, Tweardy DJ, Osman GS (1985) Increased blastogenic responses to worm antigen and loss of adherent suppressor cell activity after treatment for human infection with *Schistosoma mansoni. J. Infect. Dis., 151,* 320.
39. Rainsford KD (1985) Pharmacological manipulation of the chronic granulomatous reactions in the livers of mice infected with schistosomiasis. *Int. J. Tissue Reactions, 7,* 35.
40. Xiao S, Catto BA, Webster Jr LT (1985) Effects of praziquantel on different developmental stages of *Schistosoma mansoni* in vitro and in vivo. *J. Infect. Dis., 151,* 1130.
41. You JQ, Xiao SH, Yue WJ (1986) Effect of praziquantel in vitro on different developmental stages of *Schistosoma japonicum. Acta Pharmacol. Sin., 7,* 82.
42. Ajana F, Deicas E, Colin JJ, Poirriez J, Leduc M, Mouton Y, Caillaux M, Fourrier A, Vernes A (1986) La bilharziose humaine à *Schistosoma mekongi:* problèmes diagnostiques et thérapeutiques. *Méd. Mal. Infect., 16,* 141.
43. El-Masry NA, Farid Z, Bassily S, Trabolsi B, Stek Jr M (1985) Treatment of bilharzial colonic polyposis with praziquantel. *J. Infect. Dis., 152,* 1360.
44. Watt G, Adapon B, Long GW, Fernando M, Ranoa C, Cross JH (1986) Praziquantel in treatment of cerebral schistosomiasis. *Lancet, 2,* 529.
45. Doehring E, Ehrich JHH, Bremer HJ (1986) Reversibility of urinary tract abnormalities due to *Schistosoma haematobium* infection. *Kidney Int., 30,* 582.
46. Doehring E, Reider F, Schmidt-Ehry G, Ehrich JHH (1985) Reduction of pathological findings in urine and bladder lesions in infection with *Schistosoma haematobium* after treatment with praziquantel. *J. Infect. Dis., 152,* 807.
47. Mott KE, Dixon H, Osei-Tutu E, England EC, Davis A (1985) Effect of praziquantel on hematuria and proteinuria in urinary schistosomiasis. *Am. J. Trop. Med. Hyg., 34,* 1119.
48. Shikanai-Yasuda MA, De Carvalho SA, Yasuda PH, Del Negro G, Shiroma M, Amato Neto V (1985) Salmonelose associada à esquistossomose mansônica hépato-esplênica: açao do praziquantel. *Rev. Inst. Med. Trop. Sao Paulo, 27,* 286.
49. Kvalsvig JD (1986) The effects of *Schistosoma haematobium* on the activity of school children. *J. Trop. Med. Hyg., 89,* 85.
50. Bassily S, Farid Z, Dunn M, El-Masry NA, Stek Jr M (1985) Praziquantel for treatment of schistosomiasis in patients with advanced hepatosplenomegaly. *Ann. Trop. Med. Parasitol., 79,* 6.
51. Santos AT, Blas BL, Portillo G, Nosenas JS, Poliquit O, Papasin M (1984) Phase III clinical trials with praziquantel in *Schistosoma japonicum* infections in the Philippines. *Arzneimittelforschung, 34,* 1221.
52. Watt G, Baldovino PC, Castro JT, Fernando MT, Ranca CP (1980) Bloody diarrhoea after praziquantel therapy. *Trans. R. Soc. Trop. Med. Hyg., 80,* 345.
53. El-Raghy I, Back DJ, Osman F, Orme ML, Fathalla M (1986) Contraceptive steroid concentrations in women with early active schistosomiasis: lack of effect of antischistosomal drugs. *Contraception, 33,* 373.

54. Chen MG, Hua XJ, Wang MJ, Xu RJ, Yu CB, Jiang SB (1985) Dose finding double-blind clinical trial with praziquantel in schistosomiasis japonica patients. *Southeast Asian J. Trop. Med. Public Health, 16,* 228.
55. Kardaman MW, Fenwick A, El Igail AB, El Tayeb M, Daffalla AA, Dixon HG (1985) Treatment with praziquantel of schoolchildren with concurrent *Schistosoma mansoni* infections in Gezira, Sudan. *J. Trop. Med. Hyg., 88,* 105.
56. Rugemalila JB, Asila J, Chimbe A (1984) Randomized comparative trials of single doses of the newer antischistosomal drugs at Mwanza, Tanzania. I. Praziquantel and oxamniquine for the treatment of schistosomiasis mansoni. *J. Trop. Med. Hyg., 87,* 231.
57. De Rezende GL (1985) Survey on the clinical trial results achieved in Brazil comparing praziquantel and oxamniquine in the treatment of mansoni schistosomiasis. *Rev. Inst. Med. Trop. Sao Paulo, 27,* 328.
58. Da Silva LC, Zeitune JMR, Rosa-Eid LMF, Lima DMC, Antonelli RH, Christo CH, Saez-Alquezar A, Carboni A de C (1986) Treatment of patients with *Schistosomiasis mansoni*: a double blind clinical trial comparing praziquantel with oxamniquine. *Rev. Inst. Med. Trop. Sao Paulo, 28,* 174.
59. Kardaman MW, Fenwick A, El Igail AB, El Tayeb M, Bennett JL, Daffalla AA (1985) Field trials with oltipraz against *Schistosoma mansoni* in the Gezira Irrigated Area, Sudan. *J. Trop. Med. Hyg., 88,* 95.
60. El-Igail AB, El Tayeb M, Kardaman MW, Daffalla AA, Dixon HG, Fenwick A (1985) Dose-finding trial using oltipraz to treat schoolchildren infected with *Schistosomiasis mansoni* in Gezira, Sudan. *J. Trop. Med. Hyg., 88,* 101.
61. Homeida MMA, Ali HM (1986) Measurement of peak blood levels of oltipraz in patients infected with *S. mansoni*: correlation with the drug's antischistosomal action. *Ann. Trop. Med. Parasitol., 80,* 369.
62. Ciolo D, Pica-Mattoccia L, Rosenberg S, Archer S (1985) Evidence for the mode of antischistosomal action of hycanthone. *Life Sci., 15,* 161.
63. De Serres FJ (1986) Hycanthone: an unresolved case study in risk assessment. *Mutat. Res., 164,* 199.
64. Coles GC, Bruce JI, Kinoti GK, Mutahi WT, Dias EP, Katz N (1986) Drug resistance in schistosomiasis. *Trans. R. Soc. Trop. Med. Hyg., 80,* 347.
65. Richards HC (1985) Oxamniquine: a drug for the third world. *Chem. Britain, 21,* 1001.

CHAPTER 30

Drugs used in the treatment of toxoplasmosis

JACK S. REMINGTON and BENJAMIN J. LUFT

Infection with the intracellular protozoan, *Toxoplasma gondii*, is frequent among animals and man. *Toxoplasma* infection, which is defined as the presence of the organism in individuals with or without clinical manifestations, is much more common than toxoplasmosis, which refers specifically to disease caused by the organism. Toxoplasmosis is conveniently considered in 4 categories: postnatally acquired, congenital, ocular (may be either congenital or acquired), and in the immunocompromised host. With the advent of routine organ transplantation and more aggressive and prolonged chemotherapeutic regimens for malignant diseases, this latter category has taken on new importance as a risk factor for toxoplasmosis. In addition, patients with acquired immunodeficiency syndrome (AIDS) pose special problems with regard to diagnosis and treatment of toxoplasmosis. We review here the drugs used in the treatment of toxoplasmosis, followed by a description of their use in each of the 4 categories listed above. Since there has been little new information regarding the therapy of toxoplasmosis since the publication of *The Antimicrobial Agents Annual 2*, this discussion continues to reflect prevailing views regarding management of this disease.

Pyrimethamine

Pyrimethamine (Daraprim), a substituted phenylpyrimidine, inhibits folic acid production in the protozoal cell by selectively interfering with dihydrofolate reductase. When used alone, it is effective in production of a radical cure of mice with experimental *Toxoplasma* infection (1, 2). It has a serum half-life of 4–5 days in healthy adults (3); the half-life in newborns is not known. Although the drug appears to be concentrated in the cerebrospinal fluid of rats and dogs, spinal fluid concentrations of only 10–25% of simultaneous serum levels were found in one study of patients with meningeal leukemia (4).

The suggested oral dose of pyrimethamine in children and adults is: loading dose of 15 mg/m^2 or 1 mg/kg up to 50 mg twice a day for 2 days, followed by 15 mg/m^2 or 1 mg/kg up to 25 mg per day. After the first few weeks of therapy

Antimicrobial Agents Annual 3
P.K. Peterson and J. Verhoef, editors
© Elsevier Science Publishers BV, 1988

this dose may be given every other day or even every 3–4 days because of the drug's long half-life. Unfortunately, there are no data on which to base recommendations for dosing the seriously ill patient (e.g. the immunocompromised patient with widespread *Toxoplasma* infection of toxoplasmic encephalitis). In certain cases (see below), 50–100 mg of pyrimethamine per day is used. Pyrimethamine should not be used during the first trimester of pregnancy because of the risk of teratogenicity.

Because pyrimethamine is a folic acid antagonist, its main toxicity is a reversible, dose-related, gradual depression of the bone marrow. Most common is platelet depression, although leukopenia and anemia occur as well. Other side-effects of pyrimethamine include gastrointestinal distress, headache, and a bad taste in the mouth. Patients should have a complete blood count monitored twice a week while on this drug. The risk of bone marrow toxicity may be decreased by concomitant administration of folinic acid (leucovorin calcium). This drug has been used in doses of 5–15 mg/d (tablet or parenteral form given by mouth) in older children and adults. We use a dose of 15 mg/d in patients with AIDS, although there are no data to show that this or even lower doses in these patients prevents neutropenia or thrombocytopenia. Folinic acid does not interfere with the ability of pyrimethamine to kill *T. gondii*. In contrast, folic acid will interfere with the action of pyrimethamine on *Toxoplasma* and should not be given.

Sulfonamides

Sulfonamides have been shown to be effective in a mouse model of experimental *Toxoplasma* infection (2). Sulfadiazine was found to be as effective as trisulfapyrimidines (sulfapyrazine, sulfadimidine, sulfamerazine), and pyrimethamine was shown to act synergistically with sulfonamides in this mouse model (1, 2). Sulfadiazine has a half-life of 10–12 hours. The suggested dose of sulfadiazine (or trisulfapyrimidines) is: loading dose of 75 mg/kg (up to 4 g), followed by 100 mg/kg/d (up to 8 g/d) divided into 2 or 3 oral doses.

All other sulfonamides tested have been much less active than sulfadiazine or trisulfapyrimidines against *T. gondii*. Sulfamethoxazole (with or without trimethoprim) possesses in-vitro and in-vivo activity against *T. gondii* (5), but it is significantly less than that achieved with the combination of pyrimethamine + sulfonamide and is therefore not recommended for treatment or attempts at prevention of toxoplasmosis. Further data are needed to define its role in the treatment of any form of toxoplasmosis. Pyrimethamine + sulfadoxine (Fansidar) has been used in the long-term treatment of patients with toxoplasmic encephalitis and in infants and children with congenital infection. Each tablet contains 25 mg of pyrimethamine and 500 mg of sulfadoxine. The usual adult dosage is 2–3 tablets per week. Because of recent reports of life-threatening skin rashes, and even death, due to the long-acting sulfonamide in this preparation when used for prophylaxis of malaria, we suggest caution in its use. We have noted relapse of toxoplasmic encephalitis in an AIDS patient placed on long-term Fansidar following his having been treated with pyrimethamine and sulfadiazine in the hope of preventing relapse.

Spiramycin

Spiramycin, a macrolide antibiotic, has been demonstrated to be active against *T. gondii* in experimental animals (6). Although the actual concentration necessary to inhibit growth of, or to kill, *Toxoplasma* is unknown, high and persistent tissue levels have been found (7, 8). In one study, levels in maternal serum of 0.5–2.0 μg/ml and in placenta of 0.7–5.0 μg/m/ml were found after an oral dose of 2 g (9). The drug is supplied as a syrup or in capsule form. It is available in Western Europe, Canada, Mexico, and larger parts of South America. In the United States it can only be obtained by special request from the Food and Drug Administration.

Clindamycin

Studies in vivo have established the efficacy of clindamycin in experimental murine toxoplasmosis (10) and in ocular infection in rabbits (11). Clindamycin has been found to be concentrated in the choroid, iris, and retina of the pigmented rabbit eye after a single intramuscular injection, where, according to the authors, it remains at levels higher than the minimal concentration necessary to inhibit *Toxoplasma* for 24 hours (12). Because of the lack of controlled studies and possible untoward gastrointestinal side-effects, its use in human toxoplasmosis, particularly disease which occurs outside the eye, must be considered experimental at this time.

THERAPY OF SPECIFIC INFECTIONS

Acquired toxoplasmosis in the normal (non-immunocompromised) host

Toxoplasma infection in most immunologically normal patients is subclinical or is manifested by a mild lymphadenopathic illness and does not require specific treatment. In the rare case of severe and persistent symptoms or if there is evidence of damage to vital organs, therapy with pyrimethamine and sulfadiazine (or trisulfapyrimidines) should probably be given for 4–6 weeks. We also recommend treatment for individuals who acquire their infection by accident in the laboratory or via transfusion.

Acute *Toxoplasma* infection or toxoplasmosis acquired during pregnancy

Congenital infection is extremely rare in infants born to women who acquire their infection months or years earlier, and specific treatment in these women is not recommended. Acute, acquired *Toxoplasma* infection during pregnancy, however, results in a significant incidence of congenital infection (approximately 15% in the first trimester, 30% in the second trimester, 60% in the third trimester) (13). A lag period may exist between the onset of maternal infection and infection of the fetus. Therefore, the earlier the diagnosis is made, the more likely it is that medical therapy will be effective in prevention of infection in the fetus. Thus, it should be emphasized that treatment is administered in the hope of preventing *Toxoplasma* from invading the fetus. Early diagnosis of newly acquired infection in the pregnant woman is therefore needed.

Data which have accumulated from a variety of different groups in Europe strongly support the contention that treatment is beneficial in prevention of congenital infection. Treatment of the newly acquired infection in pregnancy with pyrimethamine + sulfadiazine (or trisulfapyrimidines) or with spiramycin has been shown to decrease the incidence of congenital infection. In a study from Germany (14), 2-week courses of sulfonamide and pyrimethamine were followed by 3-week intervals with no treatment until the time of delivery. Pyrimethamine was not used during the first trimester of pregnancy because of the concern of teratogenicity. The incidence of congenital infection was reduced from 17% in the untreated mothers to 5% in the treated group. In a series from France (15), courses of 3 weeks of oral spiramycin were alternated with 2 weeks with no treatment until term; the incidence of congenital infection was reduced from 61% to 23%. Additional studies are needed to determine the optimum drug regimen in this setting.

Once a diagnosis of the acute infection is made during pregnancy, the risks of congenital infection and the therapeutic alternatives available should be thoroughly and accurately discussed with the patient and her husband so that they can make an appropriate decision with regard to therapy. Because of the possibility of severe damage when the infection occurs early in fetal life, therapeutic abortion is an option. It should be clearly understood, however, that the vast majority of fetuses aborted in this setting will prove to be uninfected by *T. gondii* (16).

Congenital *Toxoplasma* infection and congenital toxoplasmosis

Evaluation of the efficacy of treatment of congenital *Toxoplasma* infection is hampered by the lack of controlled studies. This is understandable in light of the known high morbidity associated with this congenital infection. In addition, evaluation of treatment is difficult because of variations in severity and outcome of the infection within and between different published series, and because so many reports are anecdotal. The largest published series is that of Desmonts and Couvreur (13).

The majority of cases of congenital *Toxoplasma* infection are asymptomatic at birth but on long-term follow-up significant and often severe sequelae are frequent (17). Wilson et al (17) studied 24 children, 13 of whom were asymptomatic in the newborn period and discovered to be infected by antibody testing (Group I), and II who developed ophthalmologic or neurologic signs suggestive of congenital *Toxoplasma* infection after the neonatal period (Group II). Nine children were treated for at least 3 weeks duration before 1 year of age. Treatment, which was non-randomized, consisted of pyrimethamine plus either sulfadiazine or trisulfa-pyrimidines. Of the 22 children in Group I and II who presented with chorioretinitis in the absence of neurologic disease, major neurologic sequelae developed in 5 of 13 untreated children but in none of 9 treated children (P = 0.05). Patients in the untreated group, however, were more likely to have intracranial calcifications – risk factor for more severe neurologic sequelae. In a separate study, Remington and Desmonts (18) reported that treatment of children during the first year reduced the risk of late development of eye lesions; however, additional data are needed in this group since follow-up was relatively short.

Based on the data from uncontrolled studies in man and from studies in experimental animals (19), we recommend treatment in every case of congenital *Toxoplasma* infection (i.e. both symptomatic and asymptomatic cases). Even in cases of acute, fulminant clinical disease, early institution of therapy may prevent further invasion and destruction of vital tissues by *Toxoplasma*.

Therapy of proven or suspected congenital *Toxoplasma* infection in the United States has generally been with pyrimethamine and sulfadiazine although spiramycin has also been used in this setting (Table 1). After an initial course of spiramycin. Maisonneuve et al (20) have used pyrimethamine + sulfadoxine (Fansidar) in infants and children with congenital *Toxoplasma* infection with encouraging results. We have not had experience with this combination. Although the long half-life of the sulfadoxine makes it possible to give 1 dose every 2 weeks, concern exists regarding the possibility of serious cutaneous reactions with this drug, and its use in this setting should be considered experimental at this time.

Ocular toxoplasmosis

Patients with active chorioretinitis due to *Toxoplasma* should receive specific therapy. Controlled trials to evaluate the efficacy of systemic clindamycin, pyrimethamine + sulfadiazine, or spiramycin have not been carried out. A non-randomized study by Lakhanpal et al (21) evaluated clindamycin treatment (300 mg orally every 6 hours for a minimum of 3 weeks) in 26 consecutive patients (21). All 4 patients who received clindamycin alone, and 16 of 17 patients who received clindamycin with prednisolone showed clinical improvement. Two other patients developed diarrhea and were changed to sulfadiazine with good response. Chorioretinitis recurred in 2 (2.7%) of 26 patients during a mean follow-up period of 3 years. These results compare favorably with those reported in 2 studies in which patients were treated with sulfadiazine, pyrimethamine and corticosteroids, and in which the recurrence rate was 13%–16% (follow-up period of 1–28 months) (22,

Table 1 *Guidelines for the treatment of infants with suspected or proven congenital Toxoplasma infection*

DRUGS
Pyrimethamine + sulfadiazine: 21-day course
a.   Pyrimethamine
     (loading dose): 1 mg/kg (max. 50 mg/d) (b.i.d.) × 2 d
     (maintenance dose): 1 mg/kg/d (max. 25 mg/d)
b.   Sulfadiazine
     (loading dose): 75 mg/kg (max. 4 g).
     (maintenance dose): 100 mg/kg/d (max. 8 g/d) (b.i.d.)
Spiramycin: 30–45-day course 100 mg/kg/d (b.i.d.)
Corticosteroids: (prednisone or methylprednisolone) 1–2 mg/kg/d (b.i.d.)
Folinic acid: 5 mg/d

INDICATIONS
Congenital toxoplasmosis: Pyrimethamine + sulfadiazine for 21 days. Folinic acid to be given as soon as possible. During the first year of life, the child is given 3–4 courses of pyrimethamine + sulfadiazine separated with spiramycin courses of 30–45 days. No treatment is usually given after 12 months of age

Congenital toxoplasmosis with evidence of inflammatory process (chorioretinitis, high cerebrospinal fluid protein content, generalized infection, jaundice): As for overt congenital toxoplasmosis plus corticosteroid treatment

Subclinical congenital Toxoplasma infection: As for overt congenital toxoplasmosis

Healthy newborn in whom serological testing has not provided definitive results but definite maternal infection was acquired during pregnancy: 1 course of pyrimethamine + sulfadiazine for 21 days, followed by spiramycin. Then wait for laboratory evidence for the diagnosis

Healthy newborn born to a mother with high IgG titer – date of maternal infection undetermined: Spiramycin alone, until laboratory evidence for the diagnosis is definitive. It must be borne in mind that in certain cases the indication for treatment is difficult to define due to lack of information about the pregnancy, lack of isolation attempts from the corresponding placenta, and the fact that treatment may suppress the *Toxoplasma* antibody response of the infant

---

Adapted from Ref. 18.

23). Spiramycin has also been used in ocular toxoplasmosis, but recurrence rates as high as 30% have been reported (22, 23).

Intraocular injections of clindamycin were used by Tate and Martin (24) in 6 patients with toxoplasmic chorioretinitis. Subconjunctival injections (50–150 mg) were used in 5 patients and retrobulbar injections (75–150 mg) in 2 patients (1 patient received both). The authors concluded that subconjunctival doses of 50–75 mg were well tolerated and were a valuable adjunct in the treatment of ocular toxoplasmosis. Because retrobulbar injection led to permanent visual changes (papillitis) in both patients in whom it was used, the authors concluded that this form of therapy is contraindicated.

Because of the difficulty in making a definitive diagnosis of this infection in the eye and the lack of controlled studies, it is exceedingly difficult to know which of the above therapeutic regimens is most efficacious. When there is any real risk of significant damage to vision, we prefer to use pyrimethamine with sulfadiazine or trisulfapyrimidines. When there is macular or optic nerve involvement, corticosteroids should be added.

Toxoplasmosis in the immunocompromised host

In 1968, Vietzke et al (25) published the first thorough assessment of the problem of *Toxoplasma* infection in the immunocompromised host. Of note in this and subsequent studies has been the high incidence of central nervous system (CNS) involvement, and the high mortality associated with untreated toxoplasmosis in patients with underlying neoplastic (especially Hodgkin's disease) or collagen-vascular diseases and in recipients of organ allografts. Because of the high morbidity and mortality, no controlled trial of treatment has been performed in these high-risk groups. Ruskin and Remington reviewed data obtained in 81 cases of toxoplasmosis in patients with neoplastic or collagen-vascular disorders, or organ allografts (26). Neurologic manifestations predominated in more than half of the patients. Sixteen (80%) of 20 patients who were treated experienced either marked clinical improvement or complete remission of symptoms and signs attributable to the infection. Of the untreated patients, only 2 survived. Most treated patients were given combinations of sulfonamides and pyrimethamine. Based on the above, we recommend treatment of all immunocompromised patients with proven acute toxoplasmosis. Because data on optimal duration of treatment are not available, only guidelines can be suggested. We continue therapy for at least 4–6 weeks beyond complete resolution of all signs and symptoms of active disease. In the more severely immunosuppressed host we have treated for a minimum of 4–6 months. Careful follow-up of these patients is important since relapse may occur.

In the last several years, an epidemic of toxoplasmic encephalitis has occurred among patients with AIDS (27–29). Toxoplasmosis in this group of patients has a high mortality rate even with specific therapy aimed at *T. gondii* (29). Because AIDS patients have a striking propensity for development of toxoplasmic encephalitis, special recommendations are made for therapy in this group of patients. All patients with AIDS and CNS signs or symptoms should be studied with either computed tomography (CT) or nuclear magnetic resonance (NMR) and serological tests for toxoplasmosis. If the CT and NMR scan reveals a focal lesion, we recommend biopsy whenever medically and surgically feasible, followed by institution of empiric therapy against *T. gondii*, pending the result of the biopsy. If *T. gondii* is not visualized in biopsy specimens stained by routine hematoxylin and eosin, specific immunoperoxidase staining of tissue is necessary (28, 30). If the scan shows a focal lesion which is inaccessible for biopsy or if the patient's clinical condition is such as to preclude biopsy, presumptive therapy for *T. gondii* should be instituted. Early lesions may not be demonstrable on CT or NMR scan. If the CT is normal, NMR should be performed. If both are normal, repeat studies should be performed in 2–4 weeks in patients who are seropositive for *Toxoplasma* antibodies. At present, optimal therapy has not been defined. The following recommendations are provided as guidelines. Begin with 100 to 200 mg pyrimethamine as a loading dose and then 50–100 mg daily thereafter for primary therapy of the acute infection. This should be continued for 6 weeks. Folinic acid should be administered in a dosage of 15–50 mg daily in an attempt to prevent or reverse the bone marrow toxicity of pyrimethamine. If the sulfonamide preparation must be discontinued due to an adverse reaction, pyrimethamine may be administered alone at 100 mg/d but there are insufficient data to know if this will be effective. Patients with AIDS and toxoplasmic encephalitis have been treated with pyrimethamine plus intravenous clindamycin with apparent improvement while on therapy (31, 32). It is not clear what role clindamycin has played in the observed improvement in patients with toxoplasmic encephalitis since pyrimethamine is active against *T. gondii* when used alone. If the patient cannot tolerate sulfonamides we recommend intravenous clindamycin at a minimum dosage of 900 mg q. 6 h be administered along with pyrimethamine. Treatment with pyrimethamine and 2.4 g or more of oral clindamycin per day has been generally unsuccessful (H. Neu, personal communication). In patients placed on presumptive therapy, a therapeutic response within 10–14 days should be sought as a confirmation of the diagnosis. This response should be independent of corticosteroids when the latter are used to attempt to decrease cerebral edema. Because of the frequency of recurrence once therapy is discontinued, suppressive therapy with the pyrimethamine (25 mg/d) + sulfadiazine (2–4 g d) combination must be administered for the life of the patient. Of note, toxoplasmic encephalitis has developed in patients with AIDS who were being treated with spiramycin as well as in patients receiving 20 mg/kg/d of trimethoprim + sulfamethoxazole for therapy of *Pneumocystis carinii* pneumonia (unpublished data). Relapse had occurred in patients receiving Fansidar as maintenance therapy.

ACKNOWLEDGEMENT

We wish to thank Dr. Robert McCabe for his help in review of the manuscript.

REFERENCES

1. Eyles DE, Coleman M (1953) Synergistic effect of sulfadiazine and Daraprim against experimental toxoplasmosis in the mouse. *Antibiot. Chemother., 3*, 483.

2. Eyles DE, Coleman M (1955) An evaluation of pyrimethamine and sulfadiazine alone and in combination in experimental mouse toxoplasmosis. *Antibiot. Chemother.*, 5, 529.

3. Smith CC, Ihrig J (1959) Persistent excretion of pyrimethamine following oral administration. *Am. J. Trop. Med. Hyg.*, 8, 60.

4. Geils GF, Scott Jr CW, Baugh CM, Butterworth Jr CE (1971) Treatment of meningeal leukemia with pyrimethamine. *Blood, 38*, 131.

5. Grossman PL, Remington JS (1979) The effect of trimethoprim and sulfamethoxazole on *Toxoplasma gondii* in vitro and in vivo. *Am. J. Trop. Med. Hyg.*, 28, 445.

6. Mas Bakal P, Intveld N (1965) Postponed spiramycin treatment of acute toxoplasmosis in white mice. *Trop. Geogr. Med.*, 17, 254.

7. MacFarlane JA, Mitchell AAB, Walsh JM, Robertson JJ (1968) Spiramycin in the prevention of postoperative staphylococcal infection. *Lancet, 1*, 1.

8. Banazet F, Dubost M (1958/1959) Apparent paradox of antimicrobial activity of spiramycin. *Antibiot. Ann.*, 211.

9. Garin JP, Pellerot J, Maillard MME et al (1968) Bases théoriques de la prévention par la spiramycine de la toxoplasmose congénitale chez la femme enceinte. *Presse Méd., 76*, 2266.

10. Araujo FG, Remington JS (1974) Effect of clindamycin on acute and chronic toxoplasmosis in mice. *Antimicrob. Agents Chemother.*, 5, 647.

11. Tabbara KF, Nozik RA, O'Connor GR (1974) Clindamycin effects on experimental ocular toxoplasmosis in the rabbit. *Arch. Ophthalmol.*, 92, 244.

12. Tabbara KF, O'Connor GR (1975) Ocular tissue absorption of clindamycin phosphate. *Arch. Ophthalmol.*, 93, 1180.

13. Desmonts G, Couvreur J (1979) Congenital toxoplasmosis: a prospective study of the offspring of 542 women who acquired toxoplasmosis during pregnancy – pathophysiology disease. In: Thalhammer O, Baumgarten K, Pollak A (Eds), *Proceedings, 6th European Congress on Perinatal Medicine*, p 51. Thieme, Stuttgart.

14. Kraubig H (1963) Erste praktische Erfahrungen mit der Prophylaxe der konnatalen Toxoplasmose. *Med. Klin., 58*, 1361.

15. Desmonts G, Couvreur J (1974) Congenital toxoplasmosis: a prospective study of 378 pregnancies. *N. Engl. J. Med., 290*, 1110.

16. Desmonts G, Forestier F, Thulliez P et al (1985) Prenatal diagnosis of congenital toxoplasmosis. *Lancet, 1*, 500.

17. Wilson CB, Remington JS, Stagno S, Reynolds DW (1980) Development of adverse sequelae in children born with subclinical congenital *Toxoplasma* infection. *Pediatrics, 66*, 767.

18. Remington JS, Desmonts G (1983) Toxoplasmosis. In: Remington JS, Klein JO (Eds), *Infectious Diseases of the Fetus and Newborn Infant*, p. 143. Saunders, Philadelphia.

19. Beverly JKA, Freeman AP, Henry L, Whelan JPF (1973) Prevention of pathological changes in experimental congenital *Toxoplasma* infections. *Lyon Méd., 230*, 491.

20. Maisonneuve H, Faber C, Piens MA, Garin JP (1984) Toxoplasmose congénitale: tolérance de l'association sulfadoxine-pyrimethamine – vingt-quatre observations. *Presse Méd., 13*, 859. -

21. Lakhanpal V, Schochet SS, Nirankari VS (1983) Clindamycin in the treatment of toxoplasmic retinochoroiditis. *Am. J. Ophthalmol.*, 95, 605.

22. Canamucio CJ, Hallett JW, Leopold IH (1963) Recurrence of treated toxoplasmic uveitis. *Am. J. Ophthalmol.*, 55, 1035.

23. Ghosh M, Levy PM, Leopold IH (1965) Therapy of toxoplasmosis uveitis. *Am. J. Ophthalmol., 59*, 55.

24. Tate GW, Martin RG (1977) Clindamycin in the treatment of human ocular toxoplasmosis. *Can. J. Ophthalmol., 12*, 188.

25. Vietzke WM, Gelderman AH, Grimley DM, Valsamis MP (1968) Toxoplasmosis complicating malignancy. *Cancer, 21*, 816.

26. Ruskin J, Remington JS (1976) Toxoplasmosis in the compromised host. *Ann. Intern. Med., 84*, 193.

27. Luft BJ, Conley F, Remington JS et al (1983) Outbreak of central nervous system toxoplasmosis in Western Europe and North America. *Lancet, 1*, 791.

28. Luft BJ, Brooks RG, Conley FK et al (1984) Toxoplasmic encephalitis in patients with acquired immune deficiency syndrome. *J. Am. Med. Assoc., 252*, 913.

29. Wong B, Gold JWM, Brown AE et al (1984) Central nervous system toxoplasmosis in homosexual men and parenteral drug abusers. *Ann. Intern. Med., 100*, 36.

30. Conley FK, Jenkins KA, Remington JS (1982) *Toxoplasma gondii* infection of the central nervous system: use of the peroxidase-anti-peroxidase method to demonstrate *Toxoplasma* in formalin-fixed paraffin embedded tissue sections. *Hum. Pathol., 12*, 690.

31. Snow RB, Lavyne M (1983) CNS toxoplasmosis in a patient with AIDS. *Infect. Surg., 2*, 669.

32. Snider WD, Simpson DM, Neilson S et al (1983) Neurological complications of acquired immunodeficiency syndrome: analysis of 50 patients. *Ann. Neurol., 14*, 403.

CHAPTER 31

Drugs used in the treatment of human African trypanosomiasis

L. EYCKMANS and M. WÉRY

Since the publication of *The Antimicrobial Agents Annual 2*, unfortunately little new information has appeared in the literature regarding treatment of African trypanosomiasis. The discussion in this Chapter continues to represent current views as to management of this important parasitic disease.

The disease called 'human African trypanosomiasis' (1) is due to infection by man-adapted subspecies of *Trypanosoma brucei*, namely *T.b. gambiense* in the Western and Central part of tropical Africa, and *T.b. rhodesiense* in the Eastern part. Transmission of the infection occurs through the bite of blood-sucking flies of the genus *Glossina*, whose different species have strict life habits in relation to humidity, temperature, moist breeding places and daily feeding on man or animals. The disease is therefore restricted to the non-desert areas of tropical Africa. The western variety (*T.b. gambiense*) spreads over forest and mosaic savannah areas along forest galleries related to streams. It runs a chronic course; illness progresses over one or more years with involvement of the central nervous system (CNS) in the final stage. The eastern variety (*T.b. rhodesiense*), disseminated over grassy savannah areas, high land and valleys without relation to forest or presence of trees, is a more acute disease. It is usually fatal within a few months, and often lacks the classical somnolence seen in the western variety.

About the turn of the century, sleeping sickness, known for a long time by traders, drew attention as a major threat to the development of equatorial Africa. Early attempts at treatment with the antimony salt, tartar emetic, or the organic arsenical, atoxyl, were soon abandoned because of their relative inefficacy coupled with high toxicity (2). Therefore the search began for better arsenicals (3–7). Tryparsamide was developed and dominated the scene for a long time. It had no activity against the later stages of the eastern variety of the disease and is held responsible for many cases of blindness, through atrophy of the optic nerve. Its production was therefore stopped when other drugs such as melarsoprol (Arsobal) became available. More recently developed drugs are sometimes referred to as 'non-arsenical'! The earliest and still most widely used of these new drugs (suramin and pentamidine) have been found to have insufficient activity against trypanosomes within the CNS.

Antimicrobial Agents Annual 3
P.K. Peterson and J. Verhoef, editors
© Elsevier Science Publishers BV, 1988

Suramin

Suramin (Bayer 205, Moranyl, Germanin, Naganol, Naphuride) is the sodium salt of 8,3,3-aminobenzamido-4-methylbenzamido-naphthalene-1,3,5-trisulfonic acid. It is available as a white or pinkish powder, to be dissolved in water immediately prior to injection. It was brought into general use in the 1920s as a useful drug for the treatment of the early stages of African trypanosomiasis. It was later found to be active against the adult forms of the filaria *Onchocerca volvulus*. Its mechanisms of action are largely unknown (8), but it has been found to inhibit numerous enzyme systems including the reverse transcriptase system (9). Suramin is highly protein-bound in serum (10). Its pharmacokinetic profiles vary from one individual to another (11, 12). Serum concentrations are usually high immediately after intravenous injection but fall rapidly within the first few hours and then more slowly over ensuing days. Low concentrations are maintained for as long as 2 or 3 months. Excretion is assumed to be mainly by the renal route.

Frequent adverse effects after injection are febrile reactions, nausea and vomiting (13). These effects are more frequently observed in malnourished persons. Cases of shock have been observed after the first injection; it is therefore recommended that the susceptibility of the patient be tested by starting treatment with a small quantity of the drug. Albuminuria may develop in many patients treated with suramin, but this should not lead to the discontinuation of treatment. However, when severe renal toxicity occurs, the drug should be discontinued. Pain in the palms of the hands or the soles of the feet may represent the first signs of peripheral neuropathy and the patient should be observed carefully. Desquamation of the skin may follow the use of suramin. Since excretion of the drug is slow, desquamation may go on for weeks and become incapacitating.

Suramin is used in the treatment of the early forms of trypanosomiasis, before involvement of the CNS. Infections by *T.b. rhodesiense* are especially suited for treatment with this drug. Even after only one injection, trypanosomes are cleared very rapidly from the blood, lymph and peripheral tissues. When involvement of the CNS calls for the use of other drugs (especially arsenicals), treatment is often initiated with one injection of suramin to eliminate blood parasites (14). This should also decrease the probability of shock when arsenical treatment is started (15) and avoid infection from *Glossina* flies that may feed on the patient.

The prolonged excretion of suramin has led, in the past, to its prophylactic use (16). In view of its slow excretion, it is recommended that treatment should not be repeated within 3 months after the first course of injections.

Pentamidine

Pentamidine is one of the aromatic diamidines; it is often used as pentamidine isothionate.

Pentamidine is active against *T.b. gambiense* but less so against *T.b. rhodesiense*;

it is suited for the treatment of the early forms of these infections. The drug is active against other protozoa in experimental systems and is used for the treatment of infections by *Leishmania (L. donovani)* and *Pneumocystis carinii*. The basic action of the drug is not known, but interference with glycolysis has been suggested.

Pentamidine is rapidly absorbed from parenteral sites of administration. It appears in the blood for only brief periods and is believed to be stored in tissues (mainly liver and kidneys) for periods of weeks to months.

Adverse reactions such as a fall in blood pressure with syncope, breathlessness, tachycardia, nausea and vomiting may be dramatic but are usually of no great consequence (17). Since these reactions may be more severe after intravenous injections, it is generally advocated that the drug be administered exclusively by the intramuscular route. Hypoglycemia (18, 19), pancreatitis (20) and the onset of diabetes (21–23) have been related to the administration of pentamidine. Abortion has followed its use. Nephrotoxicity is usually manifested by reversible renal dysfunction, but severe renal failure has also been observed (24).

Pentamidine can be used as an alternative to suramin. Prophylactic use of pentamidine has also been advocated in view of its prolonged presence in the body due to storage in tissues. The drug has been used with success in mass campaigns aiming at interruption of transmission of the infection, together with other measures (16). This approach is fraught with difficulties due to side-effects (including abortion in pregnant women!) and to the masking of symptoms by the low dosage used in this treatment schedule, thus causing infected persons to go undetected, only to emerge later with severe involvement of the nervous system. The prophylactic use of pentamidine in tourists should therefore be discouraged.

Melarsoprol

Melarsoprol (Arsobal or Mel-B) is a drug containing a trivalent arsenic atom. It was introduced by Friedheim in 1949 (25) and constituted a major advantage over pentavalent arsenicals, especially in the treatment of *T.b. rhodesiense* infections, which were totally unaffected by pentavalent compounds (5). Even now, melarsoprol remains the major drug for the treatment and control of human trypanosomiasis. As the commercial name suggests, the arsenic atom is partly bound to dimercaprol (BAL), the drug used for the treatment of heavy metal or arsenical poisoning.

The mode of action of melarsoprol, as of other arsenicals, has not been completely elucidated (8, 26–28).

Surprisingly little is known about the pharmacology of melarsoprol and its pharmacokinetics are largely unknown (6, 16, 29). Although the drug is considered on empirical grounds to penetrate the CNS, this has never been established. Its side-effects include intense irritation at the site of injection, chest pain, abdominal pain, disturbance of smell, and signs of polyneuritis. The most serious side-effect, however, involves the CNS and is characterized as encephalopathy. Such encephalitic reactions occur with variable frequency but may affect up to 13% of patients (2, 5, 7, 15). Some forms of this encephalopathy are hemorrhagic and lead to irreversible brain lesions and death. Fatal encephalopathy has been reported in up to 5% of patients treated with melarsoprol. The mechanism of this complication is not known. It usually arises after 3–4 injections. Beneficial effects of adrenaline (30) or corticosteroids (31, 32) suggest that it could be allergic in nature. Some clinicians point out that the indicence of encephalopathy is lower when melarsoprol is given early in the course of the infection. It is commonly believed that encephalopathy is a consequence of massive destruction of trypanosomes in the nervous system, and that its incidence and severity are related to the stage at which the disease is treated and hence to the number of parasites present in the nervous system at the time of treatment. For this reason, an injection of suramin has been recommended prior to the administration of melarsoprol (33). Encephalopathy has been treated with dimercaprol (BAL) and corticosteroids. Administration of melarsoprol to patients with leprosy may precipitate the appearance of erythema nodosum. It is usually accepted that the drug should not be given to patients suffering from intercurrent infections such as influenza. Also, simultaneous antimalarial treatment has been advocated (34).

Melarsoprol can be used in all stages of trypanosomiasis, for *T.b. gambiense* and *rhodesiense* varieties. However, fear of its side-effects led to the recommendation to restrict its use to the later stages of the disease, when until recently no alternative was available.

In cases of relapse after a completed treatment schedule, administration of the same drug may be considered, but it would seem advisable to use an alternative drug (see below) since this type of relapse may be due to resistance of the parasite to arsenic. Indeed, the value of melarsoprol has been reduced in recent years with the appearance of resistance which has been reported in up to 50% of patients in some areas.

Alternative drugs

A number of drugs have been suggested for the treatment of trypanosomiasis (3, 35–39) based on theoretical considerations (40, 41) or experimental observations (42, 43). Their application in man has generally been disappointing (7, 44–46).

Nifurtimox

Nifurtimox (Lampit) is a nitrofuran which has been developed for the treatment of Chagas' disease or American trypanosomiasis. Although this disease has very little, if anything, in common with African sleeping sickness, the known sensitivity of trypanosomes in general to nitrofurans (47) has led to its use in the late stages of sleeping sickness in cases showing resistance to treatment with arsenicals (48).

Early results have been encouraging, but widespread experience is still lacking (49). After rapid improvement in some patients, relapses have been observed. One advantage of nifurtimox is its ready absorption after oral administration. The drug is subject to marked biotransformation.

DL-α-Difluoromethylornithine

DL-α-Difluoromethylornithine (α-DFMO) is an irreversible inhibitor of ornithine decarboxylase, an enzyme for the synthesis of polyamines. It is the product of research aimed at finding new anti-cancer drugs (50). It has been found to be active in vitro against several pathogenic protozoa (51, 52) and was tried with success in the treatment of experimental trypanosomiasis in the mouse (53–55) when used in combination with other drugs. The drug is not available commercially. Its use in a limited number of cases of human *T.b. gambiense* infection at different stages has so far given satisfactory results (56, 57). In these studies, it was possible to follow drug concentrations in the blood and spinal fluid after both oral and parenteral administration of the drug. Absorption from the gut seems to be good and diffusion into the spinal fluid is satisfactory, even if the meninges are not inflamed, although the opposite has been stated (7). Although experience is limited, the recommended daily dose is 15–30 grams, given either orally or parenterally. Pepin et al (58) treated 26 patients in Zaire with arseno-resistant *T.b. gambiense* trypanosomiasis (and thus at a late stage of the disease) by giving successive intravenous (2–3 weeks) and oral (21–24 days) administration of the drug. No relapse has been found in 16 patients followed up for 12 months or more. The most prominent side effects were anemia, diarrhea and hair loss. The drug is therefore usually well tolerated and apart from the slight gastrointestinal disturbances (59) no serious side-effects have been reported thus far. Treatment has to be protracted for a period of some 6 weeks. The amount of drug necessary to achieve this treatment schedule may be prohibitive, except in individual cases.

REFERENCES

1. Eyckmans L (1985) African sleeping sickness. In: Mandell GL, Douglas RG, Bennett JE (Eds), *Principles and Practice of Infectious Diseases, 2nd ed*, Ch 235, p 1537. Wiley, New York.
2. Williamson J (1970) Review of chemotherapeutic and chemoprophylactic agents. In: Mulligan HW (Ed), *The African Trypanosomiasis*, Ch 7, p 125. Allen and Unwin, London.
3. Meshnick SR (1984) The chemotherapy of African trypanosomiasis. In: Mansfield JM (Ed), *Parasitic Diseases, Vol 2. The Chemotherapy*, p 165. Dekker, New York.
4. Dukes P (1984) Arsenic and old taxa: subspeciation and drug sensitivity in *Trypanosoma brucei. Trans. R. Soc. Trop. Med. Hyg., 78,* 711.
5. Apted FIC (1980) Present status of chemotherapy and chemoprophylaxis of human trypanosomiasis in the Eastern Hemisphere. *Pharmacol. Ther., 11,* 391.

6. Brown JR (1983) Human trypanosomiases and their treatment. *Pharmacol. Int., 4*, 61.

7. Dumas M, Breton JC, Pestre-Alexandre M et al (1985) Etat actuel de la thérapeutique de la trypanosomiase humaine africaine. *Presse Méd., 14*, 253.

8. Williamson J (1979) Effects of trypanocides on the fine structure of target organisms. *Pharmacol. Ther., 7*, 445.

9. De Clercq E (1979) Suramin: a potent inhibitor of the reverse transcriptase of RNA tumor viruses. *Cancer Lett., 8*, 9.

10. Molyneux DH, De Raadt P, Seed J (1984) Human African trypanosomiasis. In: Gilles H (Ed), *Recent Advances in Tropical Medicine*, p 57. Churchill-Livingstone, Edinburgh.

11. Hawking F (1940) Concentrations of Bayer 205 (Germanin) in human blood and cerebrospinal fluid after treatment. *Trans. R. Soc. Trop. Med. Hyg., 34*, 37.

12. Collins JM, Yarchoan R, Fauci AS, Broder S, Klecker RW, Lane HC, Redfield RR, Myers CE (1986) Clinical pharmacokinetics of suramin in patients with HTLV-III/LAV infection. *J. Clin. Pharmacol., 26*, 22.

13. Constantopoulos G, Rees S, Barranger JA, Brady RO (1983) Suramin induced storage disease. *Am. J. Pathol., 113*, 266.

14. Foulkes JR (1981) Human trypanosomiasis in Africa. *Br. Med. J., 283*, 1172.

15. Robertson DHH (1963) The treatment of sleeping sickness (mainly due to *Trypanosoma rhodesiense*) with melarsoprol. *Trans. R. Soc. Trop. Med. Hyg., 57*, 122.

16. Neujean J (1963) Aspects pratiques de la lutte contre la trypanosomiase humaine dans la République du Congo (Léopoldville). *Bull. OMS, 28*, 797.

17. Bielenberg GW, Krieglstein J (1984) On the hypotensive effect of aromatic amidines and imidazolidines. *Arzneim.-Forsch., 34*, 958.

18. Fitzgerald DB, Young IS (1984) Reversal of pentamidine-induced hypoglycaemia with oral diazoxide. *J. Trop. Med. Hyg., 87*, 15.

19. Gauda OP (1984) Pentamidine and hypoglycemia. *Ann. Intern. Med., 100*, 464.

20. Murphey SA, Josephs AS (1981) Acute pancreatitis associated with pentamidine therapy. *Arch. Intern. Med., 141*, 56.

21. Jha TK, Sharma VK (1984) Pentamidine-induced diabetes mellitus. *Trans. R. Soc. Trop. Med. Hyg., 78*, 252.

22. Osei K, Falko JM, Nelson KP, Stephens R (1984) Diabetogenic effect of pentamidine: in vitro and in vivo studies in a patient with malignant insulinoma. *Am. J. Med., 77*, 41.

23. Naafs B (1985) Pentamidine-induced diabetes mellitus. *Trans. R. Soc. Trop. Med. Hyg., 79*, 141.

24. Limbos P (1977) Insuffisance rénale au cours du traitement de la trypanosomiase à *T. rhodesiense* par la pentamidine. *Ann. Soc. Belge Méd. Trop., 57*, 495.

25. Friedheim EAH (1949) Mel-B in the treatment of human trypanosomiasis. *Am. J. Trop. Med., 29*, 173.

26. Friedheim EAH (1959) Some approaches to the development of chemotherapeutic compounds. *Ann. Trop. Med. Parasitol., 53*, 1.

27. Sardana MK, Drummond GS, Sassa S, Kappas A (1981) The potent heme oxygenase inducing action of arsenic and parasiticidal arsenicals. *Pharmacology, 23*, 247.

28. Poltera AA, Hochmann A, Lambert PH (1981) *Trypanosoma brucei brucei*: the response to melarsoprol in mice with cerebral trypanosomiasis – an immunopathological study. *Clin. Exp. Immunol., 46*, 363.

29. Neujean G, Evens F (1958) *Diagnostic et traitement de la maladie du sommeil à Trypa-*

nosoma gambiense: bilan de dix ans d'activité au Centre de Traitement de Léopoldville. Mémoire, Académie Royale des Sciences Coloniales, Brussels.

30. Sina GC, Triolo N, Cramet B, Suh-Bandu M (1982) L'adrénaline dans la prévention et le traitement des accidents de l'arsobal-thérapie: à propos de 776 cas de trypanosomiase humaine africaine à T. *gambiense* traités dans les formations sanitaires de Fontem (R.U. du Caméroun). *Méd. Trop. (Marseille), 42,* 531.

31. Bertrand E, Rive J (1973) L'orage liquidien existe-t-il dans la trypanosomiase humaine africaine traitée par arsobal-corticoides? *Bull. Soc. Pathol. Exot., 66,* 540.

32. Pépin J, Tétrault L, Gervais C (1985) Utilisation des corticoides oraux dans le traitement de la trypanosomiase humaine africaine. *Ann. Soc. Belge Méd. Trop., 65,* 17.

33. Buyst H (1975) The treatment of *T. rhodesiense* sleeping sickness with special reference to its physio-pathological and epidemiological basis. *Ann. Soc. Belge Méd. Trop., 55,* 95.

34. Buyst H (1977) Sleeping sickness in children. *Ann. Soc. Belge Méd. Trop., 57,* 201.

35. Van der Meer C, Verluijs-Broers JAM, Opperdoes FR (1979) *Trypanosoma brucei*: trypanocidal effect of salicyl hydroxamic acid plus glycerol in infected rats. *Exp. Parasitol., 48,* 126.

36. Kinnamon KE, Steck EA, Rane DS (1979) A new chemical series active against African trypanosomes: benzyl triphenylphosphonium salts. *J. Med. Chem., 22,* 452.

37. Opperdoes FR (1980) Miconazole; an inhibitor of cyanide insensitive respiration in *Trypanosoma brucei. Trans. R. Soc. Trop. Med. Hyg., 74,* 423.

38. Ulrich PC, Grady RW, Cerami A (1982) The trypanocidal activity of various aromatic bisguanylhydrazones in vivo. *Drug. Dev. Res., 2,* 219.

39. Farrell NP, Williamson J, McLaren DJM (1984) Trypanocidal and antitumor activity of platinum-metal and platinum-metal-drug dual function complexes. *Biochem. Pharmacol., 33,* 961.

40. Arrick BA, Griffith OW, Cerami A (1981) Inhibition of glutathione synthesis as chemotherapeutic strategy for trypanosomiasis. *J. Exp. Med., 153,* 720.

41. Dumas M, Breton JC, Pestre-Alexandre M et al (1983) Réflexions sur le traitement de la trypanosomiase humaine africaine. *Bull. Soc. Pathol. Exot., 76,* 622.

42. Libeau G, Pinder M (1981) Deleterious effect of levamisole in experimental trypanosomiasis of the mouse. *Rev. Elev. Méd. Vét. Pays Trop., 34,* 399.

43. Duch DS, Bacchi CJ, Edelstein MP, Nichol CA (1984) Inhibitors of histamine metabolism in vitro and in vivo: correlation with antitrypanosomal activity. *Biochem. Pharmacol., 33,* 1547.

44. Ruppol JF, Burke J (1977) Follow-up des traitements contre la trypanosomiase expérimentée à Kimpangu (République du Zaire). *Ann. Soc. Belge Méd. Trop., 57,* 481.

45. Meshnick SR, Grady RW, Blobstein SH, Cerami A (1978) Porphyrin-induced lysis of *Trypanosoma brucei*: a role for zinc. *J. Pharmacol. Exp. Ther., 207,* 1041.

46. Meshnick SR, Blobstein SH, Grady RW, Cerami A (1978) An approach to the development of new drugs for African trypanosomiasis. *J. Exp. Med., 148,* 569.

47. Haberkorn A (1979) The effect of nifurtimox on experimental infections with Trypanosomatidae other than *Trypanosoma cruzi. Zentralbl. Bakteriol. Parasitol. Infekt.-kr., 244,* 331.

48. Janssens PG, De Muynck A (1977) Clinical trials with nifurtimox in African trypanosomiasis. *Ann. Soc. Belge Méd. Trop., 57,* 475.

49. Moens F, De Wilde M, Kola Ngato (1984) Essai de traitement au nifurtimox de la trypanosomiase humaine africaine. *Ann. Soc. Belge Méd. Trop., 64,* 37.

50. Prakash NJ, Schechter PJ, Grove J, Koch-Weser J (1978) Effect of alpha-difluoro-methylornithine, an enzyme-activated irreversible inhibitor of ornithine decarboxylase on L 1210 leukemia in mice. *Cancer Res., 38*, 3059.

51. Kinnamon KE, Steck EA, Rane DS (1979) Activity of antitumor drugs against African trypanosomes. *Antimicrob. Agents Chemother., 15*, 157.

52. Bacchi CJ, Garofalo J, Mockenhaupt D et al (1983) In vivo effects of alpha-DL-difluoromethylornithine on the metabolism and morphology of *Trypanosoma brucei brucei. Molec. Biochem. Parasitol., 7*, 209.

53. McCann PP, Bacchi CJ, Clarkson AB, Bey P, Sjoerdsma A, Schechter PJ, Walzer PD, Barlow JLR (1986) Inhibition of polyamine biosynthesis by α-difluoromethylornithine in African trypanosomes and *Pneumocystis carinii* as a basis of chemotherapy: biochemical and clinical aspects. *Am. J. Trop. Med. Hyg., 35*, 1153.

54. Karbe E, Böttger M, McCann PP et al (1982) Curative effect of alpha-difluoromethylornithine on fatal *Trypanosoma congolense* infection in mice. *Tropenmed. Parasitol., 33*, 161.

55. Clarkson AB, Bienen EJ, Bacchi CJ et al (1984) New drug combination for experimental late-stage African trypanosomiasis: DL-α-difluoromethylornithine (DFMO) with suramin. *Am. J. Trop. Med. Hyg., 33*, 1073.

56. Taelman H, Schechter PJ, Marcelis L et al (1987) Difluoromethylornithine, an effective new treatment of gambiense trypanosomiasis: results in five patients. *Am. J. Med., 82*, 607.

57. Van Nieuwenhove S, Schechter PJ, Declercq J, Boné G, Burke J, Sjoerdsma A (1985) Treatment of gambiense sleeping sickness in the Sudan with oral DFMO (DL-α-difluoromethylornithine), an inhibitor of ornithine decarboxylase: first field trial. *Trans. R. Soc. Trop. Med. Hyg., 79*, 692.

58. Pepin J, Milord F, Guern C, Schechter PJ (1987) Difluoromethylornithine for arseno resistant *Trypanosoma brucei gambiense* sleeping sickness. *Lancet, 2*, 1431.

59. Yarrington JT, Sprinkle DJ, Loudy DE et al (1983) Intestinal changes by DL-α-difluoromethylornithine (DFMO), an inhibitor of ornithine decarboxylase. *Exp. Mol. Pathol., 39*, 300.

CHAPTER 32

Acyclovir

HENRY H. BALFOUR Jr

Acyclovir (Zovirax) is the drug of choice for most forms of herpes simplex virus (HSV) and varicella-zoster virus (VZV) infections. Treatment trials of patients with cytomegalovirus (CMV) and Epstein-Barr virus (EBV) infections have yielded disappointing results, but recent data in bone marrow allograft recipients suggest that acyclovir still may prove beneficial for suppression of certain CMV syndromes. Provocative new results hint that acyclovir has an additive or even synergistic effect with zidovudine (Retrovir, formerly known as 'azidothymidine') against human immunodeficiency virus (HIV).

Acyclovir is an acyclic analog of the natural nucleoside, 2'-deoxyguanosine (Fig. 1). The initial synthesis of acyclovir focused on the key intermediate 2,6-dichloro-9-(2-benzoyloxyethoxymethyl)purine. That compound, when reacted with methanolic ammonia, nitrous acid and methanolic ammonia again, yielded a modest amount of acyclovir (1). Subsequently, acyclovir was prepared more efficiently by reacting guanine with 2-benzoyloxyethyl chloromethyl ether (3). The molecular weight of acyclovir is 225 daltons; the molecular weight of its intravenous formulation, acyclovir sodium, is 247 daltons.

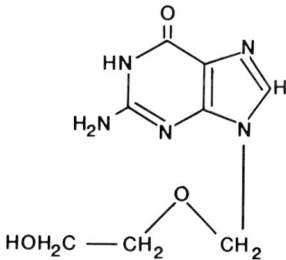

Fig. 1   Structural formula of acyclovir, chemical name 9[(2-hydroxyethoxy)methyl]guanine.

Antimicrobial Agents Annual 3
P.K. Peterson and J. Verhoef, editors
© Elsevier Science Publishers BV, 1988

ACTIVITY

Mechanism of action

Acyclovir is inactive as a nucleoside and must be phosphorylated to the nucleotide form, acyclovir triphosphate, in order to exert its antiviral activity (1, 2). The drug is selectively phosphorylated to acyclovir monophosphate by a virus-specified de-oxynucleoside kinase, commonly called thymidine kinase (TK). Viral TK is induced in cells infected by HSV or VZV.

Acyclovir monophosphate is converted to acyclovir diphosphate by cellular guanosine monophosphate (guanylate) kinase and then by additional host-cell enzymes to acyclovir triphosphate (4). Acyclovir triphosphate is both an inhibitor of and a substrate for viral DNA polymerase (1, 2, 5). Acyclovir triphosphate is a suicide inactivator of HSV DNA polymerase: once the triphosphate binds to viral DNA polymerase, enzymatic activity of the viral product is irreversibly lost (6). Very little acyclovir triphosphate is generated in uninfected host cells, and therefore acyclovir exerts minimal effects on cellular α-DNA polymerase (2). This is a major reason for the very low toxicity of the drug.

Spectrum of activity

Acyclovir inhibits replication of 5 human herpesviruses in cell culture (Table 1). HSV Type 1, HSV Type 2 and VZV code for a virus-specific TK that initiates phosphorylation of acyclovir. Large quantities of acyclovir triphosphate are produced in HSV-infected cells, accounting for the exquisite sensitivity of HSV strains (2). VZV strains are not as sensitive as HSV isolates but are more suscepti-

Table 1 *In-vitro sensitivity (ID$_{50}$)* of human herpesviruses to acyclovir*

Virus	ID$_{50}$(μM)	
	Median	Range
Herpes simplex Type 1	0.1	0.02–41.5**
Herpes simplex Type 2	0.4	0.13–83**
Varicella-zoster	2.6	1.5–17.5
Epstein-Barr	–	0.3–25+
Cytomegalovirus	63.1	18.2–200

*   ID$_{50}$ (50% inhibitory dose) is the amount of acyclovir needed to reduce the number of plaques to half those formed in control cell cultures not treated with drug. Data were compiled from the literature and our own laboratory.
**   The few herpes simplex isolates with ID$_{50}$ > 8 μM usually are thymidine-kinase-deficient mutants (see 'Resistance mechanisms' section).
+   Data from chronically-infected P3HR1 cells; patient isolates not tested.

ble to acyclovir than either EBV or CMV. EBV and CMV do not induce production of virus-specific TK, but the DNA polymerases of EBV (7, 8) and CMV (9) are inhibited by acyclovir. It is possible that the small amount of acyclovir triphosphate formed by host-cell enzymes is sufficient to halt replication of some strains of EBV and CMV. No consistent data are available to substantiate activity of acyclovir against human viruses outside the herpes group.

Resistance mechanisms

A high frequency of spontaneous mutation occurs at the acyclovir-resistance locus because 0.1–0.2% of viruses grown in the absence of acyclovir are naturally resistant (10). In addition, HSV strains resistant to acyclovir can be selected in the laboratory by passing HSV in cell cultures containing acyclovir. HSV isolates that replicate in acyclovir concentrations of 10–100 μM usually are resistant to the drug (10).

There are at least 3 mechanisms for acyclovir resistance (11, 12). The most common mechanism of resistance is decreased or absent induction of virus-specified TK. TK-deficient viruses have been the only kind of resistant HSV strains isolated from patients in any appreciable number. TK-deficient strains grow slowly in cell culture and appear to be less virulent than their wild-type parents both in vitro and in vivo (13).

A second resistance mechanism is altered substrate specificity for viral induced TK (14). Some TK is produced, but this enzyme is not efficient at phosphorylating acyclovir, although it can phosphorylate thymidine.

The third mechanism for HSV resistance is a mutation in the DNA polymerase gene, rendering the transcribed enzyme resistant to inactivation by acyclovir triphosphate (15, 16). DNA polymerase (*pol*) mutants are often resistant to other antiherpes drugs that are not biochemically related to acyclovir, e.g. phosphonoacetic acid. These *pol* mutants replicate well in the ear lobes of mice causing swelling equal to that of their wild-type parents (17). However, *pol* mutants appear to be much less neurovirulent than acyclovir-sensitive strains. Isolation of HSV *pol* mutants from patients has not been conclusively demonstrated, indicating that such mutations in a clinical setting are very uncommon.

Dekker et al (18) tested 797 HSV Type 1 and Type 2 strains collected from 301 patients during acyclovir treatment trials. These investigators showed that there was no significant change in sensitivity to acyclovir during the therapy. Considered in aggregate, clinical and laboratory data indicate that HSV resistance to acyclovir is worthy of continued monitoring but has not been an important clinical problem to date.

Laboratory strains of VZV have been shown to be resistant to acyclovir, most likely due to loss of TK (19). We tested 40 VZV strains collected from 20 patients during intravenous and oral acyclovir treatment trials and did not find any changes in the mean or median 50% inhibitory dose (ID_{50}), suggesting that emergence of VZV resistance during short-term acyclovir treatment is uncommon (20).

347

CLINICAL PHARMACOLOGY

Acyclovir has 9 formulations: 5% ointment in polyethylene glycol, 200 mg gelatin capsules, sterile lyophilized acyclovir sodium powder for intravenous administration, 5% cream in polyethylene glycol, 3% ophthalmic ointment in petrolatum, tablets in 200 mg, 400 mg and 800 mg strengths, and a 40 mg/ml pediatric oral suspension. Only the first three are licensed in the United States. The ophthalmic ointment, 200 mg tablets and topical cream are available in many countries throughout the world including the United Kingdom.

Systemic absorption of acyclovir ointment is negligible. Oral drug is poorly absorbed from the gastrointestinal tract with peak plasma concentrations being reached 1.5–2 hours after ingestion (21). The bioavailability of the oral formulations is approximately 15%.

In animal studies, intravenous acyclovir rapidly entered all tissues, including aqueous humor and brain (22, 23). The lowest amounts of drug were found in the central nervous system. The volume of distribution of acyclovir at steady state is 70% of total body weight (approx. 50 liters per 1.73 m^2), which essentially corresponds to total body water (24). Plasma protein binding averages 15% of the administered dose (25). Acyclovir levels in human cerebrospinal fluid are approximately 50% of the concomitant plasma concentrations (25).

Approximately 70% of acyclovir is excreted unchanged in the urine (23). The only significant metabolite, which is probably formed in the liver, is 9-carboxymethoxymethylguanine (26). In patients with normal renal function, approximately 10% of an acyclovir dose is recovered as this metabolite. In patients with impaired renal function, a larger portion of drug will be excreted as the 9-carboxy derivative (24).

The renal clearance of acyclovir is substantially greater than the estimated creatinine clearance, indicating that not all excretion is due to glomerular filtration (26, 27). Laskin et al (28) showed that probenicid significantly enhanced plasma concentrations of acyclovir, indicating that the drug is eliminated by renal tubular secretion at least in part via the organic acid secretory system.

Elimination of intravenous acyclovir conforms to a two-compartment model (25). The beta of terminal plasma half-life is 2.5–3.0 hours in patients older than 1 year with normal renal function (29). In infants under 3 months of age, the mean terminal plasma half-life is approximately 4 hours (30). Peak and trough levels in adults with normal renal function are given in Table 2.

Reasonable intraocular concentrations can be achieved following oral or intravenous administration of acyclovir. A 2 g total dose of oral acyclovir given during a 24-hour period produced a mean concentration of 3.26 μM in 17 adult cataract patients (31). This concentration was 37% of the simultaneously measured plasma levels. Intravitreal concentrations of 8.8–11.0 μM result from intravenous acyclovir dosages of 5 mg/kg 3 times a day (BJ Chinnock and HH Balfour Jr, unpublished observations).

Table 2   *Mean plasma acyclovir levels in adult patients with normal renal function**

Acyclovir dosage	Mean plasma levels (μM)	
	Peak	Trough
Intravenous		
5 mg/kg × 3 daily	34.7	4.2
10 mg/kg × 3 daily	73.1	7.0
Oral		
200 mg × 5 daily	2.5	1.3
400 mg × 5 daily	4.6	2.8
800 mg × 4–5 daily	7.8	3.0

*   Compiled from the literature and our own laboratory.

ADVERSE EFFECTS AND DRUG INTERACTIONS

Preclinical toxicology studies in cell cultures and animals predicted that acyclovir would be a relatively safe drug (32). This prediction was substantiated by clinical trials (33). Side-effects have been associated almost exclusively with the intravenous formulation. The only major adverse effect has been deposition of acyclovir in the kidneys of patients whose hydration and/or renal function are inadequate (34).

The maximum solubility of acyclovir in urine is 1.7 mg/ml at 37°C. When this concentration is exceeded, drug may crystalize in the renal collecting system. Deposition of acyclovir in the kidney due to inadequate hydration can be avoided by assuring that patients receive 1 liter of fluid for every gram of intravenously administered drug.

Nausea, vomiting and abdominal pain have been reported and probably are a direct toxic effect of acyclovir on the gastrointestinal tract (35). Skipping the next dose and reducing subsequent doses eliminates this side-effect.

When the intravenous formulation is reconstituted, its pH is approximately 11.0. Therefore, concentrated solutions are caustic and vesicular lesions have resulted from subcutaneous infiltration (36). Such reactions can be avoided by infusing acyclovir at a concentration no greater than 6 mg/ml through an intact intravenous line. Hypersensitivity reactions, typically transient maculopapular rashes that may erupt near infusion sites, have occurred in fewer than 1% of drug recipients.

Central nervous system toxicity is rare and has been documented mainly in bone marrow transplant recipients who had received other drugs known to affect the central nervous system, such as intrathecal methotrexate (37). Transient elevation of liver enzyme concentrations has been associated with acyclovir in some trials (38).

Patients with primary genital HSV infections treated with acyclovir had lower type-specific neutralizing antibody titers and a narrower pattern of antibody responses to viral polypeptides compared with untreated controls (39). Since the recurrence rate of genital herpes appears to be unchanged after cessation of acyclovir therapy (40), this diminished immune response to HSV probably has little or no clinical significance.

Acyclovir is eliminated in part by tubular secretion via the organic acid pathway (29). It is theoretically possible that other drugs such as the penicillins and cephalosporins, which are excreted by the same pathway, could compete with acyclovir and decrease its clearance. Conversely, acyclovir could diminish the renal clearance of drugs, such as methotrexate, that are principally eliminated by renal tubular secretion through the organic acid pathway.

CLINICAL USES

Acyclovir is currently the best drug for treatment of herpes group viral infections. My recommendations for use of the drug according to disease category follow.

Herpes simplex virus

Genital herpes   Acyclovir is an effective treatment for initial (41) and recurrent episodes of genital herpes (42). In addition, the drug can be used to suppress frequent recurrences (43, 44). The safe duration of suppressive therapy is currently under investigation. The U.S. Food and Drug Administration has approved continuous use of oral acyclovir for as long as 6 months, and a recent study indicated that the drug was safe and effective for at least 1 year (45). Intravenous acyclovir is indicated for treating patients with genital herpes who are ill enough to require hospitalization. For the remainder, oral acyclovir is the drug of choice. Topical acyclovir should be used only on external lesions because the vehicle, polyethylene glycol, is irritating to mucous membranes. Treatment during the primary episode will not prevent subsequent recurrences and, thus, acyclovir is not a cure for genital herpes.

Not every patient with genital herpes needs treatment. All patients with first episodes of genital herpes will benefit from intravenous or oral therapy. Patients whose recurrences have a sufficient medical or emotional impact to impair work or school activities should be treated.

Patients who have 6 or more recurrences per year are candidates for suppressive therapy. Acyclovir apparently does not influence the rate of recurrence once therapy is concluded (40). However, the natural history of genital herpes usually is that recurrences become less frequent and less severe with time. Therefore, it is worthwhile to prescribe acyclovir for 6 months and then discontinue it. If the patient has reached the period in the natural disease course when recurrences become infrequent, suppressive therapy will not have to be reinstituted.

Oral herpes In placebo-controlled trials, immunocompromised patients with mucocutaneous HSV lesions benefited significantly from both intravenous and topical acyclovir (46, 47). Intravenous and oral acyclovir also have been shown to suppress reactivation of oral HSV infections in bone-marrow allograft recipients (48, 49) and renal transplant patients (50). Otherwise normal patients with herpes labialis treated with acyclovir ointment experienced a significant diminution in quantity of virus cultured from lesions compared with their placebo counterparts, but rates of healing were not significantly improved (51). Nevertheless, patient-initiated therapy using oral drug may be worthwhile, especially for those who have severe recurrences. Children hospitalized because of primary herpes gingivostomatitis most likely would benefit from a short course of intravenous acyclovir. A placebo-controlled trial of acyclovir pediatric suspension for this disease is underway.

Herpes keratitis An ophthalmic ointment containing 3% acyclovir in a petrolatum base has been proved effective for herpes keratitis (52). This preparation is available in the United Kingdom but has not yet been licensed in the United States. Although efficacy against herpes keratitis is proved, topical acyclovir may not control deep stromal disease. Such patients might require oral or intravenous therapy that will provide drug concentrations in the aqueous humor greatly in excess of the ID_{50} for HSV Type 1 and Type 2 strains (31).

Herpetic whitlow Controlled trials of acyclovir therapy for herpetic whitlow have not been conducted. One case-report hints that suppressive therapy may benefit patients who have frequent recurrences (53).

Eczema herpeticum A descriptive paper on the use of intravenous acyclovir in 3 patients with eczema herpeticum has been published (54) and other anecdotal case-reports exist, but controlled trials have not been published.

Herpes encephalitis Skoldenberg et al (38) and Whitley et al (55) recently reported that intravenous acyclovir was superior to vidarabine for treatment of HSV encephalitis. Acyclovir recipients had significantly less morbidity and mortality than their vidarabine-treated counterparts. Therefore, acyclovir is the drug of choice for treatment of this serious, frequently debilitating, condition.

Neonatal herpes A multicenter controlled trial of intravenous acyclovir versus vidarabine for neonatal herpes concluded that morbidity of this disease remained high no matter which drug was given. Neither antiviral agent was a clear-cut winner, but acyclovir was associated with fewer side-effects (RS Whitley, personal communication).

Varicella-zoster virus

Varicella in immunocompromised patients   Intravenous acyclovir prevented development of pneumonitis in immunocompromised children with varicella (56). However, acyclovir should be given shortly after onset of rash to be most effective (57). Children with lymphoproliferative diseases, congenital or acquired immunodeficiencies, and organ transplant recipients should be offered acyclovir therapy as soon as possible after onset of varicella. It is unclear whether otherwise normal adults with chickenpox should be treated. I recommend intravenous acyclovir treatment for those adults who have clinical evidence of visceral varicella.

Herpes zoster in immunocompromised patients   Acyclovir halted progression of acute herpes zoster in a randomized placebo-controlled, double-blind, multicenter trial involving immunocompromised hosts (58). Acyclovir was most effective when given during the first 3 days of rash, but also significantly prevented complications of zoster for patients whose rash was more than 3 days old when acyclovir therapy was initiated. In a comparative trial by Shepp et al (59), intravenous acyclovir offered significantly greater benefit than vidarabine for treatment of early acute herpes zoster in leukemia patients, most of whom had received bone marrow allografts. The study by Shepp and colleagues combined with the information that vidarabine occasionally produces irreversible neurotoxicity (60) support my view that acyclovir is clearly superior to vidarabine for treatment of VZV infections in immunocompromised patients.

Herpes zoster in otherwise normal adults   Intravenous acyclovir shortened the duration of acute pain and accelerated healing in acute herpes zoster, but the incidence of postherpetic neuralgia was not reduced significantly (61). Because of adverse effects associated with outpatient administration in otherwise normal adults with zoster (35), intravenous acyclovir generally should not be given to outpatients. Controlled trials of oral acyclovir therapy in the United Kingdom have been published (62) and placebo-controlled U.S. trials have just concluded. Four grams of oral acyclovir taken daily for 10 days accelerated skin healing and clearance of virus from vesicles (63). The effect of therapy on incidence and severity of postherpetic neuralgia is being analyzed.

A study of 71 otherwise normal adults with herpes zoster ophthalmicus treated with either 600 mg oral acyclovir 5 times daily or placebo for 10 days has recently been published (64). Acyclovir recipients experienced a significant reduction in incidence and severity of the most common complications of herpes zoster ophthalmicus: dendritiform keratopathy, stromal keratitis, and uveitis. However, acyclovir therapy was not associated with a significant reduction in the incidence or intensity of postherpetic neuralgia.

Epstein-Barr virus

Infectious mononucleosis   The role of acyclovir for treatment of EBV disease in otherwise normal patients remains uncertain. Both intravenous and oral acyclovir have been studied for treatment of infectious mononucleosis. A trial of intravenous acyclovir (10 mg/kg 8 hourly for 7 days) performed in 31 Swedish adolescents and young adults showed that the drug significantly inhibited oropharyngeal shedding of EBV during treatment (64). However, a significant therapeutic effect could not be demonstrated unless multiple clinical parameters, such as duration of fever, weight loss, tonsillar swelling, and laryngitis, were combined.

Schooley et al (66) have described 2 patients with chronic EBV infections characterized by fever and interstitial pneumonitis. Both of these previously healthy young women appeared to benefit from relatively long-term acyclovir therapy, although one of the patients ultimately succumbed to complications of her EBV infection.

In conclusion, the role of acyclovir for treatment of EBV syndromes at the present time remains enigmatic. For diseases in which EBV replication is continuing unchecked, acyclovir therapy may be warranted. On the other hand, if the clinical manifestations result from EBV-induced immunologic aberrations, acyclovir will probably be of little benefit.

EBV-induced lymphoproliferative syndromes   EBV evokes an uncommon lymphoproliferative syndrome after transplantation which initially expresses itself as a polyclonal B-cell proliferation that may deteriorate into a disseminated, monoclonal malignancy. An uncontrolled study of 19 patients suggested that four appeared to respond to intravenous acyclovir (67). Clinical disease improved and markers of EBV infection such as oropharyngeal viral shedding and presence of EBV antigens in biopsy specimens disappeared during therapy. Since that experience was uncontrolled, the precise role of acyclovir in EBV-induced lymphoproliferative syndromes remains controversial (68).

Cytomegalovirus

CMV disease in immunocompromised hosts   Acyclovir has not been effective for treatment of CMV pneumonia in bone-marrow transplant patients (69). In a placebo-controlled, randomized, double-blind trial involving 16 immunocompromised patients, 11 of whom were renal transplant recipients, 1 week of intravenous acyclovir (500 mg/m^2/t.i.d.) significantly shortened the duration of fever and time to clinical improvement (70). Unfortunately, a second trial in renal transplant patients using 2 weeks of intravenous drug (500 mg.m^2/t.i.d.) was not associated with clinical or virologic improvement (71). Acyclovir appears at best only marginally effective for treatment of established CMV disease.

Suppression of reactivation CMV syndromes   Meyers et al (72) have just reported that a 35-day course of intravenous acyclovir (500 mg/m^2 every 8 hours) reduced the likelihood and severity of CMV infections after bone marrow transplantation among patients who were CMV-seropositive pre-transplantion. Patients were placed on acyclovir or followed as controls beginning 5 days before transplantion. Although peak levels of acyclovir achieved by this dosage were not always above the ID$_{50}$ of clinical isolates, relatively less acyclovir may be needed to halt CMV replication in the early stage of viral reactivation. Because some patients developed CMV disease after the 35-day protocol ended, additional studies are in progress to evaluate the efficacy of a longer course of acyclovir in seropositive marrow allograft recipients.

Congenital CMV infections   Plotkin et al (73) demonstrated a transient diminution in viruria in infants with congenital CMV, but urinary excretion returned to baseline levels after acyclovir was discontinued. There is no basis for using acyclovir to treat congenital CMV infections at the present time.

Infections due to viruses other than the herpes group

Preliminary experience with acyclovir in chronic hepatitis B infection has not been encouraging (74). A recent paper reported that a combination of α-interferon and intravenous acyclovir reduced serum concentrations of hepatitis B virus DNA polymerase and HBeAg (75). Controlled trials in chronic hepatitis B infections will be required to substantiate this finding. Conflicting data exist on the role of topical acyclovir in management of warts (76).

Acyclovir alone is not effective in vitro against HIV, the cause of the acquired immunodeficiency syndrome (AIDS). However, Mitsuya et al (77) have published provocative data indicating that 40 or 80 μM acyclovir combined with 3 μM zidovudine provided greater survival for HIV-infected T-cells (clone ATH8) than did either of these antiviral drugs when used alone (77). Such experiments provide a rational basis for clinical trials utilizing the combination of acyclovir and zidovudine to try to halt progression from HIV-seropositivity to full-blown AIDS.

DOSING

Ointment

Acyclovir ointment should be applied to external lesions 6 times a day for a period of 7–10 days for initial episodes of genital herpes and for 5 days for recurrent genital herpes. Immunocompromised patients with external mucocutaneous HSV should apply ointment 6 times daily until lesions are crusted, which usually occurs within 2 weeks. Because efficacy has not been proven for herpes labialis in normal patients, the number of applications per day and duration of therapy are empiric and at the discretion of the prescribing physician.

Acyclovir capsules

For initial episodes of genital herpes the recommended dose is one 200 mg capsule 5 times a day for 10 days. The same dose should be prescribed for 5 days for recurrent genital herpes. For suppressive therapy of genital herpes, one capsule 3 times a day for a period not longer than 6 months is recommended. Many patients with recurrent genital herpes can be successfully managed on 2 capsules per day. Dosage has not been established for herpes labialis as efficacy of the oral drug for that condition has not been proven. If oral drug is used to treat herpes zoster, the recommended adult dose is 800 mg 4–5 times daily for 10 days.

Intravenous acyclovir

This formulation ordinarily should be used only in hospitalized patients. Immunocompromised patients with mucocutaneous HSV and otherwise normal patients with initial genital herpes should be treated with 5 mg/kg infused over 1 hour 3 times a day for a period of 5–10 days. Patients with impaired or changing renal function should have their dose adjusted downward as indicated in the package insert. A typical 6-hour hemodialysis run will remove about 60% of the acyclovir administered. However, neither peritoneal dialysis nor exchange transfusions remove any appreciable amount of drug (78).

Patients who have less sensitive HSV isolates may require doses between 7.5 and 10 mg/kg 3 times daily. Patients with HSV encephalitis should be treated with 10 mg/kg 3 times a day for 10 days. Infants with neonatal herpes should receive 10 mg/kg 8-hourly for 10–14 days. Patients with VZV infections should receive 7.5 mg/kg 8-hourly for a least 5 days.

Any patient receiving more than 5 mg/kg/dose should have serum creatinine checked daily. If serum creatinine steadily rises, the dose should be adjusted downward. Patients with changing renal function should have plasma or serum samples tested for acyclovir levels if possible (79).

ACYCLOVIR DERIVATIVES

The structural formulae of 2 promising acyclovir derivatives are shown in Figure 2. Ganciclovir (also known as 'DHPG') is potentially useful for treatment of EBV and CMV diseases. Large amounts of ganciclovir triphosphate are formed in CMV-infected cells as compared with acyclovir (9) and, therefore, active drug is available to inhibit CMV DNA polymerase. Our clinical isolates of CMV have an ID_{50} of 2.50 $\pm$ 1.27 (SD) (80). The human pharmacokinetics in CMV-infected patients have been described (81). Preliminary uncontrolled compassionate-plea trials of ganciclovir for treatment of cytomegalovirus pneumonia in bone-marrow allograft recipients and in patients with AIDS have shown an antiviral effect without much clinical benefit (82). CMV retinitis in AIDS patients appears to respond

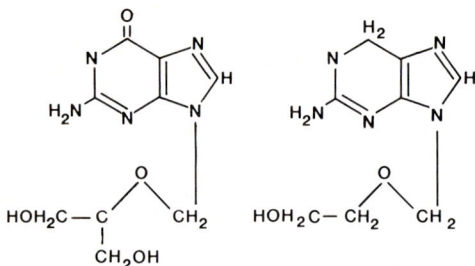

Fig. 2 Structural formulae of ganciclovir (DHPG) on the left and desciclovir on the right.

better (83, 84). An exciting prospect is the use of intravitreal ganciclovir for treatment of CMV retinitis in patients who cannot tolerate intravenous administration (85). Ganciclovir has significant toxicities in laboratory animals, including testicular atrophy in dogs and rats. The major adverse effect in clinical trials has been neutropenia that appears to be dose-related. When neutropenia develops and the drug is stopped, several weeks may elapse before the bone marrow recovers.

Another potentially valuable acyclovir-derivative is desciclovir. This compound is rapidly metabolized to acyclovir by xanthine oxidase in the intestinal tract and liver. Peak plasma concentrations are very similar to those achieved with intravenous acyclovir (86). Desciclovir may prove to be a better drug than its parent for treating infections due to EBV and possibly VZV, which are not as sensitive as HSV to acyclovir. A sustained-release formulation is now ready for clinical investigation.

Just as bacterial infections are frequently treated with combinations of antibiotics, a combination of antiviral agents, especially with different mechanisms of action, is worth investigating. A multi-drug approach might provide a greater therapeutic benefit than a single drug, especially in immunocompromised patients whose limited immune defenses cannot cope even with low levels of viral replication.

REFERENCES

1. Schaeffer HJ, Beauchamp L, De Miranda P et al (1978) 9-(2-Hydroxyethoxymethyl)-guanine activity against viruses of the herpes group. *Nature (London)*, *272*, 583.
2. Elion GB, Furman PA, Fyfe JA et al (1977) Selectivity of action of an antiherpetic agent, 9-(2-hydroxyethoxymethyl)guanine. *Proc. Natl Acad. Sci. USA*, *74*, 5716.
3. Schaeffer HJ (1982) Acyclovir chemistry and spectrum of activity. *Am. J. Med.*, *73(1A)*, 4.
4. Miller WH, Miller RL (1980) Phosphorylation of acyclovir (acycloguanosine) monophosphate by GMP kinase. *J. Biol. Chem.*, *255*, 7204.
5. Derse D, Cheng Y-C, Furman PA et al (1981) Inhibition of purified human and herpes simplex virus-induced DNA polymerases by 9-(2-hydroxyethoxymethyl)guanine triphosphate. *J. Biol. Chem.*, *255*, 11447.

6. Furman PA, St Clair MH, Spector T (1984) Acyclovir triphosphate is a suicide inactivator of the herpes simplex virus DNA polymerase. *J. Biol. Chem., 259,* 9575.

7. Datta AK, Colby BM, Shaw JE, Pagano JS (1980) Acyclovir inhibition of Epstein-Barr virus replication. *Proc. Natl Acad. Sci. USA, 77,* 5163.

8. Colby BM, Shaw JE, Elion GB, Pagano JS (1980) Effect of acyclovir [9-(2-hydroxy-ethoxymethyl)guanine] on Epstein-Barr virus DNA replication. *J. Virol., 34,* 560.

9. Biror KK, Stanat SC, Sorrell JB et al (1985) Metabolic activation of the nucleoside analog 9-[(2-hydroxy-1-(hydroxymethyl)ethoxy)methyl] guanine in human diploid fibroblasts infected with human cytomegalovirus. *Proc. Natl Acad. Sci. USA, 82,* 2473.

10. Coen DM, Schaffer PA, Furman PA et al (1982) Biochemical and genetic analysis of acyclovir-resistant mutants of herpes simplex virus type 1. *Am. J. Med., 73(1A),* 351.

11. Balfour Jr HH (1983) Resistance of herpes simplex to acyclovir. *Ann. Intern. Med., 98,* 404.

12. Larder BA, Darby G (1984) Virus drug-resistance: mechanisms and consequences. *Antiviral Res., 4,* 1.

13. Sibrack CD, Gutman LT, Wilfert CM et al (1982) Pathogenicity of acyclovir-resistant herpes simplex virus type 1 from an immunodeficient child. *J. Infect. Dis., 146,* 673.

14. Darby G, Field HJ, Salisbury SA (1981) Altered substrate specificity of herpes simplex virus thymidine kinase confers acyclovir-resistance. *Nature (London), 289,* 81.

15. Coen DM, Schaffer PA (1980) Two distinct loci confer resistance to acycloguanosine in herpes simplex virus type 1. *Proc. Natl Acad. Sci. USA, 77,* 2265.

16. Schnipper LE, Crumpacker CS (1980) Resistance of herpes simplex virus to acycloguanosine: role of viral thymidine kinase and DNA polymerase loci. *Proc. Natl Acad. Sci. USA, 77,* 2270.

17. Field HJ, Coen DM (1986) Pathogenicity of herpes simplex virus mutants containing drug resistance mutations in the viral DNA polymerase gene. *J. Virol., 60,* 286.

18. Dekker C, Ellis MN, McLaren C et al (1983) Virus resistance in clinical practice. *Antimicrob. Chemother., 12, Suppl B,* 137.

19. Biron KK, Fyfe JA, Noblin JE, Elion GB (1982) Selection and preliminary characterization of acyclovir-resistant mutants of varicella zoster virus. *Am. J. Med., 73(1A),* 383.

20. Cole NL, Balfour Jr HH (1986) Varicella-zoster virus does not become more resistant to acyclovir during therapy. *J. Infect. Dis., 153,* 605.

21. Van Dyke RB, Connor JD, Wyborny C et al (1982) Pharmacokinetics of orally administered acyclovir in patients with herpes progenitalis. *Am. J. Med., 73(1A),* 172.

22. De Miranda P, Krasny HC, Page DA, Elion GB (1981) The disposition of acyclovir in different species. *J. Pharmacol. Exp. Ther., 219,* 309.

23. De Miranda P, Krasny HC, Page DA, Elion GB (1982) Species differences in the disposition of acyclovir. *Am. J. Med., 73(1A),* 31.

24. Laskin OL, Longstreth JA, Saral R et al (1982) Pharmacokinetics and tolerance of acyclovir, a new antiherpes virus agent, in humans. *Antimicrob. Agents Chemother., 21,* 393.

25. Blum MR, Liao SHT, De Miranda P (1982) Overview of acyclovir pharmacokinetic disposition in adults and childen. *Am. J. Med., 73(1A)* 186.

26. De Miranda P, Whitley RJ, Blum MR et al (1979) Acyclovir kinetics after intravenous infusion. *Clin. Pharmacol. Ther., 26,* 718.

27. De Miranda P, Good SS, Laskin OL et al (1981) Disposition of intravenous radioactive acyclovir. *Clin. Pharmacol. Ther., 30,* 662.

28. Laskin OL, De Miranda P, King DH et al (1982) Effects of probenecid on the pharmacokinetics and elimination of acyclovir in humans. *Antimicrob. Agents Chemother., 21*, 804.

29. Laskin OL (1983) Clinical pharmacokinetics of acyclovir. *Clin. Pharmacokinet., 8*, 187.

30. Hintz M, Connor JD, Spector SA et al (1982) Neonatal acyclovir pharmacokinetics in patients with herpes virus infections. *Am. J. Med., 73(1A)*, 210.

31. Hung SO, Patterson A, Rees PJ (1984) Pharmacokinetics of oral acyclovir (Zovirax) in the eye. *Br. J. Ophthalmol., 68*, 192.

32. Tucker Jr WE, Macklin AW, Szot RJ et al (1983) Preclinical toxicology studies with acyclovir: acute and subchronic tests. *Fundam. Appl. Toxicol., 3*, 573.

33. Balfour Jr HH (1986) Acyclovir therapy for herpes zoster: advantages and adverse effects. *J. Am. Med. Assoc., 255*, 387.

34. Brigden D, Rosling AE, Woods NC (1982) Renal function after acyclovir intravenous injection. *Am. J. Med., 73(1A)*, 182.

35. Bean B, Aeppli D (1985) Adverse effects of high-dose intravenous acyclovir in ambulatory patients with acute herpes zoster. *J. Infect. Dis., 151*, 362.

36. Sylvester RK, Ogden WB, Draxler CA, Lewis FB (1986) Vesicular eruption: a local complication of concentrated acyclovir infusions. *J. Am. Med. Assoc., 255*, 385.

37. Wade JC, Meyers JD (1983) Neurologic symptoms associated with parenteral acyclovir treatment after marrow transplantation. *Ann. Intern. Med., 98*, 921.

38. Skoldenberg B, Forsgren M, Alestig K et al (1984) Acyclovir versus vidarabine in herpes simplex encephalitis. *Lancet, 2*, 707.

39. Bernstein DI, Lovett MA, Bryson YJ (1984) The effects of acyclovir on antibody response to herpes simplex virus in primary genital herpetic infections. *J. Infect. Dis., 150*, 7.

40. Mertz GJ, Critchlow CW, Benedetti J et al (1984) Double-blind placebo-controlled trial of oral acyclovir in first-episode genital herpes simplex virus infection. *J. Am. Med. Assoc., 252*, 1147.

41. Bryson YJ, Dillon M, Lovett M et al (1983) Treatment of first episodes of genital herpes simplex virus infection with oral acyclovir. *N. Engl. J. Med., 308*, 916.

42. Reichman RC, Badger GJ, Mertz GJ et al (1984) Treatment of recurrent genital herpes simplex infections with oral acyclovir: a controlled trial. *J. Am. Med. Assoc., 251*, 2103.

43. Straus SE, Takiff HE, Seidlin M et al (1984) Suppression of frequently recurring genital herpes: a placebo-controlled double-blind trial of oral acyclovir. *N. Engl. J. Med., 310*, 1545.

44. Douglas JM, Critchlow C, Benedetti J et al (1984) A double-blind study of oral acyclovir for suppression of recurrences of genital herpes simplex virus infection. *N. Engl. J. Med., 310*, 1551.

45. Mertz GJ, Eron L, Davis LG et al (1986) Suppression of frequently recurring genital herpes with oral acyclovir (ACV): long-term efficacy and toxicity. In: *Abstracts, 26th Interscience Conference on Antimicrobial Agents and Chemotherapy, New Orleans, 1986*, p 312. American Society for Microbiology, Washington, DC.

46. Meyers JD, Wade JC, Mitchell CD et al (1982) Multicenter collaborative trial of intravenous acyclovir for treatment of mucocutaneous herpes simplex virus infection in the immunocompromised host. *Am. J. Med., 73(1A)*, 229.

47. Whitley RJ, Levin M, Barton N et al (1984) Infections caused by herpes simplex virus

in the immunocompromised host: natural history and topical acyclovir therapy. *J. Infect. Dis., 150*, 323.

48. Saral R, Burns WH, Laskin OL et al (1981) Acyclovir prophylaxis of herpes simplex virus infections: a randomized, double-blind, controlled trial in bone marrow transplant recipients. *N. Engl. J. Med., 305*, 63.

49. Gluckman E, Lotsberg J, Devergie A et al (1983) Prophylaxis of herpes infections after bone marrow transplantation by oral acyclovir. *Lancet, 2*, 706.

50. Seale L, Jones CJ, Kathpalia S et al (1985) Prevention of herpesvirus infections in renal allograft recipients by low-dose oral acyclovir. *J. Am. Med. Assoc., 254*, 3435.

51. Spruance SL, Schnipper LE, Overall Jr JC et al (1982) Treatment of herpes simplex labialis with topical acyclovir in polyethylene glycol. *J. Infect. Dis., 146*, 85.

52. Jones BR, Coster DJ, Fison PN et al (1979) Efficacy of acycloguanosine (Wellcome 248U) against herpes simplex corneal ulcers. *Lancet, 1*, 243.

53. Laskin OL (1985) Acyclovir and suppression of frequently recurring herpetic whitlow. *Ann. Intern. Med., 102*, 494.

54. Swart RNJ, Vermeer BJ, Van der Meer JWM et al (1983) Treatment of eczema herpeticum with acyclovir. *Arch. Dermatol., 119*, 13.

55. Whitley RJ, Alford CA, Hirsch MS et al (1986) Vidarabine versus acyclovir therapy in herpes simplex encephalitis. *N. Engl. J. Med., 314*, 144.

56. Prober CG, Kirk LE, Keeney RE (1982) Acyclovir therapy of chickenpox in immunosuppressed children: a collaborative study. *J. Pediatr., 101*, 622.

57. Balfour Jr HH (1984) Intravenous acyclovir therapy for varicella in immunocompromised children. *J. Pediatr., 104*, 134.

58. Balfour Jr HH, Bean B, Laskin OL et al (1983) Acyclovir halts progression of herpes zoster in immunocompromised patients. *N. Engl. J. Med., 308*, 1448.

59. Shepp DA, Dandliker PS, Meyers JD (1986) Treatment of varicella-zoster virus infection in severely immunocompromised patients: a randomized comparison of acyclovir and vidarabine. *N. Engl. J. Med., 314*, 208.

60. Feldman S, Robertson PK, Lott L et al (1986) Neurotoxicity due to adenine arabinoside therapy during varicella-zoster virus infections in immunocompromised children. *J. Infect. Dis., 154*, 889.

61. Bean B, Braun C, Balfour Jr HH (1982) Acyclovir therapy for acute herpes zoster. *Lancet, 2*, 118.

62. McKendrick MW, McGill JI, Bell AM et al (1984) Oral acyclovir for herpes zoster. *Lancet, 2*, 925.

63. Bean B, Aeppli D, Huff JC et al (1986) Oral acyclovir for acute herpes zoster. *Clin. Res., 34*, 512A.

64. Cobo LM, Foulks GN, Liesegang T et al (1986) Oral acyclovir in the treatment of acute herpes zoster ophthalmicus. *Ophthalmology, 93*, 763.

65. Andersson J, Britton S, Ernberg I et al (1986) Effect of acyclovir on infectious mononucleosis: a double-blind, placebo-controlled study. *J. Infect. Dis., 153*, 283.

66. Schooley RT, Carey RW, Miller G et al (1986) Chronic Epstein-Barr virus infection associated with fever and interstitial pneumonitis. *Ann. Intern. Med., 104*, 636.

67. Hanto DW, Gajl-Peczalska KJ, Frizzera G et al (1983) Epstein-Barr virus (EBV) induced polyclonal and monoclonal B-cell lymphoproliferative diseases occurring after renal transplantation: clinical, pathologic and virologic findings and implications for therapy. *Ann. Surg., 198*, 356.

68. Sullivan JL, Medveczky P, Forman SJ et al (1984) Epstein-Barr virus induced lympho-

proliferation: implications for antiviral chemotherapy. *N. Engl. J. Med., 311*, 1163.

69. Wade JC, Hintz M, McGuffin RW et al (1982) Treatment of cytomegalovirus pneumonia with high-dose acyclovir. *Am. J. Med., 73(1A)*, 249.

70. Balfour Jr HH, Bean B, Mitchell CD et al (1982) Acyclovir in immunocompromised patients with cytomegalovirus disease: a controlled trial at one institution. *Am. J. Med., 73(1A)*, 241.

71. Balfour Jr HH (1985) Prevention and treatment of cytomegalovirus disease. In: Balfour Jr HH (Ed), *Advances in Therapy Against Herpesvirus Infections in Immunocompromised Hosts: Proceedings of a Symposium Conducted by the University of Minnesota*, p 35. University of Minnesota, Minneapolis, MN.

72. Meyers JD, Reed EC, Shepp DH et al (1986) Prevention of cytomegalovirus (CMV) infection after marrow transplant (MTx) with high-dose intravenous acyclovir (ACV). In: *Abstracts, 26th Interscience Conference on Antimicrobial Agents and Chemotherapy, New Orleans, 1986*, p 231. American Society for Microbiology, Washington, DC.

73. Plotkin SA, Starr SE, Bryan CK (1982) In vitro and in vivo responses of cytomegalovirus to acyclovir. *Am. J. Med., 73(1A)*, 257.

74. Smith CI, Scullar GH, Gregory PB et al (1982) Preliminary studies of acyclovir in chronic hepatitis B. *Am. J. Med., 73(1A)*, 267.

75. Schalm SW, Heytink RA, Van Buuren HR, DeMan RA (1985) Acyclovir enhances the antiviral effect of interferon in chronic hepatitis B. *Lancet, 2*, 358.

76. Hurwitz RM (1984) Verrucae vulgares and acyclovir ointment. *Cutis, 34*, 84.

77. Mitsuya H, Matsukura M, Broder S (1987) Rapid in vitro systems for assessing activity of agents against HTLV-III/LAV. In: Broder S (Ed), *AIDS: Modern Concepts and Therapeutic Challenges*, p 303. Marcel Dekker, Inc., New York.

78. Englund JA, Fletcher CV, Johnson D et al (1987) Effect of blood exchange on acyclovir clearance in an infant with neonatal herpes. *J. Pediatr., 110*, 151.

79. Chinnock BJ, Vicary CA, Brundage DM et al (1987) Serum is an acceptable specimen for measuring acyclovir levels. *Diagn. Microbiol. Infect. Dis., 6*, 73.

80. Cole NL, Balfour Jr HH (1987) In-vitro susceptibility of cytomegalovirus isolates from immunocompromised patients to acyclovir and ganciclovir. *Diagn. Microbiol. Infect. Dis., 6*, 255.

81. Fletcher C, Sawchuk R, Chinnock B et al (1986) Human pharmacokinetics of the antiviral drug DHPG. *Clin. Pharmacol. Ther., 40*, 281.

82. Shepp DH, Dandliker PS, De Miranda P et al (1985) Activity of 9-[2-hydroxy-1-(hydroxymethyl)ethoxymethyl]guanine in the treatment of cytomegalovirus pneumonia. *Ann. Intern. Med., 103*, 368.

83. Felsenstein D, D'Amico DJ, Hirsch MS et al (1985) Treatment of cytomegalovirus retinitis with 9-[2-hydroxy-1-(hydroxymethyl)ethoxymethyl]guanine. *Ann. Intern. Med., 103*, 377.

84. Bach MC, Bagwell SP, Knapp NP et al (1985) 9-(1,3-Dihydroxy-2-propoxymethyl)-guanine for cytomegalovirus infections in patients with the acquired immunodeficiency syndrome. *Ann. Intern. Med., 103*, 381.

85. Henry K, Cantrill H, Fletcher C et al (1987) Use of intravitreal ganciclovir (dihydroxy propoxymethyl guanine) for cytomegalovirus retinitis in a patient with AIDS. *Am. J. Ophthalmol., 103*, 17.

86. Selby P, Powles RL, Blake S et al (1984) Amino(hydroxyethoxymethyl)purine: a new well-absorbed prodrug of acyclovir. *Lancet, 2*, 1428.

CHAPTER 33

Amantadine and rimantadine

RAPHAEL DOLIN

Since the publication of *Antimicrobial Agents Annual/2*, additional information
has been generated regarding the mechanism of action and pharmacokinetics of
rimantadine. In addition, further clinical experience has been obtained in the use
of rimantadine in children and in the elderly. As of this writing, an application
for licensure for rimantadine in the United States has been submitted and is under
review by the Food and Drug Administration. The U.S. Public Health Service has
continued to recommend the use of amantadine for the prophylaxis and therapy
of influenza A in selected settings. As part of these recommendations, it has also
advised reduction of the dosage of amantadine in the elderly and in other situations where renal dysfunction may be present. Additional experience with the efficacy of lower doses of amantadine has also been obtained recently. These and
other developments are discussed below.

Amantadine (1-adamantanamine hydrochloride) and rimantadine (α-methyl-1-
adamantanemethylamine hydrochloride) are primary symmetrical amines with an
unusual 'bird-cage like' structure as illustrated in Figures 1 and 2. The structure
for the parent compound, adamantane, was first suggested by Decker in the 1920s,

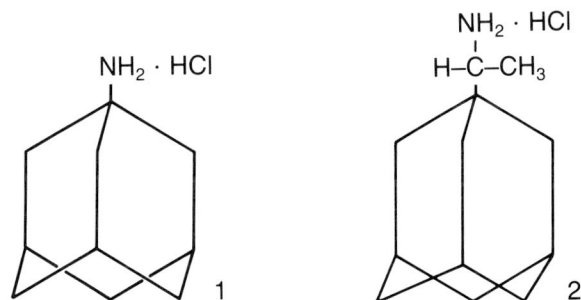

Fig. 1   Amantadine (1-adamantanamine hydrochloride).

Fig. 2   Rimantadine (α-methyl-1-adamantanemethylamine hydrochloride).

Antimicrobial Agents Annual 3
P.K. Peterson and J. Verhoef, editors
© Elsevier Science Publishers BV, 1988

who was seeking compounds with symmetrical arrays of carbon atoms, similar to those found in naturally occurring diamonds. The compound was subsequently isolated from petroleum found in Czechoslovakia, and was named 'adamantane', after the Greek word for diamond or firmness. Processes for synthesizing adamantane were developed in the 1950s, and an amino substituted compound, amantadine, was demonstrated by Davies and colleagues at DuPont Laboratories to be active against influenza A virus in vitro in 1965 (1). Despite study of many analogous compounds with substitutions in the amino group, only rimantadine has achieved clinical utility, particularly in the Soviet Union where it is used extensively for the treatment and prophylaxis of influenza A infection (2).

ACTIVITY

In practical terms, both amantadine and rimantadine are active only against influenza A virus, although some activity in vitro has been demonstrated against parainfluenza and rubella viruses, but at concentrations of 50–100 times that required for inhibition of influenza A virus (3). All subtypes of influenza A virus which have been tested have been sensitive to amantadine and rimantadine, generally at levels of 0.2–0.4 μg/ml. Although the results of in vitro sensitivity testing vary greatly depending on the techniques which are employed, rimantadine has been found to be somewhat more active than amantadine in vitro against certain influenza A virus strains (4).

The precise mechanism of activity of amantadine and rimantadine is not known on a molecular level. These compounds inhibit influenza A virus replication after attachment of the virus to the cell, most likely at a step related to uncoating of the virus and perhaps at a later step, as well. Recent studies have indicated that resistance to amantadine and rimantadine is associated with an alteration in the transmembrane portion of the M2 protein, and that single amino acid substitutions at a critical site can confer resistance (5, 6). These and other data suggest that the mechanism of action of these compounds is mediated through interaction with the M2 protein, or perhaps also through interactions between the M2 protein and the hemagglutinin. Relatively few studies of naturally occurring resistant viruses have been carried out, although occasional resistant viruses have been noted in outbreaks of influenza A where amantadine or rimantadine have not been used (7). Recently, rimantadine-resistant viruses were detected in children who had been treated with rimantadine, but the effect of the emergence of resistant virus on outcome of illness was not clear (8). Additional studies are required to determine the precise frequency and import of the emergence of viruses resistant to these compounds.

CLINICAL PHARMACOLOGY

Although the antiviral activities of the two compounds are similar, amantadine and rimantadine differ markedly in their pharmacokinetic properties (9, 10). Both compounds are available only as oral formulations. Amantadine is well absorbed after oral administration, and reaches peak levels of approximately 0.5 μg/ml, 2–4 hours after a 200 mg dose. Amantadine is not metabolized, has a serum half-life of 14 hours, and is excreted by the kidney, with 95% of a dose appearing unchanged in the urine. Amantadine has a large volume of distribution, and little is removed by hemodialysis. Penetration into pulmonary tissue appears to be extensive, and concentrations in respiratory secretions are approximately two-thirds of those in the serum.

Rimantadine is also well absorbed orally, and peak levels occur 3–8 hours after a 200 mg dose and are approximately half of those of amantadine (0.3 μg/ml). The drug is extensively metabolized to ortho-, para- and meta-hydroxylated metabolites, approximately 80% of which are excreted in the urine (11). The antiviral activity or toxic potential of these metabolites is currently unknown. The half-life of rimantadine is considerably longer than that of amantadine, being approximately 30 hours. Despite the lower blood levels of rimantadine, the drug is well concentrated in respiratory secretions, with levels that approach or exceed those found in the serum (9). Thus, rimantadine is concentrated in respiratory secretions to a greater extent than is amantadine. Rimantadine also has a large volume of distribution and little drug is removed by hemodialysis.

ADVERSE EFFECTS AND DRUG INTERACTIONS

The major toxicities of amantadine are central nervous system (CNS) side effects, probably related to its 'dopamine potentiating properties', upon which its use in Parkinson disease depends. These side effects consist largely of jitteriness, anxiety, insomnia, difficulty in concentrating, and rarely hallucinations. Such CNS side effects are generally mild and promptly reversible upon cessation of the drug. Although CNS side effects are generally dose-related and have been observed more frequently at higher plasma levels of the drug, there is a broad overlap between the levels at which toxic effects are present or absent, and thus CNS toxicity cannot be predicted directly from serum levels alone. On occasion, amantadine has also been associated with seizures with extremely high plasma levels of the compound. A variety of other side effects have also been reported, including worsening of congestive heart failure, livedo reticularis, and arrhythmias, but their causal relationship to amantadine is not established.

Although rimantadine has been less extensively studied than amantadine, the compound appears to be an exceedingly well tolerated. In a large-scale comparative study carried out in young adults in which the drugs were administered at a dose of 200 mg/d for 6 weeks, amantadine was associated with a frequency of

CNS side effects of 11%, while side effects in rimantadine recipients were no more frequent than those observed in the concurrent placebo group (Table 1) (12). In a smaller study which attempted to correlate side effects with blood levels of amantadine or rimantadine, the authors concluded that the potential for CNS toxicity was similar for either drug at similar blood levels, though no precise blood level of either drug was predictive for toxicity (9). Other observers have noted that extraordinarily high blood levels of rimantadine, even in elderly subjects with cerebrovascular dysfunction, have not been associated with CNS toxicity (13). Thus, the precise basis for the relative lack of toxicity of rimantadine remains unsettled.

Rimantadine and amantadine both have cholinergic effects and should be used cautiously, if at all, in the presence of anticholinergic drugs. Because of the potential for CNS toxicity, many clinicians avoid the use of these compounds when major tranquilizers or antidepressants are being employed as well. Rimantadine has also been reported to cause mild gastrointestinal disturbances after administration.

CLINICAL USES

Amantadine and rimantadine have been demonstrated to be effective in the prophylaxis and therapy of influenza A infections in both experimentally induced and naturally occurring influenza A infections in man in a wide variety of settings. The majority of studies of prophylaxis have demonstrated a reduction of influenza-like illness associated with influenza A infection of 50–91% (12, 14–16). In a recently conducted study in which the efficacies of rimantadine and amantadine in the pro-

Table 1 *Withdrawal rates among recipients of placebo, rimantadine and amantadine*

Treatment group (no. of subjects)	With-drawals	Reasons for withdrawal			
		CNS side-effects[*]	Non-CNS side-effects	Unrelated to side-effects	Unknown
		(no. of subjects (%))			
Placebo(148)	16(11)	6(4)	1(0.7)	8(5)	1(0.7)
Rimantadine(147)	14(10)	9(6)	1(0.7)	4(3)	0(0)
Amantadine(145)	32(22)[**]	19(13)[***]	4(3)	3(2)	6(4)

[*] Primarily insomnia, 'jitteriness', and difficulty in concentrating.
[**] $P < 0.01$ as compared with the placebo, and $P < 0.005$ as compared with rimantadine, by chi-square analysis.
[***] $P < 0.01$ as compared with placebo and $P < 0.05$ as compared with rimantadine.
Reprinted from Dolin et al (12) by courtesy of the Editors of *New England Journal of Medicine*.

phylaxis of influenza A were compared during an outbreak of influenza A/H1N1 and H3N2, both drugs were equally efficacious (Table 2) (12). Both drugs have been more effective in reduction of illness than in reduction of infection with influenza A virus, which is a potentially desirable feature of chemoprophylaxis, since subclinical infection may result in immunity (12, 16). Recently, Clover et al (17) studied the prophylaxis of influenza with rimantadine in a family setting (17). Children received rimantadine or placebo for 5 weeks after an outbreak of influenza A was recognized in the community. As noted in Table 3, all of the influenza A associated illnesses occurred in placebo recipients. The rates of influenza A infection and illness in untreated adults in families where the children received rimantadine also appeared to be reduced, although the reduction did not reach statistical significance. The majority of studies of prophylaxis have been carried out in healthy young adults, and to a lesser extent in children. Limited information is available concerning the prophylactic use of these compounds in individuals at 'high risk' for complications of influenza, although a recent study carried out in elderly nursing-home residents suggests that rimantadine is effective and safe in this setting as well (13).

Amantadine and rimantadine have also been demonstrated to be efficacious in the therapy of influenza A infections (14, 15). Controlled studies have been carried out almost exclusively in mild, self-limited disease in young adults or in normal children. The majority of such studies have shown a modest, but statistically significant effect when amantadine or rimantadine was compared to placebo. In a

Table 2 *Influenza-like illness: laboratory-documented influenza, and infection with influenza A virus among volunteers receiving placebo, rimantadine, or amantadine*

Treatment group (no. of subjects)	No. with laboratory-documented influenza[*]	No. infected with influenza A virus[**]
Placebo(132)	27(21%)	32(24%)
Rimantadine(133)	4(3%)[***]	11(8%)[***]
efficacy rate(%)[+]	85	66
Amantadine(113)	2(2%)[***]	7(6%)[***]
efficacy rate(%)[+]	91	74

[*] Defined as influenza-like illness along with virus isolation or a rise in serum antibody to influenza A virus.

[**] Defined as influenza A virus isolation or a rise in serum antibody to influenza A virus, irrespective of the presence of illness.

[***] P < 0.001 as compared with placebo by chi-square analysis.

[+] Efficacy rate as calculated by the expression:

$$\frac{\text{Rate in placebo recipients} - \text{Rate in rimantadine/amantadine recipients}}{\text{Rate in placebo recipients}} \times 100$$

Reprinted from Dolin et al (12) by courtesy of the Editors of *New England Journal of Medicine*.

Table 3   *Frequency of infection and clinical illness caused by influenza A (H1N1) virus in families in which children received rimantadine or placebo*

Drug	Children			Adults		
	No.	No.(%) infected*	No.(%) ill**	No.	No.(%) infected***	No.(%) ill
Placebo	41	13(13.7)	7 (17.0)	36	7(19.0)	1(2.9)
Rimantadine hydrochloride	35	13(31.7)	0(0.0)	34	3(8.8)	0(0.0)

* P=0.001. ** P=0.01. *** P=0.2.
Reprinted from Clover et al (17) by courtesy of the Editors of *American Journal of Diseases of Children.*

study comparing the therapeutic efficacies of the two drugs (Fig. 3), rimantadine and amantadine reduced the duration of signs and symptoms of illness by approximately 50% (18). A study by Younkin et al (19) indicated that amantadine was superior to aspirin in reducing the duration and severity of symptoms of influenza, although aspirin was more effective in reduction of fever. Two recent studies have compared the efficacy of rimantadine with that of acetaminophen in the treatment of uncomplicated influenza A infection in young children. In a study of an A/ H3N2 outbreak by Hall et al (8), children who received rimantadine showed significantly greater improvement in fever, as well as in severity of illness, compared to those who received acetaminophen (Fig. 2). In a study during an A/H1N1 outbreak by Thompson et al (20), rimantadine and acetaminophen had equivalent clinical effects on illness in children. In this latter study, relatively milder illness was observed, compared to the A/H3N2 outbreak discussed earlier, and this may have accounted for the difference in results according to the authors. Controlled studies of the efficacy of either amantadine or rimantadine in the therapy of influenza in 'high risk' subjects or in the therapy of established complications of influenza (e.g., pneumonia) have either not been carried out or have not been reported in detail. This represents a significant deficiency in our knowledge of the utility of these compounds. In the United States, National Institutes of Health (NIH) supported collaborative studies of rimantadine in these latter settings are currently underway.

Amantadine is licensed for the prophylaxis and therapy of influenza A infections in the United States and in the United Kingdom, but it has received relatively little use for these purposes. Rimantadine is being used widely in the Soviet Union and licensure for the drug is under review in the United States. Amantadine and rimantadine have been the subjects of an NIH consensus conference (21), and were also considered by the Immunization Practices Advisory Committee of the U.S. Public Health Service, as potential control measures for influenza (22). From

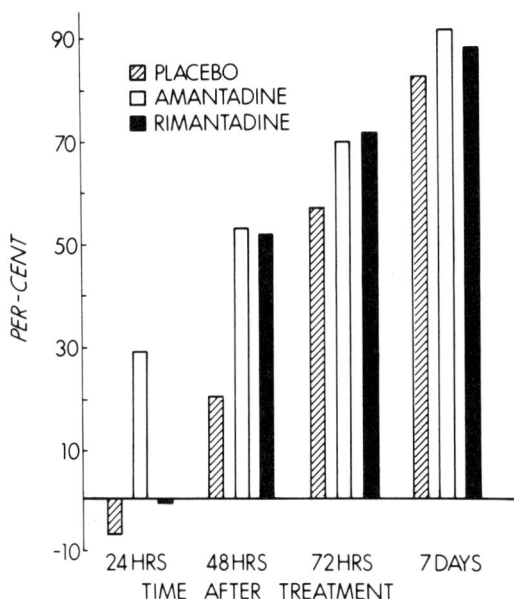

Fig. 3 Percent improvement in subjects with acute influenza A who received 200 mg of amantadine, rimantadine or placebo for 5 days. Reproduced from Van Voris et al (18) by courtesy of American Medical Association.

these and other sources, a number of recommendations regarding the use of these compounds has emerged. First, since amantadine and rimantadine are active only against influenza A viruses, it is clear that the rational use of these compounds requires that influenza A infection be present in the community, as detected by laboratory and/or epidemiologic surveillance. Once influenza A is present, prophylaxis may be considered for both adults and children at high risk for the development of serious influenza infections, particularly for those who have not received vaccine, or when the vaccine may be relatively ineffective because of major antigenic changes in the circulating virus. If an effective vaccine is available and an influenza A outbreak is underway, prophylaxis with amantadine may be begun simultaneously with vaccine administration, since amantadine is not known to interfere with antibody responses to inactivated influenza A vaccine and may thus confer protection until an immune response develops. Chemoprophylaxis with amantadine may also be considered for patients who are expected to have poor antibody responses to vaccination, such as those with immune deficiencies.

Prophylaxis may be indicated for unimmunized individuals who care for, or are in close contact with, high-risk individuals. Prophylaxis may also be considered for individuals whose activities are vital to community function and who have not been vaccinated, such as selected hospital personnel, policemen, firemen etc. Chemoprophylaxis may also be employed in those rare 'high risk' individuals with genuine hypersensitivity to influenza vaccine or to egg proteins, in whom influenza vaccination cannot be employed. Evidence also exists that prophylactic use of amantadine or rimantadine is effective during nosocomial outbreaks of influenza, or in families when an index case is first noted, and use of these compounds in those settings should be considered.

Therapy with amantadine or rimantadine has been recommended for acute influenza A in patients at high risk for the development of serious and/or complicated disease (22), although, as outlined above, the efficacy of the drug has not been demonstrated in that setting. Similarly, many physicians employ amantadine or rimantadine in the treatment of established complications of influenza such as pneumonia, although its effect on such complications is also not known. In the general population, influenza is ordinarily a self-limited illness, and the potential benefits of treatment must be weighed against other considerations such as cost, potential toxicity etc., on an individual basis for each patient. Since it is likely that the majority of cases of influenza in otherwise healthy individuals will not necessarily require treatment, therapy may be reserved for individuals who perform critical functions in the community and for whom a reduction of signs and symptoms of 24 hours may be important. Therapy may also be considered when particularly severe illness is noted in an otherwise normal individual. To be effective, therapy should be begun early, generally within 24–48 hours of the onset of illness, and should be continued until 48 hours after the resolution of signs and symptoms.

DOSING

The recommended dosage of amantadine or rimantadine for individuals above the age of 9, is 200 mg/d given once per day or in 2 divided doses. Individuals between 1 and 9 years of age should receive 4.4–8.8 mg/kg/d, not to exceed 150 mg/d. The use in children under 1 year of age has not been adequately evaluated. Because amantadine is excreted primarily by the kidney, the dosage should be reduced in the presence of renal failure, according to previously published guidelines (23). Because of concern for CNS toxicity, the U.S. Public Health Service has recommended that the dose of amantadine be lowered to 100 mg/d in elderly subjects (22), although the efficacy of this regimen has not been rigorously established in that patient population. Two recent studies have suggested that amantadine 100 mg/d was effective in the prophylaxis of influenza A in vaccinated English schoolboys (24) and in experimentally induced infection in normal volunteers (25). Investigators in the Soviet Union have suggested that lower doses of rimantadine (< 200 mg/d) may also be efficacious, but such lower doses have received little study elsewhere. Metabolites of rimantadine are also excreted by the kidney, and will likely accumulate in the presence of renal failure. Although the toxic potential of these metabolites is unknown, it would appear to be prudent to reduce the dose of rimantadine in the presence of significant renal dysfunction. Precise guidelines for dose reduction in renal failure are not yet available.

FUTURE DIRECTIONS

Additional information regarding the pharmacokinetics of amantadine, and particularly of rimantadine and its metabolites, is expected to be forthcoming in the near future. These studies should help to refine dosage regimens with these compounds. Controlled observations of the safety and efficacy of these compounds in individuals at high risk for complications of influenza are sorely needed, and large-scale trials to address this question are planned in the United States. Prospective studies to determine the frequency and significance of the emergence of virus resistant to these compounds are also planned. It is likely that studies of combinations of antiviral therapy involving amantadine or rimantadine and other anti-influenza compounds will also be carried out in the future.

REFERENCES

1. Davies WL, Grunert RR, Haff RR et al (1964) Antiviral activity of 1-adamantan-amine (amantadine). *Science, 144*, 862.
2. Zlydnikov DM, Kubar OI, Kovaleva TP et al (1981) Study of rimantadine in the USSR: a review of the literature. *Rev. Infect. Dis., 3*, 408.
3. Hoffmann CE (1973) Amantadine HCl and related compounds. In: Carter WA (Ed), *Selective Inhibitors of Viral Function*, p 199. CRC Press, Cleveland, OH.
4. Hayden FG, Cote KM, Douglas Jr RG (1980) Plaque inhibition assay for drug susceptibility testing of influenza viruses. *Antimicrob. Agents Chemother., 17*, 865.
5. Hay AJ, Wolstenholme AJ, Skehel JJ, Smith MH (1985) The molecular basis of the specific anti-influenza action of amantadine. *EMBO J., 4*, 3021.
6. Belshe RB, Hay AJ, Skehel JJ, Hall CB, Betts R (1987) The genetic basis of resistance to rimantadine emerging during treatment of influenza. In: *Abstracts, 7th International Congress of Virology, 1987*, p 217. National Research Council of Canada, Edmonton.
7. Heider H, Adamczyk B, Presber HW et al (1981) Occurrence of amantadine and rimantadine resistant influenza A virus strains during the 1980 epidemic. *Acta Virol., 25*, 395.
8. Hall CB, Dolin R, Gala CL et al (1987) Treatment of children with influenza A infection with rimantadine. *Pediatrics, 80*, 275.
9. Hayden FG, Hoffman HE, Spyker DA (1983) Differences in side effects of amantadine hydrochloride and rimantadine hydrochloride relate to differences in pharmacokinetics. *Antimicrob. Agents Chemother., 23*, 458.
10. Hayden FG, Hoffman HE (1987) Comparative single dose pharmacokinetics of amantadine HCl and rimantadine HCl in young and elderly adults. *Antimicrob. Agents Chemother., 28*, 216.
11. Wills RJ (1987) Clinical pharmacokinetics of rimantadine: a preliminary review. *J. Respir. Dis., 8*, 539.
12. Dolin R, Reichman RC, Madore HP et al (1982) A controlled trial of amantadine and rimantadine in the prophylaxis of influenza A infection. *N. Engl. J. Med., 307*, 580.
13. Dolin R, Betts RF, Treanor JJ et al (1983) Rimantadine prophylaxis in the elderly. In: *Program and Abstracts, 23rd Interscience Conference on Antimicrobial Agents and*

Chemotherapy, Las Vegas, 1983, Abstract no. 691. American Society for Microbiology, Washington, DC.

14. Couch RB, Jackson GG (1976) Antiviral agents in influenza – Summary of Influenza Workshop. VIII. *J. Infect. Dis., 134,* 516.

15. LaMontagne JR, Galasso GJ (1978) Report of a workshop on clinical studies of the efficacy of amantadine and rimantadine against influenza virus. *J. Infect. Dis., 138,* 928.

16. Monto AS, Gunn RA, Bandyk MG et al (1979) Prevention of Russian influenza by amantadine. *J. Am. Med. Assoc., 241,* 1003.

17. Clover RD, Crawford SA, Abell TD et al (1986) Effectiveness of rimantadine prophylaxis of children within families. *Am. J. Dis. Child., 140,* 706.

18. VanVoris LP, Betts RF, Hayden FG et al (1981) Successful treatment of naturally occurring influenza A/USSR/77 H1N1. *J. Am. Med. Assoc., 245,* 1128.

19. Younkin SW, Betts RF, Roth FK, Douglas Jr RG (1983) Reduction in fever and symptoms in young adults with influenza A/Brazil/78 H1N1 infection after treatment with aspirin or amantadine. *Antimicrob. Agents Chemother., 23,* 577.

20. Thompson J, Fleet W, Lawrence et al (1984) Comparison of acetaminophen and rimantadine in the treatment of influenza A infections in children. *J.Med. Virol., 21,* 249.

21. National Institutes of Health Consensus Development Symposium (1980) Amantadine: Does it have a role in the prevention and treatment of influenza? *Ann. Intern. Med., 92,* 256.

22. Anonymous (1987) Prevention and control of influenza. *Morbid. Mortal. Wkly Rep., 36,* 373.

23. Anonymous (1987) Prevention and control of influenza. *Morbid. Mortal. Wkly Rep., 33,* 253.

24. Payler DK, Purdham PA (1984) Influenza A prophylaxis with amantadine in a boarding school. *Lancet, 1,* 502.

25. Sear SD, Clements ML (1987) Protective efficacy of low dose amantadine in adults challenged with wild-type influenza A virus. *Antimicrob. Agents Chemother.,* accepted for publication.

CHAPTER 34

Interferons

KEVAN L. HARTSHORN and MARTIN S. HIRSCH

Since the publication of *Annual 2* no new information on the interferons has appeared in the literature and the discussion which follows continues to represent a current perspective regarding these agents.

Despite increasing evidence that interferons are important in natural host defenses and have potent broad-spectrum antiviral activity, their clinical future as prophylactic or therapeutic agents remains clouded. This Chapter will focus on recent developments in basic and clinical interferon research.

Interferons-α, and -β are produced principally by leukocytes and fibroblasts respectively after exposure to viruses, double-stranded RNA (dsRNA) and other stimuli. They have a common cellular receptor, extensive homology and probably a similar mechanism of action. Interferon-γ is produced mainly by lymphocytes in response to mitogenic or antigenic stimuli, has a separate receptor and has distinct immunomodulatory functions. All 3 interferons are now produced by recombinant techniques and are available in large quantity. Clinical trials in neoplastic diseases with interferon-α and increasingly with interferon-γ have proceeded at a more rapid pace than trials in viral infections, expanding our knowledge of the pharmacology and toxicity of these agents. Nevertheless, a significant potential role for interferon-α has now been defined in the prophylaxis of rhinovirus colds and potential roles in hepatitis B and papillomavirus infections are emerging.

The application of molecular biology to the study of interferon regulation and action has yielded insights which will be reviewed although their clinical significance is as yet unclear.

ACTIVITY

Mechanism of action

Interferons can induce antiviral, immunomodulatory and antiproliferative effects. The antiviral effects are believed to result largely from induction of various proteins in cells exposed to interferon. The best characterized of these proteins are

Antimicrobial Agents Annual 3
P.K. Peterson and J. Verhoef, editors
© Elsevier Science Publishers BV, 1988

the 2′,5′-oligoadenylate synthetase (2′,5′-An-synthetase) and a protein complex which phosphorylates peptide-chain initiating factor. The former leads to breakdown of viral RNAs and the latter to inhibition of viral protein formation. Detailed accounts of these pathways are available (1, 2). The antiviral effects of interferon may be exerted through other mechanisms as well. For instance, retrovirus replication is inhibited at the stage of assembly and release of viral particles (3). This effect may be mediated by interferon-induced cell membrane alterations. In this section, recent insights into the genetic mechanisms of interferon production and action will be reviewed, followed by a discussion of recent research on the mechanisms of the interferons' immunomodulatory and antiproliferative effects.

The means by which interferon production is controlled in the cell has been the subject of recent research. Regulatory sites adjacent to the interferon-β gene (4) and an interferon-α gene (5) have been identified. These cause increased transcription of the interferon genes (or even of unrelated genes placed next to them by recombinant techniques) (6) in the presence of virus or dsRNA. It has long been observed that exposing a cell to a small dose of interferon leads to enhancement of subsequent interferon production in response to virus. This is termed 'priming'. Increased transcription of the interferon gene has been shown to underlie this priming process (7).

Interferon produced and released from the cell or exogenously administered binds to specific membrane receptors and the interferon-receptor complex is then internalized and degraded in lysosomes. Recent evidence indicates that this degradation may be important in leading to antiviral effects (8). Within 30–60 minutes of the cell's exposure to interferon-α (9) or -β (10), the transcription of certain genes is markedly enhanced. For interferon-α, some of these genes have been identified (e.g. those coding for Class I HLA antigens). Interferon-γ does not induce the same genes as interferon-β in these studies. A separate study (11) has identified a gene induced in large amounts by interferon-γ but only minimally by interferon-β, coding for a protein homologous to platelet factor 4 and γ-thromboglobulin. These latter proteins are involved in inflammatory responses.

Interferons have various effects on the host immune system. They can increase antibody production and natural killer-cell activity and enhance recognition of virally infected or malignant cells by the immune system. All of the interferons lead to increases in Class I HLA antigen expression on the cell surface. This effect is evident in tumorigenic cells transformed by adenovirus Type 12 (12). Mice injected with these cells and treated with interferon have a reduced incidence of tumors (13). Hence it is possible that increased Class I HLA antigen expression facilitates immune recognition and destruction of virus-infected cells. Interferon-α also causes increased susceptibility of Burkitt lymphoma cells to complement by unclear mechanisms (14).

Interferon-γ has several distinctive immunomodulatory effects. It induces Class II HLA antigen expression in various cells. This may be important in facilitating T-cell-mediated immunity as suggested by recent studies (15, 16). It also plays a special role in the activation of macrophages. This effect is mediated by protein kinase C (17) and entails enhanced oxidative metabolism and antimicrobial activi-ty (18). In a murine in-vivo model, this effect has been shown to be critical to reso-lution of *Listeria* infection (19). The replication of a wide range of intracellular pathogens may be controlled by this mechanism.

Interferon-γ also augments antibody production through effects on helper T-cells and B-cells directly (20). It has also been shown to increase receptors for tu-mor necrosis factor leading to enhancement of tumor cell destruction by this solu-ble factor (21).

The mechanisms by which interferons exert antiproliferative effects on cells are becoming clear. Interferons have inhibitory effects on the expression of cellular oncogenes (22). Increased expression of the *c-myc* gene is probably involved in initiating cell division. The expression of the *c-myc* gene in Daudi cells is decreased by interferons-α and -β, most likely at the post-transcriptional level (23–25). This may occur through breakdown of *c-myc* mRNA by 2,5'-synthetase. The inhibitory effect of interferon-β on several oncogenes is also apparent in transfection assays (26).

Evidence is mounting that a complex interplay exists between peptide growth factors (especially platelet-derived growth factor or PDGF) and interferons in the normal control of cell growth (27). PDGF causes increased expression of the *c-myc* and *c-fos* genes and leads to cell division. Interferons-α and -β inhibit this pro-cess when added along with PDGF in vitro (28). Paradoxically PDGF also indu-ces the expression of the interferon-β and 2',5'-An-synthetase genes in a slightly delayed manner. This may provide a natural check on cell division.

Spectrum of activity

Interferons-α and -β have activity against a broad range of viruses (see below in clinical uses). Interferon-γ has antiviral activity and is important in host immunity against intracellular parasites and bacteria as well. The immunomodulatory and cell-growth regulatory effects of interferons may lead to clinical effects which are hard to predict on the basis of in-vitro antiviral testing.

Resistance mechanisms

Antibodies to interferon have been reported to develop after, and rarely before, treatment with exogenous preparations. The clinical importance of these is not yet clear, although loss of antitumor effects coincident with the development of anti-bodies has been noted (29).

PHARMACOKINETICS

Interferon-α can be administered intravenously, intramuscularly, intrathecally, in-tralesionally, as a nasal spray, or as topical cream. In most clinical situations interferons-α and -β are given intramuscularly. Previous and recent trials have provided ample data on the pharmacokinetics of leukocyte-derived and recombinant interferon-α given in this way (30–33). Peak serum levels of 15–50 U/ml for a 3 × 10^6 dose and several hundred to 2000 U/ml for a 50 × 10^6 U dose are reported. Serum half-life (t$^1/_2$) is 6–8 hours. On daily dosing, accumulation is minimal until doses of 50 × 10^6 U are reached. Penetration into cerebrospinal fluid is minimal even with intravenous doses. Degradation is believed to occur largely in the kidney, although uremic patients do not show drug accumulation (34). No major differences have been noted between the biological effects of various recombinant and non-recombinant preparations in these studies.

Recently, useful clinical data on the pharmacology of recombinant interferon-γ have been reported (35–37). Administered intravenously, it has a short t$^1/_2$ (25–35 min), leading to use of continuous infusions in recent trials. The t$^1/_2$ for intramuscular administration is 4–6 hours. Interferon activity is difficult to determine by bioassay after intramuscular (but not after intravenous) dosing, but can be measured by enzyme-linked immunosorbent assay. Intramuscular and intravenous administration lead to similar biological effects. Recent studies have begun to refer to doses in milligrams rather than antiviral units since recombinant preparations are assumed to be essentially pure. A specific activity for the preparation (i.e. antiviral units per mg protein) is generally given.

ADVERSE EFFECTS AND DRUG INTERACTIONS

Adverse effects

Extensive clinical trials in cancer patients continue to expand our knowledge of the toxicity of interferons in various doses and schedules. An excellent current review is available (29).

The nearly universal acute flu-like syndrome appears to be more severe after intravenous or intrathecal therapy and in older patients. Although this effect usually wanes with continued daily treatment, it may persist with intermittent therapy or therapy with interferon-γ. Persistent fatigue has been noted to be the most important dose-limiting side-effect of interferon therapy. There is evidence that this form of toxicity may be associated with frontal lobe abnormalities as detected by neuropsychiatric tests (38). Peripheral neuropathy can occur during interferon therapy and may be more profound when prior damage or other neurotoxic medications (e.g. *Vinca* alkaloids) are also used (39).

A study of bone marrow morphology before and after interferon treatment suggests that the mild neutropenia seen with interferon-α therapy is due to a reversible block in release of mature myeloid cells from the marrow (40). Another study of marrow granulocyte-macrophage colony formation, however, showed decreased colony formation following treatment (41). The kinetics of the neutropenia (i.e. rapid but moderate fall and rapid increase once treatment is stopped) support the notion that a reversible block in release of granulocytes is more important.

Mild anemia and thrombocytopenia on a non-immune basis are common after prolonged treatment. Recently, 2 patients with autoimmune hemolytic anemia and 5 patients with immune thrombocytopenia (42) probably secondary to interferon treatment have been described.

While proteinuria (in rare cases resulting in nephrotic syndrome) has been described with interferon-α therapy, no evidence of glomerular or tubular defects based on albumin and β_2-microglobulin excretion was noted in a recent study (43).

Three cases of hypothyroidism occurred among 13 patients with breast cancer receiving leukocyte-derived interferon-α (44). The mechanisms of this thyroid dysfunction are unclear.

Recent trials with interferon-γ (i.v. and i.m.) indicate that fever, chills, fatigue and myalgias also complicate therapy with this preparation (35–37). Elevated liver function tests and neutropenia also occur. Clinical trials with interferon inducers (synthetic dsRNA) have shown similar toxicity (45).

Drug interactions

A potentiation of radiation-induced mucositis was noted in 2 patients with epidemic Kaposi's sarcoma treated concomitantly with interferon-γ (46). Synergistic antiproliferative effects of interferon-α with either interferon-γ or cimetidine occur in vitro (47). Clinical trials combining interferon-α and cimetidine do not consistently show greater antitumor effects or toxicity (48).

CLINICAL USES

Respiratory viruses

Intranasal interferon-α has been shown to be effective in preventing rhinovirus-induced colds when given prophylactically to family members of an index case (49, 50). Two double-blind, placebo-controlled studies using 5×10^6 U/d for 7 days, starting within 48 hours of the development of cold symptoms in the index case, showed remarkably similar benefits. Rhinovirus-related illness was reduced by approximately 80% and respiratory illness in general was reduced by approximately 40%. Nasal bleeding was slightly increased in interferon recipients but did not detract substantially from symptomatic benefit. Unfortunately, respiratory illnesses induced by other viruses (with the possible exception of herpes viruses) was not significantly reduced in either study. Previous evidence of some efficacy of intranasal interferon against experimentally induced influenza A (51) and coronaviruses (52) was not confirmed. Higher interferon doses, treatment of the index case to reduce viral shedding, or prophylactic use in families during rhinoviral seasons may further increase efficacy (53). However, another study (54) demonstrates that prolonged prophylactic use (28 days in this case) in a work setting is associated with sufficient nasal side-effects to outweigh benefit. This was true despite use of a relatively low dose of 2×10^6 U/d. Thus, unless less-toxic regimens are developed, the use of topical interferons for prophylaxis of colds may be very limited.

Herpes viruses

Herpes simplex virus (HSV)   Interferons have potent activity against HSV in vitro. Herpetic keratitis has been treated with interferon with some benefit. Application of interferon continuously in low doses using therapeutic contact lenses may enhance the efficacy of such treatment (55).

Reactivation of perioral HSV lesions was noted in 7 of 19 patients receiving interferon as part of a treatment trial in chronic lymphocytic leukemia (56). This may have been secondary to interferon-induced fever. A previous trial with lower interferon doses showed inhibition of HSV reactivation after trigeminal nerve surgery (57).

Combinations of interferon with other agents are potentially promising. In-vitro and murine in-vivo data demonstrate synergistic inhibition of HSV by interferon in combination with acyclovir (58, 59). This combination has shown enhanced activity compared to acyclovir alone in the treatment of herpetic keratitis in man (60). Synergy against HSV is also noted for the combination of interferon and nonoxynol 9 in vitro (61). This combination may be of value in topical treatment of HSV infections.

Epstein-Barr virus (EBV)   Recombinant interferons-α, -β and -γ inhibit in-vitro infection of B-cells with EBV (62). This supports prior data showing activity of leukocyte-derived interferon in this context (63) and further shows a strong enhancement of viral inhibition for the combination of interferons-α and -γ. Endogenous interferon may also play a role in the resolution of acute mononucleosis due to EBV (64).

Of most clinical importance is whether interferons would benefit immunocompromised patients at risk for EBV reactivation. Among acquired immunodeficiency syndrome (AIDS) patients, EBV reactivation probably plays a role in lymphoproliferative disorders (65). EBV shedding is decreased in renal transplant recipients receiving interferon-α (66). Defective interferon-γ production has been noted in AIDS patients (67). In rheumatoid arthritis patients, defective interferon-γ production is associated with impaired cell-mediated immunity to EBV (68). Whether or not these data indicate that interferon-α or -γ therapy will prevent EBV-induced disease in immunocompromised patients is unclear. The relative importance of interferons *per se*, antiviral antibody, natural killer cells, and specific T-cell cytotoxicity in control of EBV replication in vivo has not been elucidated.

Cytomegalus virus (CMV)   Although treatment of established CMV infections with interferon has been of litle benefit, prophylactic trials in renal transplant recipients have shown significant protection (69).

Varicella zoster virus   Previous trials have shown that interferon-α confers substantial clinical benefit in immunosuppressed patients who develop varicella or herpes zoster (70, 71).

Hepatitis B virus

A group of chronic carriers of hepatitis B had a substantially greater fall in viral DNA polymerase and HBeAg levels when treated with a combination of interferon-α and acyclovir than when treated with either drug alone (72). Among 12 patients enrolled, 6 had persistent suppression of these markers of viral replication after single drug therapy (4 acyclovir, 2 interferon). Four of 5 patients who did not have a sustained response to either agent alone did so on receiving the combination. This promising early result requires confirmation in larger, controlled trials.

Comparable single-agent activity of interferon-α and a 4-week course of adenine arabinoside was seen in a randomized trial in chronic hepatitis B carriers (73). A 7- to 8-week course of adenine arabinoside resulted in diminished antiviral activity and unacceptable neurotoxicity. Acyclovir, particularly if it proves to be active in oral form against hepatitis B, may be preferable to adenine arabinoside for combination trials in hepatitis B infection.

Human papillomaviruses

A randomized trial of locally applied interferon-α cream in recurrent flat vaginal condylomatosis achieved 5 complete remissions of 8 treated patients while none of 5 placebo-treated controls responded (74). Unfortunately, histological complete remissions occurred in only 1 case, and 2 of the patients with clinical responses relapsed within 2 months of completing therapy. Interferon-α at doses of 3×10^6 U/m^2 i.m. given daily for 2 weeks, then 3 times weekly for 4–8 weeks, led to approximately 60% clinical complete responses and was well-tolerated in a similar group of patients (75). Interferon-α shows activity given intralesionally in patients with neoplasia arising in the context of epidermodysplasia verruciformis (a papillomavirus-induced condition) (76). These results support prior data indicating substantial activity of interferon-α and -β in recurrent papillomavirus-related conditions (e.g. condylomatosis or juvenile laryngeal papillomatosis). The optimal treatment regimen is yet to be established.

Retroviruses

Interferons are active against animal and human retroviruses. We have demonstrated that interferon-α and -β have in-vitro antiviral activity against human immunodeficiency virus (HIV) (77; unpublished observations). Recombinant interferon-α A (rIFNαA) synergistically inhibits HIV replication when combined with phosphonoformic acid or azidothymidine (78; in press). Multicenter clinical trials of rIFNαA in patients with AIDS are comparing patients treated with 30×10^6 U, 3×10^6 U or placebo given intramuscularly 3 times a week for 12 weeks. Results of these studies are expected during 1986. Clinical trials of interferon-α in combination with azidothymidine are planned.

Interferon-γ production is deficient in patients with AIDS and this deficiency may be predictive for disease progression among patients with AIDS-related complex (ARC) (79). In vitro, interferon-γ enhances the killing of intracellular parasites by monocytes of AIDS patients. Interleukin-2 can enhance interferon-γ production by mononuclear cells from patients with AIDS or ARC in vitro (80). A clinical trial of interferon-γ in AIDS-related Kaposi's sarcoma showed no benefit in terms of tumor size and immune parameters (81). Three of 7 patients actually appeared to have acceleration of tumor growth. Whether interferon-γ will be of value in treating other aspects of AIDS or ARC deserves further study.

Miscellaneous conditions

Six patients with subacute sclerosing panencephalitis were treated with interferon-γ given intravenously and intrathecally with only 1 patient showing slight and delayed improvement (82). Two patients with poliomyelitis demonstrated apparent clinical benefit after interferon-α treatment (83).

DOSING

The toxicity of given doses for a given duration of therapy can now be anticipated. Interferon-α given intramuscularly at 3×10^6 U daily or 3 times per week can be well tolerated for long periods. The maximally tolerated intramuscular dose is reported to be from 10 to 50×10^6 U/d. A maximally tolerated dose of interferon-γ by 6-hour infusion daily for 5 days is noted to be 10×10^6 U/d. Doses and schedules appropriate for specific viral infections are being defined.

FUTURE DIRECTIONS

Promising studies have been reported in the treatment of prophylaxis of a variety of human viral infections. Further carefully controlled clinical trials should be conducted to define dosages, routes, and length of administration in individual viral infections. Since significant numbers of patients are rarely available at single institutions, multicenter collaborative trials should be encouraged. Comparative trials between interferons and other agents (such as vidarabine and acyclovir in herpes zoster) are indicated. Combination trials in life-threatening viral infections, such as AIDS, should also be considered.

Although the history of interferon clinical studies is a frustrating one, it must be realized that we are still in the early stages of such efforts. It appears clear that important leads have been developed, requiring careful clinical follow-up in the years ahead.

REFERENCES

1. Lengyel P (1982) Biochemistry of interferons and their actions. *Am. Rev. Biochem., 51*, 251.
2. Galabru J, Hovanessian AG (1985) Two interferon-induced proteins are involved in the protein kinase complex dependent on double-stranded RNA. *Cell, 43*, 685.
3. Pitha PM, Bilello JA, Riggin CH (1982) Effect of interferon on retrovirus replication. *Texas Rep. Biol. Med., 41*, 603.
4. Goodbourn S, Zinn K, Maniatis T (1985) Human β-interferon gene expression is regulated by an inducible enhancer element. *Cell, 41*, 509.
5. Fujita T, Ohno S, Yasumitsu H, Taniguchi T (1985) Delimitation and properties of DNA sequences required for the regulated expression of human interferon-β gene. *Cell, 41*, 489.
6. Ryals J, Dierks P, Ragg H, Weissmann C (1985) A 46-nucleotide promoter segment from an IFN-α gene renders an unrelated promoter inducible by virus. *Cell, 41*, 497.
7. Nir U, Maroteaux L, Cohen B, Mory I (1985) Priming affects the transcription rate of human interferon-β gene. *J. Biol. Chem., 260*, 14242.
8. Chelbi-Alix MK, Thang MN (1985) Chloroquine impairs the interferon-induced antiviral state without affecting the 2'-5'-oligoadenylate synthetase. *J. Biol. Chem., 260*, 7960.
9. Friedman RL, Stark GR (1985) α-Interferon-induced transcription of HLA and metallothionein genes containing homologous upstream sequences. *Nature (London), 314*, 637.
10. Larner C, Janak G, Cheng YS et al (1984) Transcriptional induction of two genes in human cells by interferon. *Proc. Natl Acad. Sci. USA, 81*, 7633.
11. Luster AD, Uukeless JC, Ravetch JV (1985) Interferon γ transcriptionally regulates an early-response gene containing homology to platelet proteins. *Nature (London), 315*, 671.
12. Eager KB, Williams J, Breiding D et al (1985) Expression of histocompatibility antigens H-2K, -D, and -L is reduced in adenovirus-12-transformed mouse cells and is restored by interferon. *Proc. Natl Acad. Sci. USA, 82*, 5525.
13. Hayasaki H, Tanaka K, Jay F et al (1985) Modulation of tumorigenicity of human adenovirus-12-transformed cells by interferon. *Cell, 43*, 263.
14. Vefenof E, McConnell I (1985) Interferon amplifies complement activation of Burkitt lymphoma cells. *Nature (London), 313*, 684.
15. Preval C, Lisowska-Grospierre B, Loche M (1985) A transacting Class II regulatory gene unlinked to the MHC controls expression of HLA Class II genes. *Nature (London), 381*, 291.
16. Groenewegen G, Buurman WA, Van der Linden CJ (1985) Lymphokine dependence of in vivo expression of MHC Class II antigens by endothelium. *Nature (London), 316*, 361.
17. Hamilton TA, Becton DL, Somers SD et al (1985) Interferon γ modulates protein kinase C activity in murine peritoneal macrophages. *J. Biol. Chem., 260*, 1378.
18. Murray HW, Spitalny GL, Nathan CF (1985) Activation of mouse peritoneal macro-

phages in vitro and in vivo by interferon-*γ*. *J. Immunol.*, *134*, 1619.

19. Buchmeier NA, Schreiber RD (1985) Requirement for endogenous interferon-*γ* production for resolution of *Listeria monocytogenes* infection. *Proc. Natl Acad. Sci. USA*, *82*, 7404.

20. Frasca D, Adorini L, Landolfo S, Dorio G (1985) Enhancing effect of interferon-*γ* on helper T cell activity and IL2 production. *J. Immunol.*, *134*, 3907.

21. Aggarwal BB, Ecssalu TE, Hass PE (1985) Characterization of receptors for human tumor necrosis factor and their regulation by interferon. *Nature (London)*, *318*, 665.

22. Clemens M (1985) Interferons and oncogenes. *Nature (London)*, *313*, 531.

23. Einat M, Resnitsky D, Kimchi A (1985) Close link between reduction of *c-myc* expression by interferon and Go/G arrest. *Nature (London)*, *313*, 597.

24. Knight E, Anton ED, Fahey D et al (1985) Interferon regulates *c-myc* gene expression in Daudi cells at the post-transcriptional level. *Proc. Natl Acad. Sci. USA*, *82*, 1152.

25. Dani C, Mechti M, Piechaczyk B et al (1985) Increased rate of degradation of *c-myc* mRNA in interferon-treated Daudi cells. *Proc. Natl Acad. Sci. USA*, *82*, 4896.

26. Perucho M, Esteban M (1985) Inhibitory effect of interferon on the genetic and oncogenic transformation by viral and cellular genes. *J. Virol.*, *54*, 229.

27. Zullo JN, Cochran BH, Huang AS, Stiles CD (1985) Platelet-derived growth factor and double-stranded ribonucleic acids stimulate expression of the same genes in 3T3 cells. *Cell*, *43*, 793.

28. Einat M, Resnitsky D, Kimchi A (1985) Inhibitory effects of interferon on the expression of genes regulated by platelet-derived growth factor. *Proc. Natl Acad. Sci. USA*, *82*, 7608.

29. Quesada JR, Talpaz M, Rios A et al (1986) Clinical toxicity of interferons in cancer patients: a review. *J. Clin. Oncol.*, *4*, 234.

30. Gutterman JU, Fine S, Quesada J et al (1982) Recombinant leukocyte A interferon: pharmacokinetics, single dose tolerance, and biological effects in cancer patients. *Ann. Intern. Med.*, *98*, 598.

31. Sherwin SA, Mayer D, Ochs JJ et al (1983) A multiple dose Phase I trial of leukocyte A interferon in cancer patients. *J. Am. Med. Assoc.*, *248*, 2460.

32. Kirkwood JM, Ernstoff MS, Davis CA et al (1985) Comparison of intramuscular and intravenous recombinant alpha-2 interferon in melanoma and other cancers. *Ann. Intern. Med.*, *103*, 32.

33. Hawkins MJ, Borden EC, Merritt JA et al (1984) Comparison of the biological effects of two recombinant human interferon alpha (rA and D) in humans. *J. Clin. Oncol.*, *2*, 221.

34. Hirsch MS, Tolkoff-Rubin NE, Kelly AP, Rubin RH (1983) Pharmacokinetics of recombinant and leukocyte human interferon in patients with chronic renal failure who are undergoing hemodialysis. *J. Infect. Dis.*, *148*, 335.

35. Gutterman JN, Rosenblum MG, Rios A et al (1984) Pharmacokinetic study of partially pure *γ*-interferon in cancer patients. *Cancer Res.*, *44*, 4164.

36. Juzrock R, Rosenblum MG, Sherwin SA et al (1985) Pharmacokinetics, single dose tolerance and biological activity of recombinant interferon-*γ* in cancer patients. *Cancer Res.*, *45*, 2866.

37. Raj-Vadham S, Al-Katib A, Bhalla R et al (1986) Phase I trial of recombinant interferon gamma in cancer patients. *J. Clin. Oncol.*, *4*, 137.

38. Adams F, Quesada JR, Gutterman JU (1984) Neuropsychiatric manifestations of human leukocyte interferon therapy in patients with cancer. *J. Am. Med. Assoc.*, *252*, 938.

39. Bernsen PL, Wong-Chung RE, Janssen JT (1985) Neurologic amyotrophy and poly-radiculopathy during interferon therapy. *Lancet, 1*, 50.

40. Ernstoff M, Kirkwood J (1984) Changes in the bone marrow of cancer patients treated with recombinant interferon alpha-2. *Am. J. Med., 76*, 593.

41. Ernstoff M, Gallicchio V, Kirkwood JM (1985) Analysis of granulocyte-macrophage progenitor cells in patients treated with recombinant interferon alpha-2. *Am. J. Med., 79*, 167.

42. McLaughlin P, Talpaz M, Quesada J et al (1985) Immune thrombocytopenia following α-interferon therapy in patients with cancer. *J. Am. Med. Assoc., 254*, 1353.

43. Sumpio BE, Ernstoff MS, Kirkwood JM (1984) Urinary excretion of interferon, albumin, and β_2-microglobulin during interferon treatment. *Cancer Res., 44*, 3599.

44. Fentman IS, Thomas BS, Balkwill FR et al (1985) Primary hypothyroidism associated with interferon therapy of breast cancer. *Lancet, 1*, 1166.

45. Stevenson HC, Abrams PG, Schoenberger CS et al (1985) A Phase I evaluation of Poly (I,C)-LC in cancer patients. *J. Biol. Resp. Modif., 4*, 650.

46. Real FY, Krown SE, Nisce LZ, Oettgen HF (1985) Unexpected toxicity from radiation therapy in two patients with Kaposi's sarcoma receiving interferon. *J. Biol. Resp. Modif., 4*, 141.

47. Hirai N, Hill NO, Motoo Y, Osther K (1985) Antiviral and antiproliferative activities of human leukocyte interferon potentiated by cimetidine in vitro. *J. Interferon Res., 5*, 375.

48. Creagen ET, Ahmann DL, Green SJ et al (1985) Phase II study of recombinant leukocyte A interferon (IFN-rA) plus cimetidine in disseminated malignant melanoma. *J. Clin. Oncol., 3*, 977.

49. Douglas RM, Moore BW, Miles HB et al (1986) Prophylactic efficacy of intranasal alpha-2-interferon against rhinovirus infections in the family setting. *N. Engl. J. Med., 314*, 65.

50. Hayden FG, Albrecht JK, Kaiser DL, Gwaltney JM (1986) Prevention of natural colds by contact prophylaxis with intranasal alpha-2-interferon. *N. Engl. J. Med., 314*, 71.

51. Phillpotts RJ, Higgins PG, Willman JS et al (1984) Intranasal lymphoblastoid interferon ('Wellferon') prophylaxis against rhinovirus and influenza virus in volunteers. *J. Interferon Res., 4*, 535.

52. Higgins PG, Phillpotts RJ, Scott GM et al (1983) Intranasal interferon as protection against experimental respiratory coronavirus infection in volunteers. *Antimicrob. Agents Chemother., 24*, 713.

53. Douglas RG (1986) The common cold-relief at last? *N. Engl. J. Med., 314*, 114.

54. Douglas RM, Albrecht JK, Miles HB et al (1985) Intranasal interferon-α_2 prophylaxis of natural respiratory virus infection. *J. Infect. Dis., 151*, 731.

55. DeReccia R, DelPrete A, Benusiglio E, Orfeo V (1985) Continuous usage of low doses of human leukocyte interferon with contact lenses in herpetic kerato-conjunctivitis. *Ophthal. Res., 17*, 251.

56. Foon KA, Bottino GC, Abrams PG et al (1985) Phase II trial of recombinant leukocyte A interferon in patients with chronic lymphocytic leukemia. *Am. J. Med., 78*, 216.

57. Pazin JG, Armstrong JA, Lam MT et al (1979) Prevention of reactivated herpes simplex infection by human leukocyte interferon after operation on the trigeminal root. *N. Engl. J. Med., 301*, 225.

58. Moran DM, Kern ER, Overall JC (1985) Synergism between recombinant human in-

terferon and nucleoside antiviral agents against herpes simplex virus: examination with an automated microtiter plate assay. *J. Infect. Dis., 151,* 1116.

59. Cownell EV, Cerrati RL, Trown PW (1985) Synergistic activity of combinations of recombinant human alpha interferon and acyclovir, administered concomitantly and in sequence, against a lethal herpes simplex virus Type 1 infection in mice. *Antimicrob. Agents Chemother., 28,* 1.

60 Colin J, Chastel C, Renard G, Cantell K (1984) Combination therapy for dendritic keratitis with human leukocyte interferon and acyclovir. *Am. J. Ophthalmol., 95,* 346.

61. Rapp F, Wrzos H (1985) Synergistic effect of human leukocyte interferon and non-oxynol 9 against Herpes Simplex virus type 2. *Antimicrob. Agents Chemother., 28,,* 449.

62. Andersson JP, Andersson UG, Eruberg IT et al (1985) Effects of pure interferons on Epstein-Barr virus infection in vitro. *J. Virol., 54,* 615.

63. Garner JG, Hirsch MS, Schooley RT (1984) Prevention of Epstein-Barr virus-induced B-cell outgrowth by interferon alpha. *Infect. Immunity, 43,* 920.

64. Brewster FE, Byron KS, Sullivan JL (1985) Immunoregulation during acute infection with Epstein-Barr virus: dynamics of interferon and 2'-5'-oligoadenylate synthetase activity. *J. Infect. Dis., 151,* 1109.

65. Andiman WA, Martin K, Rubinstein A et al (1985) Opportunistic lymphoprolifera-tions associated with Epstein-Barr viral DNA in infants and children with AIDS. *Lan-cet, 2,* 1390.

66. Cheeseman SH, Henle W, Rubin RH et al (1980) Epstein-Barr virus infection in renal transplant recipients. *Ann. Intern. Med., 93,* 39.

67. Murray HW, Rubin BY, Masur H, Roberts RB (1984) Impaired production of lym-phokines and immune (gamma) interferon in the acquired immunodeficiency syn-drome. *N. Engl. J. Med., 310,* 883.

68. Hasler F, Bluestein HG, Zvaifler NJ, Epstein LB (1983) Analysis of the defects re-sponsible for the impaired regulation of Epstein-Barr virus-induced B cell prolifera-tion by rheumatoid arthritis lymphocytes. *J. Exp. Med., 157,* 173.

69. Hirsch MS, Schooley RT, Cosimi AB et al (1983) Effect of interferon-alpha on cyto-megalovirus reactivation syndromes in renal-transplant recipients. *N. Engl, J, Med. 308,* 1489.

70. Merigan TC, Rand KH, Pollard RB et al (1978) Human leukocyte interferon for the treatment of herpes zoster in patients with cancer. *N. Engl. J. Med., 298,* 981.

71. Arvin A, Kushner JH, Feldman S et al (1982) Human leukocyte interferon for the treatment of varicella in children with cancer. *N. Engl. J. Med., 306,* 761.

72. Schalm SW, Heytink RA, Van Buuren HR, DeMan RA (1985) Acyclovir enhances the antiviral effect of interferon in chronic hepatitis B. *Lancet, 2,* 358.

73. Lok AS, Novick DM, Karayiannis P et al (1985) A randomized study of the effects of adenine arabinoside 5'-monophosphate (short or long courses) and lymphoblastoid interferon on hepatitis B virus replication. *Hepatology, 5,* 1132.

74. Yesterinen E, Meyer B, Cantell K, Purola A (1984) Topical treatment of flat vaginal condyloma with human leukocyte interferon. *Obstet. Gynecol., 64,* 535.

75. Gall SA, Hughes CE, Trofatter K (1985) Interferon for the therapy of condyloma acu-minatum. *Am. J. Obstet. Gynecol., 153,* 157.

76. Lutzner A, Blanchet-Bardon C, Orth G (1984) Clinical observations, virologic studies, and treatment trials in patients with epidermodysplasia verruciformis, a disease in-duced by specific human papillomaviruses. *J. Invest. Dermatol., 83,* 18(s).

77. Ho DD, Hartshorn KL, Rota TR et al (1985) Recombinant human interferon alfa-A suppresses HTLV-III replication in vitro. *Lancet, 1*, 602.
78. Hartshorn A, Sandstrom EG, Neumeyer D et al (1986) Synergistic inhibition of human T-cell lymphotropic virus Type III replication in vitro by phosphonoformate and recombinant alfa-A interferon. *Antimicrob. Agents Chemother., 30*, 189.
79. Murray HW, Hillman JK, Rubin BY et al (1985) Patients at risk for AIDS-related opportunistic infections. *N. Engl. J. Med., 313*, 1504.
80. Murray HW, Welte K, Jacobs JL et al (1985) Production of an in vitro response to interleukin-2 in the acquired immunodeficiency syndrome. *J. Clin. Invest., 76*, 1959.
81. Krigel RI, Odajuyk CM, Laubenstein LJ et al (1985) Therapeutic trial of interferon-γ in patients with epidemic Kaposi's sarcoma. *J. Biol. Resp. Modif., 4*, 358.
82. Bye A, Balkwill F, Brigden D, Wilson J (1985) Use of interferon in the management of patients with subacute sclerosing panencephalitis. *Dev. Med. Child Neurol., 27*, 170.
83. Levin S (1985) Interferon treatment of poliomyelitis. *J. Infect. Dis., 151*, 745.

CHAPTER 35
Ribavirin

CAROLINE BREESE HALL

Although ribavirin made its debut into the antiviral world a decade and a half ago, its potential clinical use has only recently been recognized. Ribavirin appears to be singular in its broad spectrum of activity, its lack of toxicity, and its failure to induce viral resistance. Recent scientific and public attention has centered on its use in treating patients with respiratory syncytial virus (RSV) infections, influenza and Lassa fever, and its potential use in the treatment of patients with acquired immunodeficiency syndrome (AIDS) (1–9). Approval of the drug in the United States only came in December 1985 for treatment by the aerosol route of RSV infections in hospitalized children. Ribavirin currently also appears to hold promise in the treatment of Lassa fever, as well as some other arenaviruses and bunyaviruses, and influenza A and B viral infections. With the exception of influenza A virus, it is the only potential therapy for infections from these viruses.

STRUCTURE

Ribavirin (1-β-D-ribafuranosyl-1,2,4-triazole-3-carboxamide) is a synthetic purine nucleoside. Its structure is related to guanosine and inosine (Fig. 1). Among molecules of similar structure, ribavirin is the only one that has antiviral activity,

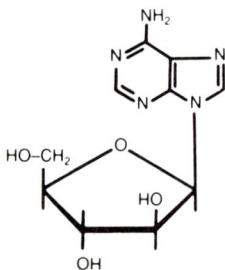

Fig. 1   Structure of ribavirin.

Antimicrobial Agents Annual 3
P.K. Peterson and J. Verhoef, editors
© Elsevier Science Publishers BV, 1988

and any alteration in the basic structure of ribavirin produces a loss of its antiviral properties (10).

ACTIVITY

Mechanism of action

Ribavirin exhibits a virustatic effect against a variety of both RNA and DNA viruses (11–15). Several different mechanisms of action of the drug appear to produce its antiviral effect, but the molecular basis of the observed effects remains arcane. Indeed, the modes of activity may vary with different viruses.

Ribavirin is quickly transported into cells where it is metabolized to the monophosphate, diphosphate and triphosphate derivatives which inhibit viral replication. Based mostly on studies of the antiviral activity against influenza virus, ribavirin appears to possess 3 major mechanisms of action (10, 15–17). First, ribavirin-5′-monophosphate, through competitive inhibition of inosine monophosphate dehydrogenase, results in decreased cellular levels of guanosine monophosphate and triphosphate (10–19). Viral enzyme systems dependent on guanosine are therefore deprived of the nutrition necessary for them to complete their own transcription. The inhibitory effect of ribavirin on many of the viral enzymes which use guanosine as a substrate may be at least partially reversed by the addition of exogenous guanosine (10, 19, 20). It should be noted, however, that adenosine kinase, which appears to be important in keeping ribavirin intracellularly and initiating its inhibitory activity, does not use guanosine as a substrate (15, 21). The diminished guanylate pools do not completely account for the effect of ribavirin, since the addition of exogenous guanosine does not entirely ablate its antiviral activity, suggesting that inhibition of viral enzymes other than inosine-5′-monophosphate (IMP) dehydrogenase occurs with the nucleotide metabolites (19). Furthermore, increasing the concentration of ribavirin in cells infected with influenza virus has been shown to produce greater inhibition of influenza replication without continued decrease in the pools of guanosine triphosphate (16).

The other 2 putative modes of action affect the production of viral messenger RNA (mRNA). Although the mechanism has not been deciphered for many viruses, experiments involving influenza, vaccinia, and vesicular stomatitis viruses indicate that ribavirin interferes with the capping and translation of mRNAs (15, 20, 22, 23). The triphosphate derivative of ribavirin appears to inhibit the enzymes involved in the capping of the 5′-end of newly produced viral mRNA. In addition, ribavirin triphosphate impairs the function of viral RNA polymerases responsible for the initiation and elongation of the mRNA, both of which require guanosine (15, 17).

Since ribavirin is a nucleoside, there has been concern about whether it might be incorporated into host cell DNA or RNA. Although it is technically difficult to rule out minor incorporation, studies utilizing high-specific-activity substrate indicate that ribavirin is not significantly incorporated into DNA and only slightly, if at all, into RNA (10, 24, 25).

Inhibition of host cell DNA and RNA synthesis by ribavirin has been cited in older reports as occurring at low concentrations, although little toxicity of the drug has been observed in cell culture, animals or man (26, 27). However, more recent studies have shown that tritiated thymidine incorporation, as used in previous studies, does not measure DNA synthesis in human cells treated with ribavirin. It is thymidine phosphorylation which is suppressed at low concentration (2 μM) of ribavirin and not DNA synthesis (26, 27). DNA synthesis is only inhibited at high concentrations (200 μM) of ribavirin, which are generally 100–200 times the concentrations necessary to inhibit viral DNA synthesis or viral replication, and is reversible once the drug is removed.

Spectrum of activity

Ribavirin has shown inhibitory activity against a wide spectrum of viruses in tissue culture, in animal models and, to a lesser extent, in trials in humans (Tables 1 and 2). Among the RNA viruses which are pathogenic for man, besides RSV, the activity of ribavirin against the influenza viruses, the parainfluenza viruses, measles, the arenaviruses, the bunyaviruses, the herpes viruses, hepatitis A virus and human immunodeficiency virus (HIV) are considered of potential therapeutic importance (9, 14, 28–30). The enteroviruses, poliovirus, Coxsackie viruses and echoviruses, have generally not appeared to be as sensitive to ribavirin as the respiratory viruses. One possible explanation for this is that these viruses do not contain a cap structure on their RNA. However, ribavirin does appear to inhibit the closely related encephalomyocarditis (EMC) virus in the severe myocarditis of mice (14).

Of particular interest is the potential use of ribavirin in treatment of the severe, often fatal, diseases in other parts of the globe caused by the arenaviruses and bunyaviruses (7, 9, 28, 31). The activity in vitro of ribavirin against the arenaviruses has been expanded to show effectiveness in the rodent and primate models, as well as in man for Lassa fever. In these animal models for Junin virus, the agent of Argentine hemorrhagic fever, and for Machupo virus, the agent of Bolivian hemorrhagic fever, ribavirin is effective in ameliorating the hemorrhagic signs, decreasing the viremia, and initially prolonging the survival. Subsequently, however, the animals develop encephalitis which is eventually fatal. Without treatment, however, the animals tend to die earlier from the hemorrhagic part of the disease. In monkeys infected with Junin virus, treatment did result in survival in some animals; 28% survived in the treated group compared to 0% in the untreated controls (28, 31).

Recent studies by Huggins et al (32) using a suckling mouse model have shown encouraging results for the treatment of Hantaan virus, the agent of Korean hemorrhagic fever. Animals treated with ribavirin 50 mg/kg/d, beginning on the 10th day after inoculation, when clinical signs and virus in the organs were already present, resulted in the survival and complete recovery of 55% of the animals, compared to no survival in the 70 controls.

Most of the Togaviruses show some degree of inhibition in vitro with ribavirin. However, in the animal models the effect of ribavirin on the experimental encephalitis has generally been disappointing. The one possible exception is West Nile infections in the mouse which have been treated with intraperitoneal ribavirin. Studies of the treatment of yellow fever in rodents similarly were unaffected by ribavirin, but in rhesus monkeys some therapeutic effect was observed (31).

Of the DNA viruses examined for their sensitivity to ribavirin herpes simplex virus has perhaps received the most attention and study (Table 2). Both Types 1 and 2 viruses have exhibited inhibition in vitro and in animal models. In some preliminary human studies ribavirin appeared to exert some beneficial activity (13). The observed effectiveness of ribavirin, however, for many of the herpes viruses, especially herpes simplex and vaccinia, appears to be greatly influenced by the conditions of the laboratory assay. The degree of sensitivity of some of these viruses is highly variable according to which cell line is employed, the concentration of virus inoculated, and the time at which the drug is added to the infected cells. Furthermore, various strains of herpes simplex demonstrate variability in their sensitivity to different concentrations of ribavirin. Nevertheless, ribavirin has been shown to have antiviral activity against viruses from each of the 3 families, the Adenoviridae, Herpesviridae and Poxviridae.

The development of resistance to ribavirin by any RNA or DNA virus has not been observed. Studies in vitro of repeated passage and cloning of virus exposed to low concentrations of ribavirin has not produced a resistant virus (13, 33). More importantly, resistance has not been observed to develop during prolonged clinical use. RSV isolates obtained prior to treatment and after treatment with aerosolized ribavirin or placebo obtained from hospitalized infants showed no change in their degree of sensitivity to ribavirin (4). The various mechanisms of inhibition of viral replication of ribavirin may account for this lack of development of resistance, which has occurred with other antiviral drugs possessing a very specific mechanism of action. Furthermore, viruses which have been shown in vitro to develop resistance to other antiviral drugs, do not show cross-resistance to ribavirin (11, 34).

CLINICAL PHARMACOLOGY

Ribavirin may be administered by mouth, by the intravenous route or by small-particle aerosol. Plasma and serum levels vary greatly depending on the route of administration, the dose, and, at least in the case of aerosol administration, the number of days of therapy. After an oral dose of 1000 mg/day or 15 mg/kg/day divided into 3 doses, the mean plasma level $2^1/_2$ hours after the dose had been administered was 0.8 μg/m (35). The pharmacokinetics of ribavirin given intravenously have been studied in African patients with Lassa fever (35). In these studies

Table 1   *RNA viruses for which the effect of ribavirin has been examined in vitro and/or in vivo*

	Inhibitory activity of ribavirin			
	In vitro (MIC in μg/ml)	In animal model	In man (type of infection affected)	Route
Orthomyxoviruses Influenza A and B	+ (0.01–8.5)	+ mouse ferret monkey	experimental (A/H3N2) natural A/H3N2 A/H1N1 influenza B	aerosol oral
Paramyxoviruses Parainfluenza 1,3	+ (3.2–32)	+ mouse hamster	natural infection in immunodeficient infants	aerosol
Respiratory syncytial virus	+ (3–32)	+ cotton rat	experimental, and lower respiratory tract disease in infants	aerosol
Mumps	+ (0.1–10)			
Measles	+ (0.003–10)	+ mouse	natural infection	oral
Coronaviruses	+*	+ mouse		
Picornaviruses Rhinoviruses 1,1A,8,13,56	+ (10–100) (most 10–32)			
2,42	–			
Foot and mouth disease	+	+ mouse		
Enteroviruses Polio, Coxsackie	±* (20–1000)	– mouse		
Encephalomyo- carditis virus		+ myocarditis of mice		
Hepatitis A virus	+		natural infection	oral
Arenaviruses Lassa fever	+ (1–10)	+ guinea-pig, monkey	natural infection	oral i.v.
Pinchinde	+	+ hamster, guinea-pig		

* Sensitivity of virus to ribavirin varies with cell line used in assay.

Table 1   (*continued*)

	Inhibitory activity of ribavirin			
	In vitro (MIC in μg/ml)	In animal model	In man (type of infection affected)	Route
Junin	+	+ guinea-pig, primates		
Macupo	+	+ guinea-pig, monkey		
Bunyaviruses				
Rift Valley fever	+	+ mouse, hamster monkey		
Hantaan virus (Korean hemorrhagic fever)	+	+ mouse		
Punta Toro	+	+ hamster		
Togaviruses				
Alphaviruses	+ (1.5–32)	− mouse, hamster monkey		
Flaviviruses	+	+ mouse (West Nile) + monkey (yellow fever) − mouse (Bonzi, Japanese encephalitis)		
Ebola virus		− guinea-pig, monkey		
Reoviruses				
Reovirus 1, 2, 3 Animal rotaviruses	+ (0.32–10)	± mouse		
Colorado tick fever virus	+ (3.2)			
Rhabdoviruses				
Vesicular stomatitis	+ (1.5–320)	+ mouse (tail lesions)		
Retroviruses	+	+ mouse (Friend leukemia virus)		
Human immunodeficiency virus	+ (10–100)			

Table 2 *DNA viruses for which the effect of ribavirin has been examined in vitro and/or in vivo*

	Inhibitory activity of ribavirin			
	In vitro (MIC in μg/ml)	In animal model	In man (type of infection affected)	Route
Adenoviruses				
Types 2, 3, 5, 19	+ (3,5*, 19) (3–32)			
Type 12	+	+ mouse tumor		
Herpes viruses				
Herpes simplex				
Type 1	+* (0.32–100) (most 0.32–3.2)	+ guinea-pig, mouse rabbit, hamster	gingivostomatitis	oral
Type 2	+. (1–100) (most 0.32–3.2)	+ guinea-pig, mouse	genital	oral
Cytomegalovirus				
Human	+ (10–32)			
Murine	+ (3.2–32)	– mouse		
Varicella-zoster	±		zoster	topical
Infectious bovine rhinotracheitis	+ (10)			
Feline rhinotracheitis	± (320)			
Pseudorabies	– ($\geq$1000)			
Marek's disease	+ (10)	± chicken tumor		
Pox viruses				
Vaccinia	+* (0.1–50) (most 0.1–3.2)	+ rabbit, mouse		
Myxoma	+ (3.2)			
Papovaviruses				
Shope fibroma	+	+		
Hepatitis B virus	+	chimpanzees (chronic infection)	no effect on antigen production	

* Sensitivity of virus to ribavirin varies with cell lines used in this assay.

the patients received an initial intravenous dose of 1 g followed by 4 g/d in 4 doses for 4 days. For the next 6 days the dose was reduced to 1500 mg/d in 3 divided doses. The mean peak plasma level after the 1 g dose was 23.5 μg/ml with a range of 22.8–25 μg/ml. After the 500 mg dose the mean peak plasma level was 17 μg/ml with a range of 13–21 μg/ml.

Recent studies have administered ribavirin by small-particle aerosol, which appears to be the most promising method of therapy for respiratory viruses (1–5). Lung scans have shown that the small aerosolized particles are distributed uniformly from the upper respiratory tract to the distal alveoli. The studies of Connor et al (35, 36) indicate that a major advantage of this route of administration is that very high levels of ribavirin may be obtained in the respiratory secretions, theoretically at the site of viral replication, with little systemic absorption, resulting in relatively low plasma levels. The dose of ribavirin administered by small-particle aerosol has been estimated for adults by Knight, McClung and co-workers (1, 2) as 0.82 mg/kg body weight per hour of administration for a solution of ribavirin at a concentration of 20 mg/ml, which is the concentration used in recent clinical studies. For infants, however, the dose is likely to be greater. Although the proportion and distribution of the deposited particles appears to be similar for adults and children, the minute volume ventilation per kilogram is greater in infants, and has been estimated by Knight (personal communication) to be about 1.4 mg/kg/h ribavirin therapy. The dose will, nevertheless, vary in patients with different lung function and pathology.

The levels of ribavirin in plasma and in respiratory secretions after varying durations of aerosol therapy in patients studied by Connor et al (35, 36) are shown in Table 3. The average plasma $t_{1/2}$ after aerosol administration is about 9.5 hours and about 2 hours in the tracheal secretions. This long plasma $t_{1/2}$ suggests a 3-compartment type of distribution with slow release into the serum (35). Accumulation of ribavirin appears to occur if the duration of treatment per day is longer than 8 hours, with plasma levels being almost twice as high on the 3rd day of treatment as on the 1st day. In one ventilated patient the mean plasma level after 4–6 days of therapy was approximately 1.8 μg/ml, but after 26 days of continuous aerosol therapy, the plasma level reached 15–17 μg/ml (35).

The levels of ribavirin in the respiratory secretions with small-particle aerosol administration are hundreds to thousands times higher than in the plasma. At the end of 20 hours of aerosol therapy the mean level in the secretions in the patients studied by Connor et al (35) was approximately 3000 μg/ml. However, the levels in the secretions, and to a lesser extent in the plasma, depend on the means by which the aerosol is administered. If the aerosol is delivered directly into an endotracheal tube, the levels in the secretions are much higher than if the aerosol is administered by mask or mist tent. Although the concentration in the secretions is high, indeed many times the minimum inhibitory concentration (MIC) for most viruses, they are still well below the solubility of ribavirin, which is 200 mg/ml physiologic solution.

Ribavirin is rapidly absorbed after oral administration and is metabolized in

Table 3 *Levels of ribavirin in plasma and respiratory secretions after aerosol administration**

Duration of treatment (h/d)	Estimated dose (mg/kg/d)**	Mean peak plasma level (µg/ml)	Plasma half-life (h)	Mean peak level in tracheal secretions (µg/ml)	Half-life in tracheal secretions (h)
2.5	2.1	0.19	9–10	–	–
5	4.1	0.28	6.5– 11	250–1375	1.4–2.5
8	6.6	1.1	–	1925	2.0
20	16.4	0.68–3.3	–	312–28,250	–

* Adapted from Connor et al (35).
** Estimated dose for ribavirin at 20 mg/ml in reservoir = 0.82 mg/kg/h (2).

man to the deribosylated form, 1,2,4-triazole carboxamide. Ribavirin is excreted mainly via the kidney unchanged or as the deribosylated product. Approximately one-third of an oral dose is excreted in the urine in the first 24 hours. At 72 hours 53% of ^{14}C-ribavirin can be recovered in the urine and 15% in the feces. Studies in humans and baboons have indicated that some accumulation of ribavirin and its metabolites occurs in the red blood cells, reaching a peak after 4 days and then declining with an apparent $t_{1/2}$ of 40 days. Although ribavirin was initially thought not to penetrate the blood-brain barrier based on animal studies, recent evidence has shown that in man ribavirin does penetrate into the cerebrospinal fluid, reaching approximately 70% of the concurrent plasma ribavirin levels (37).

ADVERSE EFFECTS

Ribavirin has generally been well tolerated in clinical studies with only transient hematologic effects noted after oral administration; no toxicity or side effects were noted with aerosol administration in any of the controlled studies. The hematologic effects, which generally have been a mild and rapidly reversible decrease in the red cell mass, have been noted with high oral dosage (13–17 mg/kg/d) given for extended periods of 2–4 weeks (38). Anemia related to ribavirin therapy has not been noted during aerosol administration. Similarly, transient increases in serum bilirubin, aspartate aminotransferase (AST) and alanine aminotransferase (ALT) concentrations have occurred during use of oral and intravenous, but not aerosol, therapy.

The long-term effect of aerosol administration of ribavirin on the lung, particularly on the infant's lung, is still unknown. However, no acute adverse effects on the lung have been detected by serial pulmonary function tests in volunteer subjects (39).

The effects of ribavirin versus water aerosol have been examined in a small number of patients with chronic lung disease, 6 patients with asthma and 6 with chronic obstructive pulmonary disease (COPD), all of whom required chronic bronchodilators (40). The bronchodilator therapy was stopped 24 hours prior to the ribavirin or water aerosol therapy, and forced expiratory volumes (FEV) and flows were obtained at 5 intervals, up to 215 minutes of cumulative aerosol exposure. In the 6 COPD subjects slight, but significant, decreases during ribavirin therapy occurred only in the $FEV_{1.0}$ at 35 and 95 minutes. In the 6 asthmatic subjects, variable reductions in the spirometric values occurred with ribavirin therapy at 35 or 95 minutes. The reductions were not, however, of a clinically important magnitude, and were transient in all COPD and asthmatic subjects. At 215 minutes the spirometric values were not significantly different between patients receiving ribavirin and water aerosol therapy. An inhalation of a bronchodilator was able to ablate any of the observed changes. This study suggests that in patients with chronic lung disease, ribavirin aerosol therapy was generally well tolerated, but may produce some measurable reductions in lung function if bronchodilator therapy is discontinued.

CLINICAL USES

Currently the most promising use of ribavirin in the United States is in the treatment of acute viral respiratory tract infections with aerosol administration (1–5). At the end of December 1985 the Food and Drug Administration approved ribavirin administered as an aerosol for the treatment of RSV infections in hospitalized infants and young children. Similar approval was recently obtained in Canada and is expected soon in the United Kingdom.

Studies initiated in 1981 at Baylor and the University of Rochester have indicated a beneficial effect on the signs, symptoms and viral shedding of infants with bronchiolitis and pneumonia from RSV infection (4, 5). RSV is the major respiratory pathogen of infants and young children, accounting for an appreciable proportion of the pediatric hospitalizations and intensive care admissions each year. No vaccine or other means of protection or treatment has been available.

In these studies, hospitalized infants with lower respiratory tract disease from RSV infection were randomized in a double-blind manner to receive either ribavirin or placebo (water) by aerosol which was administered essentially continuously for 12–20 hours each day. The concentration of ribavirin in the liquid reservoir was 20 mg/ml and the mean duration of treatment was 5 days (4, 5). A more rapid rate of improvement was observed in the treated infants within the first 3 days, and the severity of illness by the 4th day was significantly less than in infants treated with placebo. Arterial oxygen saturation determinations, obtained as an objective measurement of improvement, were significantly better in the infants receiving ribavirin. The duration and quantity of viral shedding in the nasal washes in the treated infants was also less. In all the children the aerosol therapy was well tolerated with no adverse effects noted.

Currently 7 double-blind, placebo-controlled studies of ribavirin therapy for RSV infections in humans have been reported in the United States and England (4, 5, 39, 41, 44). All of these controlled studies demonstrated, first, a significant beneficial effect on the severity of illness and, second, no toxicity or adverse effects. Amelioration of severe RSV lower respiratory tract disease was shown, not only in normal infants, but also in those with underlying cardiopulmonary conditions which place them at highest risk for fatal or complicated RSV infection. Preliminary studies have also indicated that this mode of therapy may be particularly useful in treating the overwhelming and often fatal viral infections seen in infants with severe combined immunodeficiency disease (SCID) and other children with immunocompromised states (45, 46). Two reports suggest that ribavirin may be useful in controlling parainfluenza virus, as well as RSV, in these immunocompromised patients (45, 46).

The effectiveness of ribavirin in the prophylaxis and treatment of influenza infections when given orally has been variable (47–49). In contrast, small-particle aerosol administration of ribavirin to adults with natural influenza A and influenza B has been uniformly beneficial (1–3, 50). In these double-blind, controlled studies patients who had been ill for usually no more than 24 hours were treated with ribavirin aerosol for 12–16 h/day. Those receiving ribavirin experienced significantly more rapid improvement in their signs and symptoms, in the height and duration of fever, and had diminished viral shedding. No side effects or toxicity were noted with the aerosol therapy in any of these patients. Several double-blind, placebo-controlled trials of ribavirin treatment of rubeola have been conducted in children in Brazil, Mexico, and the Philippines (30). In these studies in which ribavirin was administered orally at a dose of 10 mg/kg for 5–7 days the length and severity of the signs and symptoms of the illness were more rapidly reduced in the treated groups. In patients receiving ribavirin, fever disappeared within 1 day in most and by 3 days in all, in comparison to the persistence of fever in the placebo-treated groups for 3–7 or more days (30). Ribavirin treatment appeared to be most effective if initiated during the pre-exanthem phase of the disease, but even if first administered once, the rash was evident and clinical benefit remained significant. No adverse effects were noted in any of the trials.

Oral ribavirin therapy has also been shown to have a beneficial effect on the clinical and laboratory course of hepatitis A viral infection in double-blind placebo-controlled studies in several other countries (51, 52).

Clinical experience with ribavirin therapy for adenoviral infections is limited. Aerosolized ribavirin has been used for adenoviral pneumonia in a few young children and has appeared to be beneficial in the clinical manifestations and has led to diminished viral shedding (53). However, no studies have evaluated ribavirin therapy for adenoviral infections in a controlled manner.

One of the most exciting recent clinical uses of ribavirin has been in the treatment of Lassa fever (6, 7, 9, 54). Studies by McCormick et al (6, 7, 9) in Sierra Leone have demonstrated remarkable success in the treatment of this severe and often fatal arenaviral disease using ribavirin either orally or intravenously. In patients identified to be at high risk by having a serum AST level of 150 IU/l or more the fatality rate without treatment was 55%, compared to 5% in those who received 10 days of intravenous ribavirin, begun within 6 days of the onset of fever. If treatment was delayed to 7 or more days after the onset of fever, the fatality rate was 26% (9). In the cynomolgus monkey model combined therapy with immune serum + ribavirin allowed successful treatment even of monkeys in whom treatment was delayed for 10 days. Treatment with convalescent plasma did not significantly add benefit or reduce the mortality in the Sierra Leone patients.

Of recent interest is the effect of ribavirin on HIV, the agent associated with AIDS (8, 5, 6). Recent studies in vitro demonstrated that the replication of HIV in cultures of adult human T-lymphocytes was suppressed by ribavirin in doses of 30–50 μg/ml. Clinical studies using daily oral ribavirin therapy in patients with AIDS-related complex (ARC) are currently underway.

DOSING

Oral doses of ribavirin in clinical trials have been generally about 10–15 mg/kg/d, with the adult dose being about 1 g/d divided into 3 or 4 doses. The experience with intravenous ribavirin is limited, but in the Lassa fever studies the dose for the first few days was approximately 4 g/d or 60 mg/kg/d. At this high dosage the hematocrit was noted to decline by 3–5% (7).

For administration by aerosol, ribavirin is dissolved in water at a concentration of 20 mg/ml. The small-particle aerosol is produced by a device employing a type of Collison generator which runs from compressed air. The mist produced contains approximately 190 μg of ribavirin per liter with the aerosolized particles having a median mass diameter of 1.3 μm, and 95% have a mass diameter of <5 μm. The nebulized solution then passes through a drying chamber before passing into tubing which can be attached to a face mask, oxygen hood, tent or ventilator. The actual dose of ribavirin which the patient receives will depend not only on the concentration of the drug actually aerosolized, but also upon the patient's minute volume, how much drug is retained in the lung (the pulmonary retention factor, which has been estimated to be 0.70) and the duration of exposure to the aerosol (1, 2). Thus, the calculated retained dose for a drug concentration of 20 mg/ml is 50–55 mg/h exposure. In the clinical trials of the treatment of influenza and respiratory syncytial virus the minimal amount of exposure has been approximately 12 h/d for 3 days, and for RSV the usual duration of therapy has been 18–20 h/day for 3–5 days. In severely ill patients extended periods of therapy, lasting 1–4 weeks, have been utilized without observed adverse effect (45, 46).

FUTURE DIRECTIONS

Investigations in the near future within the realm of clinical medicine will hopefully better define the use of ribavirin in the treatment, not only of the arenaviruses, bunyaviruses and HIV, but also of hepatitis, the herpes viruses, parainfluenza virus, adenovirus, and measles. Among the more plebian respiratory viruses the impact of ribavirin needs to be better defined. Of particular importance is the delineation of ribavirin's long-term effect on the lung of young infants with RSV. The enduring effect of ribavirin on the developing lung of these infants could be adverse, although there is no evidence currently to suggest this, or it could be beneficial. If the treatment of the acute primary infection could diminish the high rate of sequelae observed after RSV lower respiratory tract disease in infancy, the worth of acute treatment would be greatly enhanced.

The clinical use of ribavirin in the United States currently centers around the aerosolized form of therapy for serious viral respiratory disease in hospitalized patients. Future technology, however, could result in outpatient aerosol treatment, which might be particularly useful for influenza and RSV infections. The oral and intravenous forms appear to be particularly promising for treatment of infections with the arenaviruses and bunyaviruses, and the potential for treatment of AIDS is being explored. A use outside of clinical medicine may also exist in the veterinarian and agricultural worlds, considering its spectrum of activity. As an example, ribavirin has been recently reported as effective in eliminating foot-and-mouth-disease virus infection in tissue culture (57).

Thus, at this time it is difficult to envision what the pharmacologic crystal ball holds for ribavirin. However, the potential of ribavirin may lie in its piquant characteristics of low toxicity and a broad spectrum of antiviral activity.

REFERENCES

1. Knight V, Wilson SZ, Quarles JM, Greggs SE, McClung HW, Waters BK, Cameron RW, Zerwas JM, Couch RB (1981) Ribavirin small-particle aerosol treatment of influenza. *Lancet, 1*, 945.
2. McClung HW, Knight V, Gilbert BE, Wilson SZ, Quarles Jr JM, Divine GW, Couch RB, Gordon WH, Thurston JM, Almar RL, Schlautt WR (1983) Ribavirin aerosol treatment of influenza B virus infection. *J. Am. Med. Assoc., 249*, 2671.
3. Wilson SZ, Gilbert BE, Quarles JM, Knight V, McClung HW, Moore RV, Couch RB (1984) Treatment of influenza A (H1N1) virus infection with ribavirin aerosol. *Antimicrob. Agents Chemother., 26*, 200.
4. Hall CB, McBride JT, Walsh EE, Bell DM, Gala CL, Hildreth SW, TenEyck LG, Hall WJ (1983) Aerosolized ribavirin treatment of infants with respiratory syncytial virus infection: a randomized double blind study. *N. Eng. J. Med., 308*, 1443.
5. Taber LH, Knight V, Gilbert BE, McClung HW, Wilson SZ, Norton HJ, Thurston JM, Gordon WH, Atmar RL, Schlaudt Jr WR (1983) Ribavirin aerosol treatment of bronchiolitis due to respiratory syncytial virus infection in infants. *Pediatrics, 72*, 613.

6. McCormick JB, Webb PA, Johnson KM (1980) Lassa immune plasma and ribavirin in the therapy of acute Lassa fever. In: Smith RA, Kirkpatrick W (Eds), *Ribavirin: A Broad Spectrum Antiviral Agent*, p 213. Academic Press, New York.

7. McCormick JB, Webb PA, Johnson KM, Scribner CS (1984) Chemotherapy of acute Lassa fever with ribavirin. In: Smith RA, Knight V, Smith JAD (Eds), *Clinical Applications of Ribavirin*, p 187. Academic Press, Orlando, FL.

8. McCormick JB, Getchell JP, Mitchell SW, Hicks DR (1984) Ribavirin suppresses replication of lymphadenopathy associated virus in cultures of human adult T lymphocytes. *Lancet, 2*, 1367.

9. McCormick JB, King IJ, Webb PA, Scribner CL, Craven RB, Johnson KM, Elliott LH, Belmont-Williams R (1984) Lassa fever: effective therapy with ribavirin. *N. Engl. J. Med., 314*, 20.

10. Smith RA (1984) Background and mechanisms of action of ribavirin. In: Smith RA, Knight V, Smith JAD (Eds), *Clinical Applications of Ribavirin*, p1. Academic Press, Orlando, FL.

11. Sidwell RW (1980) Ribavirin: in vitro antiviral activity. In: Smith RA, Kirkpatrick W (Eds), *Ribavirin: A Broad Spectrum Antiviral Agent*, p 32. Academic Press, New York.

12. Allen LB (1980) Review of in vivo efficacy of ribavirin. In: Smith RA, Kirkpatrick W (Eds), *Ribavirin: A Broad Spectrum Antiviral Agent*, p 43. Academic Press, New York.

13. Sidwell RW (1984) In vitro and in vivo inhibition of DNA viruses by ribavirin: In: Smith RA, Knight V, Smith JAD (Eds), *Clinical Applications of Ribavirin*, p 19. Academic Press, Orlando, FL.

14. Crumpacker CS (1984) Overview of ribavirin treatment of infection caused by RNA viruses. In: Smith RA, Knight V, Smith JAD (Eds), *Clinical Applications of Ribavirin*, p 33. Academic Press, Orlando, FL.

15. Gilbert BE, Knight V (1986) Biochemistry and clinical applications of ribavirin (Mini-review). *Antimicrob. Agents Chemother., 30*, 206.

16. Wray SK, Gilbert BE, Noall MW, Knight V (1985) Mode of action of ribavirin: effect of nucleotide pool alterations on influenza virus ribonucleoprotein synthesis. *Antiviral Res., 5*, 29.

17. Wray SK, Gilbert BE, Knight V (1985) Effect of ribavirin triphosphate on primer generation and elongation during influenza virus transcription in vitro. *Antiviral Res., 5*, 39.

18. Stridh S (1983) Determination of ribonucleoside triphosphate pools in influenza A virus-infected MDCK cells. *Arch. Virol., 77*, 223.

19. Robins RK, Revankar GR, McKernan PA, Murray BK, Kirsi JJ, North JA (1985) The importance of IMP dehydrogenase inhibition in the broad spectrum antiviral activity of ribavirin and selenazofurin. *Adv. Enzyme Regul., 24*, 29.

20. Toltzis P, Huang AS (1986) Effect of ribavirin on macromolecular synthesis in vesicular stomatitis virus-infected cells. *Antimicrob. Agents Chemother., 29*, 1010.

21. Willis RC, Carson DA, Seegmiller JE (1978) Adenosine kinase initiates the major route of ribavirin activation in a cultured human cell line. *Proc. Natl Acad. Sci., 75*, 3042.

22. Canonico PG (1983) Ribavirin: a review of efficacy, toxicity and mechanisms of antiviral activity. *Antibiotics, 4*, 161.

23. Goswami BB, Borek E, Sharma OK, Fujitaki J, Smith RA (1979) The broad spectrum antiviral agent ribavirin inhibits capping of mRNA. *Biochem. Biophys. Res. Commun., 89*, 830.

24. Smith RA, Wade M (1986) Ribavirin: a broad spectrum antiviral agent. In: Stapleton T (Ed), *Studies with a Broad Spectrum Antiviral Agent*, p 3. Royal Society of Medicine Services Ltd., London.

25. Zimmerman TP, Deeprose RD (1978) Metabolism of 5-amino-2-beta-D-ribofurano-syl-imidazole-4-carboxamide and related five-membered heterocytes to 5'-triphosphates in human blood and L 5178Y cells. *Biochem. Pharmacol., 27*, 709.

26. Drach JC, Barnett JW, Thomas MA et al (1980) Inhibition of viral and cellular DNA synthesis by ribavirin. In: Smith RA, Kirkpatrick W (Eds), *Ribavirin: a Broad Spectrum Antiviral Agent*, p 119. Academic Press, New York.

27. Drach JC, Thomas MA, Barnett JW, Smith SC, Shipman Jr C (1981) Tritiated thymidine incorporation does not measure DNA synthesis in ribavirin treated human cells. *Science, 212*, 549.

28. Weissenbacher MC, Calello MA, Merani MS, McCormick JB, Rodriguez M (1986) Therapeutic effect of the antiviral agent ribavirin in Junin virus infection of primates. *J. Med. Virol., 20*, 261.

29. Canonicol PG (1985) Efficacy, toxicology and clinical applications of ribavirin against virulent RNA viral infections. *Antiviral Res., Suppl 1*, 75.

30. Banks G, Fernandez H (1984) Clinical use of ribavirin in measles: a summarized review. In: Smith RA, Knight V, Smith JAD (Eds), *Clinical Applications of Ribavirin*, p 203. Academic Press, Orlando, FL.

31. Huggins W, Jahrling P, Kende M, Canonico PG (1984) Efficacy of ribavirin against virulent RNA virus infections. In: Smith RA, Knight V, Smith JAD (Eds), *Clinical Applications of Ribavirin*, p 49. Academic Press, Orlando, FL.

32. Huggins JW, Kim GR, Brand OM, McKee Jr KR (1986) Ribavirin therapy for Hantaan virus infection in suckling mice. *J. Infect. Dis., 153*, 489.

33. Huffman JH, Allen LB, Sidwell RW (1977) Comparison of the development of resistant strains of type 1 Herpes simplex virus to in vitro activity of 5-iodo-2-deoxyuridine or ribavirin. *Ann. NY Acad. Sci., 284*, 233.

34. Connor CS (1984) Ribavirin (Editorial). *Drug Intell. Clin. Pharm., 18*, 137.

35. Connor JD, Hintz M, VanDyke R, McCormick JB, McIntosh K (1984) Ribavirin pharmacokinetics in children and adults during therapeutic trials. In: Smith RA, Knight V, Smith JAD (Eds), *Clinical Applications of Ribavirin*, p 107. Academic Press, Orlando, FL.

36. Connor JD, Van Dyke R, Hintz M, DeVinney R, McIntosh K (1983) Pharmacokinetics of ribavirin small particle aerosol therapy in children and adults. In: Abstracts, 23rd Interscience Conference on Antimicrobial Agents and Chemotherapy, Las Vegas, 1983, p 256. American Society for Microbiology, Washington, DC.

37. Crumpacker C, Bubley G, Lucey D, Hussey S, Connor J (1986) Ribavirin enters cerebrospinal fluid (Letter to Editor). *Lancet, 2*, 45.

38. Shulman NR (1984) Assessment of hematologic effects of ribavirin in humans. In: Smith RA, Knight V, Smith JAD (Eds), *Clinical Applications of Ribavirin*, p 79. Academic Press, Orlando, FL.

39. Hall CB, Walsh EE, Hruska JF, Betts RF, Hall WJ (1983) Ribavirin treatment of experimental respiratory syncytial viral infection: a controlled double blind study in young adults. *J. Am. Med. Assoc., 249*, 2666.

40. Light B, Aoki FY, Serrette C (1984) Tolerance of ribavirin aerosol inhaled by normal volunteers and patients with asthma or chronic obstructive airways disease. In: Smith RA, Knight V, Smith JAD (Eds), *Clinical Applications of Ribavirin*, p 97. Academic Press, Orlando, FL.

41. Rodriguez WJ, Kim HW, Brandt CD, Fink RJ, Getson PR, Arrobio J, Murphy TM, McCarthy V, Parrott RH (1987) Aerosolized ribavirin in the treatment of patients with respiratory syncytial virus infection. *Pediatr. Infect. Dis., 6*, 159.

42. Chiardullo-Geraci K, Rosner I, Palumbo P, Laskin O et al (1985) IgE anti-RSV secretory immune response in infants treated with ribavirin aerosol (Abstract). *Pediatr. Res., 19*, 290 A.

43. Hall CB, McBride JT, Gala CL, Hildreth SW, Schnabel KC (1985) Ribavirin aerosol treatment of respiratory syncytial viral infection in infants with underlying cardiac and pulmonary disease. *J. Am. Med. Assoc., 254*, 3047.

44. Barry W, Cockburn F, Cornall R, Price JF, Sutherland G, Vardag A (1986) Ribavirin aerosol for acute bronchiolitis. *Arch. Dis. Child., 6*, 593.

45. Gelfand EW, McCurdy D, Rab P, Middleton PJ (1983) Ribavirin treatment of viral pneumonitis in severe combined immunodeficiency disease. *Lancet, 2*, 732.

46. McIntosh K, Kurachek SC, Cairns LM, Burns JC, Barrett G (1984) Treatment of respiratory viral infection in an immunodeficient infant with ribavirin aerosol. *Am. J. Dis. Child., 138*, 305.

47. Magnussen CR, Douglas Jr RG, Betts RF, Roth FK, Meagher MP (1977) Double blind evaluation of oral ribavirin (Virazole) in experimental influenza A virus infection in volunteers. *Antimicrob. Agents Chemother., 12*, 498.

48. Smith CB, Charette RP, Fox JP, Cooney MK, Hall CE (1980) Lack of effect of oral ribavirin in naturally occurring influenza A virus (H1N1) infection. *J. Infect. Dis., 141*, 548.

49. Salido-Rengell F, Nasser-Quinones H, Briseno-Garcia B (1977) Clinical evaluation of 1β-D-ribafuranosyl-1,2,4-triazole-3-carboxamide (ribavirin) in a double blind study during an outbreak of influenza. *Ann. NY Acad. Sci., 284*, 272.

50. Gilbert BE, Wilson SZ, Knight V, Couch RB, Melhoff TL, McClung HW, Divine GW, Bartlett DD, Cohan LC, Gallior TL (1984) Ribavirin small-particle aerosol treatment of influenza in college students, 1981–1983. In: Smith RA, Knight V, Smith JAD (Eds), *Clinical Applications of Ribavirin*, p 125. Academic Press, Orlando, FL.

51. Sanchez FA, Sosa IRG, Vargas GM, Nunez EA (1984) Treatment of type A hepatitis with ribavirin. In: Smith RA, Knight V, Smith JAD (Eds), *Clinical Applications of Ribavirin*, p 193. Academic Press, Orlando, FL.

52. Patki SA, Gupta P (1982) Evaluation of ribavirin in the treatment of acute hepatitis. *Chemotherapy (Basel), 28*, 298.

53. Buchdahl RM, Taylor P, Warner JD (1985) Nebulised ribavirin for adenovirus pneumonia (Letter to Editor). *Lancet, 2*, 1070.

54. Jahrling PB, Peters CJ, Stephen EL (1984) Enhanced treatment of Lassa fever by immune plasma combined with ribavirin in cynomolgus monkeys. *J. Infect. Dis., 149*, 420.

55. De Clerq E (1986) Chemotherapeutic approaches to the treatment of the acquired immune deficiency syndrome (AIDS). *J. Med. Chem., 29*, 1561.

56. Sandstrom E (1986) Antiviral drugs for AIDS: current status and future prospects. *Drugs, 31*, 463.

57. De la Torre JC, Alarcon B, Martinez-Salas E, Carrasco L, Domingo E (1987) Ribavirin cures cells of a persistent infection with foot-and-mouth disease virus in vitro. *J. Virol., 61*, 233.

CHAPTER 36

Vidarabine

GEORGE J. GALASSO

The success of vidarabine in treating an ongoing, life-threatening disease caused by the herpesvirus (1) led to an increased interest in developing more specific and effective antiviral agents. Previously, some antiviral drugs were being developed and used, but their anticipated toxicity dampened enthusiasm. Vidarabine was found to be effective and relatively non-toxic at therapeutic levels for the indicated diseases. This success led to a rapid increase in antiviral agent research. Newer drugs, such as acyclovir, are now proving to be more effective than vidarabine (2–4). In the future, the preferred drug will probably not be vidarabine, due to more effective drugs, and its relative insolubility. Its importance will be as an effective back-up drug should drug resistance occur. The potential for drug resistance may become a major problem with the increasing usage of antiviral agents by the medical profession and with several viral infections having the propensity for recurrence. Drug resistance to acyclovir has already been reported during treatment of herpes simplex (5). Vidarabine will therefore remain an important component of the clinical armamentarium.

Current research on vidarabine is directed toward comparing its therapeutic effects against other newer antiviral agents as well as testing it in combination with other drugs to enhance its efficacy, reduce toxicity, and reduce potential drug resistance. Synergy has been observed in tissue culture, in animal studies, and in clinical studies between vidarabine and various other drugs, including acyclovir and interferon (6–15). The clinical research efforts on combination therapy must be increased and as the role of vidarabine as a single agent decreases, its role in combination therapy may increase.

All currently available antiviral agents have been developed through serendipity; vidarabine (adenine arabinoside, ara-A, Vira-A) is no exception. It was not the antiviral properties of vidarabine, however, that first drew notice but its mild antibacterial action. In the early 1960s routine screening procedures at Parke-Davis detected some activity in the supernatant fluid of *Streptomyces antibioticus* isolated from a soil sample. With some difficulty, the material was crystallized, but the antibacterial properties were lost. Fortunately, the material was submitted

Antimicrobial Agents Annual 3
P.K. Peterson and J. Verhoef, editors
© Elsevier Science Publishers BV, 1988

to the company's new antiviral section, where it was found to have activity against herpes simplex (16).

Subsequently, work with the sponge *Cryptotethia crypta* elsewhere yielded arabinosyl nucleosides, which were studied in the hope that they might inhibit cancer cell growth. When one of the resultant nucleosides, adenine arabinoside – the same compound crystallized by Parke-Davis – was found to have antiviral activity, preclinical work on the compound began in earnest (17).

Vidarabine (Fig. 1) is a purine nucleoside with antiviral activity against herpes, pox, and rhabdoviruses (17). Tissue culture studies indicate that it can reduce herpes simplex virus plaque formation by 90% at 10 μg/ml and by 60% at 4 μg/ml. It is most effective against herpes simplex 1 and 2, varicella-zoster, vaccinia and cytomegalovirus.

ACTIVITY AND CLINICAL PHARMACOLOGY

The mechanism of action, pharmacology and preclinical studies of vidarabine are discussed in Annual 1 (18). Thirty minutes after intravenous administration of the radiolabeled drug, 70% of the tritium could be detected in the plasma (19). Tritium's half-life in adult plasma is 3–5 hours. Its concentration declines more slowly with time and remains at a relatively high level for several days. The half-life in infants and children is essentially half that in adults. Appropriate plasma levels of the labeled drug were more difficult to achieve when administered intramuscularly. This fact considered together with poor patient tolerance of this route of administration led to termination of intramuscular studies. Maximum urinary excretion occurred in the first 4 hours after dosing, with mean recovery of about 45% within 24 hours. Urinary excretion accounted for 50% of the dose. Most of the drug is excreted as hypoxanthine arabinoside (ara-Hx). In patients given slow-drip infusions over 4–10 days, vidarabine showed a rapid rise of plasma levels but remained constant over the period of administration with rapid decline when infusion was terminated. The distribution of ara-Hx between plasma and erythrocytes

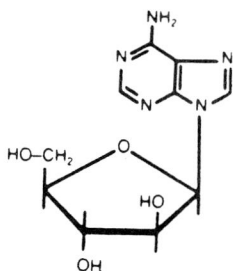

Fig. 1   Structure of vidarabine (9-β-D-arabinofuranosyladenine, adenine arabinoside, ara-A, Vira-A).

indicate parallel levels. Detectable (although variable) levels could be found in the cerebrospinal fluid, indicating penetration of the blood-brain barrier and potential for treatment of herpes encephalitis. These studies demonstrated rapid distribution of the drug into the tissues, rapid metabolization to ara-Hx, excretion through the urinary tract, and no potential for drug accumulation. However, in patients with impaired renal function, some accumulation was observed indicating that extra care must be exercised in treating these patients. One principle disadvantage of the drug is its low solubility and the necessity of administering it by slow-drip infusion over a 12-hour period daily.

When administered at levels of 5–15 mg/kg/d intravenously in man, vidarabine produced few or no observed toxic effects (20). The principal adverse reactions (incidence, 10–15%) involve the gastrointestinal tract and are anorexia, nausea, vomiting, and diarrhea. These reactions are mild to moderate and seldom require termination of treatment. Some central nervous system (CNS) disturbances – tremors, dizziness, hallucination, confusion, psychosis, and ataxia – have been occasionally reported at doses exceeding those previously mentioned. This is particularly true in adults. Liver function and hematologic tests are recommended because elevated SGOT and bilirubin levels and/or decreased hemoglobin, hematocrit, and white blood cell counts sometimes have been associated with therapy.

Increased neurotoxicity has been observed in patients receiving allopurinol and vidarabine. This may result from the accumulation of ara-Hx due to xanthine oxidase inhibition by allopurinol. Increased neurotoxicity has also been observed when the drug is given in combination with interferon, although the mechanism is not understood.

CLINICAL USES

Ophthalmic use

Herpes simplex 1, a leading cause of corneal blindness, is a relatively common infection of the eye affecting 1 per 1000 individuals yearly. It can be readily diagnosed by the characteristic dendritic lesion visualized with fluorescein stain. Characteristic of herpes viruses, a latent infection that causes periodic recurrences, is readily established, probably through incorporation in the trigeminal ganglion. Vidarabine was approved for the treatment of acute and recurrent keratoconjunctivitis and keratitis in 1977. Much of the data was presented in a symposium (17) and summarized by Buchanan and Hess (19). The drug is not effective in preventing recurrences, nor is it effective against stromal keratitis and uveitis.

The drug is available as a 3% ophthalmic ointment in a petrolatum base. Approximately 0.5 inches of ointment should be placed into the lower conjunctival sac 5 times daily at 3–4 hour intervals. An average of 7–9 days of treatment is required to achieve corneal re-epithelialization. In controlled trials, 3 weeks of treatment were required for complete re-epithelialization. If there are no signs of improvement after 1 week, or if complete re-epithelialization has not occurred by 3 weeks, other forms of therapy should be considered.

Combinations of antiviral drugs and antiviral drugs with interferon are being evaluated for enhanced activity. As yet no treatment for stromal disease has been found, but it is anticipated that combination drugs will result in improved therapy.

Herpes simplex encephalitis (HSE)

Encephalitis is a rare complication of herpes simplex infection. Since it is only one of several causes of encephalitis, the exact incidence is unknown and may range from 3 to 50 cases per million per year. Attempts at non-invasive diagnosis are being tried, but presently only a brain biopsy can confirm diagnosis. The mortality rate of HSE is 70% with severe residual effects in a large percentage of survivors. It has been demonstrated in a placebo-controlled and follow-up study (1, 21) that parenteral administration of vidarabine can reduce the mortality to half with a concomitant reduction in debilitating neurological sequelae. Optimal effects are obtained in patients in the early stages of the disease and in those less than 30 years old. Little benefit can be expected in comatose patients.

To treat HSE, vidarabine must be given by intravenous infusion at a dosage of 15 mg/kg/d. The drug must be diluted in an appropriate intravenous solution; each liter will solubilize a maximum of 450 mg of drug. The solution should be administered at a constant rate over a 12–24 hour period.

Because of the large amounts of fluid required for the administration of vidarabine and the demonstrated efficacy of acyclovir, a study was performed to compare the relative merits of these two drugs (2). The dosage of vidarabine was as before, 15 mg/kg/d for 10 days. The dosage of acyclovir was 30 mg/kg/d, divided into 3 daily doses at 8 hour intervals in a minimum volume of 100 ml of standard intravenous fluid over a period of 1 hour. The mortality rate in vidarabine-treated patients was 54% overall (greater than the earlier study explained by the inclusion of older patients with a lower level of consciousness at time of therapy initiation); the mortality rate in a comparable patient population treated with acyclovir was 28%. A 6-month morbidity analysis indicated that 14% of vidarabine-treated survivors were functioning normally compared to 38% of those treated with acyclovir. A study (4) in Sweden using 53 patients with confirmed HSE showed a similar pattern of results indicating acyclovir as the drug of choice in this disease.

Varicella-zoster (VZV)

Diseases caused by this virus are usually self-limiting (chickenpox and shingles) and easily controlled in an otherwise healthy individual, but they can be a serious problem in patients treated with immunosuppressive drugs or who are otherwise immunocompromised. In a double-blind, placebo-controlled study vidarabine proved effective in accelerating healing of cutaneous lesions and in decreasing cutaneous dissemination and zoster-related complications. It has also been reported that the duration of post-herpetic neuralgia was reduced and no serious drug toxicity was observed. Treatment was most effective when started within the first 3 days and administered for 5 days (22). A similar double-blind placebo-controlled study was performed in immunocompromised patients with varicella (chickenpox) with comparable results. Drug therapy accelerated cessation of new lesion formation and resolution of fever, and reduced varicella-related complications (23). In both instances the drug should be initiated as soon as possible after the appearance of lesions and be continued for 5 days at a dosage of 10 mg/kg/d.

Results comparing the efficacy of vidarabine and acyclovir in severely immunocompromised patients are still equivocal. In Seattle 22 patients were randomly assigned to treatment with vidarabine, 10 mg/kg/d, by 12-hour infusion or with acyclovir, 500 mg/m² body surface every 8 hours as a 1-hour infusion (3). They were treated for 7 days or for at least 2 days beyond the last day of new lesion formation, whichever was longer. Treatment was initiated within 72 hours of onset of infection. Cutaneous dissemination of infection occurred in none of the 10 acyclovir recipients and in 5 of the 10 vidarabine recipients who had begun the study with localized dermatomal disease. Acyclovir compared favorably to vidarabine in all parameters examined, such as: new lesion formation, time to decrease in pain, pustulation of all lesions, crusting, healing, and reduction of fever.

In Paris, researchers have reported that they found no difference in the efficacy of vidarabine and acyclovir in immunocompromised patients with severe VZV infections (24). Thirty-eight patients were given 10 mg/kg/d of vidarabine or 30 mg/kg/d of acyclovir according to a computer-generated random code for 5 days. There were no significant differences in the time required for the disappearance of fever or the cessation of lesion formation. No statistically significant differences were found in the number of patients with VZV isolated in cultures taken on day 5. Although there appeared to be no difference in the efficacy of acyclovir and vidarabine, the study recommended acyclovir as the preferred drug when treating patients with a high risk of cardiopulmonary failure due to the large amounts of fluids needed to administer vidarabine.

The efficacy of 2'-fluoro-5-iodoarabinosylcytosine (FIAC), a pyrimidine nucleotide analogue, was compared to vidarabine in immunosuppressed patients recently (25). Thirty-four patients were treated in a randomized double-blind study using 400 mg/m²/d of FIAC and 400 mg/m²/d of vidarabine for 5 days. The time for the cessation of new lesions was less in patients taking FIAC. Pain was also reduced and initial crusting within 72 hours of treatment was accelerated for FIAC patients. However, there was no significant difference in the distribution of positive varicella cultures between the two groups. FIAC compared favorably with vidarabine, but more controlled studies need to be conducted. Acceleration of complete healing time, which is essential for lessening pain, was not measured (20).

Mucocutaneous herpes simplex

HSV-1 also causes serious problems in immunocompromised individuals. A simple fever blister can lead to facial disfigurement, weight loss and even death through dissemination to the lung, liver, or brain in an immunocompromised host. Studies have shown that 10 mg/kg/d of vidarabine administered for 7 days accelerated loss of pain and defervescence. This therapy did not accelerate healing in the total population but it did clear the virus more rapidly in patients over 40 years of age (26). The U.S. Food and Drug Administration has not yet approved the drug for this indication.

Neonatal herpes

Although relatively uncommon (incidence, 1–3 per 30,000 live births), this disease has a relatively high mortality (approximately $1/3$ of infected infants) and morbidity (severe retardation in another $1/3$). Infection can be manifested by localized infection (eye, mouth, and/or skin), localized to the CNS only, or disseminated with multiple organ involvement. Mortality is associated with only the latter two manifestations, which account for over 75% of all neonatal herpes, and is 40% and 82%, respectively.

A placebo-controlled study demonstrated that the 75% mortality rate in the population studied could be reduced to 38% when vidarabine was given intravenously at a dose of 15 mg/kg/d. The prognosis was best in infants with CNS localized disease (mortality reduced from 50% to 10%) as opposed to that in those with disseminated disease (86% to 57%). In infants with localization to skin, eye, or mouth, severe sequelae occurred in 38% of placebo recipients and in none of those on drug therapy (27). Subsequent studies (28) indicated that infants can tolerate dosages of 30 mg/kg/d, and the beneficial effects of this dosage increase strikingly (disease progression reduced from 22% to 4%).

Since acyclovir proved more effective than vidarabine in the treatment of herpes encephalitis and varicella-zoster, a comparison was made in neonatal herpes (29). A study in 182 infants with herpes simplex infections was recently completed; 87 received vidarabine (V) and 95 acyclovir (A). They were divided into 3 categories: 64 with CNS involvement, 43 with disseminated disease (DIS), and 75 with infection localized to the skin, eye or mouth (SEM). None of the SEM babies died at 1 year; 85% V and 93% A were developing normally 1 year post-infection. The mortality in neonates with CNS infection was 13% V and 8% A, and 37% V and 34% A were developing normally at 1 year. The highest mortality was in DIS disease: 50% V and 65% A, with only 23% V and 29% A developing normally at 1 year. Therefore, unlike with the previous two indications, there is no advantage for either drug; both drugs appeared equally effective.

Other clinical studies

Currently, vidarabine is not being used for the treatment of chronic hepatitis B (30, 31). A study (31) using vidarabine monophosphate showed some beneficial results while patients were in treatment, but these results were transient and returned to pretreatment levels after treatment was terminated. Since vidarabine monophosphate could be administered on an outpatient basis, there was some hope that this drug would be effective. However, in addition to its lack of efficacy, vidarabine monophosphate proved to be highly toxic. Severe and prolonged neuropathic syndrome developed in some patients when the drug was given systemically over a prolonged period.

Studies performed with vidarabine and the more soluble vidarabine monophosphate to test their topical efficacy against oral and genital herpes have yielded mostly negative results.

FUTURE DIRECTIONS

Vidarabine as a single agent against herpes infections is slowly being replaced either by more effective drugs or more soluble comparable drugs. The low solubility of vidarabine and hence the inability to administer it to outpatients is a severe drawback. Research with prodrugs which can be readily administered with similar or improved efficacy is to be encouraged. Results with the analog cyclaradine, which is readily soluble, appears to have a wider range of activity than vidarabine, and is effective when given parenterally, topically, or orally, are anxiously awaited.

Several clinical studies with antiviral agents as single agents versus placebo, or in comparison to other antiviral agents, continue to be published. What needs to be done is to use effective drugs in combination in hopes of a synergistic effect. Combination therapy may also result in reduction of drug resistance and reduced toxicity through reduced dosage. It is expected that more soluble forms, such as cyclaradine, and vidarabine in combination with other drugs, will prove even more useful in the quest for more effective antiviral treatment.

REFERENCES

1. Whitley RJ, Soong S-J, Dolin R, Galasso GJ, Ch'ien LT, Alford Jr CA (1977) Adenine arabinoside therapy of biopsy-proven herpes simplex encephalitis. *N. Engl. J. Med., 297*, 289.
2. Whitley RJ, Alford CA, Hirsch MS, Schooley RT, Luby JP, Aoki FY, Hanley D, Nahmias AJ, Soong S-J (1986) Vidarabine versus acyclovir therapy in herpes simplex encephalitis. *N. Engl. J. Med., 314*, 144.
3. Shepp DH, Dandliker PS, Meyers JD (1986) Treatment of varicella-zoster virus infection in severely immunocompromised patients. *N. Engl. J. Med., 314*, 208.

4. Skoldenberg B, Forsgren M (1985) Acyclovir versus vidarabine in herpes simplex encephalitis. *Scand. J. Infect. Dis., 47, Suppl.,* 89.

5. Crumpacker CS, Schnipper LE, Marlowe SI, Kowalsky PN, Hershey BJ, Levin MS (1982) Resistance to antiviral drugs of herpes simplex virus isolated from a patient treated with acyclovir. *N. Engl. J. Med., 306,* 343.

6. Moran DM, Kern ER, Overall Jr JC (1985) Synergism between recombinant human interferon and nucleoside antiviral agents against herpes simplex virus: examination with an automated microtiter plate assay. *J. Infect. Dis., 151,* 1116.

7. Kaufman HE, Varnell ED, Centifanto-Fitzgerald YM (1984) Virus chemotherapy: antiviral drugs and interferon. *Antiviral Res., 4,* 333.

8. Baba M, Ito M, Snigeto S, DeClerq E (1984) Synergistic antiviral effects of antiherpes compounds and human leukocyte interferon on varicella-zoster virus in vitro. *Antimicrob. Agents Chemother., 25,* 515.

9. Omura S, Imamura N, Kuga H, Ishikawa H, Yamazaki Y, Okano K, Kimura K, Takahashi Y, Tanaka H (1985) Adechlorin, a new adenosine deaminase inhibitor containing chlorine production, isolation and properties. *J. Antibiol., 39,* 1008.

10. Karim MR, Marks MI, Benton DC, Rollerson W (1985) Synergistic antiviral effects of acyclovir and vidarabine on herpes simplex infection in newborn mice. *Chemotherapy, 31,* 310.

11. Spector SA, Kelley E (1985) Inhibition of human cytomegalovirus by combined acyclovir and vidarabine. *Antimicrob. Agents Chemother., 27,* 600.

12. Allen LB, Vanderslice LK, Fingal CM, McCright FH, Harris EF, Cook PD (1982) Evaluation of the anti-herpesvirus drug combination: virazole plus arabinofuranosyl hypoxanthine and virazole plus arabinofuranosyl adenine. *Antiviral Res., 2,* 203.

13. Crane LR, Milne DA, Sunstrum JC, Lerner AM (1984) Comparative activities of selected combinations of acyclovir, vidarabine, arabinosyl hypoxanthine, interferon, and polyriboinosinic acid-polyribocytidylic acid complex against herpes simplex virus type 2 in tissue culture and intravaginally inoculated mice. *Antimicrob. Agents Chemother., 26,* 557.

14. Schinazi RF, Peters J, Sokol MK, Nahmias AJ (1983) Therapeutic activities of 1-(2-fluoro-2-deoxy-β-D-arabinofuranosyl)-5-iodocytosine and -thymine alone and in combination with acyclovir and vidarabine in mice infected intracerebrally with herpes simplex virus. *Antimicrob. Agents Chemother., 24,* 95.

15. Park N-H, Callahan JG, Pavan-Langston D (1984) Effect of combined acyclovir and vidarabine on infection with herpes simplex virus in vitro and in vivo. *J. Infect. Dis., 149,* 757.

16. Eron C (1981) *The Virus that Ate Cannibals,* p 159, McMillan, New York.

17. Pavan-Langston D, Buchanan RA, Alford Jr CA (Eds) (1975) *Adenine Arabinoside: An Antiviral Agent.* Raven Press, New York.

18. Galasso GJ (1986) Vidarabine. In: Peterson PK, Verhoef J (Eds), *The Antimicrobial Agents Annual 1,* p 370. Elsevier, Amsterdam.

19. Buchanan RA, Hess F (1980) Vidarabine (Vira A) pharmacology and clinical experience. *Pharmacol. Ther., 8,* 143.

20. Whitley RJ (1985) Therapy for human herpesvirus infection: a perspective. *Ala. J. Med. Sci., 22,* 193.

21. Whitley RF, Soong S-J, Hirsch MS, Karchmer AW, Dolin R, Galasso GJ, Dunnick JK, Alford Jr CA (1981) Herpes simplex encephalitis – vidarabine therapy and diagnostic problems. *N. Engl. J. Med., 304,* 313.

22. Whitley RJ, Soong S-J, Dolin R, Betts R, Linneman Jr C, Alford Jr CA (1982) Early vidarabine therapy to control the complications of herpes zoster in immunosuppressed patients. *N. Engl. J. Med., 308,* 971.

23. Whitley RJ, Hilty M, Haynes R, Bryson Y, Connor JD, Soong S-J, Alford Jr CA (1982) Vidarabine therapy of varicella in immunosuppressed patients. *J. Pediatr., 101,* 125.

24. Vilde JL, Bricaire F, Leport C, Renaudie M, Brun-Vezinet F (1986) Comparative trial of acyclovir and vidarabine in disseminated varicella-zoster virus infections in immunocompromised patients. *J. Med. Virol., 20,* 127.

25. Leyland-Jones B, Donnelly H, Groshen S, Myskowski P, Donner AL, Fanucchi M, Fox J (1986) 2′-Fluoro-5-iodoarabinosylcytosine, a new potent antiviral agent: efficacy in immunosuppressed individuals with herpes zoster. *J. Infect. Dis., 154,* 430.

26. Whitley RJ, Spruance S, Hayden FG, Overall J, Alford Jr CA, Gwaltney JM, Soong S-J (1984) Vidarabine therapy for mucocutaneous herpes simplex virus infections in immunocompromised host. *J. Infect. Dis., 149,* 1.

27. Whitley RJ, Nahmias AJ, Soong S-J, Galasso GJ, Fleming CL, Alford Jr CA (1980) Vidarabine therapy of neonatal herpes simplex virus infection. *J. Pediatr., 66,* 495.

28. Whitley RJ, Yeager A, Kartus P, Bryson Y, Connor JD, Alford Jr CA, Nahmias A, Soong S-J (1983) Neonatal herpes simplex infection: follow up evaluation of vidarabine therapy. *J. Pediatr., 72,* 778.

29. Whitley RJ, Arvin A, Corey L, Powell D, Plotkin S, Starr S, Alford Jr CA, Connor J, Nahmias AJ, Soong S-J, and NIAID Collaborative Study Group (1986) Vidarabine versus acyclovir therapy of neonatal herpes simplex virus infection. In: *Abstracts, Annual Meeting of the Society for Pediatric Research*, Abstract No. 987, Washington, DC.

30. Garcia G, Smith CI, Weissberg JI, Eisenberg M, Bissett J, Nair PV, Rosno S, Roskamp D, Waterman K, Pollard RB, Tong MJ, Brown BW, Robinson WS, Gregory PB, Merigan TC (1987) Adenine arabinoside monophosphate in combination with human leukocyte interferon in the treatment of chronic hepatitis B: a randomized, double-blind, placebo-controlled trial. *Ann. Intern. Med., 107,* 278.

31. Hoofnagel JH, Hanson RG, Minuk GY, Pappas SC, Schafer DF, Fusheiko M, Straus SE, Popper H, Jones EA (1984) Randomized controlled trial of adenine arabinoside monophosphate for chronic type B hepatitis. *Gastroenterology, 86,* 150.

CHAPTER 37

Penicillin-binding proteins

NAFSIKA H. GEORGOPAPADAKOU

Over the past decade, penicillin-binding proteins (PBPs) have emerged as a unique prokaryotic protein family and an important quantifiable parameter of β-lactam susceptibility and resistance. Studies on PBPs have contributed significantly to our understanding of the mode of action of β-lactam antibiotics and of newly recognized mechanisms of antibiotic resistance. Most importantly, studies on PBPs have provided a framework for structure-activity relationships, which may eventually lead to the rational design of new antibiotics.

PBPs are bacterial proteins which bind selectively and covalently penicillin and other β-lactam antibiotics. They vary from species to species in number, size, abundance, and affinity for β-lactam antibiotics, usually following taxonomic lines (1). Generally they are 4–8, of molecular weights 35–120 kD, and comprise about 1% of the membrane proteins. Some PBPs catalyze essential reactions in bacterial cell-wall biosynthesis and control such fundamental processes as cell growth and division (2). Their binding to β-lactams may trigger autolysins, thereby causing cell death (3–5). Enzymatic activities associated with PBPs (sensitive to penicillin; hence the term, penicillin-sensitive enzymes (PSEs)) are transpeptidase, DD-carboxypeptidase, endopeptidase, and β-lactamase, sometimes two or more activities residing on the same protein. For example, PBP-4 of *Staphylococcus aureus* has transpeptidase, DD-carboxypeptidase, and β-lactamase activity (6). Despite their diversity and versatility, PBPs share several structural and functional similarities, including sequence homology in their active sites (2).

This review considers the role of PBPs in: (a) bacterial physiology and biochemistry; (b) antibacterial action of β-lactams; (c) bacterial resistance to β-lactams. The effects of β-lactam structure on binding to PBPs and the implications for drug design will also be discussed. As much as possible, clinically important bacteria will be used as examples. Other features of PBPs and PSEs are discussed in several recent reviews (2, 7–16). Background topics, such as peptidoglycan biosynthesis (17, 18), penicillin action (19, 20), β-lactam antibiotics (21–23), β-lactamases (24–27) and autolysins (4, 5) have also been reviewed recently and will be discussed only briefly in this review.

Antimicrobial Agents Annual 3
P.K. Peterson and J. Verhoef, editors
© Elsevier Science Publishers BV, 1988

PENICILLIN-BINDING PROTEINS AND PENICILLIN ACTION

The discovery of PBPs was preceded by extensive studies on the structure and bio-synthesis of the bacterial cell wall and the mechanism of action of penicillin. The effects of penicillin on cell-wall structure and morphology were shown soon after its introduction, and by the late 1950s penicillin was reported to be a specific inhi-bitor of bacterial cell-wall biosynthesis. During the following decade, the structure of the bacterial cell wall and the mechanism of its synthesis were elucidated. Fol-lowing on from these studies in the early 1970s came the identification of the 2 types of bacterial enzymes sensitive to penicillin, peptidoglycan transpeptidase and DD-carboxypeptidase. Also at that time, multiple PBPs were discovered in several bacteria. These developments are detailed in a classical review (28).

Bacterial cell-wall structure and biosynthesis

Peptidoglycan, the major component of the bacterial cell wall, is a rigid, bag-like macromolecule which surrounds, in one or more layers, the cytoplasmic mem-brane. It consists of linear sugar chains substituted with short peptide strands which are crosslinked at a D-alanine residue either directly or via a peptide bridge. The sugar chains are composed invariably of alternating *N*-acetylglucosamine and *N*-acetylmuramic acid residues, while the amino acid composition of the peptide strands varies from species to species (29). Peptidoglycan biosynthesis is believed to proceed in 3 distinct stages: (a) the synthesis of the *N*-acetylmuramic acid-pen-tapeptide monomer in the cytoplasm; (b) its transfer to the cytoplasmic mem-brane, the addition *N*-acetylglucosamine (and species-specific modifications); (c) the transfer of the disaccharide-peptide unit outside the cytoplasmic membrane and its crosslinking, through both sugar and peptide moieties, to sugar and peptide groups in the growing peptidoglycan.

Penicillin action

Penicillin inhibits the crosslinking of peptide strands in the growing peptidogly-can, a reaction catalyzed by specific transpeptidase(s). The mechanism of inhibi-tion, first proposed in 1965 (30), involves the formation of a stable penicilloyl-enzyme complex with peptidoglycan transpeptidase, very similar to the transition-state complex formed between the peptide strand of the growing peptidoglycan and the enzyme.

Detection of penicillin-binding proteins

The finding of multiple proteins that bound penicillin covalently in several bacte-ria led to the suggestion of multiple penicillin targets (28). However, it was the subsequent introduction of a specific and convenient PBP labeling assay (31) that made possible the characterization of PBPs from a variety of bacteria. The assay involves incubating whole cells or bacterial membranes for 10 minutes with radio-labeled penicillin G at 30°C (or lower temperature if enzymatic release of bound radioactivity is a concern (32)). Proteins are solubilized with detergent, fractionated on sodium dodecylsulfate (SDS)-polyacrylamide gels, and fluorographed. Detection of a particular PBP depends on the amount of PBP present, its affinity for the labeled penicillin, and the specific activity of the label. Differences in binding between whole cells and membranes have been reported (33). Binding of a given β-lactam is usually measured indirectly, as decreased binding of labeled penicillin G. Significant differences in binding between β-lactam enantiomers have been reported (34, 35), arguing against using racemic mixtures. Binding of β-lactam antibiotics can also be measured directly, using radiolabeled β-lactam of specific activity comparable to that of penicillin G (36). Binding results have been correlated with minimal inhibitory concentrations (MICs) and cell morphology. Causal relations are difficult to establish when: (a) binding occurs to more than one PBP at near-MIC concentration (37); (b) PBP binding is not associated with discrete morphologic changes (38); and (c) more than one PBP is responsible for a given function (39). Resolving these complications experimentally can be a major challenge.

Recently, a more sensitive PBP detection method has been introduced, involving reaction with antibodies against the penicilloyl determinant (40). However, the observed variability in PBPs on immunoblots, which is sometimes independent of the amount of the penicilloyl-protein present, and the lack of commercial antibodies preclude widespread use of this method.

Properties of penicillin-binding proteins

PBP assays, being population measurements, give no intrinsic spatial or temporal resolution. Consequently, little is known about the spatial distribution of PBPs in the cell or their regulation during the cell cycle. Minor PBPs associated with localized functions, such as septum formation, are probably concentrated at specific regions in the cytoplasmic membrane (41). Studies with synchronously growing *Escherichia coli* have uncovered transpeptidase activity associated with septation but not cell elongation (42), although there was no corresponding increase in the amount of PBP-3 during septation (43). Another factor, just beginning to be appreciated, is the effect of growth conditions on PBP expression (44). In *S. aureus*, for example, pH has a significant effect on the expression of PBP-2a (45) and possibly PBP-2 (Georgopapadakou and Cummings, unpublished data).

PBPs have been found in all bacteria so far examined, with the exception of mycoplasma, which lack cell wall (46). Typically, an organism contains 4–8 PBPs of molecular weights 35–120 kD. They are numbered by convention in the order of decreasing molecular weight. Once the number of PBPs for a given organism is established, additional PBPs are numbered as derivatives of established ones even though they are not related to them. This is done to avoid renumbering the PBPs and thereby causing confusion with the older literature. Thus, PBP-1 (91 kD) of *E. coli* was resolved into 2 components, termed PBP-1a and -1b (47); a 78-kD protein, detected using a radiolabeled ampicillin derivative, was termed PBP-1c (48). In methicillin-resistant *S. aureus*, a novel 78-kD PBP, unrelated by peptide analysis to PBP-2 of that organism and associated with resistance, has been termed PBP-2′ (49) or PBP-2a (45).

Essential PBPs are generally minor proteins of molecular weights 60–120 kD. They have been identified in several bacteria, but specific biochemical and physiologic functions have so far been assigned only for the PBPs of *E. coli* (50). Analogous functions have been inferred for the PBPs of related bacteria (51–54). Information on other bacteria, whose PBPs are not correlatable to those of *E. coli*, is sketchy. For example, specific physiologic functions have been tentatively assigned to PBP-2 and -3 of *S. aureus* and PBP-1 and -2 of *Bacteroides fragilis* based on morphology data (55, 56).

Purification of PBPs is usually accomplished by affinity chromatography on Sepharose, the *β*-lactam ligand being selected on the basis of PBP affinity. PBPs are subsequently eluted with neutral hydroxylamine, which cleaves the covalent bond between the *β*-lactam and the PBP (1, 12, 28). Most of the purified PBPs are devoid of enzymatic activity, a fact variously attributed to inactivation during purification, loss of lipid environment, or inappropriate assay conditions, especially substrate (57). Obviously, retention of the penicillin-binding activity does not necessarily imply retention of carboxypeptidase or transpeptidase activity.

PENICILLIN-BINDING PROTEINS IN GRAM-NEGATIVE BACTERIA

Escherichia coli

In the *E. coli* cytoplasmic membrane 7 PBPs have been consistently found (Table 1). They are coded by specific genes which are dispersed in the *E. coli* chromosome (39, 58). PBP-1 (a and b), -2, and -3 are essential and are involved, respectively, in elongation, shape and septation. All three are bifunctional enzymes with transpeptidase and transglycosylase activities (59–63) which probably reside in the amino- and carboxy-terminal half of the protein, respectively (2, 64–67). The genes coding for PBP-1a, 1b, -2, and -3 have recently been sequenced (68–70). *β*-Lactam antibiotics which bind to PBP-1 cause lysis, while those binding to PBP-2 produce giant spherical-shaped cells, and those binding to PBP-3 result in filamentation (50).

PBP-1 has been resolved into 2 genetically distinct components, 1a and 1b, with similar biochemical and physiological functions although different affinities toward *β*-lactam antibiotics. PBP-1a is sensitive to most *β*-lactam antibiotics; their binding simultaneously to PBP-1a and -3 has been suggested to lead to cell death (71). However, monobactams bind to PBP-3 only and are still bacteriocidal (72). Other evidence also suggests that binding to PBP-3 is sufficient for cell death (73) and that additional binding to PBP-1a may be antagonistic (74). PBP-1b is rela-

Table 1   *Properties of Escherichia coli PBPs*

PBP	MW	Copies/cell	Enzyme activity	Physiologic function
1a	92	200	transpeptidase/	cylindrical cell wall
1b	90	250	transglycosylase	synthesis (elongation)
2	66	20	transpeptidase	cylindrical cell wall synthesis (initiation)
3	60	50	transpeptidase/ transglycosylase	cross-wall synthesis (septation)
4	49	110	DD-carboxypeptidase/ endopeptidase	autolysin?
5	42	1800	DD-carboxypeptidase/	regulation of cross-
6	40	600	penicillinase	linking?

tively resistant to β-lactam antibiotics. It has been further resolved into 3 genetically indistinguishable proteins, α, β, and γ (75–77). While mutants lacking PBP-1a have no phenotypic defect, those lacking PBP-1b are hypersensitive to β-lactam antibiotics, reflecting the high sensitivity of PBP-1a (78). PBP-1b mutants have been successfully used in the discovery of naturally-occuring β-lactam antibiotics (79). Mutants lacking both PBP-1a and -1b are not viable (80). PBP-2 is highly sensitive to mecillinam (amdinocillin), to some penicillins, and to a lesser extent thienamycin and clavulanic acid. It is generally resistant to cephalosporins and to monobactams. Simultaneous binding to PBPs-2 and -3 has been reported to cause cell lysis (81). PBP-2 has been suggested to initiate peptidoglycan biosynthesis (82). PBP-3 is sensitive to most β-lactam antibiotics, being generally less affected by structural changes on the β-lactam nucleus than are PBP-1 and -2. It is the target of most β-lactamase-stable antibiotics, such as tetrazolyl amoxycillin (CP-35587) (83), ceftazidime (84), and the monobactams carumonam (85) and aztreonam (72). Mutants resistant to cefalexin were found to have altered PBP-3, with reduced affinity to cefalexin though still functional in septation (86, 87). On the other hand, changing the active-site serine residue to a cysteine resulted in loss of physiologic function (cells grew as filaments) but retention of the ability to bind to penicillin (88, 89). In addition to being a septation-associated transpeptidase/ transglycosylase, PBP-3 may interact with FtsA protein, also involved in septation (90).

The low-molecular-weight PBP-4, -5 and -6 appear not to be essential, as binding of β-lactam antibiotics causes no growth defects (50). PBP-4 is generally sensitive to β-lactam antibiotics and has DD-carboxypeptidase, endopeptidase,

Table 2   *Binding of β-lactam antibiotics to Escherichia coli PBPs**

Compound	Concentration (μg/ml) required for 90% inhibition of binding of [^{14}C]penicillin G						MIC (μg/ml)
	PBP-1a	PBP-1b	PBP-2	PBP-3	PBP-4	PBP-5/6	
Penicillins							
Benzylpenicillin	2.0	10	2.0	0.5	0.1	100	12
Ampicillin	2.0	10	0.5	2.0	0.1	100	0.4
Amoxycillin	2.0	10	2.0	2.0	0.1	100	0.2
Piperacillin	10	10	0. 5	0.1	10	100	0.05
Carbenicillin	10	30	30	2.0	2.0	>100	0.8
Azlocillin	10	10	2.0	0.1	2.0	100	0.2
Mezlocillin	10	10	0.1	0.1	10	100	0.05
Amdinocillin	>100	>100	0.1	>100	>100	>100	0.1
Cephalosporins							
Cefaloridine	0.5	30	>100	0.5	2.0	>100	1.6
Cefalotin	0.5	100	100	2.0	100	10	1.6
Cefalexin	10	>100	>100	30	30	>100	6.3
Cefaclor	30	30	>100	2.0	2.0	>100	1.6
Cefoperazone	0.5	100	100	0.1	100	>100	1.6
Cefamandole	0.1	100	100	0.5	10	>100	0.2
Cefoxitin	0.5	10	100	2.0	0.5	10	3.1
Cefuroxime	0.5	10	10	0.1	10	>100	0.2
Cefotaxime	0.5	2.0	10	0.1	10	>100	0.4
Ceftriaxone	0.5	2.0	10	0.1	100	>100	0.4
Ceftazidime	10	10	>100	0.5	100	>100	0.4
Other β-lactams							
Moxalactam	2.0	10	>100	0.1	0.5	30	0.8
Imipenem	2.0	10	0.1	2.0	0.1	30	0.8
Aztreonam	10	>100	>100	0.1	>100	>100	0.1
Carumonam	30	>100	>100	0.1	>100	>100	0.1

* Data from the author's laboratory.

and 'model' transpeptidase activity, all 3 activities occuring at the same active site (91–93). Mutants with defective PBP-4 are viable, but have reduced peptidoglycan crosslinking (94). PBP-5 and -6 are moderately sensitive to β-lactam antibiotics and have DD-carboxypeptidase and weak penicillinase activity (95). The major DD-carboxypeptidase activity is associated with PBP-5 (96). Mutants defective in both PBP-5 and -4 have increased peptidoglycan crosslinking (94). Mutants over-producing PBP-5 are spherical (98), possibly reflecting decreased availability of pentapeptide substrate for cell elongation (98). Complete loss of PBP-5 and -6 has been associated with hypersensitivity to β-lactam antibiotics (99, 100). Two additional PBP, -7 and -8, appear in some preparations. Based on their amounts and mobilities on SDS gels, they seem to be degradation products of PBP-5 and -6 (Georgopapadakou and Smith, unpublished data). Recently, PBP-7 (30 kD) has been proposed to be a penem target (101).

Enterobacteria and *Pseudomonas*

Enterobacter, Klebsiella, and *Salmonella* have PBPs very similar to those of *E. coli* (1, 51, 54). In *Proteus,* PBPs are almost identical from species to species and somewhat different from, though still correlatable to, *E. coli* PBPs (52, 54). *Serratia* PBPs, on the other hand, vary from strain to strain, ranging from almost identical to *E. coli* to substantially different (Georgopapadakou and Smith, unpublished data). Like *E. coli,* both *Proteus* and *Serratia* possess a 36-kD PBP with DD-carboxypeptidase and weak penicillinase activity (52).

The PBP pattern of *Pseudomonas aeruginosa* is also correlatable to that of *E. coli,* and binding of β-lactam antibiotics results in morphologic changes similar to those observed in *E. coli* (53, 54). α-Sulfocephalosporins are an exception, in that PBP-3 of *P. aeruginosa* is very sensitive to them while PBP-3 of *E. coli* is resistant (102). Consequently, these compounds induce filamentation and lysis in *P. aeruginosa* but only lysis in *E. coli.* Clinical isolates resistant to β-lactams have been reported, in which binding to PBP-3 was reduced (103).

Other aerobic bacteria

In *Neisseria gonorrhoeae* 3 PBPs have been detected, of molecular weights 87 (PBP-1), 59 (PBP-2), and 44 (PBP-3) kD (104, 105). PBP-1 is the least sensitive to β-lactam antibiotics and is probably the major peptidoglycan transpeptidase; binding of cefaloridine and penicillin results in spheroplasts (106). PBP-2 is the killing site for most β-lactam antibiotics, but is not a major peptidoglycan transpeptidase, since binding is not associated with inhibition of peptidoglycan crosslinking (107). It has been implicated in the *O*-acetylation of peptidoglycan (107, 108). Binding to PBP-2 causes an increase in cell size and thickening of the septum (104). PBP-3 may be a DD-carboxypeptidase similar to PBP-4 (39 kD) of the related *Branhamella catarrhalis* (1). Specific resistance to β-lactam antibiotics is associated with decreased binding to PBP-1 and -2 (104), while non-specific resistance appears to correlate more closely with decreased outer-membrane permeability (109).

In *Haemophilus influenzae* there are 8 PBPs of molecular weights 27–90 kD (110). PBP-2 (80 kD) and PBP-3 (75 kD) correspond, on the basis of sensitivity to β-lactam antibiotics, to PBP-1a and -2 of *E. coli.* Resistance to β-lactams in clinical isolates has been associated with decreased affinity of PBP-5 (59 kD) for β-lactams (111, 112).

Anaerobic bacteria

B. fragilis has 4 PBPs of molecular weights 32–100 kD (56). PBP-1 (100 kD) may be the major peptidoglycan transpeptidase in this organism, as binding to β-lactam antibiotics results in cell lysis. PBP-2 (86 kD) is the target for most β-lactam antibiotics and may be involved in septation. PBP-4 (32 kD) has weak penicillinase activity and may be a DD-carboxypeptidase. Other *Bacteroides* species have similar PBP patterns (113). Resistance to β-lactams has been associated with decreased binding to PBP-1 and -2 (56, 114).

PENICILLIN-BINDING PROTEINS IN GRAM-POSITIVE BACTERIA

Aerobic bacteria

In *S. aureus*, 4 PBPs of molecular weights 41–87 kD have been observed (115, 116). Pharmacologic and microbiologic studies have suggested that PBPs-2 (80 kD) and -3 (75 kD) are the killing sites for β-lactam antibiotics in this organism (116–119), and are probably involved, respectively, in peptidoglycan growth and septation. Methicillin-resistant organisms overproduce a novel 78-kD PBP, variously termed PBP-2′ (120, 49) or PBP-2a (121, 122). Its induction is strongest under conditions favoring methicillin resistance such as acidic pH, low temperature, and high salt (49, 123). PBP-4 (42 kD) is a DD-carboxypeptidase with transpeptidase and weak penicillinase activities (6). Mutants lacking it grow normally suggesting that it is not essential (118). However, mutants overproducing it are β-lactam-resistant (Georgopapadakou and Cummings, unpublished data). PBP-4 has been implicated in the secondary crosslinking of peptidoglycan (124). The related *Staphylococcus epidermidis* has a similar PBP pattern (1), and a similar mode of methicillin resistance (125). The use of PBP profile as a means to classify staphylococci (126) and enterococci (127) has been suggested recently.

In *Streptococcus faecalis* 5 PBPs with molecular weights 42–105 kD have been observed (116, 128, 129). Pharmacologic studies, using several structurally unrelated β-lactam antibiotics, have suggested that the killing sites are PBP-1 (105 kD) and PBP-3 (79 kD) (116). The related *Streptococcus faecium* has a very similar PBP pattern (129). In this organism, a 79-kD PBP (referred to as PBP-5) is also a killing site and mutants overproducing it are resistant to β-lactam antibiotics (130–132). PBP-6 (42 kD) is a DD-carboxypeptidase with penicillinase and transpeptidase activities (131).

In *Streptococcus pneumoniae* 5 PBPs have been detected, of molecular weights 52–100 kD (134). Studies with penicillin-resistant clinical isolates suggest that PBP-1 and -2 are the killing sites for β-lactam antibiotics (135–137). PBP-3 (43 kD) is a DD-carboxypeptidase and has been recently purified by affinity chromatography (138).

Table 3   *Binding of β-lactam antibiotics to Staphylococcus aureus PBPs**

Compound	Concentration (μg/ml) required for 90% inhibition of binding of [^{14}C]penicillin G				MIC (μg/ml)
	PBP-1	PBP-2	PBP- 3	PBP-4	
Penicillins					
Benzylpenicillin	0.1	0.1	0.1	>100	<0.05
Ampicillin	0.1	2.0	0.1	>100	1.6
Methicillin	0.1	2.0	0.1	>100	0.8
Piperacillin	0.1	0.1	0.1	>100	0.4
Azlocillin	0.5	0.5	0.5	>100	0.4
Mezlocillin	0.1	0.1	0.1	>100	0.4
Amdinocillin	100	>100	2.0	>100	12.5
Cephalosporins					
Cefaloridine	0.1	0.1	0.1	100	<0.05
Cefalotin	0.5	0.5	0.5	100	0.1
Cefalexin	0.5	>100	0.1	>100	0.8
Cefaclor	0.1	>100	0.1	>100	0.2
Cefoperazone	0.5	0.5	0.5	>100	0.8
Cefamandole	0.1	0.5	0.5	100	0.1
Cefoxitin	10	2.0	10	0.5	0.8
Cefuroxime	100	0.5	>100	>100	6.2
Cefotaxime	0.5	0.5	10	>100	1.6
Ceftriaxone	0.5	2.0	0.5	>100	1.6
Ceftazidime	0.1	2.0	100	100	12.5
Other β-lactams					
Moxalactam	0.1	2.0	10	0.1	3.1
Imipenem	0.1	>100	10	0.1	3.1
Aztreonam	>100	>100	>100	>100	>100
Carumonam	>100	>100	>100	>100	>100

* Data from the author's laboratory.

Anaerobic bacteria

In *Clostridium perfringens* 6 PBPs have been observed, of molecular weights 42–100 kD (139, 140). PBP-1 (125 kD) and PBP-2 (103 kD) are relatively insensitive to β-lactam antibiotics. PBP-3 (90 kD) and PBP-4 (81 kD) have been suggested to be the killing sites and to be involved in septation. β-Lactam-resistant mutants, isolated by in vitro selection, had decreased affinity of PBP-1 for β-lactams (141).

PENICILLIN-BINDING PROTEINS AS PENICILLIN-SENSITIVE ENZYMES

The major enzymatic activities associated with the PBP family are DD-carboxy-peptidase and peptidoglycan transpeptidase. A dynamic interplay may exist between the two enzymes regulating the degree of peptidoglycan crosslinking, quite similar to that postulated for topoisomerase I and DNA gyrase in DNA supercoiling (142). The fact that both DD-carboxypeptidase and topoisomerase I mutants are viable, in the latter case due to compensatory changes (143), is consistent with the suggested similarity.

DD-Carboxypeptidase and peptidoglycan transpeptidase are mechanistically similar; they act on the same pentapeptide substrate, and form the same covalent intermediate involving a serine residue (144). The similarity extends to their amino-acid sequences in the active site; the amino-terminal half of a peptidoglycan transpeptidase has been reported to have some homology to that of a DD-carboxypeptidase (2).

Peptidoglycan transpeptidases

Peptidoglycan transpeptidases are associated with high-molecular-weight (60–120 kD) PBPs. Individual enzymes have been purified from the membranes of PBP-overproducing *E. coli* strains by affinity chromatography and identified as PBP-1a, -2, and -3 (Table 1). With the exception of PBP-2, these PBPs are bifunctional enzymes, acting both as transpeptidases and transglycosylases. Inhibition constants (IC_{50}s) for several β-lactam antibiotics have been determined with individual transpeptidases from that organism (145). Transglycosylase activity is not inhibited by β-lactam antibiotics, but is sensitive to the glycophospholipid monoemycin (146).

In other bacteria, peptidoglycan transpeptidases have been associated with high-molecular-weight PBPs on the basis of microbiologic rather than biochemical studies. Biochemical studies have been limited to cell-wall preparations (147, 148) and permeabilized cell systems (98, 149). In these assays the sum of transpeptidase activities minus the sum of DD-carboxypeptidase and endopeptidase activities is actually being measured. Inhibition data obtained from such studies can be quite misleading. For example, transpeptidase activity in permeabilized *E. coli* cells corresponds to activity associated with PBP-1b only (145). Furthermore, inhibition of PBP-5 can result in an apparent stimulation of transpeptidase activity (150).

DD-Carboxypeptidases

The enzymes from a variety of species have been isolated and studied extensively (9). They are 25–50 kD proteins possessing exopeptidase, esterase, endopeptidase, transpeptidase, and penicillinase activities. All 5 activities most likely occur at the same active site (9, 151). The physiologic role of the exopeptidase activity may be to regulate the availability of pentapeptide substrates for transpeptidation, while endopeptidase may function as an autolysin. Transpeptidase activity is usually confined to 'model substrates' (UDP-MurNAc pentapeptide, small peptides, glycine) and is probably of little physiologic consequence. Notable exceptions are *Gaffkya homari*, which uses tetrapeptide substrates (152), and *S. aureus*, where DD-carboxypeptidase (PBP-4) has been associated with secondary peptidoglycan crosslinking (118, 124) and β-lactam resistance (Georgopapadakou and Cummings, unpublished data).

Most DD-carboxypeptidases are membrane-bound, probably anchored to the outer side of the cytoplasmic membrane through their carboxy terminus (153). The extensively studied enzymes from *Streptomyces* R61, *albus* G, and *Actinomadura* R39, are excreted into the growth medium in their final form (14), which undoubtedly has contributed to their research appeal. Most DD-carboxypeptidases studied thus far are readily inhibited by penicillins, 7α-methoxy cephalosporins (cephamycins) (9, 154), and to a lesser degree non-methoxylated cephalosporins and monobactams (36, 155). With a single exception (the *albus* G enzyme), inhibition is through covalent binding to a serine residue on the enzyme (9). This serine residue appears to be conserved in the amino-acid sequence of several carboxypeptidases and is also present in peptidoglycan transpeptidases and β-lactamases (2), underlining the relatedness of the 3 enzymes. Bound penicillins are released by DD-carboxypeptidases as penicilloic acids (fast release), or as phenylacetyl glycine and penicillamine (slow release) (14). With a few exceptions, DD-carboxypeptidases and PBPs in general lack significant cephalosporinase activity (14, 156).

The unavailability of peptidoglycan transpeptidases, coupled with their similarity to DD-carboxypeptidases, has made the latter attractive models of the former. As such, DD-carboxypeptidases have provided valuable mechanistic insights into the interaction of β-lactam antibiotics with their targets. However, accumulating evidence points to their limitations and strengthens the case for using the PBP assay as a guide to drug design. For example, *Streptomyces* R61 DD-carboxypeptidase has a β-lactam inhibition profile very similar to that of *E. coli* PBP-4, also a DD-carboxypeptidase (Georgopapadakou and Smith, unpublished data). Unfortunately, both are different from the β-lactam binding profiles of the 3 target PBPs in *E. coli*.

CLINICAL IMPLICATIONS

Susceptibility to β-lactam antibiotics reflects the combined effects of essential PBP binding, stability to β-lactamases and, in the case of gram-negative bacteria, permeability (23, 157, 158). These factors can sometimes present conflicting structural requirements. For example, the anionic side chain of ceftazidime contributes to its greater β-lactamase stability and, in *P. aeruginosa*, increased outer-membrane permeability relative to cefotaxime. It also contributes to its reduced PBP binding (Tables 2 and 3).

Resistance to β-lactam antibiotics may develop as a result of a change in any of the above factors. In addition, resistance may result from reduced autolysin activity, in which case it is called 'tolerance' (159). So far, PBP-associated resistance is less common than resistance associated with β-lactamases or permeability. Nevertheless, it has been reported in clinical isolates of several common gram-negative and gram-positive pathogens (Table 4), and could become more common as single-target β-lactam antibiotics are increasingly used. Examples of such compounds are ceftazidime, temocillin, and the monobactams. Generally, they are very stable to β-lactamases, but have reduced intrinsic activity, number of killing sites, and antibacterial spectrum.

A functional classification of β-lactam antibiotics based on PBP-binding profiles may be useful, particularly as the structural diversity of these compounds increases. For example, the PBP-binding profiles of carumonam and cefalotin, cefoxitin and moxalactam, thienamycin and Sch-34343, and other pairs of structurally unrelated β-lactam antibiotics are similar. A functional classification could extend to include outer-membrane permeability and β-lactamase stability considerations and thus have the added advantage of predicting cross-resistance.

FUTURE DIRECTIONS

The development of β-lactam antibiotics has not always followed a rational, pre-

Table 4   *PBP-associated resistance to β-lactams*

Organism	PBP altered	Type of alteration
Gram-positive		
Staphylococcus aureus	3	reduced affinity
	2' (2a)	novel PBP, induced
	4	overproduced[*]
Staphylococcus pneumoniae	1, 3	reduced affinity
Clostridium perfringens	1	reduced affinity
Gram-negative		
Escherichia coli	2	overproduced[*]
	3	reduced affinity[*]
Pseudomonas aeruginosa	3	reduced affinity
Neisseria gonorrhoeae	1, 2	reduced affinity
Haemophilus influenzae	4	reduced affinity
Bacteroides fragilis	2	reduced affinity

[*] Laboratory strains; all other are clinical isolates.

420

dictable path. Serendipity has played a major role, not only in the discovery of naturally occurring β-lactams (thienamycin, clavulanic acid), but of synthetic compounds as well (mecillinam, cefuroxime). The situation is now changing as the individual factors contributing to β-lactam susceptibility become quantified: the structural requirements for outer-membrane permeability, the substrate profiles of various β-lactamases, and PBP binding profiles for β-lactams. Thus, the stage is set for the rational design of new β-lactam antibiotics.

Essential to the understanding of the interaction between β-lactams and their target PBPs is the structural and functional characterization of these proteins. To this end, investigators have been addressing 3 complementary sets of questions: (a) the specific physiologic functions of PBPs in different bacteria; (b) the molecular basis for the remarkable differences in affinity of PBPs for β-lactams with different side chains; (c) the common molecular mechanisms of transpeptidases, DD-carboxypeptidases, and β-lactamases. Exploitable similarities among PBPs in different bacteria could broaden the antibacterial spectrum of β-lactams, while exploitable differences between PBPs and β-lactamases could circumvent β-lactamases.

Detailed crystallographic studies of water-soluble DD-carboxypeptidases and the related β-lactamases are in progress (160, 161). Similar studies on peptidoglycan transpeptidases, or enzymatically active fragments of them, are certain to follow. The complementary approach, site-specific mutagenesis, has been successfully used with PBP-3 of *E. coli* and has been instrumental in elucidating the penicillin-binding site in that enzyme. This approach will undoubtedly be used with other target PBPs once their amino acid sequences are known. The challenge is to define the structural elements of β-lactams that enable them to interact with the target PBP(s). An important step in that direction has been the finding that a bicyclic β-lactam nucleus is not necessary for the interaction with PBPs (155, 162).

Unfortunately, our optimism must be tempered by the proven resourcefulness of the bacterial pathogens. Evolving in a true Darwinian sense against the constant onslaught of β-lactam antibiotics, they have been able to find the Achilles heel for every new agent. It is unlikely that this will change in the future. Gram-negative bacteria, especially enterobacteria and *Pseudomonas*, will probably continue to use the combination of decreased outer-membrane permeability and increased β-lactamase production as their first line of defense. Gram-positive bacteria, not being endowed with such an effective gate-keeper, will use the β-lactamase alone to search and destroy. This might be difficult with the newer β-lactamase-stable compounds. Thus, PBP-associated resistance, including PBP induction, might become more common, its frequency increasing with decreasing number of PBP targets.

REFERENCES

1. Georgopapadakou NH, Liu FY (1980) Penicillin-binding proteins in bacteria. *Antimicrob. Agents Chemother., 18*, 834.
2. Spratt B (1983) Penicillin-binding proteins and the future of β-lactam antibiotics. *J. Gen. Microbiol., 129*, 1247.
3. Kitano K, Tomasz A (1979) Triggering of autolytic cell-wall degradation in *Escherichia coli* by beta-lactam antibiotics. *Antimicrob. Agents Chemother., 16*, 838.
4. Tomasz A (1979) From penicillin-binding proteins to the lysis and death of bacteria: a 1979 view. *Rev. Infect. Dis., 1*, 434.
5. Shockman GD, Daneo-Moore L, Cornett JB, Mychajlonka M (1979) Does penicillin kill bacteria? *Rev. Infect. Dis., 1*, 787.
6. Kozarich JW, Strominger JL (1978) A membrane enzyme from *Staphylococcus aureus* which catalyzes transpeptidase, carboxypeptidase, and penicillinase activities. *J. Biol. Chem., 253*, 1272.
7. Ghuysen JM, Frere JM, Leyh-Bouille M, Coyette J, Dusart G, Nguyen-Distéche M, Mauquet A, Duez C (1979) Interaction between penicillin and its enzyme target. In: Matsuhashi S (Ed), *Microbial Drug Resistance, Vol. 2*, p 287. University Park Press, Tokyo.
8. Spratt BG (1980) Biochemical and genetical approaches to the mechanism of action of penicillin. *Philosoph. Trans. R. Soc. London, Ser. B., 289*, 273.
9. Ghuysen JM, Frere JM, Leyh-Bouille M, Dideberg O, Lamotte-Brasseur J, Perkins H, De Coen JL (1981) Penicillins and Δ^3-cephalosporins as inhibitors and mechanism-based inactivators of D-alanyl-D-alanine peptidases. In: Burgen ASV, Roberts GCK (Eds), *Topics in Molecular Pharmacology*, p 63. Elsevier/North-Holland Biomedical Press, Amsterdam.
10. Waxman DJ, Strominger JL (1982) β-Lactam antibiotics: biochemical mode of action. In: Morin RB, Gorman M (Eds), *The Chemistry and Biology of β-Lactam Antibiotics, Vol 3*, p 209. Academic Press, New York.
11. Georgopapadakou NH, Sykes RB (1983) Bacterial enzymes interacting with β-lactam antibiotics. In: Demain AL, Solomon NA (Eds), *Handbook of Experimental Pharmacology, Vol 67/II*, p 1. Springer-Verlag, Heidelberg.
12. Waxman DJ, Strominger JL (1983) Penicillin-binding proteins and the mechanism of action of β-lactam antibiotics. *Annu. Rev. Biochem., 52*, 825.
13. Georgopapadakou NH (1983) Bacterial penicillin-binding proteins. *Annu. Rep. Med. Chem., 18*, 119.
14. Ghuysen JM, Frere JM, Leyh-Bouille M et al (1984) Bacterial wall peptidoglycan, DD-peptidases and β-lactam antibiotics. *Scand. J. Infect. Dis., Suppl 42*, 17.
15. Tomasz A (1984) Penicillin-binding proteins: their role in β-lactam action and resistance. In: Root RK, Sande MA (Eds), *New Dimensions in Antimicrobial Therapy*, p 1. Churchill Livingstone, New York.
16. Frere JM, Joris B (1985) Penicillin-sensitive enzymes in peptidoglycan biosynthesis. *CRC Crit. Rev. Microbiol., 11*, 299.
17. Shockman GD, Barrett JF (1983) Structure, function, and assembly of cell walls of gram-positive bacteria. *Ann. Rev. Microbiol., 37*, 501.
18. Ward JB (1984) Biosynthesis of peptidoglycan: points of attack by wall inhibitors. *Pharmacol. Ther., 25*, 327.

19. Lamotte-Brasseur J, Dive G, Ghuysen JM (1984) On the structural analogy between D-alanyl-D-alanine terminated peptides and β-lactam antibiotics. *Eur. J. Med. Chem.-Chim. Ther., 19*, 319.

20. Tipper DJ (1985) Mode of action of β-lactam antibiotics. *Pharmacol. Ther., 27*, 1.

21. Page MI (1984) The mechanisms of reactions of β-lactam antibiotics. *Acc. Chem. Res., 17*, 144.

22. Durckheimer W, Blumbach J, Lattrell R, Scheunemann KH (1985) Recent developments in the field of β-lactam antibiotics. *Angew. Chem. Int. Ed. Engl., 24*, 180.

23. Neu HC (1986) β-Lactam antibiotics: structural relationships affecting in vitro activity and pharmacologic properties. *Rev. Infect. Dis., 8*, S237.

24. Fisher JF, Knowles JR (1978) Bacterial resistance to β-lactams: the β-lactamases. *Annu. Rep. Med. Chem., 13*, 239.

25. Ambler RP (1980) The structure of β-lactamases. *Phil. Trans. R. Soc. London, B289*, 321.

26. Fink AL (1985) The molecular basis of β-lactamase catalysis and inhibition. *Pharm. Res., 2*, 55.

27. Bush K, Sykes RB (1987) Characterization and epidemiology of β-lactamases. In: Peterson PK, Verhoef J (Eds), *The Antimicrobial Agents Annual 2*, p 371. Elsevier, Amsterdam.

28. Blumberg PM, Strominger JL (1974) Interaction of penicillin with the bacterial cell: penicillin-binding proteins and penicillin-sensitive enzymes. *Bacteriol. Rev., 38*, 291.

29. Schleifer KH, Kandler O (1972) Peptidoglycan types of bacterial cell walls and their taxonomic implications. *Bacteriol. Rev., 36*, 407.

30. Tipper DJ, Strominger JL (1965) Mechanism of action of penicillins: a proposal based on their structural similarity to acyl-D-alanyl-D-alanine. *Proc. Natl Acad. Sci. USA, 72*, 4162.

31. Spratt BG (1977) Properties of the penicillin-binding proteins of *Escherichia coli* K12. *Eur. J. Biochem., 72*, 341.

32. Labia R, Baron P, Masson JM, Hill G, Cole M (1984) Affinity of temocillin for *Escherichia coli* K-12 penicillin-binding proteins. *Antimicrob. Agents Chemother., 26*, 335.

33. Berenguer J, DePedro MA, Vazquez DV (1982) Interaction of nocardicin-A with the penicillin-binding proteins of *Escherichia coli* in intact cells and in purified cell envelopes. *Eur. J. Biochem., 126*, 155.

34. Georgopapadakou NH, Liu FY, Ondetti MA (1979) Comparison of D and L isomers in 7-substituted cephalosporins. In: *Program and Abstracts, 19th Interscience Conference on Antimicrobial Agents and Chemotherapy, Boston 1979*, No. 567. American Society for Microbiology, Washington, DC.

35. Shigi Y, Kojo H, Wakasugi M, Nishida M (1981) Differences between ceftizoxime and its stereoisomer in antibacterial activity and affinity for penicillin-binding proteins. *Antimicrob. Agents Chemother., 19*, 393.

36. Georgopapadakou NH, Smith SA, Cimarusti CM, Sykes RB (1983) Binding of monobactams to penicillin-binding proteins of *Escherichia coli* and *Staphylococcus aureus*: relation to antibacterial activity. *Antimicrob. Agents Chemother., 23*, 98.

37. Coyette J, Ghuysen JM, Fontana R (1978) Solubilization and isolation of the membrane-bound DD-carboxypeptidase of *Streptococcus faecalis* ATCC 9790. *Eur. J. Biochem., 88*, 297.

38. Murphy T, Barza M, Park JT (1981) Penicillin-binding proteins in *Clostridium perfringens*. *Antimicrob. Agents Chemother., 20*, 809.

39. Suzuki H, Nishimura I, Hirota Y (1978) On the process of cellular division in *Escherichia coli*: a series of mutants of *E. coli* altered in the penicillin-binding properties. *Proc. Natl Acad. Sci. USA, 75*, 664.

40. Hakenbeck R, Briese T, Ellerbrook H (1986) Antibodies against the benzylpenicilloyl moiety as a probe for penicillin-binding proteins. *Eur. J. Biochem., 157*, 101.

41. Buchanan CE (1981) Topographical distribution of penicillin-binding proteins in the *Escherichia-coli* membrane. *J. Bacteriol., 145*, 1293.

42. Botta GA, Park JT (1981) Evidence for involvement of penicillin-binding protein 3 in murein synthesis during septation but not during cell elongation. *J. Bacteriol., 145*, 333.

43. Wientjes FB, Olijhoek TJM, Schwarz U, Nanninga N (1983) Labeling pattern of major penicillin-binding proteins of *Escherichia coli* during the division cycle. *J. Bacteriol., 153*, 1287.

44. Mendelman PM, Chaffin DO (1985) Two penicillin-binding proteins of *Haemophilus influenzae* are lost after cells enter stationary phase. *FEMS Microbiol. Lett., 30*, 399.

45. Chambers HF, Hartman BJ, Tomasz A (1985) Increased amounts of a novel penicillin-binding protein in a series of methicillin-resistant *Staphylococcus aureus* exposed to nafcillin. *J. Clin. Invest., 76*, 325.

46. Martin HH, Schilf W, Schiefer HG (1980) Differentiation of mycoplasmatales from bacterial protoplast L-forms by assay for penicillin-binding proteins. *Arch. Microbiol., 127*, 297.

47. Spratt BG, Jobanputra V, Schwarz U (1977) Mutants of *Escherichia coli* which lack a component of penicillin-binding protein 1 are viable. *FEBS Lett., 79*, 374.

48. Schwarz U, Seeger K, Wengenmayer F, Strecker H (1981) Penicillin-binding proteins of *Escherichia coli* identified with a ^{125}I-derivative of ampicillin. *FEMS Microbiol. Lett., 10*, 107.

49. Utsui Y, Yokota T (1985) Role of an altered penicillin-binding protein in methicillin- and cephem-resistant *Staphylococcus aureus*. *Antimicrob. Agents Chemother., 28*, 397.

50. Spratt BG (1975) Distinct penicillin-binding proteins involved in the division, elongation and shape of *Escherichia coli* K12. *Proc. Natl Acad. Sci. USA, 72*, 2999.

51. Shepherd JT, Chase HA, Reynolds PE (1977) The separation and properties of two penicillin-binding proteins from *Salmonella typhimurium*. *Eur. J. Biochem., 78*, 521.

52. Ohya S, Yamazaki M, Sugawara S, Mitsuhashi S (1979) Penicillin-binding proteins in *Proteus* species. *J. Bacteriol., 137*, 474.

53. Noguchi H, Matsuhashi M, Mitsuhashi S (1979) Comparative studies of penicillin-binding proteins in *Pseudomonas aeruginosa* and *Escherichia coli*. *Eur. J. Biochem., 100*, 41.

54. Curtis NAC, Orr D, Ross GW, Boulton MG (1979) Competition of β-lactam antibiotics for the penicillin-binding proteins of *Pseudomonas aeruginosa, Enterobacter cloacae, Klebsiella aerogenes, Proteus rettgeri*, and *Escherichia coli*: comparison with antibacterial activity and effects upon bacterial morphology. *Antimicrob. Agents Chemother., 16*, 325.

55. Georgopapadakou NH, Dix BA, Mauriz YR (1986) Possible physiological functions of penicillin-binding proteins in *Staphylococcus aureus*. *Antimicrob. Agents Chemother., 29*, 333.

56. Georgopapadakou NH, Smith SA, Sykes RB (1983) Penicillin-binding proteins in *Bacteroides fragilis*. *J. Antibiot., 36*, 907.

57. Kleppe G, Strominger JL (1979) Studies of the high-molecular-weight penicillin-binding proteins of *Bacillus subtilis. J. Biol. Chem., 254*, 4856.

58. Tamaki S, Matsuzawa H, Matsuhashi M (1980) Cluster of *mrd* A and *mrd* B genes responsible for the rod shape and mecillinam sensitivity of *Escherichia coli. J. Bacteriol., 141*, 52.

59. Ishino F, Mitsui K, Tamaki S, Matsuhashi M (1980) Dual enzyme activities of cell wall peptidoglycan transglycosylase and penicillin-sensitive transpeptidase, in purified preparations of *Escherichia coli* penicillin-binding protein 1A. *Biochem. Biophys. Res. Commun., 97*, 287.

60. Nakagawa U, Tamaki S, Matsuhashi M (1979) Purified penicillin-binding proteins 1Bs from *Escherichia coli* membranes showing activities of both peptidoglycan polymerase and peptidoglycan crosslinking enzyme. *Agric. Biol. Chem., 43*, 1379.

61. Ishino F, Tamaki S, Spratt BG, Matsuhashi M (1982) A mecillinam-sensitive peptidoglycan crosslinking reaction in *Escherichia coli. Biochem. Biophys. Res. Commun., 109*, 689.

62. Ishino F, Park W, Tomioka S, Tamaki S, Takase I, Kunugita K, Matsuzawa H, Asoh S, Ohta T, Spratt BG, Matsuhashi M (1986) Peptidoglycan synthetic activities in membranes of *Escherichia coli* caused by overproduction of penicillin-binding protein 2 and RodA protein. *J. Biol. Chem., 261*, 7024.

63. Ishino F, Matsuhashi M (1981) Peptidoglycan synthetic enzyme activities of highly purified penicillin-binding protein 3 in *Escherichia coli*: a septum-forming reaction sequence. *Biochem. Biophys. Res. Commun., 101*, 905.

64. Hedge P, Spratt BG (1984) A gene fusion that localizes the penicillin-binding domain of penicillin-binding protein 3 of *Escherichia coli. FEBS Lett., 176*, 179.

65. Keck W, Glauner B, Schwarz U et al (1985) Sequences of the active-site peptides of three of the high-M_r penicillin-binding proteins of *Escherichia coli* K-12. *Proc. Natl Acad. Sci. USA, 82*, 1999.

66. Nicholas RA, Strominger JL, Suzuki H, Hirota Y (1985) Identification of the active site in penicillin-binding protein 3 of *Escherichia coli. J. Bacteriol., 164*, 456.

67. Nicholas RA, Suzuki H, Hirota Y, Strominger JL (1985) Purification and sequencing of the active site tryptic peptide from penicillin-binding protein 1b of *Escherichia coli. Biochemistry, 24*, 3448.

68. Broome-Smith JK, Edelman A, Yousif S, Spratt BG (1985) The nucleotide sequence of the *pon*A and *pon*B genes encoding penicillin-binding proteins 1A and 1B of *Escherichia coli* K12. *Eur. J. Biochem., 147*, 437.

69. Asoh S, Matsuzawa H, Ishino F, Strominger JL, Matsuhashi M, Ohta T (1986) Nucleotide sequence of the *pbp*A gene and characteristics of the deduced amino acid sequence of penicillin-binding protein 2 of *Escherichia coli* K12. *Eur. J. Biochem., 160*, 231.

70. Nakamura M, Maruyama IN, Soma M, Kato J, Suzuki H, Hirota Y (1983) On the process of cellular division in *Escherichia coli*: nucleotide sequence of the gene for penicillin-binding protein 3. *Mol. Gen. Genet., 191*, 1.

71. Chase HA, Fuller C, Reynolds PE (1981) The role of penicillin-binding proteins in the action of cephalosporins against *Escherichia coli* and *Salmonella typhimurium. Eur. J. Biochem., 117*, 301.

72. Georgopapadakou NH, Smith SA, Sykes RB (1982) Mode of action of azthreonam. *Antimicrob. Agents Chemother., 21*, 950.

73. Curtis NAC, Eisenstadt RL, Turner KA, White AJ (1985) Inhibition of penicillin-binding protein 3 of *Escherichia coli* K-12. Effects upon growth, viability and outer membrane barrier function. *J. Antimicrob. Chemother., 16*, 287.

74. Tuomanen E, Gilbert K, Tomasz A (1986) Modulation of bacteriolysis by cooperative effects of penicillin-binding proteins 1a and 3 in *Escherichia coli. Antimicrob. Agents Chemother., 30*, 659.

75. Rojo F, Ayala J, De Pedro MA, Vazquez D (1984) Analysis of the different molecular forms of penicillin-binding protein 1B in *Escherichia coli ponB* mutants lysogenized with specialized transducing (*ponB*$^+$) bacteriophages. *Eur. J. Biochem., 144*, 571.

76. Kato J, Suzuki H, Hirota Y (1984) Overlapping of the coding regions for α and γ components of penicillin-binding protein 1b in *Escherichia coli. Mol. Gen. Genet., 196*, 449.

77. Suzuki H, Kato JI, Sakagami Y, Masaaki M, Suzuki A, Hirota Y (1987) Conversion of the α-component of penicillin-binding protein 1b to the β component in *Escherichia coli. J. Bacteriol., 169*, 891.

78. Kato J, Suzuki H, Hirota Y (1985) Dispensability of either penicillin-binding protein-1a or -1b involved in the essential process for cell elongation in *Escherichia coli. Mol. Gen. Genet., 200*, 272.

79. Aoki H, Kunugita K, Hosoda J, Imanaka H (1977) Screening of new and novel β-lactam antibiotics. *J. Antibiot., 30*, S207.

80. Yousif SY, Broome-Smith JK, Spratt BG (1985) Lysis of *Escherichia coli* by β-lactam antibiotics: deletion analysis of the role of penicillin-binding proteins 1A and 1B. *J. Gen. Microbiol., 131*, 2839.

81. Gutmann L, Vincent S, Billot-Klein D, Acar JF, Mrena E, Williamson R (1986) Involvement of penicillin-binding protein 2 with other penicillin-binding proteins in lysis of *Escherichia coli* by some β-lactam antibiotics alone and in synergistic lytic effect of amdinocillin (mecillinam). *Antimicrob. Agents Chemother., 30*, 906.

82. De la Rosa EJ, De Pedro MA, Vazquez D (1985) Penicillin-binding proteins: role on initiation of murein synthesis in *Escherichia coli. Proc. Natl Acad. Sci. USA, 82*, 5632.

83. Presslitz JE (1978) Mode of action of a structurally novel beta-lactam. *Antimicrob. Agents Chemother., 14*, 144.

84. O'Callaghan CH, Acred P, Harper PB, Ryan DM, Kirby SM, Harding SM (1980) GR 20263, a new broad-spectrum cephalosporin with anti-pseudomonal activity. *Antimicrob. Agents Chemother., 17*, 876.

85. Then RL, Kohl I (1985) Affinity of carumonam for penicillin-binding proteins. *Chemotherapy, 31*, 246.

86. Hedge PJ, Spratt BG (1985) Amino acid substitutions that reduce the affinity of penicillin-binding protein 3 of *Escherichia coli* for cephalexin. *Eur. J. Biochem., 151*, 111.

87. Hedge PJ, Spratt BG (1985) Resistance of β-lactam antibiotics by remodeling the active site of an *E. coli* penicillin-binding protein. *Nature (London), 318*, 478.

88. Broome-Smith JK, Hedge PJ, Spratt BG (1985) Production of thiol-penicillin-binding protein 3 of *Escherichia coli* using a two primer method of site-directed mutagenesis. *EMBO J., 4*, 231.

89. Huba-Harin N, Hara H, Inoue M, Hirota Y (1985) Binding of penicillin to thiol-penicillin-binding protein 3 of *Escherichia coli*: identification of its active site. *Mol. Gen. Genet., 201*, 499.

90. Tormo A, Ayala JA, De Pedro MA, Aldea M, Vicente M (1986) Interaction of FtsA and PBP 3 proteins in *Escherichia coli* septum. *J. Bacteriol., 166*, 985.

91. Nguyen-Disteche M, Ghuysen JM, Pollock JJ, Reynolds PE, Perkins HR, Coyette J, Salton MRJ (1974) Enzymes involved in wall peptide crosslinking in *Escherichia coli* K12, strain 44. *Eur. J. Biochem., 41*, 447.

92. Nguyen-Disteche M, Pollock JJ, Ghuysen JM, Puig J, Reynolds PE, Perkins HR, Coyette J, Salton MRJ (1974) Sensitivity to ampicillin and cephalothin of enzymes involved in wall peptide crosslinking in *Escherichia coli* K12, strain 44. *Eur. J. Biochem., 41*, 457.

93. Pollock JJ, Nguyen-Disteche M, Ghuysen JM, Coyette J, Linder R, Salton MRJ, Kim KS, Perkins HR, Reynolds PE (1974) Fractionation of the DD-carboxypeptidase-transpeptidase activities solubilized from membranes of *Escherichia coli* K12, strain 44. *Eur. J. Biochem., 41*, 439.

94. De Pedro MA, Schwarz U, Nishimura U, Hirota Y (1980) On the biological role of penicillin-binding proteins 4 and 5. *FEMS Microbiol. Lett., 9*, 219.

95. Tamura T, Imae Y, Strominger JL (1976) Purification to homogeneity and properties of two D-alanine carboxypeptidases I from *Escherichia coli*. *J. Biol. Chem., 251*, 414.

96. Matsuhashi M, Tamaki S, Curtis SJ, Strominger JL (1979) Mutational evidence for identity of penicillin-binding protein 5 in *Escherichia coli* with the major D-alanine carboxypeptidase IA activity. *J. Bacteriol., 137*, 644.

97. Markiewicz Z, Broome-Smith JK, Schwarz U, Spratt BG (1982) Spherical *E. coli* due to elevated levels of D-alanine carboxypeptidase. *Nature (London), 297*, 702.

98. Mirelman D, Yashouv-Gan Y, Schwarz U (1976) Peptidoglycan biosynthesis in a thermosensitive division mutant of *Escherichia coli*. *Biochemistry, 15*, 1781.

99. Tamaki S, Nakagawa J, Maruyama IN, Matsuhashi M (1978) Supersensitivity to β-lactam antibiotics in *Escherichia coli* caused by D-alanine carboxypeptidase 1A mutation. *Agric. Biol. Chem., 42*, 2147.

100. Broome-Smith JK (1985) Construction of a mutant of *Escherichia coli* that has deletions of both the penicillin-binding protein 5 and 6 genes. *J. Gen. Microbiol., 131*, 2115.

101. Tuomanen E, Gilbert K, Tomasz A (1986) A low molecular size (LMS) penicillin-binding protein (PBP) in *E. coli*: a new physiologically important target. In: *Program and Abstracts, 26th Interscience Conference on Antimicrobial Agents and Chemotherapy, New Orleans, 1986*, No. 122. American Society for Microbiology, Washington, DC.

102. Curtis NAC, Boulton MG, Orr D, Ross GW (1980) The competition of α-sulfocephalosporins for the penicillin-binding proteins of *Escherichia coli* K12 and *Pseudomonas aeruginosa* – comparison with effects upon morphology. *J. Antimicrob. Chemother., 6*, 189.

103. Godfrey AJ, Bryan LE, Rabin HR (1981) β-Lactam resistant *Pseudomonas aeruginosa* with modified penicillin-binding proteins emerging during cystic fibrosis treatment. *Antimicrob. Agents Chemother., 19*, 705.

104. Dougherty TJ, Koller AE, Tomasz A (1980) Penicillin-binding proteins of penicillin-susceptible and intrinsically resistant *Neisseria gonorrhoeae*. *Antimicrob. Agents Chemother., 18*, 730.

105. Barbour AG (1981) Properties of the penicillin-binding proteins in *Neisseria gonorrhoeae*. *Antimicrob. Agents Chemother., 19*, 316.

106. Dougherty TJ, Koller AE, Tomasz A (1981) Competition of β-lactam antibiotics for the penicillin-binding proteins of *Neisseria gonorrhoeae*. *Antimicrob. Agents Chemother., 20*, 109.

107. Dougherty TJ (1983) Peptidoglycan biosynthesis in Neisseria gonorrhoeae strains sensitive and intrinsically resistant to β-lactam antibiotics. *J. Bacteriol., 153*, 429.

108. Blundell JK, Perkins HR (1981) Effects of β-lactam antibiotics on peptidoglycan synthesis in growing *Neisseria gonorrhoeae*, including changes in the degree of O-acetylation. *J. Bacteriol., 147*, 633.

109. Lysko PG, Morse SA (1981) *Neisseria gonorrhoeae* cell envelope: permeability to hydrophobic molecules. *J. Bacteriol., 145*, 946.

110. Makover SD, Wright R, Telep E (1981) Penicillin-binding proteins in *Haemophilus influenzae. Antimicrob. Agents Chemother., 19*, 584.

111. Mendelman PM, Chaffin DO, Stull TL, Rubens CE, Mack KD, Smith AL (1984) Characterization of non-β-lactamase-mediated ampicillin resistance in *Haemophilus influenzae. Antimicrob. Agents Chemother., 26*, 235.

112. Serfass DA, Mendelman PM, Chaffin DO, Needham CA (1986) Ampicillin resistance and penicillin-binding proteins of *Haemophilus influenzae. J. Gen. Microbiol., 132*, 2855.

113. Piddock LJV, Wise R (1986) Properties of the penicillin-binding proteins of four species of the genus *bacteroides. Antimicrob. Agents Chemother., 29*, 825.

114. Piddock LJV, Wise R (1986) Cefoxitin resistance in *Bacteroides* species: evidence indicating two mechanisms causing decreased susceptibility. *J. Antimicrob. Chemother., 19*, 161.

115. Suginaka H, Blumberg PM, Strominger JL (1972) Multiple penicillin-binding components in *Bacillus subtilis, Bacillus cereus, Staphylococcus aureus* and *Escherichia coli. J. Biol. Chem., 247*, 5279.

116. Georgopapadakou NH, Liu FY (1980) Binding of β-lactam antibiotics to penicillin-binding proteins of *Staphylococcus aureus* and *Streptococcus faecalis* – relation to antibacterial activity. *Antimicrob. Agents Chemother., 18*, 834.

117. Hayes MV, Curtis NA, Wyke AW, Ward JB (1981) Decreased affinity of a penicillin-binding protein for β-lactam antibiotics in a clinical isolate of *Straphylococcus aureus* resistant to methicillin. *FEMS Microbiol. Lett., 10*, 119.

118. Curtis NAC, Hayes MV, Wyke AW, Ward JB (1980) A mutant of *Staphylococcus aureus* H lacking penicillin-binding protein 4 and transpeptidase activity in vitro. *FEMS Microbiol. Lett., 9*, 263.

119. Curtis NA, Hayes MV (1981) A mutant of *Staphylococcus aureus* H deficient in PBP 1 is viable. *FEMS Microbiol. Lett., 10*, 227.

120. Ubukata K, Yamashita N, Konno M (1985) Occurence of a β-lactam-inducible penicillin-binding protein in methicillin-resistant staphylococci. *Antimicrob. Agents Chemother., 27*, 851.

121. Rossi L, Tonin E, Cheng YR, Fontana R (1985) Regulation of penicillin-binding protein activity: description of a methicillin-inducible penicillin-binding protein in *Staphylococcus aureus. Antimicrob. Agents Chemother., 27*, 828.

122. Tonin E, Tomasz A (1986) β-Lactam-specific mutants of *Staphylococcus aureus. Antimicrob. Agents Chemother., 30*, 577.

123. Reynolds PE, Brown DFJ (1985) Penicillin-binding proteins of β-lactam resistant strains of *Staphylococcus aureus*: effect of growth conditions. *FEBS Lett., 192*, 28.

124. Wyke AW, Ward JB, Hayes MV, Curtis NAC (1981) A role in vivo for penicillin-binding protein 4 of *Staphylococcus aureus. Eur. J. Biochem., 119*, 389.

125. Reynolds PE, Fuller C (1986) Methicillin-resistant strains of *Staphylococcus aureus*: presence of identical additional penicillin-binding protein in all strains examined. *FEMS Microbiol. Lett., 33*, 251.

126. Canepari P, Varaldo PE, Fontana R, Satta G (1985) Different staphylococcal species contain various numbers of penicillin-binding proteins ranging from four (*Staphylococcus aureus*) to only one (*Staphylococcus hyicus*). *J. Bacteriol., 163*, 796.

127. Williamson R, Gutmann L, Horaud T, Delbos F, Acap GF (1986) Use of penicillin-binding proteins for the identification of enterococci. *J. Gen. Microbiol., 132*, 1929.

128. Coyette J, Ghuysen JM, Fontana R (1980) The penicillin-binding proteins in *Streptococcus faecalis* ATCC 9790. *Eur. J. Biochem., 110*, 445.

129. Williamson R, Calderwood SB, Moellering RC, Tomasz A (1983) Studies on the mechanism of intrinsic resistance to β-lactam antibiotics in group D streptococci. *J. Gen. Microbiol., 129*, 813.

130. Fontana R, Bertoloni G, Amalfitano G, Canepari P (1984) Characterization of penicillin-resistant *Streptococcus faecium* mutants. *FEMS Microbiol. Lett., 25*, 21.

131. Fontana R, Grossato A, Rossi L, Cheng YR, Satta G (1985) Transition from resistance to hypersusceptibility to β-lactam antibiotics associated with loss of a low-affinity penicillin-binding protein in a *Streptococcus faecium* mutant highly resistant to penicillin. *Antimicrob. Agents Chemother., 28*, 678.

132. Canepari P, Del Mar Lleo M, Cornaglia G, Fontana R, Satta G (1986) In *Streptococcus faecium* penicillin-binding protein 5 alone is sufficient for growth at submaximal but not at maximal rate. *J. Gen. Microbiol., 132*, 625.

133. Williamson R, Le Bouguenec C, Gutmann L, Horaud T (1985) One or two low affinity penicillin-binding proteins may be responsible for the range of susceptibility of *Enterococcus faecium* to benzylpenicillin. *J. Gen. Microbiol., 131*, 1933.

134. Williamson R, Hakenbeck R, Tomasz A (1980) The penicillin-binding proteins of *Streptococcus pneumoniae* grown under lysis-permissive and lysis-protective (tolerant) conditions. *FEMS Microbiol. Lett., 7*, 127.

135. Hakenbeck RH, Tarpay M, Tomasz A (1980) Multiple changes of penicillin-binding proteins in penicillin-resistant clinical isolates of *Streptococcus pneumoniae*. *Antimicrob. Agents Chemother., 17*, 364.

136. Handwerger S, Tomasz A (1986) Alterations in kinetic properties of penicillin-binding proteins of penicillin-resistant *Streptococcus pneumoniae*. *Antimicrob. Agents Chemother., 30*, 57.

137. Zighelboim S, Tomasz A (1980) Penicillin-binding proteins of multiply antibiotic resistant South African strains of *Streptococcus pneumoniae*. *Antimicrob. Agents Chemother., 17*, 434.

138. Hakenbeck R, Kohiyama M (1982) Purification of penicillin-binding protein 3 from *Streptococcus pneumoniae*. *Eur. J. Biochem., 110*, 445.

139. Murphy TF, Barza M, Park JT (1981) Penicillin-binding proteins in *Clostridium perfringens*. *Antimicrob. Agents Chemother., 20*, 809.

140. Williamson R, Ward JB (1982) Benzylpenicillin-induced filament formation of *Clostridium perfringens*. *J. Gen. Microbiol., 128*, 3025.

141. Williamson R (1983) Resistance of *Clostridium perfringens* to β-lactam antibiotics mediated by decreased affinity of a single essential penicillin-binding protein. *J. Gen. Microbiol., 129*, 2339.

142. Wang JC (1985) DNA topoisomerases. *Annu. Rev. Biochem., 54*, 665.

143. Pruss GJ, Manes SH, Drlica K (1982) *Escherichia coli* DNA topoisomerase I mutants: increased supercoiling is corrected by mutations near gyrase genes. *Cell, 31*, 35.

144. Amanuma H, Strominger JL (1984) Trapping of the substrate-derived acyl intermediate of purified penicillin-binding protein 1a of *Escherichia coli*. *J. Bacteriol., 160*, 824.

145. Matsuhashi M, Ishino F, Tamaki S, Nakajima-Iijima S, Tomioka S, Nakagawa JI, Hirata A (1982) Mechanism of action of β-lactam antibiotics: inhibition of peptidoglycan transpeptidases and novel mechanisms of action. In: Umezawa H, Demain A, Hata T, Hutchinson CR (Eds), *Trends in Antibiotic Research*, p 99. Japan Antibiotics Research Association, Tokyo.

146. Van Heijenoort Y, Derrien M, Van Heijenoort J (1978) Polymerization by transglycosylation in the biosynthesis of the peptidoglycan of *Escherichia coli* K 12 and its inhibition by antibiotics. *FEBS Lett., 89*, 141.

147. Anderson JS, Meadow PM, Haskin MA, Strominger JL (1966) Biosynthesis of the peptidoglycan of bacterial cell walls. *Arch. Biochem. Biophys., 116*, 487.

148. Mirelman D, Sharon N (1972) Biosynthesis of peptidoglycan by a cell wall preparation of *Staphylococcus aureus* and its inhibition by penicillin. *Biochem. Biophys. Res. Commun., 46*, 1909.

149. Beck BD, Park JT (1976) Activity of three murein hydrolases during the cell division cycle of *Escherichia coli* K 12 as measured in toluene-treated cells. *J. Bacteriol., 126*, 1250.

150. Oka T, Fujita H (1978) Effect of β-lactam antibiotics on in vitro peptidoglycan cross-linking by a particulate fraction from *Escherichia coli* K-12 and *Bacillus megaterium* KM. *Antimicrob. Agents Chemother., 14*, 625.

151. Georgopapadakou NH, Liu FY, Ryono DE, Neubeck R, Ondetti MA (1981) Chemical modifications of the active site of *Streptomyces* R61 DD-carboxypeptidase. *Eur. J. Biochem., 115*, 53.

152. Wrenzel PW, Ellis LF, Neuhaus FC (1986) *In vivo* target of benzylpenicillin in *Gaffkya homari*. *Antimicrob. Agents Chemother., 29*, 432.

153. Pratt JM, Holland IB, Spratt BG (1981) Precursor forms of penicillin-binding proteins 5 and 6 of *E. coli* cytoplasmic membrane. *Nature (London), 293*, 307.

154. Curtis NAC, Ross GW, Boulton MG (1979) Effect of 7-α methoxy substitution of cephalosporins upon their affinity for the penicillin-binding proteins of *E. coli* K12: comparison with antibacterial activity and inhibition of membrane-bound model transpeptidase activity. *J. Antimicrob. Chemother., 5*, 391.

155. Georgopapadakou NH, Smith SA, Cimarusti CM (1982) Interaction between monobactams and *Streptomyces* R61 DD-carboxypeptidase. *Eur. J. Biochem., 124*, 507.

156. Faraci WS, Pratt RF (1986) Interactions of cephalosporins with the *Streptomyces* R61 DD-transpeptidase/carboxypeptidase. *Biochem. J., 238*, 309.

157. Sykes RB, Georgopapadakou NH (1981) Bacterial resistance to β-lactam antibiotics: an overview. In: Salton MRJ (Ed), *β-Lactam Antibiotics: Mode of Action, New Developments and Future Prospects*, p 199. Academic Press, New York.

158. Malouin F, Bryan LE (1986) Modification of penicillin-binding proteins as mechanisms of β-lactam resistance. *Antimicrob. Agents Chemother., 30*, 1.

159. Handwerger S, Tomasz A (1985) Antibiotic tolerance among clinical isolates of bacteria. *Annu. Rev. Pharmacol. Toxicol., 25*, 349.

160. Kelly JA, Knox JR, Moews PC, Hite GJ, Bartolone JB, Zhao H, Joris B, Frere JM, Ghuysen JM (1985) 2.8-A Structure of penicillin-sensitive D-alanyl carboxypeptidase-transpeptidase from *Streptomyces* R61 and complexes with β-lactams. *J. Biol. Chem., 260*, 6449.

161. Samraoui B, Sutton BJ, Todd RJ, Artymiuk RJ, Waley SG, Phillips DC (1986) Tertiary structural similarity between a class A β-lactamase and a penicillin-sensitive D-alanyl carboxypeptidase-transpeptidase. *Nature (London), 320*, 378.

162. Nozaki Y, Katayama N, Ono H, Tsubotani S, Harada S, Okazaki H, Nakao Y (1987) Binding of a non-*β*-lactam antibiotic to penicillin-binding proteins. *Nature (London),* *325*, 179.

CHAPTER 38

Human immunodeficiency virus: prospects for antiviral therapy

H. TAELMAN, G. VAN DER GROEN and P. PIOT

The acquired immunodeficiency syndrome (AIDS) was first identified in 1981 as a clinical entity characterized by life-threatening opportunistic infections and Kaposi's sarcoma suggestive of an underlying immunodeficiency. Initially restricted to the United States, AIDS has readily been recognized on all continents. The ever-increasing incidence of the disease constitutes at the present time a major public health problem and a threat to all populations. There is therefore an urgent need for effective prevention and therapy of AIDS. From early epidemiologic studies it soon became obvious that AIDS was an infectious disease transmitted by semen and blood. In 1983 and 1984 clear evidence has been provided that the etiologic agent of AIDS is a human retrovirus variously called lymphadenopathy-associated virus (LAV) (1), human T-cell lymphotropic virus type III (HTLV-III) (2), AIDS-associated retrovirus (ARV) (3) or human immunodeficiency virus (HIV) as recently recommended by the International Committee on the Taxonomy of Viruses for purposes of uniformity (4).

Prior to the demonstration of HIV as the causative agent of AIDS, the treatment of AIDS and AIDS-related conditions was essentially directed at the therapy of opportunistic infections and malignancies and at enhancement of immune function with immunomodulating agents. The result of this approach was at best a transient improvement of the patients' condition but with the persistence of the underlying immune defect and consequently the recurrence of new opportunistic infections or malignancies.

Over the last 3 years a large amount of knowledge has been accumulated on the replication mechanisms and molecular biology of HIV, resulting in the identification of well-defined virus-specific replication sites that may serve as appropriate targets for antiviral strategies.

This Chapter discusses the various aspects relevant to the antiviral therapy of HIV infection. It includes the life cycle of HIV, the rationale and potential limitations of antiviral therapy, the targets and strategies for antiviral therapy, the anti-

Antimicrobial Agents Annual 3
P.K. Petersen and J. Verhoef, editors
© Elsevier Science Publishers BV, 1988

HIV drugs screening system, the properties of anti-HIV agents for use in man, the clinical use of anti-HIV agents and future directions.

THE LIFE CYCLE OF HUMAN IMMUNODEFICIENCY VIRUS

The life cycle of HIV (Fig. 1) starts with the binding of the virus to an appropriate cell-membrane receptor. There is now clear evidence that the CD4/T4 antigen is an essential component of the HIV receptor (5–7) and that it specifically interacts with the viral glycoprotein gp110/120 (8, 9). The CD4/T4 antigen characterizes

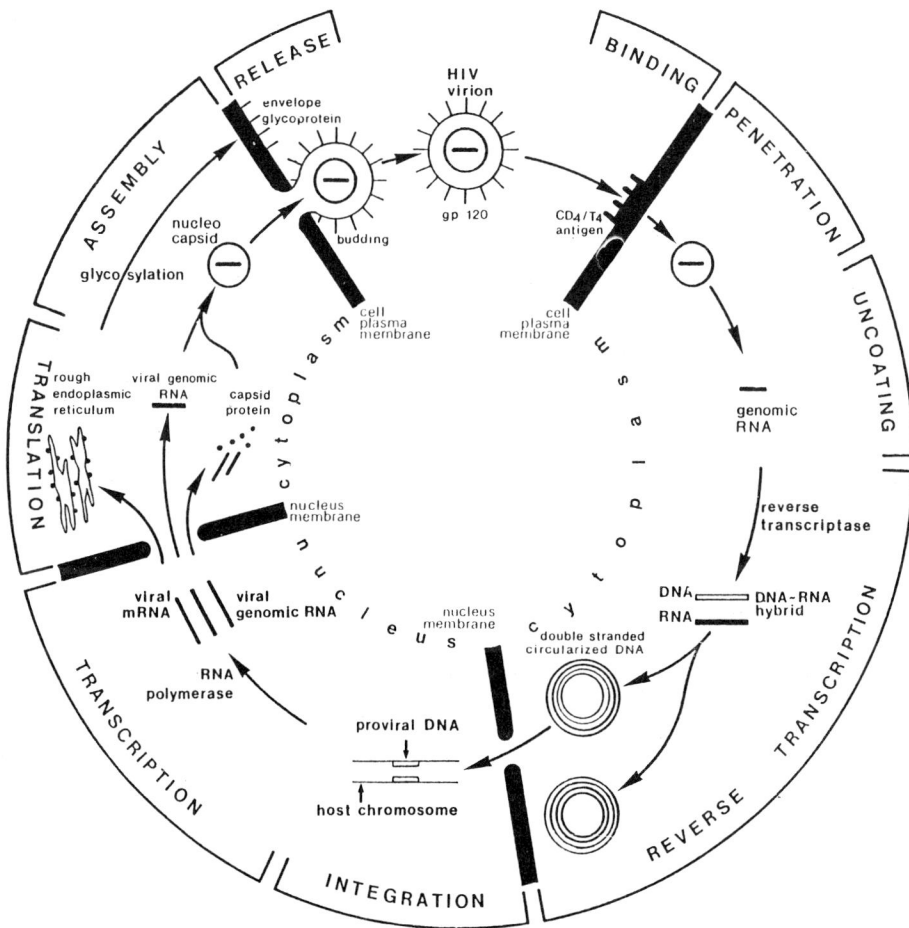

Fig. 1   The life cycle of human immunodeficiency virus (HIV).

the T-helper cells but is also found in some cells of the brain (10). It has also been shown that monocyte/macrophage cells and Epstein-Barr virus (EBV) trans-formed lymphocytes might be permissive for HIV (11–16). Entry of the HIV vi-rion into the cell is poorly understood but might proceed via the endocytic path-way (17).

After penetration, the virion is uncoated and a viral single-stranded RNA is re-leased in the cytoplasm. Further on, an RNA-dependent DNA polymerase com-plexed to the RNA genome, known as 'reverse transcriptase', forms an initial complementary single-stranded DNA copy (cDNA) using a host lysyl transfer-RNA as primer (18, 19). In addition, it catalyses the production of a DNA copo-lymer and generates a linear double-stranded proviral DNA. This proviral DNA is then circularized and subsequently either remains in the cytoplasm or becomes integrated into the host cell genome. Expression of the provirus, which might re-sult from activation of the infected cell, first proceeds by transcription of integrat-ed DNA into viral messenger RNA (mRNA) and viral genomic RNA using host RNA polymerases. During the posttranscriptional processing the mRNAs under-go splicing at both ends: the 5′-end is capped by guanosine residues and the 3′-end is polyadenylated (18). Messenger RNAs are then translated into viral precursor proteins. Using the host cell enzymes as well as the viral enzymes, some proteins further undergo proteolytic cleavage or glycosylation and produce viral capsid proteins, envelope glycoproteins and enzymes.

A feature of HIV is that one of its genes (*tat*-III) encodes for a transactivating factor, the so-called *tat*-III protein. This retroviral protein is thought to be capable of markedly enhancing the production of viral proteins by activating the expres-sion of other genes and by increasing translation of viral RNA (20, 21).

Recently, it has been shown that the specific *art* or *trs* gene of HIV also produ-ces a protein that probably acts as an essential transacting regulator factor in viral protein synthesis (22, 23).

The life-cycle ends with the assembly of the viral particles and their release by budding through the plasma cell membrane at areas where viral glycoproteins have congregated.

ANTIVIRAL THERAPY FOR AIDS: RATIONALE AND POTENTIAL LIMITATIONS

The rationale of the treatment of AIDS with antiviral agents is based on the as-sumption that persistent replication of HIV plays a major role in the genesis of AIDS-related disorders. The predominant target cells for HIV are the helper/in-ducer subset of T-lymphocytes referred to as the 'T4 cells' (24) and the monocyte/ macrophage cells (11–15). HIV infection of the T4 cells at an advanced stage pro-duces numerous abnormalities of both cellular and humoral immunity, eventually resulting in complete collapse of the cellular immune system (24).

Recently, evidence has been provided that cells with the characteristics of monocytes/macrophages are predominantly infected in HIV-associated central nervous system (CNS) (25–30) and lung disease (31).

It has been suggested that the monocyte/macrophage cell of the CNS may play a major role in HIV infection as a productive reservoir and as the cell that initiates the disease process (13, 14). It is generally admitted that progressive infection of T4 cells with HIV results in the death of these cells due to the cytopathic effect of HIV. The precise mechanisms of the cytopathic effect of HIV are unclear. The depletion of T4 cells cannot be totally explained by the direct killing of the cells by HIV. Indeed, only a small percentage of peripheral blood mononuclear cells contain and express HIV at any given time (32, 33).

Therefore, several alternative mechanisms of lymphodepletion have been suggested (34) including: (a) selective depletion of a subset of T4 cells critical to the propagation of the entire T-cell pool; (b) induction by HIV of viral products or lymphokines with toxic effects on T4 lymphocytes (35, 36); (c) autoimmune reaction (37); (d) induction by the HIV envelope protein expressed in infected cells of fusion and syncytium formation followed by subsequent lysis of T4-dependent infected and uninfected cells (38–40).

As mentioned above, HIV is also able to integrate into the host genome and to establish an infection in T4 cells for an undetermined time (41, 42).

Following stimulation of the cells, the latent infection can develop into an active infection (43, 44). It may therefore be necessary to administer any drug effective on HIV for long periods of time — perhaps lifelong — to maintain a protective effect against HIV infection.

Since HIV infection at an advanced stage causes immune dysfunction, no synergism can be anticipated between an anti-HIV agent and the immune system.

POTENTIAL TARGETS AND STRATEGIES FOR ANTIVIRAL THERAPY OF HIV INFECTION

In general, all major stages in the HIV replication cycle may serve as targets for therapeutic intervention (45–49). These targets include cell binding, penetration, uncoating, reverse transcription, integration of viral DNA into host chromosome DNA, transcription of DNA to mRNA, translation of mRNA, transactivation by *tat*-III protein, viral protein production and assembly, budding and release of viral particles.

Cell binding

The first step in HIV cell infection may be prevented by blocking or modifying the cell membrane receptor for HIV or by neutralization of the HIV particles or immunoreactive HIV proteins.

Blocking of the receptor may be achieved with specific monoclonal antibodies to the CD4/T4 antigen or by synthetic oligopeptides with amino acid sequences homologous to certain regions of the virus envelope. Recently, Pert et al (50) have found that an octapeptide, designated 'peptide T', which is an amino acid sequence corresponding to one sequence maintained in the HIV envelope glycoprotein gp-120 of the various AIDS virus isolates, was able to inhibit HIV-T cell infectivity in vitro by blocking the binding of the viral envelope to the CD4-related receptor. However, other investigators (51) have failed to confirm this observation.

Diphenylhydantoin (52) and AL-721 (53) are both compounds able to inhibit HIV infection in vitro by attaching to or modifying the cell membrane of lymphocytes.

Because of the long incubation period of clinical AIDS, neutralization of HIV virions or proteins by inducing antibodies involved in antibody-dependent cell cytotoxicity or antibodies directed against immunoreactive HIV proteins could be an alternative strategy to prevent the entry of HIV or its products into the host cell (54). These antibodies could exert their activity as soon as the infected cells start expressing the viral proteins, e.g. the envelope glycoprotein at the time of the budding and release of the viral particles.

Another possible approach is the neutralization of the envelope glycoprotein by the use of anti-idiotypic antibodies against CD4/T4 antigen (55, 56).

Penetration and uncoating

Penetration of the virus into the cell, although not well known, probably proceeds through an endocytic process during which fusion of the virus requires an acidic environment. Inhibition of intracytoplasmic acidification may therefore be another approach to halt viral replication.

Ammonium chloride and amantadine, both inhibitors of intracytoplasmic acidification, appear to reduce the infectivity of HIV (17). Uncoating of the virus is another theoretical means of intervention, but so far no agent active at that site has been developed.

Reverse transcription

Reverse transcription is a very specific and essential step in the replication cycle of HIV and therefore constitutes a prime target for anti-HIV therapy. There are actually different steps in this enzymatic reaction, all of which could be targets for pharmacologic agents. Reverse transcriptase is an RNA-dependent DNA polymerase that uses host transfer-RNA as primer to catalyze the synthesis of cDNA with viral genomic RNA as template. It requires a divalent cation such as Mn^{2+} or Mg^{2+} for optimal activity. Reverse transcriptase inhibitors can be classified into 5 main groups (49): (a) enzyme-binding compounds, e.g. suramin, HPA23, rifamycins; (b) template/primer-binding compounds, e.g. actinomycine D; (c) substrate or product analogues, e.g. phosphonoformate, 2′,3′-dideoxynucleoside triphosphates; (d) template analogues, e.g. 2′-substituted polynucleotide derivatives; (e) divalent-cation binding agents, e.g. thiosemicarbazones.

Integration into the host genome

So far, no pharmacologic agent has been reported to be active at this stage of the HIV life cycle, but theoretically agents capable of interfering with the enzyme mediating the integration phase might also reveal inhibitors of viral replication.

Transcription of DNA to RNA, translation of mRNA and *tat*-III transactivation

Transcription of HIV DNA to mRNA and genomic RNA, and translation of mRNA are other potential targets. It has been shown that nuclease-resistant phosphorothioate analogs of several 'anti-sense' oligodeoxynucleotides, made of short sequences of DNA complementary to HIV genome (57) or to viral RNA (58), exhibit an inhibitory effect in vitro on HIV replication and cytopathogenicity. Recently, mismatched double-stranded RNA has been found to exert anti-HIV activity by stimulating enzymes which promote cleavage of viral RNA and interruption of viral protein synthesis (59). It has been hypothesized that ribavirin might be active at these sites as a guanosine analog interfering with the 5'-capping of viral RNA (60).

The *tat*-III gene product is able to amplify considerably the generation of new virions by exerting a positive feedback on the virus, and may thus constitute a target of choice for an anti-HIV strategy. As yet the development of an agent active at this site is still awaited. The same is true for the *art* or *trs* gene product.

Production and assembly of viral proteins and release of virions

Since this step is under the control of viral proteases and host glycosylating enzymes, any pharmacologic agent active on them might have an inhibiting effect on viral replication. In this respect, castanospermine, a potent competitive inhibitor of glucosidase I involved in the processing of glycoproteins, has shown itself to be capable of dramatically inhibiting syncytium formation, presumably by interfering with the function of the HIV envelope (61).

Ho et al (61) have demonstrated that recombinant human α-interferon suppresses HIV replication (62). If interferons act against HIV as they do against other retroviruses, it is possible that they may interfere with budding. The release of virions could also constitute a target for anti-gp120 antibodies (see above).

ANTI-HIV DRUG SCREENING SYSTEM

In 1984, as soon as there was evidence that HIV was the causative agent of AIDS and that large quantities of virus were available, Mitsuya et al (63) developed an anti-HIV drug screening system allowing rapid and sensitive evaluation of potential inhibitors of HIV replication. The strategy of this screening system proceeds through 6 stages (64):

1. Assessment of the protective effect of the drug against the cytopathic effect of HIV, using normal or immortalized target T-cells (e.g. ATH8 cells).
2. Assessment of the protective effect of the drug against the cytopathic effect of different HIV strains in target T-cells as an additional control of HIV-isolate variability.
3. Determination of the inhibitory effect of the drug on the viral p24 *gag* protein expression in susceptible T-cells (e.g. H9 cells) following exposure to HIV, by an indirect immunofluorescence assay using monoclonal antibodies (e.g. anti-p24 antibodies).
4. Determination of the inhibitory effect of the drug on HIV DNA synthesis and RNA expression in susceptible T-cells exposed to the virus in the presence of drugs, using hybridization techniques.
5. Determination of the inhibitory effect of the drug on viral reverse transcriptase production and release by peripheral blood mononuclear cells exposed to the virus.
6. Evaluation of the potential effect of the drug on immune reactivity of normal T-cells in vitro.

To be declared effective in vitro, a drug should at least fulfil two criteria: potency for complete inhibition of viral infectivity and replication, and minimal toxicity for the host cells, in particular the immunoreactive cells.

PROPERTIES OF ANTI-HIV AGENTS FOR USE IN MAN

The aim of anti-HIV therapy is the inhibition or elimination of the virus with safe and effective drugs. To achieve this objective, two features of HIV should particularly be taken into consideration: the integration of HIV into the host genome and its possible persistence in a latent proviral DNA form for many years, probably for a life-time (41, 42), and the tropism of HIV for the CNS (25–30) which results in the formation of a virus reservoir in the brain. Hence, the ideal properties of an anti-HIV agent should include (47): (a) effective inhibition of HIV replication at drug levels attainable in vivo; (b) acceptable toxicity, particularly after long-term usage; (c) penetration into the CNS; (d) suitability for oral administration; (e) long half-life; (f) low cost.

ASSESSMENT OF ANTI-HIV DRUGS IN PATIENTS WITH HIV DISEASE

Assessment of the efficacy of an anti-HIV drug in patients with HIV disease is based on the follow-up of three kinds of parameters: clinical, immunologic and virologic.

Clinical parameters to be followed should include mortality rates, occurrence of opportunistic infections, development of Kaposi sarcoma or modifications of Kaposi sarcoma lesions, changes in body weight, AIDS-related symptom scores, and CNS symptomatology. Clinical assessment must also carefully monitor any side effect of the drug.

Immunologic parameters suitable for monitoring are the absolute number of T4 cells, the blastogenic responses of lymphocytes to mitogens and antigens, the cytotoxic responses to virally infected autologous cells and delayed-type cutaneous hypersensitivity reactions.

Virologic assessment is based on co-culture of the patient's lymphocytes with allogenic mononuclear cells from a normal donor or with a susceptible cell line. Production of HIV is monitored by repeated examination of the cells for the presence of a cytopathic effect, for viral protein expression using indirect immunofluorescence, and by measuring reverse transcriptase activity and HIV-specified antigen in culture fluids. Some authors measure the HIV load by determining the 'co-culture titre' defined as the average optical density of the ELISA assay, after subtraction of the negative control value (65).

HIV activity in blood cells has also been determined by quantifying HIV RNA directly in blood mononuclear cells by *in situ* molecular hybridization using molecularly cloned HIV probes (65, 66).

Recently, repeated simultaneous determinations of HIV core antigenemia and serum antibody reactivity to p24 have been proposed as a possible assessment of viral replication (67).

At the present time, one must be aware that there is no reliable method of evaluating changes in viral load. The currently available methods are designed to maximize the growth of cells and consequently to replicate the virus artificially. Therefore, they cannot clearly differentiate between cells actively producing virus and cells with latent virus.

CLINICAL USES OF ANTI-HIV AGENTS *(Table 1)*

Suramin

Suramin is a 'hexasodium salt' derivative of naphthaleine trisulfonic acid with a molecular weight of 1 429, known for many years as an effective drug in the treatment of the early phase of African trypanosomiasis and of onchocerciasis.

In 1979, De Clercq reported that suramin was a potent inhibitor of reverse transcriptase of a variety of animal retroviruses (68). Soon after the discovery of HIV in 1983 and 1984, suramin was screened for anti-HIV activity. In vitro studies conducted at the National Cancer Institute showed suramin at a concentration of 25–50 μg/ml to be able to block the cytopathic effect of HIV on ATH8 cells as well as the expression of p24 *gag* proteins in H9 cells (69). At 100 μg/ml it also exhibits an inhibitor effect on lymphocyte proliferation; thus, the safety margin (toxicity/activity ratio) of suramin is narrow.

Suramin is also known to inhibit other enzymes, e.g. DNA α-polymerase at HIV inhibitory concentrations and it could be that its mechanism of action on HIV is not necessarily restricted to inhibition of reverse transcriptase activity. Su-

Table 1 Characteristics of drugs with anti-HIV activity used in clinical trials

Drug	Mode of action	Inhibitory concentration in vivo	Selectivity index*	Routes of administration	In vivo effects	Adverse effects	CSF penetration
Suramin	RT inhibition	25–50 μM	5	i.v.	virostatic, no clinical or immunologic improvement	fever, rash, dysesthesia, renal and adrenal insufficiency	0
HPA-23	RT inhibition	>15 μM	< 0.1	i.v.	virostatic, no clinical or immunologic improvement	thrombocytopenia, liver dysfunction	?
Phosphonoformate	RT inhibition	132–680 μM	> 1	i.v.	virostatic, no clinical or immunologic improvement	headache, phlebitis, anemia, renal failure	good
Ribavirin	interference with 5'-mRNA capping	100 μg/ml (partial)	< 0.3	i.v./p.o.	virostatic, delay of progression to AIDS	anemia, leukopenia	excellent

	Mechanism	Concentration	Selectivity index*	Route	Activity	Side effects	Rating
Zidovudine	DNA chain termination	1–10 μM	> 50	i.v./p.o.	virostatic, short-term clinical and immunologic improvement	nausea, myalgia, insomnia, headache, anemia, neurologic disorders	excellent
Interferon-α	inhibition of budding?	4-64 U/ml (partial) 256–1 024 U/ml (total)	–	i.m./s.c.	active only against KS	fever, bone marrow suppression	poor
Ampligen	stimulation of IFN associated natural killer activity	50 μg/ml	–	i.v.	virostatic, clinical improvement of ARC/LAS patients, immunological improvement	none	?

* Selectivity index: ratio of compound concentration required to reduce the growth of normal uninfected ATH8 cells by 50% to the compound concentration (MIC) required for achieving full protection of ATH8 cells against HIV, according to De Clercq (49) and Balzarini et al (83).

ARC = AIDS-related complex; KS = Kaposi sarcoma; LAS = lymphadenopathy syndrome; RT = reverse transcriptase; i.v. = intravenous; i.m. = intramuscular; s.c. = subcutaneous; p.o. = per os.

ramin has an exceptionally long half-life ranging from 44 to 54 days due to its extensive binding (99.7%) to proteins (70). It is administered weekly at doses of 20 mg/kg (max. 1 g/dose) intravenously, preferably in slow infusion over 2 or more hours. On this regimen, suramin may reach plasma levels of 100 μg/ml or more after 6 injections (71).

Several clinical trials have been conducted in the United States and in Europe. HIV was no longer detected in cultures of peripheral blood lymphocytes (71, 72) in a substantial number of patients at plasma levels of 100 μg/ml or lower. However, HIV replication reappeared soon after interruption of suramin treatment.

In spite of a virustatic effect, no immunologic reconstitution or any real clinical benefit was observed (71–76).

Side effects frequently observed during suramin treatment included rash, fever, and paresthesias in the extremities. Toxic keratopathy (77) and adrenal insufficiency (75, 78) have also been described.

Common laboratory abnormalities were proteinuria, pyuria and granular casts in urine sediment; neutropenia and rise in hepatic transaminases were occasionally reported.

The results of these trials led to the conclusion that suramin should not be given as a single agent in the treatment of AIDS or AIDS-related diseases. Another reason to reject suramin as a single drug for HIV infection is its lack of penetration into the CNS, which is known to constitute a major target for HIV and a virus reservoir.

HPA-23

HPA-23 (antimoniotungstate) is a mineral-condensed polyanion of ammonium 21-tungsto-9-antimoniate with a molecular weight of 6 800. The drug is a competitive inhibitor of RT of oncornaviruses (79) and is active in vivo against a broad spectrum of tumor viruses (80). It exhibits a potent inhibition of HIV reverse transcriptase (81, 82). However, in the HIV-ATH8 cell system, HPA-23 at a concentration of 100 μg/ml had no protective effect against the cytopathogenicity of HIV, while being toxic for the uninfected cells at a concentration of 10 μg/ml (83). In the H9 cell system, HPA-23 proved only weakly inhibitory to HIV replication, bringing about only a partial reduction in p24 *gag* expression at a concentration of 10 μg/ml (83).

HPA-23 has a half-life of 20 minutes and is administered daily either in intravenous bolus injection or slow infusion. In a pilot study (84), 4 patients — 3 with AIDS and 1 with AIDS-related complex (ARC) — who were treated with HPA-23 at daily doses ranging from 1 to 3.3 mg/kg given intravenously showed no immunologic improvement, although a decrease in reverse transcriptase activity was noted. The clinical condition remained stable or had improved in the 4 patients. Platelet counts fell in 3 cases and hepatic transaminases were slightly increased in 3 cases, but these abnormalities returned to pre-treatment values within 3–6$\frac{1}{2}$ weeks.

In a second clinical trial (85), in 15 patients with HIV infection (AIDS, ARC, seropositive patients) who received daily intravenous doses of 50 mg of HPA-23 for 4–15 months, no significant effect on T4 lymphocyte counts was noted, although there was some indication of inhibition of viral replication. The treatment was well tolerated but in each case there was a decrease in platelet count.

Phosphonoformate

Trisodium phosphonoformate (PFA, foscarnet) is an analog of pyrophosphate. It inhibits the replication and the RT of the visna lentivirus (86), DNA polymerases of herpes simplex virus, cytomegalovirus, hepatitis B virus and the RNA polymerase of influenza virus (87).

PFA is thought to interact with DNA polymerase at the site where pyrophosphate is split off during DNA polymerization (88). PFA inhibits 100% of reverse transcriptase activity of cell-free HIV particles at a concentration as low as 5 μM (89). However, to provide complete protection of ATH8 cells against the cytopathic effect of HIV, concentrations of 350 μM were required, and to completely inhibit HIV replication in H9 cells a concentration of 680 μM was necessary (89–91).

The drug has a half-life of 1–3 hours. To achieve a steady-state plasma concentration of 250–500 μM (75–150 μg/ml) PFA has to be administered as a continuous infusion at a dose of 0.05–0.11 mg/kg/min after an initial intravenous injection of 20 mg/kg given over 10–30 minutes. The results of two pilot studies with PFA (92, 93) given over a 3 week-period in AIDS and ARC did not show clinical or immunologic improvement despite the failure to isolate the virus or to detect HIV antigen in blood in some patients who had positive HIV cultures and/or circulating HIV antigens prior to treatment. PFA is also able to penetrate into the CNS and cerebrospinal fluid (CSF) levels 25–80% of serum levels have been attained (92). Anemia and a rise in serum creatinine levels were observed as toxic effects of the drug in some patients, particularly in those with severe disease.

Ribavirin

Ribavirin (see Chapter 35) is a synthetic nucleoside guanosine analog, active against a wide range of DNA and RNA viruses in vitro (94).

One of the mechanisms of action of the drug is thought to be reduction of viral protein synthesis through interference with the 5′-capping of viral mRNA by competitive inhibition of both guanyltransferase and methyltransferase enzymes (94, 95). Ribavirin has been shown to suppress the replication of HIV in cultures of adult T-lymphocytes at a concentration of 50 μg/ml or more (96). However, at this concentration the drug does not protect ATH8 cells against the cytopathic effect of HIV and shows toxicity for the host cells (83).

Ribavirin can be administered orally or intravenously. Its plasma half-life is 24 hours. It crosses the blood-brain barrier (97). Ribavirin has been given to infants with HIV infection at doses ranging from 35–70 mg/kg/d. The tolerance of the drug was excellent, but no clinical or immunologic improvement was observed (98).

In another open trial (99) ribavirin was administered intravenously to 10 adult patients at doses of 4 g/d for 7 days and 2 g/d for the next 14 days followed by 4 g/d orally. Side effects observed included hypocalcemia, leukopenia and anemia. No beneficial clinical effects of the drug were observed in this study.

However, in a randomized, double-blind, placebo-controlled trial including 163 patients with the lymphadenopathy syndrome treated with placebo or oral ribavirin at daily doses of 600 or 800 mg, prolonged ribavirin therapy appeared to be well tolerated and to delay progression to AIDS (100). In another similar trial but conducted in ARC patients, no effect was found on serum HIV Ag levels but a significant difference in culture positivity between placebo and drug groups was seen (101).

Zidovudine

Zidovudine (3'-azido-3'-deoxythymidine, BW-A509U, azidothymidine, AZT, Retrovir) is a 2',3'-dideoxynucleoside derivative. It is an analog of naturally occurring thymidine in which the 3'-hydroxy (-OH) is replaced by an azido ($-N_3$) group (102).

AZT is a very potent in vitro inhibitor of the infectivity and cytopathic effect of HIV in susceptible target cells at 1–3 μM without affecting lymphocyte proliferation (103, 104). Following cellular uptake, AZT undergoes anabolic phosphorylation and is converted by host cell kinases to a triphosphate form (AZT-TP) (105). This form competes with the naturally produced thymidine-5' triphosphate and is efficiently and selectively utilized by HIV reverse transcriptase (105). Because of the azido substituent at the 3'-carbon of the ribose moiety, further 5',3'-phosphodiester linkages, which are necessary for DNA elongation in the transcription of the virus from a RNA form to a DNA form, cannot be formed. AZT-TP thus acts as a DNA-chain terminator in viral DNA synthesis. Other 2',3'-dideoxynucleosides that can be metabolized by mammalian kinases to 5'-triphosphate forms such as 2',3'-dideoxycytidine and 2',3'-dideoxyadenosine show a similar anti-HIV pattern of activity (106, 107).

Additional studies conducted by Furman et al (105) have shown that cellular DNA α-polymerase, assumed to be the key DNA enzyme for DNA replication during cell growth, is 100 times less susceptible to inhibition by AZT-TP than HIV reverse transcriptase.

However, AZT can bring about reduction of pyrimidine pools and it is likely that this reduction is responsible for the bone-marrow suppression observed in some patients treated with the drug. In vitro studies have shown that AZT activity can be potentiated by acyclovir (43), α-interferon (108), dextran sulfate (109) and Ampligen (110). In contrast, ribavirin antagonizes the anti-HIV activity of AZT (111).

Results of a Phase I trial of AZT (112) in 19 patients with AIDS or ARC showed that the drug has an oral bioavailability of 65% and penetrates into CSF, the levels being 15–70% those of plasma. Peak plasma levels of 1.5–2, 4–6 and 6–10 μM are attained with oral doses of 2, 5 and 10 mg/kg respectively. The half-life of AZT is approximately 1 hour. Twenty-five percent of the drug is eliminated unchanged by renal excretion and 60% by conversion to the glucuronide metabolite. Among the 19 patients treated for 14 days with 1–5 mg/kg i.v. every 4–8 hours, followed by 4 weeks of oral therapy with twice the intravenous dosage, 13 increased their weight, 2 cleared a mycotic infection of the nail-bed and 6 other improved clinically; 15 had increases in the absolute number of circulating T-helper lymphocytes; 6 who were anergic at entry developed positive delayed hypersensitivity skin tests. A virostatic effect was obtained at the dose of 60 mg/kg/d p.o.

In February, 1986, a randomized, double-blind, placebo-controlled trial of orally administered AZT (113, 114) was started in 282 patients with AIDS or ARC at 12 centers in the United States. A total of 145 (85 AIDS and 60 ARC patients) received AZT and 137 (75 AIDS and 67 ARC patients) placebo. AIDS patients entered the trial only if they had experienced their first episode of *Pneumocystis carinii* pneumonia within 120 days before enrolment.

The dosage of AZT initially was 250 mg 4-hourly, but in some patients the drug was discontinued or the dosage decreased because of bone-marrow toxicity. On 18 September, 1986 (at which time the mean duration of the treatment was 120 days) there were 19 deaths (13 AIDS and 6 ARC patients) in the placebo group and only one in the AZT group (1 AIDS patient).

The incidence of opportunistic infections was reduced in the treated group, compared with the placebo recipients (24 *vs* 45). The opportunistic infections were also less severe or more responsive to therapy in the treated group than in the placebo group. Kaposi sarcoma developed in 6 AZT-treated patients and in 10 placebo-treated patients. Other evidence of clinical improvement in the treated patients was provided by maintenance of the initial Karnofsky score, weight gain and reduction of frequency and severity of AIDS-related symptoms. Recently Yarchoan et al (115) have reported clinical improvement in 3 of 4 patients with AIDS-associated neurologic disease treated with AZT, as shown by clinical examination, psychometric tests, nerve conduction studies and/or positron tomography.

Immunologic benefit was observed in some treated patients as evidenced by increase in T4 lymphocyte numbers (+ 37.4 *vs* − 26.3). Patients with AIDS who received AZT showed an initial sharp increase in T4 count up to week 4, which gradually declined with time. This decrease appeared to be related to the development of leukopenia. In patients with ARC who received AZT, increases in the number of T4 cells persisted throughout the study. In addition, 29% of AZT recipients developed reactivity to at least one of a battery skin test antigens compared with 9% of the placebo recipients.

Data on the antiviral effect of the drug by assessment of reverse transcriptase acitivity determinations were inconclusive but measurements of HIV antigen levels in serum indicated highly significant differences in antigenemia (116). At week

16, patients receiving AZT showed a decline in core antigen while placebo patients exhibited a significant increase in core antigen.

Nausea, myalgia and insomnia were the only events reported significantly more often in the AZT-treated group. Moderate and severe headaches also appeared to occur more often in AZT-treated patients but not significantly (43 *vs* 24%). Focal epilepsy unresponsive to anticonvulsants and Wernicke's encephalopathy were observed in one occasion each (117, 118). Neutropenia of less than 750 cells/mm^3, leukopenia of less than 2 500 cells/mm^3 and anemia with hemoglobin levels below 7.5 g/100 ml developed more frequently in AZT-treated patients than in placebo recipients (39 *vs* 7%; 27 *vs* 7%; 24 *vs* 4% respectively). Changes resulting in red blood cell suppression led to a significantly greater number of blood transfusions in the AZT-treated group than in the placebo group (31 *vs* 11%).

Severe neurologic adverse events have been described in 2 patients: one developed headache, confusion, convulsions and died; the other developed signs of Wernicke's encephalopathy.

Potential drug interactions may result from the concurrent use of nephrotoxic or bone-marrow-suppressive drugs or of drugs interfering with hepatic glucuronidation. However, so far only acetaminophen has been associated with an increased risk of marrow suppression. Interaction of AZT with acyclovir has been reported (119).

Overall, AZT reduced mortality and the incidence and severity of opportunistic infections. In addition, improvement in general condition and partial immunologic restoration were seen in treated patients.

Although clear demonstration of the in vivo antiviral effect of the drug is lacking, partly because of inadequate techniques, the decrease in HIV antigenemia in AZT recipients suggests that the drug has some anti-HIV activity in vivo. Use of AZT is associated with marked but reversible depression of white and red blood cells. This hematologic toxicity appears to be proportional to pre-existing marrow damage and the severity of the disease.

In patients with hemoglobin levels of 7.5–9 g/100 ml or granulocyte counts of 750–1 000/mm^3, AZT should be reduced to 200–300 mg every 8 hours. AZT should be temporarily discontinued when hemoglobin levels or granulocyte counts reach values of 7.5 g/100 ml and 750/mm^3 respectively. Recovering of bone-marrow function usually occurs rapidly and may allow re-initiation of dosing within 2 weeks.

Interferons

Interferons have been shown to inhibit effectively a wide range of viruses, including animal retroviruses (see Chapter 34). Inhibition of transcription, translation, assembly and release of virions are various mechanisms that have been implicated in interferon-mediated antiviral acitivity.

In 1985, Ho et al (62) provided data showing recombinant human interferon-αA (rIFN-αA) had a dose-related suppressive effect on HIV replication in vitro in normal peripheral blood lymphocytes. Partial inhibition of viral replication was obtained at concentrations of 4–64 U/ml while complete inhibition required concentrations of 256–1 024 U/ml. Such concentrations were not toxic to peripheral blood lymphocytes.

Pharmacokinetic studies from earlier trials have shown that doses of 50.10^6 U of rIFN-αA produced peak serum levels of 100–200 U/ml, but penetration of the drug into the CSF was low.

From a double-blind placebo-controlled study on interferon-α2 administered subcutaneously at doses of 10.10^6 U/d, 3 days per week for 6 months in 18 patients with benign reactive lymphadenopathic syndrome, Abrams and co-workers concluded that the drug may not be particularly effective in the setting of the AIDS-related lymphadenopathic syndrome (120). Recently, Friedland et al (121), in a randomized, double-blind, placebo-controlled trial of rIFN-α-2A were unable to demonstrate any effectiveness of the drug in unselected AIDS patients without Kaposi sarcoma. However, because of its acceptable toleration, it might play a role in therapy of AIDS patients in combination with other drugs such as AZT. Indeed, in vitro studies have demonstrated synergistic inhibition of HIV replication by the combination of phosphonoformate and rIFN-αA (122) as well as AZT and rIFN-αA (108). Other double-blind, placebo-controlled trials of rIFN-αA in patients with AIDS are currently underway.

Ampligen

Ampligen is a non-toxic, mismatched double-stranded (ds) RNA polymer of the form *poly rIn.r(C12,U)n*. It is a derivative of the highly toxic *rIn.Cn* in which a mismatched region consisting of uracil residues is periodically inserted into the polypyrimidine strand to accelerate dsRNA hydrolysis and thus to prevent its toxicity without loosing its immunologic inductive potential. The drug belongs to the class of the biologic response modifiers and is thought to enhance antiviral activity by promoting production of lymphokines, including tumor necrosis factor and interferons. It also stimulates the IFN-associated natural killer activity by activating the dsRNA-dependent 2′,5′-oligoadenylate synthetase and dsRNA-dependent kinase, enzymes which promote respectively the cleavage of viral RNA and the interruption of viral protein synthesis.

Ampligen has been shown to inhibit HIV replication in vitro (59) and to reduce by at least 5-fold the concentration of zidovudine required for virostatic activity against HIV (110). As the modes of action of the two drugs are totally different, synergistic toxicity is unlikely.

Recently, ampligen has been administered intravenously at doses of 200 or 250 mg twice a week to 10 patients with AIDS, ARC or lymphadenopathy syndrome (LAS) for up to 18 weeks (65) and clinical, immunologic and virologic effects were monitored. Nine patients who were positive for HIV RNA in peripheral blood mononuclear cells before Ampligen administration became negative during treatment. In 6 of 7 patients with ARC or LAS, reduction of HIV load, as measured by co-culture assays, was observed. All 10 patients had augmentation of delayed-type hypersensitivity skin reactions. Increase or maintenance of numbers of T4 lymphocytes, improvement in HIV-related symptoms and signs, rise in levels of neutralizing antibodies against HIV and restoration of proper function of the natural lymphocyte antiviral RNA-dependent pathway were documented. No side effects or toxicity were noted.

Thus, the results indicate that ampligen is active in patients with various stages of HIV infection, and probably works as both an antiviral and immunorestorative drug.

Other potential drugs

Among the potential drugs effective against HIV, the most promising seem to be the *2',3'-dideoxynucleoside derivatives*. Several of these agents show an inhibitory effect in vitro on infectivity and on replication of HIV (64, 106, 107, 123, 124), the most potent being 2',3'-dideoxycytidine (45, 46, 64, 106, 107). Phase I clinical trials with this agent are currently underway.

D-Penicillamine (3-mercapto-D-valine, DPA), a chelating agent of heavy metals, has been shown to produce selective inhibition of the replication of HIV in vitro (125), possibly by cross-linking with disulfide groups of HIV and inactivation of essential viral proteins such as the cystein-rich nucleic binding protein.

DPA has been given on an escalating dose schedule to reach a maximal dose of 2 g/d p.o., to 13 HIV-infected homosexuals with persistent generalized lymphadenopathy and altered T-helper lymphocytes (126). All patients treated for at least 2 weeks showed evidence of HIV inhibition. Treatment with DPA was associated with a decrease in lymph node size, a 20% drop in absolute lymphocyte count and diminished T-cell lymphoproliferative responses without changes in T4/T8 ratios. One of the 13 patients developed opportunistic infections during the study. Skin rashes and mild transient elevations in hepatocellular enzymes were observed in 3 and 2 patients respectively.

Peptide T (106) is an octapeptide corresponding to a segment of the envelope glycoprotein gp120 of HIV, capable of inhibiting T-cell infectivity. It has been administered on a compassionate basis to 4 near-terminal AIDS patients by intravenous infusion at a dose of 1 mg twice daily for 1 week followed by 2 mg twice daily for the next 3 weeks (127). During the treatment period, there was no clinical deterioration, the drug appeared to be non-toxic and lymphocyte counts improved. The results justify further investigations with this drug.

AL-721 (33) is a lipid compound composed of neutral glycerides, phosphatidylcholine, and phosphatidylethanolamine in a 7:2:1 ratio. The compound is able to extract cholesterol from cellular membranes both in vitro and in vivo. A reduction in viral infectivity was observed when peripheral blood lymphocytes or H9 cell lines were exposed to HIV in presence of AL-721 at a concentration of 100 μg/ml, achievable in vivo without adverse reactions.

Rifabutin (ansamycin), a rifamicin-S derivative used in atypical mycobacterial infections, has been shown to block the in vitro infectivity and replication of HIV (128). Drug levels required for 99% inhibition of viral activity in vitro are achievable by regimens known to be essentially non-toxic in patients with AIDS-related *Mycobacterium avium complex* infection. Recently, rifabutin has been shown to cross the blood-brain barrier (129). Phase I trials with the drug in patients with AIDS are underway.

Amphotericin B methyl ester, a water-soluble derivative of amphotericin B (130), and *Avarol* and *Avarone* (131), two antimitotic and antimutagenic agents, also exhibit an inhibitory activity on the replication of HIV in vitro and thus deserve further evaluation as potential anti-HIV agents.

Recently, Wong et al (132) have reported very interesting in vitro results with the combination of two cytokines: *tumor necrosis factor-α* and *interferon-γ*. This combination not only protected cells against HIV infection but also was capable to kill cells acutely infected with HIV and to inhibit the production of HIV mRNA in chronically infected H9 cells.

Finally, *sodium diethyldithiocarbamate (Imuthiol)* and *inosine prabonex (Isoprinosine)*, both agents with immunomodulatory properties (133), have been shown to partially inhibit HIV expression and reverse transcriptase activity. In January 1987, a randomized, double-blind, placebo-controlled trial of 92 patients with ARC was started in France and seems to be producing promising results (134).

FUTURE DIRECTIONS

Because HIV is a virus that may exist in a latent proviral DNA form, integrated in the host genome for prolonged periods, probably for a life-time, prolonged therapy will be required to control the disease. Combination antiviral therapy may therefore prove to be very useful in reducing long-term drug toxicity.

In addition, combination of antiviral agents by allowing simultaneous interference at two or more sites of HIV replication may be more efficient than the use of one drug alone.

Combination drug therapy also decreases the possibility of emergence of drug resistance. Of great importance is the necessity for the drug to cross the blood-brain barrier in order to stop replication of the virus in the CNS. It is probable that regimens combining antiviral agents and immunomodulators or immune reconstitution procedures will be required to achieve effective treatment of HIV disease. Because of the lethal potential of the disease all reasonable approaches to therapy should be explored, provided ethical rules are respected. As Samuel Broder says (135), if we carefully absorb what the disciplines of human retrovirology, molecular biology, and biochemical pharmacology have to teach us and if we build a foundation of carefully controlled clinical trials, the various strategies for dealing with the virus should succeed and, at least at certain stages, infections with the virus may become curable.

REFERENCES

1. Barré-Sinoussi F, Chermann JC, Rey F, Nugeyre MT, Chamaret S, Gruest J, Dauguet C, Axler-Blin C, Brun-Vézinet F, Rouzioux C, Rozenbaum W, Montagnier L (1983) Isolation of a T-lymphotropic retrovirus from a patient at risk for the acquired immune deficiency syndrome (AIDS). *Science, 220*, 868.
2. Gallo RC, Salahuddin SZ, Popovic M, Shearer GM, Kaplan M, Haynes BF, Palker TJ, Redfield R, Oleske J, Safai B, White G, Foster P, Markham PD (1984) Frequent detection and isolation of cytopathic retroviruses (HTLV-III) from patients with AIDS and at risk for AIDS. *Science, 224*, 500.
3. Levy JA, Hoffman AD, Kramer SM, Landis JA, Shimabukuro JM, Oshiro LS (1984) Isolation of lymphocytopathic retroviruses from San Francisco patients with AIDS. *Science, 225*, 840.
4. Coffin J, Haase A, Levy JA, Montagnier L, Oroszlan S, Teich N, Temin H, Toyoshima K, Varmus HJ, Vogt P, Weiss R (1986) Human immunodeficiency viruses. *Science, 232*, 697.
5. Dalgleish AG, Beverly PCL, Clapham PR, Crawford DH, Greaves MF, Weiss RA (1984) The CD4 (T4) antigen is an essential component of the receptor for the AIDS retrovirus. *Nature (London), 312*, 763.
6. Klatzmann D, Champagne E, Chamaret S, Gruest J, Guetard D, Hercend T, Gluckman JC, Montagnier L (1984) T-Lymphocyte T4 molecule behaves as the receptor for human retrovirus LAV. *Nature (London), 312*, 767.
7. Popovic MR, Gallo RC, Mann DL (1984) OKT4 bearing molecule is a receptor for the human retrovirus HTLV-III. *Clin. Res., 33*, 560.
8. McDougal JS, Kennedy MS, Sligh J, Cort SP, Mawle A, Nicholson JKA (1986) Binding of HTLV-III/LAV to $T_4 + T$ cells by a complex of the 110 K viral protein and the T4 molecule. *Science, 231*, 382.
9. McDougal JS, Nicholson JKA, Cross GD, Cort SP, Kennedy MS, Mawle AC (1986) Binding of the human retrovirus HTLV-III/LAV/ARV/HIV to the CD4 (T4) molecule: conformation dependence, epitope mapping, antibody inhibition and potential for idiotype mimicry. *J. Immunol., 138*, 2937.
10. Maddon PJ, Dalgleish AG, McDougal JS, Clapham PR, Weiss RA, Axel R (1986) The T4 gene encodes the AIDS virus receptor and is expressed in the immune system and the brain. *Cell, 47*, 333.
11. Ho D, Rota T, Hirsch MS (1986) Infection of monocyte/macrophages by human T-lymphotropic virus type III. *J. Clin. Invest., 77*, 1712.
12. Levy JA, Schimabukuro J, McHugh T, Casavant C, Stites DP, Oshiro LS (1985) AIDS-associated retroviruses (ARV) can productively infect other cells besides human T helper cells. *Virology, 147*, 441.
13. Gartner S, Markovits P, Markowitz DM, Kaplan MH, Gallo RC, Popovic M (1986) The role of mononuclear phagocytes in HTLV-III/LAV infection. *Science, 233*, 215.
14. Streicher MZ, Joynt RJ (1986) HTLV-III/LAV and the monocyte/macrophage. *J. Am. Med. Assoc., 256*, 2390.
15. Gyorkey F, Melnick JL, Sinkovics JG, Gyorkey P (1985) Retrovirus resembling HTLV in macrophages of patients with AIDS. *Lancet, 1*, 106.
16. Montagnier L, Gruest J, Chamaret S, Dauget C, Axler C, Guetard D, Nugeyre MT, Barré-Sinoussi FC, Chermann JC, Brunet JB, Klatzmann D, Gluckman JC (1984) Adaptation of lymphadenopathy-associated virus (LAV) to replication in EBV-transformed B lymphoblastoid cell line. *Science, 225*, 63.

17. Dalgleish AG (1986) Antiviral strategies and vaccines against HTLV-III/LAV. *J. R. Coll. Physicians London, 20,* 258.
18. Wong-Staal F, Gallo RC (1985) Human T-lymphotropic retroviruses. *Nature (London), 317,* 395.
19. Verma I (1977) The reverse transcriptase. *Biochim. Biophys. Acta, 473,* 1.
20. Sodroski J, Rosen C, Wong-Staal F, Salahuddin SZ, Popovic M, Aryn S, Gallo R, Haseltine WA (1985) Transacting transcriptional regulation of human T-cell leukemia virus type III long terminal repeat. *Science, 227,* 171.
21. Rosen CA, Sodroski JG, Goh WC, Dayton AI, Lippke J, Haseltine WA (1986) Post-transcriptional regulation accounts for the transactivation of the human T-lymphotropic virus type III. *Nature (London), 319,* 555.
22. Sodroski J, Goh WC, Rosen C, Dayton A, Tergwilliger E, Haseltine W (1986) A second post-transcriptional transactivator gene required for HTLV-III replication. *Nature (London), 321,* 412.
23. Feinberg MB, Jarrett RF, Aldovini A, Gallo RC, Wong-Staal F (1986) HTLV-III expression and production involve complex regulation of the levels of splicing and translation of viral RNA. *Cell, 46,* 807.
24. Bowen DL, Lane HV, Fauci AS (1985) Immunopathogenesis of the acquired immunodeficiency syndrome. *Ann. Intern. Med., 103,* 704.
25. Shaw GM, Harper ME, Hahn BH, Epstein LE, Gajdusek DC, Price RW, Navia BH, Petito CK, O'Hara CJ, Groopman JC, Cho ES, Oleske JM, Wong-Staal F, Gallo RC (1985) HTLV-III infections in brains of children and adults with AIDS encephalopathy. *Science, 227,* 177.
26. Levy JA, Shimabukuro J, Hollander H, Mills J, Kaminsky L (1985) Isolation of AIDS-associated retroviruses from cerebrospinal fluid and brain of patients with neurological symptoms. *Lancet, 2,* 586.
27. Ho DD, Rota TR, Schooley RT, Kaplan JC, Allan JD, Groopman J, Resnick L, Felsenstein D, Andrews CA, Hirsch MS (1985) Isolation of HTLV-III from cerebrospinal fluid and neural tissues of patients with neurological syndromes related to the acquired immunodeficiency syndrome. *N. Engl. J. Med., 313,* 1493.
28. Gartner S, Markovits P, Markovitz DM, Betts RF, Popovic M (1986) Virus isolation from and identification of HTLV-III/LAV-producing cells in brain tissue from a patient with AIDS. *J. Am. Med. Assoc., 256,* 2365.
29. Koenig S, Gendelman HC, Orsenstein JM, Dal Canto MC, Yungbluth M, Janotta F, Aksamit A, Martin MA, Fauci AS (1986) Detection of AIDS virus in macrophages in brain tissue from AIDS patients with encephalopathy. *Science, 233,* 1089.
30. Stoler MH, Eskin TA, Benn S, Angerer RC, Angerer LM (1986) Human T-cell lymphotropic virus type III infection of the central nervous system. *J. Am. Med. Assoc., 256,* 2360.
31. Chayt KJ, Harper ME, Marselle LM, Lewin EB, Roser RM, Oleske JM, Castein LG, Wong-Staal F, Gallo RC (1986) Detection of HTLV-III RNA in lungs of patients with AIDS and pulmonary involvement. *J. Am. Med. Assoc., 256,* 2356.
32. Shaw G, Hahn BH, Arya SK, Groopman JE, Gallo RC, Wong-Staal F (1984) Molecular characterization of human T-cell leukemia (lymphotropic) virus type III in the acquired immunodeficiency syndrome. *Science, 226,* 1165.
33. Harper ME, Marselle LM, Gallo RC, Wong-Staal F (1986) Detection of lymphocytes expressing human T-lymphotropic virus type III in lymph nodes and peripheral blood from infected individuals by in situ hybridisation. *Proc. Natl Acad. Sci. USA, 83,* 772.

34. Fauci AS (1986) Current issues in developing a strategy for dealing with the acquired immunodeficiency syndrome. *Proc. Natl Acad. Sci. USA, 83*, 9278.

35. Laurence J, Gottlieb AB, Kuinkel HG (1983) Soluble suppressor factors in patients with acquired immunodeficiency syndrome and its prodrome: elaboration in vitro by T-lymphocyte adherent cell interactions. *J. Clin. Invest., 72*, 2072.

36. Pahwa S, Pahwa R, Saxinger C, Gallo RC, Good RA (1985) Influence of the human T-lymphotropic virus/lymphadenopathy-associated virus on functions of human lymphocytes: evidence for immunosuppressive effects and polyclonal B-cell activation by bonded preparations. *Proc. Natl Acad. Sci. USA, 82*, 8198.

37. Klatzmann D, Montagnier L (1986) Approaches to AIDS therapy. *Nature (London), 319*, 10.

38. Sodroski J, Goh WC, Rosen C, Campbell K, Haseltine WA (1986) Role of the HTLV-III/LAV envelope in syncytium formation and cytopathogenicity. *Nature (London), 322*, 470.

39. Lifson JD, Feinberg MB, Reyes GR, Rabin L, Banapour B, Chakrabarti S, Moss B, Wong-Staal F, Steimers KS, Engelman EG (1986) Induction of CD4-dependent cell fusion by the HTLV-III/LAV envelope glycoprotein. *Nature (London), 323*, 725.

40. Yoffe B, Lewis DE, Petrie BL, Noonan CA, Melnick JL, Hollinger FB (1987) Fusion as a mediator of cytolysis in mixtures of uninfected CD_4+ lymphocytes and cells infected by human immunodeficiency virus. *Proc. Natl Acad. Sci. USA, 84*, 1429.

41. Folks T, Powell DM, Lightfoot MM, Benn S, Martin MA, Fauci AS (1986) Induction of HTLV-III/LAV from a non-virus producing T-cell line: implications for latency. *Science, 231*, 600.

42. Hoxie JA, Haggarty BS, Rackowski JL, Pillsbury N, Levy JA (1985) Persistent noncytopathic infection of normal human T-lymphocytes with AIDS-associated retrovirus. *Science, 229*, 1400.

43. McDougal JS, Mawle A, Cort SP, Nicholson JKA, Cross GD, Scheppler-Campbell JA, Hicks D, Sligh J (1985) Cellular tropism of the human retrovirus HTLV-III/LAV. I. Role of T cell activation and expression of the T4 antigen. *J. Immunol., 135*, 3151.

44. Zagury O, Bernard J, Leonard R, Cheynier R, Feldman M, Sarin PMS, Gallo RC (1986) Long-term cultures of HTLV-III-infected T-cells, a model of cytopathology of T-cell depletion in AIDS. *Science, 321*, 850.

45. Yarchoan R, Broder S (1987) Development of antiretroviral therapy for the acquired immunodeficiency syndrome and related disorders. *N. Engl. J. Med., 316*, 557.

46. Mitsuya H, Broder S (1987) Strategies for antiviral therapy in AIDS. *Nature (London), 325*, 773.

47. Yarchoan R, Broder S (1987) Strategies for the pharmacological intervention against HTLV-III/LAV. In: Broder S (Ed), *AIDS. Modern Concepts and Therapeutic Challenges*, p 335. Marcel Dekker, New York-Basel.

48. Vogt M, Hirsch MS (1986) Prospects for the prevention and therapy of infections with the human immunodeficiency virus. *Rev. Infect. Dis., 8*, 991.

49. De Clercq E (1986) Chemotherapeutic approaches to the treatment of the acquired immune deficiency syndrome (AIDS). *J. Med. Chem., 29*, 1561.

50. Pert CB, Hill JM, Ruff MR, Berman RM, Robey WG, Arthur LO, Ruscetti FW, Farkar WL (1986) Octapeptides deduced from the neuropeptide receptor-like pattern of antigen T4 in brain potently inhibit human immunodeficiency virus receptor-binding and T-cell infectivity. *Proc. Natl Acad. Sci. USA, 23*, 9254.

51. Sodroski J, Kowalski M, Dorfman T, Basiripour L, Rosen C, Haseltine W (1987) HIV

envelope-CD4 interaction not inhibited by synthetic octapeptides. *Lancet, 1*, 1428.

52. Zimmer JP, Lehr HA, Kornhuber MC, Breitig D, Montagnier L, Gietzen K (1986) Diphenylhydantoin (DPH) blocks HIV receptor on T-lymphocyte surface. *Blut, 53*, 447.

53. Sarin PS, Gallo RC, Scheer DI, Crews F, Lippa AS (1985) Effects of a novel compound (AL 721) on HTLV-infection in vitro. *N. Engl. J. Med., 313*, 1289.

54. Salk J (1987) Prospects for the control of AIDS by immunizing seropositive individuals. *Nature (London), 327*, 473.

55. Chanh TC, Aldrete BE, Zhou EM, Kennedy RC (1987) Anti-idiotypic antibodies against OKT4 bind to human immunodeficiency virus (Abstract). *Fed. Proc., 46*, 1352.

56. Sattentau QJ, Weber JN, Weiss RA, Beverley PCL (1987) Antisera to Leu 3A with anti-idiotypic activity react with gp110/130 of HIV-1 and LAV-2. In: *Abstracts. Proceedings, III International Conference on AIDS, Washington, 1987*, TH.9.4, p 160.

57. Matsukura M, Shinozuka K, Zon G, Mitsuya H, Cohen JS, Broder S (1987) Phosphorothioate analogs of oligodeoxynucleotides: novel inhibitory of replication and cytopathic effects of HTLV-III/LAV (Human Immunodeficiency Virus) in vitro. In: *Abstracts, III International Conference on AIDS, Washington, 1987*, T4.4, p 54.

58. Zamecnik PC, Goodchild J, Taguchi Y, Sarin PS (1986) Inhibition of replication and expression of human T-cell lymphotropic virus type III in cultured cells by exogenous synthetic oligonucleotides complementary to viral RNA. *Proc. Natl Acad. Sci. USA, 83*, 4143.

59. Montefiori DC, Mitchell WM (1987) Antiviral activity of mismatched double-stranded RNA against human immunodeficiency virus in vitro. *Proc. Natl Acad. Sci. USA, 84*, 2985.

60. Goswami BB, Borek E, Sharma OK, Fujitaki J, Smith RA (1979) The broad spectrum antiviral agent ribavirin inhibits capping of RNA. *Biochem. Biophys. Res. Commun., 89*, 830.

61. Walker BD, Kowalski M, Wei Chun GOH, Rohrschneider L, Haseltine WA, Sodroski J (1987) Anti-HIV properties of castanospermine. In: *Abstracts, III International Conference on AIDS, Washington, 1987*, T4.3, p 54.

62. Ho DD, Hartshorn KL, Rota TR, Andrews CK, Kaplan JC, Schooley RT, Hirsch MS (1985) Recombinant human interferon alpha suppresses HTLV-III replication in vitro. *Lancet, 1*, 602.

63. Mitsuya H, Matsushita S, Harper ME, Broder S (1985) Pharmacological inhibition of infectivity of HTLV-III in vitro. *Cancer Res., 45, Suppl.*, 4583.

64. Mitsuya H, Matsukura M, Broder S (1987) Rapid in vitro systems for assessing activity agents against HTLV-III/LAV. In: Broder S (Ed), *AIDS. Modern Concepts and Therapeutic Challenges*, p 303. Marcel Dekker, New York-Basel.

65. Carter WA, Strayer DR, Brodsky I, Lewin M, Pellegrino MG, Einck L, Henriques HF, Simon GL, Parenti DM, Scheir RG, Schulof RS, Montefiori DC, Robinson WE, Mitchell WM, Volsky DJ, Paul D, Paxton H, Meyer III WA, Kariko K, Reichenbach N, Suhadolnick RJ, Gillespie DH (1987) Clinical, immunological, and virological effects of ampligen, a mismatched double-stranded RNA, in patients with AIDS or AIDS-related complex. *Lancet, 1*, 1286.

66. Rasheed S, Cooper RE, Shu Su (1987) Quantitation of the human immunodeficiency virus in patients treated with antiviral drugs. In: *Abstracts, III International Conference on AIDS, Washington, 1987*, T4.6, p 54.

67. Lange JMA, Paul DA, Huisman HG, De Wolf F, Van den Bergh H, Coutinho RA,

Danner SA, Van der Noordaa J, Goudsmit J (1986) Persistent HIV antigenaemia and decline of HIV core antibodies associated with transition to AIDS. *Br. Med. J., 293,* 1495.

68. De Clercq E (1979) Suramin: a potent inhibitor of the reverse transcriptase of RNA tumor viruses. *Cancer Lett., 8,* 9.
69. Mitsuya H, Popovic M, Yarchoan R, Matsushita S, Gallo RC, Broder S (1984) Suramin protection of T cells in vitro against infectivity and cytopathic effect of HTLV-III. *Science, 226,* 173.
70. Collins JM, Klecker RW, Yarchoan R, Lane HC, Fauci AS, Redfield RR, Broder S, Myers CE (1986) Clinical pharmacokinetics of suramin in patients with HTLV-III/LAV infection. *J. Clin. Pharmacol., 26,* 22.
71. Broder S, Yarchoan R, Collins JM, Lance HC, Markham PD, Mitsuya H, Hoth DF, Gelmann E, Groopman JE, Resnick L, Gallo RC, Myers CE, Fauci AS (1985) Effects of suramin on HTLV-III/LAV infection presenting as Kaposi's sarcoma or AIDS-related complex: clinical pharmacology and suppression of virus replication in vivo. *Lancet, 2,* 627.
72. Taelman H, Sprecher S, Teirlynck O, Bogaert MG, Demedts P, Gigase P, Piot P, Thiry L (1986) Suramin treatment in patients with AIDS or AIDS-related complex: preliminary results. In: Staquet M, Hemmer R, Baert A (Eds), *Clinical Aspects of AIDS and AIDS-Related Complex,* p 182. Oxford Medical Press, Oxford.
73. Saimot AG, Matheron S, Le Port C, Michon C, Katlama C, Morinière B, Dousset-Faure I, Leibowitch J, Kernbaum S, Bricaire F, Vachon F, Vilde JL, Coulaud JP, Zagury D (1986) An open trial of suramin in AIDS patients: suppression of HTLV-III/LAV replication and clinical outcome. In: Staquet M, Hemmer R, Baert A (Eds), *Clinical Aspects of AIDS and AIDS-Related Complex,* p 188. Oxford Medical Press, Oxford.
74. Cheson BD, Levine A, Mardvan D, Kaplan L, Rios A, Wolfe P, Groopman J, Hawkins MJ (1986) Suramin therapy in AIDS and related diseases: initial report of the U.S. Suramin Working Group. In: *Abstracts, II International Conference on AIDS, Paris, 1986,* p 35.
75. Levine AP, Gill PS, Cohen J, Hawkins JG, Forment SC, Aguilar S, Meyer PR, Krailo M, Parker J, Rasheed S (1986) Suramin antiviral therapy of acquired immunodeficiency syndrome: clinical, immunologic and virologic results. *Ann. Intern. Med., 105,* 32.
76. Busch W, Brodt R, Ganser A, Helm EB, Stille W (1985) Suramin treatment for AIDS. *Lancet, 2,* 1247.
77. Teich SA, Handwerger S, Mathur-Waugh U, Yancovitz S, Desnick RJ, Milvan D (1986) Toxic keratopathy associated with suramin therapy. *N. Engl. J. Med., 314,* 1455.
78. Stein CA, Saville W, Yarchoan R, Broder S, Gelmann E (1986) Suramin and function of the adrenal cortex. *Ann. Intern. Med., 104,* 286.
79. Chermann JC, Sinoussi FC, Jasmin C (1975) Inhibition of RNA-dependent DNA polymerase of murine oncornaviruses by ammonium-5-tungsto-2-antimoniate. *Biochem. Biophys. Res. Commun., 65,* 1229.
80. Jasmin C, Chermann JC, Herve G, Teze A, Souchay P, Boy-Loustiau C, Raybaud N, Sinoussi F, Raynaud M (1974) In vivo inhibition of murine leukemia and sarcoma viruses by the heterpolyanion 5-tungsto-2-antimoniate. *J. Natl Cancer Inst., 53,* 469.
81. Dormont D, Spire B, Barré-Sinoussi FC, Montagnier L, Chermann JC (1985) Inhibition of RNA-dependent DNA polymerases of AIDS and S AIDS retroviruses by

HPA-23 (antimonio-21-tungsto-9-antimoniate). *Ann. Inst. Pasteur/Virol., 136E,* 75.

82. Chermann JC, Spire B, Barré F, Montagnier L, Dormont D (1985) Mechanism of inhibition of LAV replication in patients treated with antimoniotungstate (HPA 23). In: *Abstracts, I International Conference on AIDS, Atlanta, 1985,* p 72.

83. Balzarini J, Mitsuya H, De Clercq E, Broder S (1986) Comparative inhibitory effects of suramin and other selected compounds on the infectivity and replication of human T-lymphotropic virus (HTLV-III)/lymphadenopathy-associated virus (LAV). *Int. J. Cancer, 37,* 451.

84. Rozenbaum W, Dormont D, Spire B, Vilmer E, Gentilini M, Griscelli C, Montagnier L, Barré-Sinoussi FC, Chermann JC (1985) Antimoniotungstate (HPA 23) treatment of three patients with AIDS and one with prodrome. *Lancet, 1,* 450.

85. Dormont D, Maillet T, Di Maria H, Gardere M, Barré-Sinoussi FC, Chermann JC (1986) Virologic and immunologic follow-up of 15 patients with AIDS or AIDS-related complex, and 4 LAV/HTLV-III seropositive patients treated with daily IV doses of HPA 23 during 4 to 15 months. In: *Abstracts, II International Conference on AIDS, Paris, 1986,* p 34.

86. Sundquist B, Larner E (1979) Phosphonoformate inhibition of visna virus replication. *J. Virol., 30,* 847.

87. Larsson A, Oberg B (1981) Selective inhibition of herpes virus DNA synthesis by foscarnet. *Antiviral Res., 1,* 55.

88. Öberg B (1983) Antiviral effects of phosphonoformate (PFA, foscarnet sodium). *Pharmacol. Ther., 19,* 387.

89. Sandstrom EG, Kaplan JC, Byington RE, Hirsch MS (1985) Inhibition of human T-cell lymphotropic virus type III in vitro by phosphonoformate. *Lancet, 1,* 1480.

90. Sarin PS, Taguchi Y, Sun J, Thornton A, Gallo RC, Öberg B (1985) Inhibition of HTLV-III/LAV replication by foscarnet. *Biochem. Pharmacol., 34,* 4075.

91. Beldekas JC, Levy EM, Black P, Von Krogh G, Sandstrom E (1985) In vitro effect of foscarnet on expansion of T-cells from people with LAS and AIDS. *Lancet, 2,* 1128.

92. Farthing CF, Dalgleish AG, Clark AL, McClure M, Chanas A, Gazzard BG (1987) Phosphonoformate (foscarnet): a pilot study in AIDS related complex. *AIDS, 1,* 21.

93. Gaub J, Pedersen C, Poulsen AG, Mathiesen LR, Ulrich K, Lindhardt BØ, Faber V, Gerstoft J, Hofman B, Lernested JO, Nielsen CM, Nielsen JO, Platz P (1987) The effect of foscarnet (phosphonoformate) on human immunodeficiency virus isolation, T-cell subsets and lymphocyte function in AIDS patients. *AIDS, 1,* 27.

94. Fernandez H, Banks G, Smith R (1986) Ribavirin: a clinical overview. *Eur. J. Epidemiol., 2,* 114.

95. Smith RA (1984) Background and mechanism of action of ribavirin. In: Smith RA, Knight V, Smith JAD (Eds), *Clinical Applications of Ribavirin,* p 1. Academic Press, Orlando, FL.

96. McCormick JB, Getchell JP, Mitchell SW, Hicks DR (1984) Ribavirin suppresses replication of lymphadenopathy-associated virus in cultures of human adult T lymphocytes. *Lancet, 2,* 1367.

97. Crumpacker C, Bubley G, Lucey D, Hussey S, Connor J (1986) Ribavirin enters cerebrospinal fluid. *Lancet, 2,* 45.

98. Blanche S, Fischer A, Le Deist F, Griscelli C, Guetard D, Favier V, Montagnier L (1986) Ribavirin in HTLV-III/LAV infection of infants. *Lancet, 1,* 863.

99. Matheron S, Katlama C, Leport C, Brun-Vézinet F, Wolff M, Dournon E (1986) A ribavirin open trial in AIDS. In: *Abstracts, II International Conference on AIDS, Paris, 1986,* p 68.

100. Mansell PWA, Heseltine ANR, Roberts RB, Dickinson GM, Leedom JM (1987) Ribavirin delays progression of the lymphadenopathy syndrome (LAS) to the acquired immune deficiency syndrome (AIDS). In: *Abstracts, III International Conference on AIDS, Washington, DC, 1987*, T8.5, p 58.

101. Vernon A, Schulof RS, Ribavirin ARC Study Group (1987) Serum HIV core antigen in symptomatic patients taking oral ribavirin. In: *Abstracts, III International Conference on AIDS, Washington, DC, 1987*, T8.6, p 58.

102. Lin TS, Prusoff WH (1978) Synthesis and biological activity of several amino acid analogues of thymidine. *J. Med. Chem., 21*, 109.

103. Mitsuya H, Weinhold KY, Furman PA, St Clair MH, Nusinoff-Lehrman S, Gallo RC, Bolognesi D, Barry DW, Broder S (1985) 3′-Azido-3′-deoxythymidine (BWA509U): an antiviral agent that inhibits the infectivity and cytopathic effect of human T-lymphotropic virus type III/lymphadenopathy-associated virus in vitro. *Proc. Natl Acad. Sci. USA, 82*, 7096.

104. Nakashima H, Matsui T, Harada S, Kobayashi N, Matsuda A, Ueda T, Yamamoto N (1986) Inhibition of replication and cytopathic effect of human T-cell lymphotropic virus type III/lymphadenopathy-associated virus by 3′-azido-3′-dideoxythymidine in vitro. *Antimicrob. Agents Chemother.; 30*, 933.

105. Furman PA, Fyfe JA, St Clair MH, Weinhold K, Rideout JL, Freeman GA, Nusinoff Lehrman S, Bolognesi DP, Broder S, Mitsuya H, Barry DW (1986) Phosphorylation of 3′-azido-3′-deoxythymidine and selective interaction of the 5′-triphosphate with human immunodeficiency virus reverse transcriptase. *Proc. Natl Acad. Sci. USA, 83*, 8333.

106. Mitsuya H, Broder S (1986) Inhibition of the in vitro infectivity and cytopathic effect of human T-lymphotropic virus type III/lymphadenopathy-associated virus (HTLV-III/LAV) by 2′,3′-dideoxynucleosides. *Proc. Natl Acad. Sci. USA, 93*, 1911.

107. Mitsuya H, Jarrett J, Matsukura M, Di Marzo Veronese F, De Vico AL, Sarangadharan MG, Johns DG, Reitz MS, Broder S (1987) Long-term inhibition of human T-lymphotropic virus type III/lymphadenopathy-associated virus (human immunodeficiency virus) DNA synthesis and RNA expression in T cells protected by 2′, 3′-dideoxynucleosides in vitro. *Proc. Natl Acad. Sci. USA, 84*, 2033.

108. Hartshorn KL, Vogt MW, Chou TC, Blumberg RS, Byington R, Schooley RT, Hirsch MS (1987) Synergistic inhibition of human immunodeficiency virus in vitro by azidothymidine and recombinant alpha-A interferon. *Antimicrob. Agents Chemother., 31*, 168.

109. Veno R, Kuno S (1987) Dextran sulphate, a potent anti-HIV agent in vitro having synergism with zidovudine. *Lancet, 1*, 1379.

110. Mitchell WM, Montefiori DC, Strayer DR, Carter WA (1987) Mismatched double-stranded RNA (Ampligen) reduces concentration of zidovudine (azidothymidine) required for in vitro inhibition of human immunodeficiency virus. *Lancet, 1*, 890.

111. Vogt MW, Hartshorn KL, Furman PA, Chou TC, Fyfe JA, Coleman LA, Crumpacker C, Schooley RT, Hirsch MS (1987) Ribavirin antagonizes the effect of azidothymidine on HIV replication. *Science, 235*, 1376.

112. Yarchoan R, Klecker RW, Weinhold KJ, Markham PD, Lyerly HK, Durack DT, Gelmann E, Lehrman SN, Blum RM, Barry DW, Shearer GM, Fischl MA, Mitsuya H, Gallo RC, Collins JM, Bolognesi DP, Myers CE, Broder S (1986) Administration of 3′-azido-3′-deoxythymidine, an inhibitor of HTLV-III replication, to patients with AIDS or AIDS-related complex. *Lancet, 1*, 575.

113. Fischl MA, Richman DD, Grieco MH, Gottlieb MS, Volberding PA, Laskin OL, Leedom JM, Groopman JE, Mildvan D, Schooley RT, Jackson GG, Durack DT, King D, AZT Collaborative Working Group (1987) The efficacy of azidothymidine (AZT) in the treatment of patients with AIDS and AIDS-related complex: a double-blind, placebo-controlled trial. *N. Engl. J. Med., 317*, 185.
114. Richman DD, Fischl MA, Grieco MH, Gottlieb MS, Volberding PA, Laskin OL, Leedom JM, Groopman JE, Mildvan D, Hirsch MS, Jackson GG, Durack DT, Nusinoff-Lehrman S, AZT Collaborative Working Group (1987) The toxicity of azidothymidine (AZT) in the treatment of patients with AIDS and AIDS-related complex: a double-blind, placebo-controlled trial. *N. Engl. J. Med., 317*, 192.
115. Yarchoan R, Berg G, Brouwers P (1987) Response of human immunodeficiency virus-associated neurological disease to 3'-azido-3'-deoxythymidine. *Lancet, 1*, 132.
116. Chaisson RE, Allain JP, Volberding PA (1986) Significant changes in HIV antigen level in the serum of patients treated with azidothymidine. *N. Engl. J. Med., 315*, 1610.
117. Hagler DN, Frame PT (1986) Azydothymidine neurotoxicity. *Lancet, 2*, 1932.
118. Davtyan DG, Vinters HV (1987) Wernicke's encephalopathy in AIDS patients treated with zidovudine. *Lancet, 1*, 919.
119. Bach MC (1987) Possible drug interaction during therapy with azidothymidine and acyclovir for AIDS. *N. Engl. J. Med., 316*, 547.
120. Abrams DI, Andes WA, Kisner DL, Golando JP, Volberding PA (1986) A trial of alpha-2 interferon in a benign reactive lymphadenopathic syndrome. In: *Abstracts, II International Conference on AIDS, Paris, 1986*, p 34.
121. Friedland GH, Landesman SH, Crumpacker CS, Hirsch MS, Handsfield HH, Pizzuti DJ (1987) A clinical trial of recombinant alpha interferon in patients with AIDS. In: *Abstracts, III International Conference on AIDS, Washington, DC, 1987*, TH.4.6, p 156.
122. Hartshorn KL, Sandstrom EG, Neumeyer D, Paradis TJ, Chou TC, Schooley RT, Hirsch MS (1986) Synergistic inhibition of human T-cell lymphotropic virus type III replication in vitro by phosphonoformate and recombinant alpha-A-interferon. *Antimicrob. Agents Chemother., 30*, 189.
123. Balzarini I, Mitsuya H, De Clercq E, Cooney DH, Kang CI, Dalal M, Johns DG, Broder S (1987) Potent and selective anti HTLV-III/LAV activity of 2', 3'-dideoxycytidinene, the 2', 3'-unsaturated derivative of 2', 3'-dideoxycytidine. *Biochem. Biophys. Res. Commun., 140*, 735.
124. Hamamoto Y, Nakashima H, Matsui T, Matsuda A, Ueda T, Yamamoto N (1987) Inhibitory effect of 2', 3'-didehydro-2', 3'-dideoxy nucleosides on infectivity, cytopathic effects, and replication of human immunodeficiency virus. *Antimicrob. Agents Chemother., 31*, 907.
125. Chandra P, Sarin PS (1986) Selective inhibition of replication of the AIDS-associated virus HTLV-III/LAV by synthetic D-penicillamine. *Arzneim. Forsch./Drug Res., 36*, 184.
126. Schulof RS, Scheib RG, Parenti DM, Simon GL, Digioia RA, Paxton HM, Sztein MB, Chandra P, Courtless JW, Taguchi YT, Sun DK, Goldstein AL, Sarin PS (1986) Treatment of HTLV-III/LAV-infected patients with D-penicillamine. *Arzneim. Forsch./Drug Res., 36*, 1531.
127. Wetterberg L, Alexius B, Sääf J, Sönnerborg A, Britton S, Pert C (1987) Peptide T in treatment of AIDS. *Lancet, 1*, 159.
128. Anand R, Moore J, Feorino P, Curran J, Srinivasan A (1986) Rifabutin inhibits HTLV-III. *Lancet, 1*, 87.

129. Davidson BP, Siegal FP, Reife RA, Gehan K, Burger H, Weiser B, Anand R (1987) Ansamycin (Rifabutin), an inhibitor of HIV in vitro, crosses the blood-brain barrier. In: *Abstracts, III International Conference on AIDS, Washington, DC*, THP.228, p 209.

130. Schaffner CP, Plescia OJ, Pontani D, Sun D, Thornton A, Pandey RC, Jarin PS (1986) Anti-viral activity of amphotericin B methyl ester: inhibition of HTLV-III replication in cell culture. *Biochem. Pharmacol., 35*, 4110.

131. Sarin PS, Sun D, Thornton A, Müller WEG (1987) Inhibition of replication of the etiologic agent of acquired immune deficiency syndrome (human T-lymphotropic retrovirus/lymphadenopathy-associated virus) by Avarol and Avarone. *J. Natl Cancer Inst., 78*, 663.

132. Wong GWH, Krowka J, Stites DP, Goeddel DV (1987) Tumor necrosis factor-α and interferon-γ have an anti-HIV activity. In: *Abstracts, III International Conference on AIDS, Washington, DC, 1987*, T4.5, p 54.

133. Pompidou A, Zagury D, Gallo RC, Sun D, Thornton A, Sarin PS (1985) In vitro inhibition of LAV/HTLV-III infected lymphocytes by dithiocarb and inosine pranobex. *Lancet, 2*, 1423.

134. AIDS-Imuthiol French Study Group (1987) Treatment of ARC patients with sodium diethyldithiocarbamate (DTC, Imuthiol®). In: *Abstracts, III International Conference on AIDS, Washington, DC, 1987*, MP.227, p 47.

135. Broder S (1987) Identification of therapies against the retroviruses. *Ann. Intern. Med., 106*, 568.

CHAPTER 39

Management of urinary tract infections

I.M. HOEPELMAN

Urinary tract infections (UTI) are second only to respiratory tract infections as problems encountered by practicing physicians and are probably the most common treatable infectious disease. During the last few years, several traditional concepts regarding diagnosis and treatment have been reconsidered. The evaluation and treatment of patients with UTI used to depend on the type of infection, the setting in which it occurred, the pathogen, and the severity of the patient's symptoms. It has become evident, however, that one cannot locate the type and site of infection on the basis of the symptoms and physical signs. Moreover, resistance patterns have changed and the duration of treatment has been re-evaluated; probably the most important change has been in definitions of uncomplicated UTI. These new definitions and the therapeutic principles are discussed below.

DIAGNOSIS OF URINARY TRACT INFECTIONS

Symptoms are notoriously unreliable for the diagnosis and localization of UTI (1–3) and even the 'gold standard' urine culture ($\geqslant 10^5$ CFU/ml) has become a subject of debate (4).

The most important variable in the prediction of infection is pyuria. However, there is still controversy about the best way to measure this. The most commonly used method — determination of cells per high-power field in centrifuged urine — is not reproducible and does not correlate well with the leukocyte excretion rate (5), which is a highly reproducible but time-consuming technique to differentiate patients with symptomatic bacteriuria from asymptomatic patients without bacteriuria (6). Measuring pyuria with a hemocytometer (7) seems a convenient way of detecting pyuria and avoids the errors which can be introduced by examination of the sediment (8). Symptomatic men and women with UTI can be separated by this method from those with colonization alone or with other diseases (5, 7, 9). However, a more rapid screening method for detecting pyuria has recently become available. Chemical detection by a dipstick method to detect esterases, en-

Antimicrobial Agents Annual 3
P.K. Peterson and J. Verhoef, editors
© Elsevier Science Publishers BV, 1988

zymes normally not present in serum, urine or kidney tissue, seems attractive (10). The false-positive rate of this test is 6–10%, and the false-negative rate approximately 12% (10, 11). A disadvantage of the last two methods is that bacteriuria itself remains undetected. Hence, the measurement of pyuria can be combined with the ability of freshly voided urine to reduce nitrate to nitrite (Griess nitrate reduction assay). Although most uropathogens are able to reduce nitrate, false-negative results may be caused by (a) lack of dietary nitrate, (b) reduction of nitrate concentration due to frequent diuresis or (c) infections due to enterococci and *Acinetobacter* that do not reduce nitrate as well as some *Pseudomonas* strains that reduce nitrate to nitrogen gas (12). However, in UTI with low bacterial counts (see below), in patients with UTI caused by the novobiocin-resistant coagulase-negative strain *Staphylococcus saprophyticus* — a frequent cause of uncomplicated infection (7, 13) — and in UTI caused by other gram-positive micro-organisms the nitrate reduction test yields negative results and patients may therefore be falsely categorized as having 'chlamydial' urethritis.

The diagnosis of UTI by culture has undergone some major changes and it has become clear that the criteria applied depend on the clinical setting. The criterion for detecting significant bacteriuria, originally described by Kass (14) as 100,000 or more organisms per milliliter urine ($\geqslant 10^5$ CFU/ml), remains valid after 30 years for patients with asymptomatic infection or acute pyelonephritis, although a recently published trial used $\geqslant 10^4$ CFU/ml as a diagnostic criterion in acute bacterial pyelonephritis (15). Symptomatic lower UTI may result in lower colony counts (10^2–10^5 CFU/ml) (4). The original criterion identified only 51% of symptomatic women whose bladder urine (suprapubic aspirates) contained coliforms (4).

Stamm et al (4) suggested that the best diagnostic criterion is $\geqslant 10^2$ CFU/ml in ambulant symptomatic women: the sensitivity using this criterion is 0.95 and the specificity 0.85. However, this is still a matter of debate (16). Indirect proof for the validity of their criteria is that treatment of symptomatic patients with this 'low count bacteriuria' results in prompt clinical and bacteriologic cure, as compared with placebo (17). For infections with *S. saprophyticus* the best criterion of infection is $\geqslant 10^4$ CFU/ml (4).

Patients with symptoms, pyuria and a positive nitrate assay can be treated without culturing the urine. In the case of single-dose trimethoprim sulfamethoxazole therapy as primary treatment, compared to obtaining an initial culture, the latter reduced average symptom days by 10% but increased costs by 39% (18). If the patient has pyuria without a positive nitrate assay, chlamydial urethritis, gonococcal urethritis or UTI with one of the organisms mentioned above seems more likely. This management strategy only applies to symptomatic ambulatory *women*, because, when all urine specimens presented to the laboratory are examined, the sensitivity of pyuria is lower (19).

Because it is well recognized that, in women, upper UTI is more difficult to treat than lower UTI and because all women who have renal infection should be investigated with an intravenous pyelogram, localization of the infection is important. Several methods are available to help distinguish upper from lower UTI (20).

However, most are invasive techniques and are therefore not easy to use in routine practice. Two methods — the antibody-coated bacteria test (ACB) and the response to single-dose treatment — may be used for localization in general practice.

In the ACB test, bacteria in urine sediments from patients with upper UTI demonstrate antibody binding on their surface when they have been exposed to a fluorescein-labeled antihuman globulin (21). False-negative results occur in 12–20% of patients who have upper UTI as assessed by direct localization procedures (22). These false-negatives probably result in most cases from inadequate or delayed antibody production, particularly in women with first-time coliform infections (23). Experiments in animals appear to confirm this hypothesis (24). Another explanation is the inability of antibody, once formed, to attach to the bacteria due to its mucoid coating, e.g. *Pseudomonas aeruginosa* (22). False-positive results occur in 24% of patients with lower UTI (22) and are due to technical problems, autofluorescence of yeast and *Pseudomonas* strains, staphylococci which can bind immunoglobulin non-specifically, and certain urologic diseases (22). Probably the ACB test does not have sufficient sensitivity and specificity to be of value in the routine clinical management of patients.

In 1976, Ronald et al (25) proposed that a single-dose therapeutic regimen could be a useful method of diagnosing renal infections in patients with bacteriuria but without renal symptoms. Of their patient population 92% of patients with infection confined to the bladder were cured with a single intramuscular injection of kanamycin (500 mg) compared to 30% of patients with upper UTI diagnosed by a modified Fairley bladder washout technique. Rubin et al (23) demonstrated the same with a single oral dose of amoxicillin (3 g). Women with ACB-positive infections responded in 30%, compared to 90% in the ACB-negative group.

Thus, a urinary culture obtained 2 weeks after single-dose therapy, if positive with the same micro-organism, localizes the infection to the kidneys and can therefore identify patients in whom additional investigations (e.g. IVP or cystoscopy) will only occasionally provide information that is important in management (uncomplicated UTI or reinfection) and patients in whom these investigations should be performed (complicated UTI) (26).

UNCOMPLICATED URINARY TRACT INFECTION IN ADULT WOMEN

About 20% of adult women experience an episode of acute dysuria each year (27). Stamm et al (7) categorized these patients into 4 groups: (a) patients with bacterial cystitis traditionally defined as symptomatic patients with pyuria and $\geqslant 10^5$ CFU/ ml in midstream urine; (b) women who have lower colony counts but by other criteria bacterial urethrocystitis (low-count bacteriuria + pyuria); (c) women with pyuria but sterile cultures, and evidence of recent infection with *Chlamydia trachomatis* (urethral and cervical cultures); and (d) a group of patients in whom no abnormalities are found but who may have 'interstitial cystitis' (28).

461

Since a surprising proportion of women (10–80%) who have only dysuria and no signs or symptoms of acute pyelonephritis nevertheless have upper UTI (1, 3, 7), it would seem logical to regard these patients as a fifth subgroup (subclinical pyelonephritis). Two other groups can be added to this list: patients with vaginitis or genital herpes simplex virus who generally present with vaginal discharge, irritation and 'external' dysuria (2) and patients with other forms of urethritis, e.g. gonorrhea. Since the first and second groups of Stamm can be taken together, patients with acute dysuria can be classified into 6 categories (29).

The optimal therapy regimen for patients with lower UTI has been re-evaluated during the last few years. After the first publication of efficacy of single-dose therapy in this group by Gruneberg and Brumfitt (30), single oral-dose therapy (1, 23, 31–34) or parenteral therapy (25) has been extensively studied and recommended as effective by many authorities (29, 35, 36). Single-dose treatment regimens have several advantages such as lower cost, better patient compliance, and fewer side effects; they can probably identify uncomplicated from complicated UTI and possibly have less effect on the gastrointestinal flora. A major disadvantage could be that if used in a patient with unrecognized upper UTI they might not only fail to treat the infection adequately, but, by delaying definitive therapy or by transiently masking progression of the infection, might result in progressive pyelonephritis (23, 37, 38). Indeed, there is some evidence that failures of single-dose therapy are more difficult to treat (23), but not everyone agrees (37). Another minor disadvantage could be that periurethral and vaginal flora is not eradicated, which could lead to a higher rate of reinfection (15).

The oral single-dose treatment regimens that have been best studied are amoxicillin (3 g), trimethoprim + sulfamethoxazole (TMP + SMZ) (1920 mg) and sulfonamides (sulfisoxazol 1 g).

In studies in which treatment was based on symptoms and only the detection of pyuria, the cure rates were lower (1, 34) and small differences in outcome, although not statistically significant, have been reported (1, 23, 34, 39). However, when 14 randomized controlled trials on this subject were pooled, it appeared that single-dose amoxicillin was significantly less effective than conventional multidose therapy (69 *vs* 84%) while single-dose TMP + SMZ was undistinguishable from multidose (87 *vs* 90%) regimens (39). Also, a more recent large-scale study showed that higher cure rates can be expected in patients who receive a standard 10-day course of therapy than in those who receive single-dose therapy with TMP + SMZ (37).

Also important is the report by Hooton et al (38). Their randomized investigator-blinded comparison of the effectiveness of single-dose regimens of TMP + SMZ, amoxicillin and cyclacillin was prematurely stopped because of frequent treatment failures and the development of pyelonephritis in 1 patient. When the code was broken, cure rates at 2 weeks were 85% for TMP + SMZ, 50% for amoxicillin and 30% for cyclacillin. Moreover, 1 patient in the cyclacillin group developed pyelonephritis and in 2 patients treated with amoxicillin the ACB test results were converted from negative to positive after therapy; in 1 patient in the

TMP + SMZ group the test results were also converted but the patient probably had a reinfection.

Another study that enrolled adequate numbers of patients to avoid a Type II error (inadequate number of patients enrolled in an individual study) demonstrated that single-dose therapy was as effective as a 3-day or a 10-day treatment course with TMP + SMZ. In this study 3 patients in the single dose (n = 93) and 3 in the 3-day therapy group (n = 91) developed symptoms of upper UTI due to a relapse (40). Therefore, given the available data, single-dose therapy with TMP + SMZ appears at the moment the best drug regimen to use for treatment of acute bacterial cystitis. However, a large randomized controlled trial in general practice is necessary before it can be concluded that the small differences that have been reported are not statistically significant (29).

Limited data indicate that 'the low count bacteriuria + pyuria' syndrome can be treated by single-dose antimicrobial therapy (34, 41). UTI in males by definition are complicated and should not be treated with single-dose therapy. Data on children and pregnant women are incomplete and will be discussed below.

One of the questions that remains unresolved is whether patients treated with a single dose should return for follow-up cultures. Ronald (42) in his excellent review suggests that they should and gives two reasons: (a) some patients with asymptomatic renal infections will be treated inadequately by a single dose; (b) after single-dose treatment some women may have symptoms for 24–48 hours and may be concerned that treatment has been ineffective. In my opinion the second reason can be overcome by explaining to the patient that her symptoms may last for 2 days, even if she is cured. The first issue can be addressed in the following way: What proportion of untreated renal infections is asymptomatic and what are the consequences of not treating asymptomatic bacteriuria in these patients?

In an early study 70% of patients with a relapse after single-dose therapy were asymptomatic (1). More recent studies, however, have shown that about 85% were symptomatic and almost all of the relapses occurred in the first 14 days after treatment (34, 37).

In a clinical study addressing the clinical significance of asymptomatic bacteriuria, many patients had evidence of renal damage and there was a high recurrence rate even after adequate treatment (43). In a 3–5-year follow-up of this group there was no evidence that asymptomatic bacteriuria leads to a rise in blood pressure, serum urea concentration, or kidney scarring (44). Moreover, many infections that are positive for the ACB test resolve after 1 day of treatment with TMP + SMZ (37). Hence, unless obstruction, diabetes mellitus or analgesic abuse complicates infection in this group of patients, renal failure does *not* ensue from asymptomatic bacteriuria and *follow-up cultures may not be necessary* (45).

Do the newer quinolones (see Chapter 15) deserve a place in the treatment of uncomplicated UTI? Some experts advise against the use of these drugs in uncomplicated UTI because other established agents are available and they reserve quinolones for the treatment of more complicated infections. However, the fluoroquinolones are characterized by very good activity against uropathogens such as

Neisseira gonorrhoeae and some also have activity against *Chlamydia trachomatis* (46, 47). They are very well absorbed and provide good urinary and renal concentrations (46, 47). Therefore, these drugs seem to be excellent candidates for the initial treatment of the dysuria + pyuria syndrome; however, their efficacy remains to be proven in this setting.

Norfloxacin (200 and 400 mg) is effective for the treatment of uncomplicated UTI, when given twice daily for 7 days (48–50). Norfloxacin, ofloxacin and ciprofloxacin are effective in single doses for the treatment of gonococcal urethritis and in multidoses for the treatment of chlamydial urethritis (46, 47).

Probably more important in this setting is the fact that ciprofloxacin and norfloxacin in preliminary studies when given in a *single* dose proved effective in the treatment of uncomplicated UTI (51, 119). Especially promising in single-dose treatment are pefloxacin, ofloxacin and a new fluoroquinolone, fleroxacin (Ro 23–6240), because all have half-lives of 8–14 hours (47, 52), a property which seems important for successful single-dose therapy (38).

ACUTE BACTERIAL PYELONEPHRITIS

The clinical findings associated with acute bacterial pyelonephritis are familiar: recurrent rigors and fever, back and loin pain (usually unilateral), abdominal pain, nausea and vomiting, dysuria and frequency. However, these findings occur in only about half of the patients (3). *Escherichia coli* strains responsible for pyelonephritis cluster into a few O-serogroups, exhibit mannose-resistant hemagglutination, usually possess Gal-Gal binding adhesins, elaborate β-hemolysin, and have adhesins specific for P-blood group; even when not expressed on initial testing, *E. coli* has the genetic material to encode for these phenotypic properties (53–55).

On the other hand, several host factors are very important clinically in predisposing the kidney to infection (56): urinary tract obstruction, vesicoureteral reflux, instrumentation, pregnancy, several non-infectious renal disorders (e.g. analgesic nephropathy) and probably diabetes mellitus. However, genetic factors such as an increase in glycolipid receptors (57) or simply the possession of B blood group may also predispose to the development of pyelonephritis (58), which could explain the occurrence of pyelonephritis in otherwise healthy women (59).

Most experts advise that patients should be hospitalized and given parenteral antibacterial treatment with an aminoglycoside + ampicillin as initial treatment (42). However, monotherapy with newer wider-spectrum penicillin derivatives and the new third-generation cephalosporins have been used in several studies for the initial treatment of both community-acquired and nosocomial-acquired acute bacterial pyelonephritis. Also, in experimental studies little evidence was found in favor of combination therapy in the initial treatment of pyelonephritis in rats (60). Moreover, a recently published study showed that an *oral* 2-week course of TMP + SMZ is sufficient to manage acute mild pyelonephritis in women (15).

The optimal duration of treatment is unknown, although most patients are treated for a total of 10–14 days. This regimen frequently does not sterilize the renal parenchyma as indicated by a relapse 1–2 weeks after antimicrobial therapy has been discontinued (31, 34, 61). It has been postulated that bacterial variants or L-forms persisted during treatment with β-lactam agents in hyperosmotic renal tissue and re-emerged after treatment (62).

There is some evidence to show that extending the duration (6 weeks) of drug treatment in most women achieves a higher cure rate (34, 63). However, this approach is controversial (15, 59, 61), especially when most recurrences in at least mild pyelonephritis were noted to be reinfections (15). Men have been shown to benefit from more prolonged courses (64, 65).

Except in individuals with papillary necrosis, urinary obstruction, and intrarenal or perinephritic abscess, the manifestations of acute pyelonephritis usually subside within a few days, even without specific antibacterial therapy (66). When fever and symptoms persist after 72 hours of treatment, a careful search must be made for complications which require special management (67, 68).

Again, as noted in the discussion on single-dose therapy, a recent study has cast doubt on the use of ampicillin or amoxicillin for the treatment of UTI (15). Not only was a high resistance rate found in the community and in hospital (69), but also in the oral treatment of mild pyelonephritis, ampicillin was less effective (cure rate 56%) than TMP + SMZ (88%). Moreover, it was ineffective in eliminating rectal carriage of Enterobacteriaceae and even caused selection of ampicillin-resistant strains (15).

URINARY TRACT INFECTION IN PREGNANCY

Depending on the socioeconomic status, asymptomatic bacteriuria is detected in 2–10% of pregnant women; 30% of pregnant women with asymptomatic bacteriuria subsequently develop acute pyelonephritis (70). Since pyelonephritis can have serious consequences for both mother and fetus, screening for and treatment of bacteriuria of pregnancy would appear to be justified. Both symptomatic and asymptomatic bacteriuria have repeatedly been accused of having adverse effects on the fetus such as an increased prevalence of prematurity and newborn mortality; however, the data are contradictory (71).

In pregnant women it is clearly beneficial to administer the lowest effective dose of a drug for the shortest possible duration to avoid toxicity to the fetus. Although single-dose therapy with amoxicillin may not be as successful as multidose therapy in non-pregnant women (38, 39), we agree that a single dose of 3 grams amoxicillin with follow-up cultures is a safe, effective and acceptable method of treating bacteriuria in pregnancy and the puerperium (72). However, attention must be paid to symptomatic infections due to the high rate of resistance to amoxicillin in Enterobacteriaceae (69). Pyelonephritis should not be treated with amoxicillin as monotherapy (15); third-generation cephalosporins are a good alternative.

Cure rates with single-dose streptomycin, sulfadoxine, cefaloridine, nitrofurantoin and a combination of streptomycin and sulfamethopyrazine have been somewhat lower (40–70%) than these reported for a single dose (84%) or for two doses (65%) of amoxicillin (73–76).

TMP+SMZ also seems to be effective (75), but since the teratogenicity of this combination in man is not clearly defined, it is not recommended for use in pregnancy at the present time (77).

URINARY TRACT INFECTION IN CHILDREN

The rate of bacteriuria is 1% in newborns at term, 2–3% in those born prematurely, 1% in preschool infants and 2–5% at school age (78). The neonatal period is the only period, besides old age, in which UTI is more common in males than in females.

Clinical manifestations, especially in children under 2 years of age, are non-specific and they often present with fever, vomiting, diarrhea, septicemia etc. (79).

All infants and children with their first-documented UTI should have radiologic studies, since malformations of the urinary tract are found in a high percentage (78). 'Bacteriuria' in early childhood in girls defines a group at great risk for recurrent symptomatic UTI and renal scars, and at low risk for reduced renal function (80). Gillenwater et al (80) conducted a long-term case-control study of bacteriuria in 60 school girls and 38 controls and showed that the patients were at risk for considerable morbidity from recurrent infection, especially in pregnancy. Follow-up radiologic studies were normal in 60% of girls with recurrent UTI; moreover, 20% of subjects developed abnormalities after having a normal primary X-ray. The Newcastle Covert Bacteriuria Research Group reported after 5 years of follow-up that prophylactic chemotherapy for 2 years significantly reduced the prevalence of bacteriuria at the 5-year follow-up but conferred no discernible advantage in terms of clinical history, progression of renal abnormalities or renal growth (81). When these girls were re-examined at 18 years and during subsequent pregnancies, only the renal fractional reabsorption of glucose was significantly reduced in those with renal scars whether or not they received prophylaxis (82). Chemoprophylaxis seems indicated, therefore, in patients with substantial reflux and in patients with recurrent UTI regardless of their primary X-ray.

As yet we have no adequate information to allow us make a definite assessment of single-dose therapy for UTI in children. Studies are complicated by the fact that a high percentage of children with UTI have vesicoureteral reflux or renal abnormalities. The study referred to most, claiming that short-course therapy is less effective, is that by McCracken et al (83). However, in this study a regimen (cefadroxil 30 mg/kg in two doses) was used which also proved to be inadequate in adults (36).

Three studies have been published on amoxicillin (single dose 50–100 mg/kg) claiming efficacy rates of 63–78% compared to 56–92% in the conventional treatment group (84–86). In one study (84) more complicated infections were included in the control group than in the single-dose group, probably explaining the low cure rate (56%) in the former.

The most effective treatment regimen in adults (TMP + SMZ) has also been evaluated. The efficacy of single dose (70–100%) treatment was comparable to cure rates in the conventional treatment group (80–100%) (87–89).

Two well-designed studies, excluding children with complicated UTI, both showed the same cure rate for children treated for 3 days (74–91%) with the chosen drug (nitrofurantoin, ampicillin, sulfisoxazole and cefalexin) compared with the control group treated for 10 days (80–92%) (90, 91).

The results of short-course therapy (3 days) therefore seem promising, but more studies, also in children with uncomplicated UTI, are needed.

RECURRENT URINARY TRACT INFECTION

Many adult women experience an episode of acute dysuria each year and about 50% of these have UTI diagnosed by the standard criteria (7). Some have recurrent infections.

The course in women with recurrent UTI was described by Kraft and Stamey (92). In 23 adult women with uncomplicated recurrent UTI treated for 10 days with an appropriate antibiotic for each infection, the attack rate was 0.17 per month, 94% of infections has associated symptoms, and 66% of all infections recurred within 6 months. Repeated infections in women may be either a relapse or a reinfection, and because both require a different approach, it is important to discriminate between these entities. Relapses refer to recurrences of bacteriuria with the same infecting micro-organism which was present before therapy was initiated. Reinfection is recurrence of bacteriuria with a micro-organism different from the original one and accounts for nearly all cases of recurrence in women.

Escherichia coli is by far the most common urinary pathogen in uncomplicated UTI. When structural abnormalities of the urinary tract are present, the relative frequency of infection caused by *Proteus*, *Pseudomonas* and *Klebsiella/Enterobacter* species, and by enterococci and staphylococci increases greatly. As already mentioned, bacterial virulence factors are important in the pathogenesis of pyelonephritis. However, despite these virulence factors, host factors are at least as important in recurrent infection.

E. coli appears to adhere more easily to the uroepithelial cells of girls and women who are prone to recurrent infections even when these patients are uninfected. This increased adherence is probably due to a genetically determined increase in uroepithelial cell receptors (57). Besides the genetic factors mentioned above, there is a clear relationship to sexual intercourse, shown by the fact that a single-dose antibiotic taken prophylactically after intercourse is effective in decreasing infection episodes (93). Cost-benefit studies indicate that a cluster of 3 or more acute UTIs within 1 year is an indication for a 6-month course of antibiotic prophylaxis (94). Also, single-dose therapy administered by the patients themselves at the onset of urinary symptoms is effective and more economical than conventional therapy or prophylaxis (95). It may even have the advantage of fewer resistant strains present in the gastrointestinal tract than with continous prophylaxis. Also, more often than not, UTIs recur after prophylactic treatment is discontinued. Intravenous pyelography rarely reveals an important and surgically correctable lesion in women with a recurrence due to a reinfection. However, cystoscopy detects correctable lesions in 4% and may therefore be recommended in these patients (26).

Women with a relapse of a UTI often have a renal infection (25, 31). Since these infections require a longer period of treatment than cystitis, it is important to differentiate between upper and lower UTI.

Therapy in patients with relapsing infection should be given for at least 10–14 days with cure rates between 85 and 93% (15, 23). However, an earlier study by the same group showed that half the women with renal infection also experienced recurrences after completion of a 10-day regimen (31). In these patients extension of therapy may therefore be useful (34, 63) (see above).

The prevalence of bacteriuria in adult males is low, and frequently associated with anatomic abnormalities. In males with dysuria a urine culture should be performed to differentiate between true bacteriuria and urethritis (gonococcal and non-specific) because symptoms and the presence of urethral discharge are not always reliable (96). Men with recurrent UTI very often have a prostatic focus and the prostatic localization method described by Meares and Stamey is useful in this setting, especially when urinary cultures are negative (64, 97). In sexually active men, homosexual or bisexual contacts seem to predispose to UTI (96). Men treated for UTI with a conventional 10–14 day course of an antibiotic often have recurrent infections (64, 65). Most have a relapse (65) and 50% will have a prostatic focus (64). A course of extended therapy to 6–12 weeks is more efficacious than a conventional period of treatment in this patient population (64, 65).

ASYMPTOMATIC BACTERIURIA

Asymptomatic bacteriuria is likely to occur in pregnant women, in about 3% of non-pregnant women, in patients with indwelling catheters, in patients with urologic abnormalities, and in the elderly. The first two categories have already been discussed and the current consensus is that asymptomatic bacteriuria does not require treatment in non-pregnant women but does in pregnant women. Bacteriuria in patients with indwelling catheters will be discussed below.

Bacteriuria is common in the elderly (98, 99) and the prevalence of bacteriuria increases with advancing age (98, 100). There is a lack of association between bacteriuria and symptoms in the elderly and bacteriuria may be transient with frequent spontaneous cure, reinfection or relapse (101, 102).

Bacteriuria in elderly men and women seems to be related to mortality (98, 99, 103–105), but it may be a marker for other diseases that are the primary causes of increased mortality rather than being itself the direct cause (98). The only study that took into account the transient nature of bacteriuria in the elderly, by obtaining urine samples monthly, did not show any difference in survival between non-bacteriuric, intermittently bacteriuric or continuously bacteriuric elderly institutionalized men (120). However, studies are difficult to compare since different populations have been examined.

Therapy for bacteriuria in elderly hospitalized persons, in the absence of obstructive uropathy, is neither necessary nor effective since it is asymptomatic, may be transient in nature, and does not reduce mortality (101–103). However, in elderly ambulatory, non-hospitalized women, antimicrobial therapy may be effective, may prevent the development of symptomatic urinary tract infection, and can eliminate bacteriuria in most elderly women for at least 6 months (121).

CATHETER-ASSOCIATED URINARY TRACT INFECTIONS

About 10% of all patients admitted to a general hospital are treated with an indwelling catheter (106, 107). Bacteriuria occurs in at least 25% of them and the risk factors associated with acquisition of infection include duration of catheterization, lack of systemic antibiotics during short periods of catheterization, lack of urinemeter drainage (the use of an urinemeter is *protective*), female sex, diabetes mellitus, microbial colonization of the drainage bag, serum creatinine $> 180 \mu$mol, the reason for catheterization, and the use of catheters with an unsealed collection junction when no antibiotics are administered (106–108).

Genitourinary tract manipulation and especially catheterization are closely related to bloodstream infections in hospitalized patients (109) and have been associated with a 3-fold increase in mortality (104).

Infection can occur by two routes. In transurethral infections, the infecting bacteria migrate from the rectum, establish periurethral colonization and then ascend between the catheter and the urethral mucosa to the bladder, especially in women (110). The importance of intraluminal ascending infections is suggested by the fact that closed collecting systems have markedly reduced the incidence of catheter-associated bacteriuria (106, 108), by the observation that opening the sterile collection system increases the risk of bacteriuria (107, 108), by the demonstration of proximal migration of bacteria from the collection bag to the bladder in some patients (107), and by the protective role of the urinemeter (108). Moreover, patients with an indwelling catheter show a significant increase in bacterial adherence to uroepithelial cells in the bladder 2–4 days before the onset of bacteriuria (111), which may be an important early event in the development of catheter-associated bacteriuria.

It is not well defined what quantitative level of bacteriuria is relevant in the catheterized patient. There is a discrepancy in cultures taken from catheters in situ over 30 days and those from newly inserted catheters (112); this is probably due to intraluminal growth which is enhanced by a decrease in flow often seen with long-term indwelling catheters (113). Moreover, in most instances low-level bacteriuria or candiduria will progress to concentrations above 10^5 CFU/ml (114).

Prevention of infection is very important. As already mentioned, the advantage of a closed sterile drainage system has clearly been established. The catheter should never be disconnected from the system, either on insertion or for culture, as this is likely to result in contamination.

Data on the use of antiseptics instilled directly into the bladder or added to the drainage bag have yielded conflicting results. For example, irrigation of the bladder with a polymyxin B+neomycin solution did not significantly reduce the rate of contamination (115). Attempts have also been made to sterilize the contents of drainage systems using antiseptic solutions. Gillespie et al (116) have shown that chlorhexidine can maintain sterility in drainage bags, but the frequency of UTI was no different from the control group. Others (117) have shown that periodic instillation of hydrogen peroxide into the drainage reservoir prevented bacterial growth in the collecting bag and delayed the onset of bacteriuria. More recently, however, a controlled study of this method was unable to demonstrate the efficacy of hydrogen peroxide instillation (118).

A recent study by Kunin et al (113) has shown that although the catheter appeared to be functioning well according to the nursing staff, 40% were either completely blocked or showed a delayed flow, and there appeared to be a subgroup of patients, with a decreased 'catheter half life', who would benefit from regular catheter inspection and change.

Antibiotics have an even smaller part in the management of patients with long-term indwelling catheters. Prophylactic antibiotics may delay, but will not prevent, bacteriuria. Bacteriuria should not be treated with antibiotics unless there is evidence that the infection has extended to the kidneys or bloodstream.

CONCLUSIONS

Further investigation is needed into the predictive value of diagnostic tests. The efficacy of single-dose treatment regimens to detect renal infections, in comparison with established techniques, should be determined.

Single-dose treatment of uncomplicated UTI, the duration of treatment of relapsing UTI, and the optimal duration of treatment for pyelonephritis remain issues for further study.

It will also be important to determine the optimal treatment regimen for chlamydial urethritis, with regard to both recurrent infections and immediate cure, especially since new quinolones will continue to appear on the market in the near future. The exact place and role, however, of the quinolones in the treatment of both uncomplicated and complicated UTI remains to be determined.

REFERENCES

1. Sarvard-Fenton M, Fenton BW, Reller LB, Lauer BA, Byyny RL (1982) Single dose amoxicillin therapy with follow up urine culture. *Am. J. Med., 73,* 808.
2. Komaroff AL, Pass TM, McCue JD, Cohen AB, Hendricks YM, Friedland G (1978) Management strategies for urinary and vaginal infections. *Arch. Intern. Med., 138,* 1069.
3. Fairley KF, Carson NE, Gutch RC, Leighton P, Grounds AD, Laird EC, McCallum PHG, Sleeman RL (1971) Site of infection in acute urinary tract infection in general practice. *Lancet, 2,* 615.
4. Stamm WE, Counts GW, Running KR, Fihn S, Turck M, Holmes KK (1982) Diagnosis of coliform infection in acutely dysuric women. *N. Engl. J. Med., 307,* 463.
5. Stamm WE (1983) Measurement of pyuria and its relation to bacteriuria. *Am. J. Med., 75, Suppl 1B,* 53.
6. Brumfitt W (1965) Urinary cell counts and their value. *J. Clin. Pathol., 18,* 550.
7. Stamm WE, Wagner KF, Amsel R, Alexander ER, Turck M, Counts GW, Holmes KK (1980) Causes of the acute urethral syndrome in women. *N. Engl. J. Med., 303,* 409.
8. Gadeholt H (1964) Quantitative estimation of urinary sediment, with special regard to sources of error. *Br. Med. J., 1,* 1.
9. Musher DM, Thornsteinsson SB, Airola VM (1976) Quantitative urinalysis: diagnosing UTI in men. *J. Am. Med. Assoc., 236,* 2069.
10. Kusumi RK, Grover PJ, Kunin CM (1981) Rapid detection of pyuria by leucocyte esterase activity. *J. Am. Med. Assoc., 245,* 1653.
11. Scheer WD (1987) The detection of leucocyte esterase activity in urine with a new reagent strip. *Am. J. Clin. Pathol., 87,* 86.
12. Verhoef J (1973) Detection of bacteriuria. *Lancet, 1,* 1066.
13. Maskell R (1974) Importance of coagulase-negative staphylococci as pathogens in the urinary tract. *Lancet, 1,* 1155.
14. Kass EH (1956) Asymptomatic infections of the urinary tract. *Trans. Assoc. Am. Physicians, 69,* 59.
15. Stamm WE, McKevitt M, Counts GW (1987) Acute renal infection in women: treatment with TMP/SMZ or ampicillin for two or six weeks. *Ann. Intern. Med., 106,* 341.
16. Smith GW, Brumfitt W, Hamilton-Miller J (1983) Diagnosis of coliform infections in acutely dysuric women. *N. Engl. J. Med., 309,* 1393.
17. Stamm WE, Running KR, Mc Kevitt M, Counts GW, Turck M (1981) Treatment of the acute urethral syndrome. *N. Engl. J. Med., 304,* 956.
18. Carlson KJ, Mulley AG (1985) Management of acute dysuria. *Ann. Intern. Med., 102,* 244.
19. Latham RH, Wong ES, Larson A, Coyle M, Stamm WE (1985) Management of UTI in ambulatory women. *J. Am. Med. Assoc., 254,* 3333.
20. Sheldon CA, Gonzalez R (1984) Differentiation of upper and lower UTI. *Med. Clin. North Am., 68,* 321.
21. Thomas VL, Shelokov A, Forland M (1974) Antibody coated bacteria in the urine and the site of urinary tract infection. *N. Engl. J. Med., 290,* 588.
22. Thomas VL, Forland M (1982) Antibody coated bacteria in urinary tract infections. *Kidney Int., 21,* 1.
23. Rubin RH, Fang LST, Jones SR, Munford RS, Slepack JM, Varga PA, Onheiber L,

Hall C, Tolkoff-Rubin NE (1980) Single dose amoxicillin therapy for UTI. *J. Am. Med. Assoc., 244*, 561.

24. Smith JW, Jones SR, Kaijser B (1977) Significance of antibody coated bacteria in urinary sediment in experimental pyelonephritis. *J. Infect. Dis., 135*, 577.

25. Ronald AR, Boutros P, Montada H (1976) Bacteriuria localization and response to single dose therapy in women. *J. Am. Med. Assoc., 235*, 1854.

26. Fowler JE, Pulaski ET (1981) Excretory urography, cystography and cystoscopy in the evaluation of women with UTI. *N. Engl. J. Med., 304*, 462.

27. Waters WE (1969) Prevalence of symptoms of urinary tract infection in women. *Br. J. Prev. Soc. Med., 23*, 263.

28. Messing EM, Stamey TA (1978) Interstitial cystitis: early diagnosis, pathology and treatment. *Urology, 12*, 381.

29. Komaroff AL (1984) Acute dysuria in women. *N. Engl. J. Med., 310*, 368.

30. Gruneberg RN, Brumfitt W (1967) Single dose treatment of acute UTI. *Br. Med. J., 3*, 649.

31. Fang LS, Tolkoff-Rubin NE, Rubin RH (1978) Efficacy of single and conventional amoxicillin therapy in UTI localized by the ACB technique. *N. Engl. J. Med., 298*, 413.

32. Tolkoff-Rubin NE, Weber D, Fang LS, Kelly M, Wilkinson R, Rubin RH (1982) Single-dose therapy with TMP-SMZ for UTI in women. *Rev. Infect. Dis., 4*, 444.

33. Buckwold FJ, Ludwig P, Harding GKM, Thompson L, Slutchuk M, Shaw J, Ronald AR (1982) Therapy for acute cystitis in adult women. *J. Am. Med. Assoc., 247*, 1 839.

34. Tolkoff-Rubin NE, Wilson ME, Zuromskis P, Jacoby I, Martin AR, Rubin RH (1984) Single-dose amoxicillin therapy for acute UTI in women. *Antimicrob. Agents Chemother., 25*, 626.

35. Kunin C (1981) Duration of treatment of urinary tract infection. *Am. J. Med., 71*, 849.

36. Souney P, Pok BF (1982) Single dose antimicrobial therapy for UTI in women. *Rev. Infect. Dis., 4*, 29.

37. Schultz HJ, McCaffrey LA, Keys TF, Nobrega FT (1984) Acute cystitis: a prospective study of laboratory tests and duration of therapy. *Mayo Clin. Proc., 59*, 391.

38. Hooton TM, Running K, Stamm WE (1985) Single-dose therapy for cystitis in women. *J. Am. Med. Assoc., 253*, 387.

39. Philbrick JT, Bracikowski JP (1985) Single-dose antibiotic treatment for uncomplicated UTI: less for less? *Arch. Intern. Med., 145*, 1672.

40. Gossius G, Vorland L (1984) A randomized comparison of single-dose *vs* three day and ten day therapy with TMP/SMZ for acute cystitis in women. *Scand. J. Infect. Dis., 16*, 373.

41. Cardenas J, Quinn EL, Rooker G, Bavinger J, Pohlod D (1986) Single-dose cephalexin therapy for acute bacterial UTI and acute urethral syndrome with bladder bacteriuria. *Antimicrob. Agents Chemother., 29*, 383.

42. Ronald AR (1984) Current concepts in the management of urinary tract infections in adults. *Med. Clin. North Am., 68*, 335.

43. Asscher AW, Sussmann M, Waters WE, Evans JAS, Campbell H, Evans KT, Williams JE (1969) The clinical significance of ASB in the nonpregnant women. *J. Infect. Dis., 120*, 17.

44. Asscher AW, Chick S, Radford N, Waters WE, Sussmann M, Evans JS, McLachlan MSF, Williams JE (1973) Natural history of ASB in non-pregnant women. In: Brum-

fitt W, Asscher AW (Eds), *Urinary Tract Infections*, p 51. Oxford University Press, London.

45. Winickoff RN, Wilner SI, Gall G, Laage T, Barnett O (1981) Urine culture after treatment of uncomplicated cystitis in women. *South. Med. J., 74*, 165.

46. Bergan T (1986) Quinolones. In: Peterson PK, Verhoef J (Eds), *The Antimicrobial Agents Annual 1*, p 164. Elsevier, Amsterdam.

47. Bergan T (1987) Quinolones. In: Peterson PK, Verhoef J (Eds), *The Antimicrobial Agents Annual 2*, p 169. Elsevier, Amsterdam.

48. Goldstein EJC, Alpert ML, Ginsberg BP (1985) Norfloxacin vs. TMP-SMZ in the therapy of uncomplicated community acquired UTI. *Antimicrob. Agents Chemother., 27*, 422.

49. The Urinary Tract Infection Study Group (1987) Coordinated multicenter study of norfloxacin vs. TMP-SMZ treatment of symptomatic UTI. *J. Infect. Dis., 155*, 170.

50. Haase DA, Harding GKM, Thomson MJ, Kennedy JK, Urias BA, Ronald AR (1984) Comparative trial of norfloxacin and TMP-SMZ in the treatment of women with localized acute, symptomatic UTI and antimicrobial effect on periurethral flora and fecal microflora. *Antimicrob. Agents Chemother., 26*, 481.

51. Garlando F, Reitiker S, Tauber MG, Flepp M, Meier B, Luthy R (1987) Single-dose ciprofloxacin at 100 versus 250 mg for treatment of uncomplicated urinary tract infections in women. *Antimicrob. Agents Chemother., 31*, 354.

52. Manek N, Andrews JM, Wise R (1986) In vitro activity of Ro 23-6240, a new difluoroquinolone derivative, compared with that of other antimicrobial agents. *Antimicrob. Agents Chemother., 30*, 330.

53. Turck M, Petersdorf RG (1962) The epidemiology of non-enteric *Escherichia coli* infection: prevalence of serological groups. *J. Clin. Invest., 41*, 1760.

54. O'Hanley P, Low D, Romero I, Lark D, Vosti K, Falkow S, Schoolnik G (1985) Gal-Gal binding and hemolysin phenotypes and genotypes associated with uropathogenic *E. coli. N. Engl. J. Med., 313*, 414.

55. Källenius G, Svenson SB, Hultberg H, Mollby R, Helin I, Cedergren B (1981) Occurrence of P-fimbriated *Escherichia coli* in urinary tract infections. *Lancet, 2*, 1189.

56. Sobel JD, Kaye D (1984) Host factors in the pathogenesis of UTI. *Am. J. Med., 76*, 122.

57. Lomberg H, Hanson LA, Jacobsson B, Jodal U, Leffler H, Svanborg-Eden C (1983) Correlation of P blood group, vesicoureteral reflux and bacterial attachment in patients with recurrent pyelonephritis. *N. Engl. J. Med., 308*, 1189.

58. Ratner JJ, Thomas VL, Forland M (1986) Relationship between human blood groups, bacterial pathogens, and UTI. *Am. J. Med. Sci., 292*, 87.

59. Gleckmann R, Bradley P, Roth R, Hibert D, Pelletier C (1985) Therapy of symptomatic pyelonephritis in women. *J. Urol., 133*, 176.

60. Meylan PR, Braoudakis G, Glauser MP (1986) Influence of inflammation on the efficacy of antibiotic treatment of experimental pyelonephritis. *Antimicrob. Agents Chemother., 29*, 760.

61. Little PJ, Wardener HE (1966) Acute pyelonephritis incidence of reinfection in 100 patients. *Lancet, 2*, 1277.

62. Gutman LT, Turck M, Petersdorf RG, Wedgwood RJ (1965) Significance of bacterial variants in urine of patients with chronic bacteriuria. *J. Clin. Invest., 44*, 1945.

63. Turck M, Anderson KN, Petersdorf RG (1966) Relapse and reinfection in chronic bacteriuria. *N. Engl. J. Med., 275*, 70.

64. Smith JW, Jones SR, Reed WP, Tice AD, Deupree RH, Kaijser B (1979) Recurrent UTI in men. *Ann. Intern. Med., 91*, 544.

65. Gleckman R, Crowley M, Natsios GA (1979) Therapy of recurrent invasive UTI of men. *N. Engl. J. Med., 301*, 878.

66. Lindemeyer RI, Turck M, Petersdorf RG (1963) Factors determining the outcome of chemotherapy in infections of the urinary tract. *Ann. Intern. Med., 58*, 201.

67. Thorley JD, Jones SR, Sanford JP (1974) Perinephric abscess. *Medicine, 53*, 441.

68. Costello AJ, Blandy JP, Hately W (1983) Percutaneous aspiration of renal cortical abscess. *Urology, 21*, 201.

69. Gruneberg RN (1984) Antibiotic sensitivities of urinary pathogens. *J. Antimicrob. Chemother., 14*, 17.

70. Williams JD, Reeves DS, Brumfitt W, Condie AP (1973) The effects of bacteriuria in pregnancy on maternal health. In: Brumfitt W, Asscher AW (Eds), *UTI*, p 103. Oxford University Press, London.

71. Anonymous (1985) UTI during pregnancy (Editorial). *Lancet, 2*, 190.

72. Masterton RG (1985) Single dose amoxicillin in the treatment of bacteriuria in pregnancy and the puerperium — a controlled clinical trial. *Br. J. Obstet. Gynaecol., 92*, 498.

73. Williams JD, Smith EK (1970) Single dose therapy with streptomycin and sulfametopyrazine for bacteriuria during pregnancy. *Br. Med. J., 4*, 651.

74. Brumfitt W, Faiers MC, Franklin INS (1970) The treatment of UTI by means of single dose of cephaloridine. *Postgrad. Med. J., 46, Suppl*, 65.

75. Bailey RR (1984) Single dose antibacterial treatment for bacteriuria in pregnancy. *Drugs, 27*, 183.

76. Brumfitt W, Hamilton-Miller JMT, Franklin INS, Anderson FM, Brown GM (1982) Conventional and two dose amoxicillin treatment of bacteriuria in pregnancy and recurrent bacteriuria: a comparative study. *J. Antimicrob. Chemother., 10*, 239.

77. Chow AW, Jewsson PJ (1985) Pharmacokinetics and safety of antimicrobial agents during pregnancy. *Rev. Infect. Dis., 7*, 287.

78. McCracken GH (1984) Recurrent UTI in children. *Pediatr. Infect. Dis., 277*, S28.

79. Ginsburg CM, McCracken GH (1982) Urinary tract infections in young infants. *Pediatrics, 69*, 409.

80. Gillenwater JY, Harrison RB, Kunin CM (1979) Natural history of bacteriuria in schoolgirls. *N. Engl. J. Med., 301*, 396.

81. Newcastle Covert Bacteriuria Research Group (1981) Covert bacteriuria in school girls in Newcastle upon Tyne. *Arch. Dis. Child., 56*, 585.

82. Davison JM, Sprott MS, Selkon JB (1984) The effect of covert bacteriuria in schoolgirls on renal function at 18 years and during pregnancy. *Lancet, 2*, 651.

83. McCracken GH, Ginsburg CM, Namasonthi V, Petruska M (1981) Evaluation of short-term antibiotic therapy in children with uncomplicated UTI. *Pediatrics, 67*, 796.

84. Bailey RR, Abott GD (1977) Treatment of UTI with a single dose of amoxicillin. *Nephron, 18*, 316.

85. Shapiro ED, Wald ER (1981) Single dose amoxicillin treatment of UTI. *J. Pediatr., 99*, 989.

86. Avner ED, Ingelfinger JR, Herrin JT, Link DA, Marcus E, Tolkoff-Rubin NE, Russell-Getz L, Rubin RH (1983) Single-dose amoxicillin therapy of uncomplicated pediatric UTI. *J. Pediatr., 102*, 623.

87. Bailey RR, Abbott GD (1978) Treatment of UTI with a single dose MP-SMZ. *Can. Med. Assoc. J., 118*, 551.

88. Pitt WR, Dyer SA, McNee JL, Burke JR (1982) Single dose TMP-SMZ treatment of symptomatic UTI. *Arch. Dis. Child., 57*, 229.

89. Stahl GE, Topf P, Fleisher GR, Norman ME, Rosenblum HW, Gruskin AB (1984) Single dose treatment of uncomplicated UTI in children. *Ann. Emergency Med., 13*, 705.

90. Lohr JA, Hayden GF, Kesler RW (1981) Three-day therapy of lower UTI with nitrofurantoin macrocrystals: a randomized clinical trial. *J. Pediatr., 99*, 980.

91. Khan AJ, Kumar K, Evans HE (1981) Three-day antimicrobial therapy of UTI. *J. Pediatr., 99*, 992.

92. Kraft JK, Stamey TA (1977) The natural history of symptomatic recurrent bacteriuria in women. *Medicine, 56*, 55.

93. Vosti KL (1975) Recurrent urinary tract infections. *J. Am. Med. Assoc., 231*, 934.

94. Stamm WE, Counts GW, Wagner KF, Martin D, Gregory D, McKevitt M, Turck M, Holmes KK (1980) Antimicrobial prophylaxis of recurrent urinary tract infections: a double-blind, placebo controlled trial. *Ann. Intern. Med., 92*, 770.

95. Wong ES, McKevitt M, Running K, Turck M, Stamm WE (1985) Management of recurrent urinary tract infections with patient-administered single-dose therapy. *Ann. Intern. Med., 102*, 302.

96. Barnes RC, Roddy RE, Daifuku R, Stamm WE (1986) Urinary-tract infection in sexually active homosexual men. *Lancet, 1*, 171.

97. Meares EM, Stamey TA (1968) Bacteriologic localization patterns in bacterial prostatitis and urethritis. *Invest. Urol., 5*, 492.

98. Nordenstamm GR, Brandberg A, Oden AS, Svanborg Eden CM, Svanborg A (1986) Bacteriuria and mortality in an elderly population. *N. Engl. J. Med., 314*, 1152.

99. Nicolle LE, Bjornson J, Harding GKM, MacDonell JA (1983) Bacteriuria in elderly institutionalized men. *N. Engl. J. Med., 309*, 1420.

100. Brocklehurst JC, Dillane JB, Griffiths L, Fry J (1968) Prevalence of UTI in an aged population. *Gerontol. Clin., 10*, 242.

101. Boscia JA, Kobasa WD, Abrutyn E, Levison ME, Kaplan AM, Kaye D (1986) Lack of association between bacteriuria and symptoms in the elderly. *Am. J. Med., 81*, 979.

102. Boscia JA, Kobasa WD, Knight RA, Abrutyn E, Levison ME, Kaye D (1986) Epidemiology of bacteriuria in an elderly ambulatory population. *Am. J. Med., 80*, 208.

103. Dontas AS, Kasviki-Charvati P, Panayiotis CL, Marketos SG (1981) Bacteriuria and survival in old age. *N. Engl. J. Med., 304*, 939.

104. Platt R, Polk BF, Murdock B, Rosner B (1982) Mortality associated with nosocomial UTI. *N. Engl. J. Med., 307*, 637.

105. Evans DA, Hennekens CH, Miao L, Miall WE, Kass EH, Rosner B, Kendrick MI, Stuart KL (1982) Bacteriuria and subsequent mortality in women. *Lancet, 1*, 156.

106. Kunin CM, McCormack RC (1966) Prevention of catheter induced UTI by sterile closed drainage. *N. Engl. J. Med., 274*, 1155.

107. Garibaldi RA, Burke JP, Dickmann ML, Smith CB (1974) Factors predisposing to bacteriuria during indwelling urethral catheterization. *N. Engl. J. Med., 291*, 215.

108. Platt R, Polk BF, Murdock B, Rosner B (1986) Risk factors for nosocomial UTI. *Am. J. Epidemiol., 124*, 977.

109. Krieger JN, Kaiser DL, Wenzel RP (1983) Urinary tract etiology of bloodstream infections in hospitalized patients. *J. Infect. Dis., 148*, 57.

110. Daifuku R, Stamm WE (1984) Association of rectal and urethral colonization with UTI in patients with indwelling catheter. *J. Am. Med. Assoc., 252*, 2028.

111. Daifuku R, Stamm WE (1986) Bacterial adherence to uroepithelial cells in catheter associated UTI. *N. Engl. J. Med., 314*, 1208.
112. Grahn D, Norman DC, White ML, Cantrell M, Yoshikave TT (1985) Validity of urinary catheter specimens for diagnosis of UTI in the elderly. *Arch. Intern. Med., 145*, 1858.
113. Kunin CM, Chin QF, Chamber S (1987) Indwelling urinary catheter in the elderly. *Am. J. Med., 82*, 405.
114. Stark RD, Mali DG (1984) Bacteriuria in the catheterized patient. *N. Engl. J. Med., 311*, 560.
115. Warren JW, Platt R, Thomas RJ, Rosner B, Kass EH (1978) Antibiotic irrigation and catheter associated UTI. *N. Engl. J. Med., 299*, 570.
116. Gillespie WA, Simpson R, Jones J, Teardale C, Speller DCE (1983) Does the addition of disinfectant to urinary bags prevent infection in catheterized patients? *Lancet, 2*, 1037.
117. Maizels M, Schaeffer AJ (1980) Decreased incidence of bacteriuria associated with periodic instillation of hydrogen peroxide into urethral drainage bag. *J. Urol., 123*, 841.
118. Thompson RL, Haley CE, Searcy MA, Guenther SM, Kaiser DL, Groschel DHM, Gillenwater JY, Wenzel RP (1984) Catheter associated bacteriuria. *J. Am. Med. Assoc., 251*, 747.
119. Vevey P, Darioli R, Bille J, Glauser MP (1987) Etude comparative du traitement de l'infection urinaire simple par une dose unique de norfloxacine versus co-trimoxazole. *Schweiz. Med. Wochenschr., 117*, 968.
120. Nicolle LE, Henderson E, Bjornson J, McIntyre M, Harding GKM, MacDonell JA (1987) The association of bacteriuria with resident characteristics and survival in elderly institutionalized men. *Ann. Intern. Med., 106*, 682.
121. Boscia JA, Kobasa WD, Knight RA, Abrutyn E, Levison ME, Kaye D (1987) Therapy versus no therapy for bacteriuria in elderly ambulatory non-hospitalized women. *J. Am. Med. Assoc., 257*, 1067.

CHAPTER 40

Prophylaxis in abdominal surgery

RONALD LEE NICHOLS

The use of effective antimicrobial prophylaxis has among other scientific and technical developments led to an ever increasing scope of modern-day surgery. This technique specifically refers to the perioperative use of an antibiotic to lessen the effect of exogenous and endogenous bacterial contamination occurring during operation, with a resultant end-point of reduced postoperative wound and deep-space infections. The economic, physical and psychologic impact of these postoperative infections mandates the clinical use of all preventive methods which have been proven to decrease their incidence (1, 2).

The use of properly chosen and appropriately administered prophylactic antibiotics has had its greatest success in abdominal operations where almost all procedures are at high risk for postoperative infections due to the escape of the luxuriant endogenous microflora that colonizes the gastrointestinal and gynecologic organs (3). Recent improvements in antibiotic prophylaxis including the timing of initial administration, appropriate choice of antibiotic agents in each clinical setting and short duration of administration have allowed for the more clearly defined value of this technique by authoritative groups (4, 5).

HISTORICAL DEVELOPMENTS

Soon after the discovery of the sulfonamides in the 1930s a report of the apparent efficacy of the preoperative oral administration of sulfanilamide before colorectal operations was published (6). In this report 21 patients given up to 15 grams of sulfanilamide per day were noted to have less postoperative morbidity and peritonitis than usually observed, but also developed a peculiar cyanosis not seen in patients not receiving the sulfonamide. Other early non-randomized trials conducted in the 1950s utilizing prophylactic penicillin, chloramphenicol or streptomycin in abdominal operations failed to show efficacy (5). The failure of the prophylactic regimens in these early studies was largely due to the helterskelter fashion in which they were prescribed. There was little information available concerning the antibiotic sensitivity of the potentially infecting micro-organisms and no criteria avail-

Antimicrobial Agents Annual 3
P.K. Petersen and J. Verhoef, editors
© Elsevier Science Publishers BV, 1988

able concerning the choice of agents, routes of administration or timing of the doses.

In 1964, Bernard and Cole (7) were the first investigators to report on the successful use of prophylactic antibiotics in a randomized, prospective placebo-controlled study in abdominal operations on the gastrointestinal tract or pancreaticobiliary system. Their study design utilized a total of 3 doses of intramuscularly administered penicillin, methicillin and chloramphenicol given in appropriate doses shortly before, during and shortly after operation. Sixty-six patients receiving the antibiotics had a significantly reduced postoperative infection rate of 8% compared to the 27% infection rate observed in 79 placebo patients. The success of antibiotic prophylaxis noted in this early study was clearly due to the authors' appropriate patient selection and wise choice of available agents, as well as appropriate timing of administration. Not limiting antibiotic prophylaxis to the high-risk patients as defined by Bernard and Cole appears to be the primary reason a similarily designed study published in 1966 failed to show the value of antibiotic prophylaxis (8).

In the early 1960s several studies were published that helped to better clarify our understanding of antimicrobial prophylaxis. Burke (9) utilizing experimental design demonstrated the crucial relationship between the timing of antibiotic administration and its prophylactic efficacy. His experimental studies showed that in order to greatly reduce experimental skin infection produced by penicillin-sensitive *Staphylococcus aureus*, the penicillin must be in the skin shortly before or at the time of bacterial inoculation. Critical delays after bacterial inoculation of 3–4 hours before antibiotic administration resulted in infected lesions that were indistinguishable in size and histology from those in animals who had received

Table 1   *Risk factors for the development of wound infection*

Patient factors
Poor nutritional status
Malignancy and/or chemotherapy
Underlying chronic disease (cardiac, renal, pulmonary, metabolic)
Exogenous obesity
Corticosteroid therapy
Diabetes mellitus

Surgical risk factors
Duration of preoperative hospitalization
Preoperative cleansing with antiseptic solution
Timing and type of hair removal
Use of prophylactic drains
Insertion of foreign bodies (implants)
Duration of the surgical procedure
Elective operation done in the face of an active remote infection (urine, pulmonary or soft tissue)

no prophylaxis. This experimental study and others provided clear data which gradually helped to curb the common clinical practice error of administering the initial dose of prophylactic antibiotics in the recovery room during the early postoperative course (10, 11). These studies also helped to develop the attitude that in order to prevent subsequent infection the antibiotic must be in the tissues before or at the time of bacterial contamination.

Further advances in our understanding of antibiotic prophylaxis in abdominal surgery occurred in the 1970s. It was during this decade that the qualitative and quantitative nature of the endogenous gastrointestinal flora in health and disease was appropriately defined (12–15). This knowledge allowed surgeons to pick the prophylactic regimen which had maximum effect against the most likely infecting micro-organisms, thus alleviating the need to include drugs active against every potential pathogen.

NON-ANTIBIOTIC FACTORS THAT INFLUENCE THE POSTOPERATIVE INFECTION RATE

Many factors besides prophylactic antibiotics may exert an influence on the development of postoperative wound sepsis (2). Generally, these factors have their greatest influence on non-abdominal clean surgical procedures, where antibiotic prophylaxis is of varying importance. Most critical to a successful outcome in all operations are proper operative technique and sound judgment exercised by the responsible surgeon and his/her team. A list of patient and surgical risk factors is included in Table 1. Very little change in *patient risk factors* can be accomplished preoperatively other than recommending weight loss or improvement in the nutritional status prior to elective abdominal operation. However, preoperative attention to *surgical risk factors* will decrease subsequent infections in elective abdominal procedures.

Surgical risk factors

Elective abdominal procedures should not be done during the same hospital stay after prolonged hospitalizations for workup or treatment of another disease state. Whenever possible, the preoperative workup should be conducted in outpatient facilities with hospital admission occurring on the day prior to major surgery. The risk of skin colonization with hospital-acquired antibiotic-resistant micro-organisms increases daily in hospitalized patients, especially those who are located in critical care units (16), while the postoperative infection rate directly relates to the duration of preoperative hospital stay (17).

The presence of an active remote infection at the time of elective operation also increases the postoperative wound infection rate (17). A careful search should be conducted in all patients prior to hospital admission for elective surgery, and if such an infection is identified, it should be actively treated. These remote infections most commonly involve skin and the respiratory or urinary tracts. Parenteral antibiotics started the night before the elective procedure to treat these remote infections are not effective in diminishing the increased postoperative infection rate observed in these patients (18).

Showering or bathing with an antiseptic solution or soap on the night prior to operation decreases the skin microflora and also has been shown to decrease post-operative infections (17). Areas of dirt and soilage should be removed from the body surface at this time with special attention to cleansing of the umbilicus. The archaic ritual of extensive razor shaving of the skin surrounding the operative field on the night before operation frequently causes skin damage and bacterial growth, which also may result in increased postoperative wound sepsis (17). It is postulated that even skillful razor preparation causes microscopic injury, thus providing portals of exit from and entry to injured tissue which serves as a substrate for bacterial growth. Appropriate hair removal when necessary should be done just prior to operation in a limited fashion with either a razor or an electric clipper (17, 19).

The chance of developing a postoperative wound infection also *almost doubles* with each hour of operation time (17). Shapiro et al (20) have reported that an increasing duration of operative time in hysterectomy was associated with a decreasing effect of antibiotic prophylaxis in preventing infection at the operative site. The statistically significant benefit of antibiotic prophylaxis in decreasing wound sepsis in these operations lasting 1 hour was lost in operations lasting over $3^1/_3$ hours. This finding undoubtedly relates to the pharmacokinetics of the antibiotic prophylaxis employed by these authors as well as to increased bacterial wound colonization which occurs in lengthy, complicated operative procedures.

The use of 'prophylactic' latex Penrose drainage in abdominal surgery also increases the likelihood of subsequent infection (21, 22). This finding is most likely due to the contamination of the tissues at the interior aspect of the abdominal drain with exogenous skin bacteria (21). The presence of this type of foreign body also has been shown in experimental wound models to enhance dramatically the infection rate even in the presence of subinfective doses of bacteria (23). It appears safe to conclude, therefore, that the prophylactic use of abdominal drains is unwarranted and, indeed, may be a dangerous practice. Drains, when required to empty localized collections, should be placed through sites other than the primary surgical incision and should be of a closed suction drainage type.

Many other factors are considered, without convincing evidence, to influence postoperative wound infection, including preoperative scrub techniques, surgical glove damage, barrier materials, suture selection and 'laminar flow' air-blowing systems in the operating room. Anecdotal experience and commercial interests rather than scientific studies usually account for these associations.

BASIC PRINCIPLES — SURGICAL ANTIBIOTIC PROPHYLAXIS

Many authoritative reviews of countless clinical studies concerning surgical prophylaxis have classified those patients who may be expected to benefit from perioperative antibiotics (4, 5, 24, 25). In *clean operations* which account for about 75% of all surgical procedures, prophylactic antibiotics are presently advocated only in those cases that utilize a foreign-body implant. The chance of infection in these cases is generally reported to be 1–3% and results from exogenous contamination with gram-positive organisms such as staphylococci during the course of operation. Recently however, a study has been reported which analyzed 10 risk factors for infections with stepwise multiple logistic regression techniques in 58,498 surgical patients (26). The developed index formula utilizing 4 of the risk factors was then found to be valid as a predictor of surgical wound infection in 59,352 surgical patients. The results of this study showed that the overall infection rate in *clean* surgical procedures was 2.9%; however, low-risk patients had a 1.1% infection rate while those in the high-risk category had 15.8%. Similar findings were noted in the other categories of surgical procedures including *clean-contaminated, contaminated* and *dirty*. These findings appear to indicate that the control of surgical infections might be enhanced if efforts could be focused on the high-risk patient groups in each category of surgical procedures in which almost all the infections occur.

Most abdominal surgical procedures fall into the categories of clean-contaminated, contaminated and dirty. Dirty procedures, which account for about 5% of all surgical cases, imply active infection where *therapeutic* antibiotics are required. Therefore, a discussion of prophylactic antibiotics in abdominal surgery would include about 20% of all surgical procedures which fall into the categories of *clean-contaminated* (elective genitourinary or biliary and gastrointestinal procedures) and contaminated (penetrating or blunt abdominal trauma with hollow viscus injury or early viscus perforation due to a disease state).

Choice of antibiotics

No single antibiotic agent or combination should be relied on for effective prophylaxis in all abdominal operations. The agent or agents employed should be chosen primarily on the basis of their efficacy against the endogenous micro-organisms that usually cause the infectious complications in each clinical setting, as well as their safety profile and cost. Where multiple drugs or regimens have been proven equally efficacious and safe, local hospital cost analyses and utilization studies may result in choosing the agent that will result in the greatest savings (27). The usual infecting micro-organisms in each abdominal procedure and the prophylactic antibiotic recommendations are listed in Table 2. It has been stressed that covering all the potential pathogens is not a desired feature of a prophylactic antibiotic regimen (5). However, it is important to maintain a local hospital up-to-date analysis of the antimicrobial susceptibilities of wound isolates in order to detect important shifts in patterns of resistance.

The cephalosporin agents because of their proven efficacy and low toxicity remain the parenterally administered drugs of choice in surgical antibiotic prophylaxis (4, 5). In abdominal surgery cephalosporins are utilized in antibiotic prophyla-

Table 2 *Micro-organisms most commonly implicated in postoperative sepsis in abdominal surgery and prophylactic antibiotic recommendations*

Surgical procedure	Endogenous organisms		Recommended agents	Route	Dose	Alternative agents
	Aerobic	Anaerobic				
Gastroduodenal	streptococci coliforms	*Bacteroides* (other than *B. fragilis*) peptostreptococci	1st generation cephalosporins*	i.v.	1 gr	2nd or 3rd generation cephalosporin (i.v.)
Elective colon resection	coliforms	*B. fragilis* peptostreptococci clostridia	Neomycin + erythromycin base**	p.o.	1 gr each × 3	aminoglycoside (p.o.) + metronidazole (p.o.) or tetracycline (p.o.)
Appendectomy	coliforms	*B. fragilis* peptostreptococci clostridia	2nd or 3rd generation cephalosporin+	i.v.	1 g	clindamycin (i.v.) + aminoglycoside (i.v.) or metronidazole (i.v.) + aminoglycoside (i.v.) or piperacillin (i.v.)
Penetrating abdominal trauma	coliforms	*B. fragilis* peptostreptococci clostridia	2nd or 3rd generation cephalosporin+	i.v.	1 g	clindamycin (i.v.) + aminoglycoside (i.v.) or metronidazole (i.v.) + aminoglycoside (i.v.) or piperacillin (i.v.)

Cholecystectomy	coliforms	clostridia	1st generation cephalosporin*	i.v.	1 g	2nd or 3rd generation cephalosporin (i.v.) *or* aminoglycoside (i.v.)
Hysterectomy	coliforms	*B. fragilis* and other species peptostreptococci clostridia	1st generation cephalosporin*	i.v.	1 g	2nd or 3rd generation cephalosporin (i.v.)
Prostatectomy (infected urine)	coliforms Group D streptococci	none	1st generation cephalosporin*,++	i.v.	1 g	based on sensitivity of infecting organisms

* Choice should be based on lowest cost to hospital cefazolin (Ancef, Kefzol), cefalotin (Keflin) or cephapirin (Cefadyl).
** Some recommendations include an additional single preoperative dose of i.v. antibiotic with efficacy against aerobic coliforms and anaerobic *Bacteroides*.
+ Agent with *B. fragilis* activity.
++ If preoperative urine shows sensitive organism.

xis as the primary approach in all but elective colorectal operations where oral antibiotic bowel preparation appears to be preferred (28). A recent study reviewing published studies which compare older first-generation cephalosporins with newer second- and third-generation agents in surgical prophylaxis have failed to disclose any significant differences (29). The authors have therefore cautioned against adoption of the newer, more expensive cephalosporins as the agents of choice in surgical prophylaxis until evidence of superiority is available.

Timing of antibiotic prophylaxis

The effective use of prophylactic antibiotics depends to a great extent on the appropriate timing of their administration (28). However, the most common errors of prophylaxis in the past, which undoubtedly dulled the lustre of this technique, were the faulty timing of the initial administration and the common practice of continuing the antibiotic beyond 72 hours (30). A recent paper reporting a multi-hospital education program on 'Antibiotic Prophylaxis in Surgery' showed a significant improvement in physician timing of prophylactic antibiotics following the course (31).

Current recommendations indicate that the parenteral antibiotic used in prophylaxis should be given in sufficient dosage within 30 minutes of incision (4, 5). This can be facilitated by having the anesthesiologist give the antibiotic when the intravenous lines are started within the operating room shortly before operative incision. This timing replaces the old approach of giving the antibiotic 'on-call' to the operating room, a technique that frequently resulted in delays of 3–4 hours and low or absent serum and tissue levels of antibiotic at the start of operation. Starting the antibiotic agent within 30 minutes of incision results in therapeutic drug levels in the wound and related tissues during the operation. Evidence from clinical trials is accumulating that this single preoperative dose of antibiotic results in the same efficacy as multiple doses of prophylactic antibiotics given during the perioperative course (32). Those that advocate single-dose prophylaxis generally recommend that another dose be given in operations lasting over 3 hours. It appears at this time that no benefit can be achieved from longer courses of antibiotic prophylaxis (over 24 hours) which may allow for the development of bacterial resistance.

When prophylaxis is accomplished with orally administered antibiotics, as is frequently practiced in elective colon resection, the agents should be given during the 24 hours before operation. Longer periods of preoperative preparation are not necessary and have been associated with the isolation of resistant organisms within the colonic lumen at the time of resection (5).

Route of administration of prophylactic antibiotics

Intravenous administration of the selected prophylactic antibiotic is preferred in most patients undergoing abdominal surgery. When this is accomplished with a relatively small volume of diluent over a short period of time, one can expect high serum and tissue levels of the antibiotic. Administration of equivalent doses of antibiotics either by continuous intravenous infusion or intermittent intramuscular injection produces lower blood levels and retarded entry of the antibiotics into wound fluid (33). Oral administration of antibiotics plays a major role only in the elective preparation of patients before elective colon operations (4, 5).

PROPHYLAXIS IN GASTROINTESTINAL TRACT SURGERY

Operations on the gastrointestinal tract most frequently involve an incision through the luminal mucosa, which harbors a luxuriant endogenous bacterial flora. As a result, such procedures are associated with a high risk of postoperative infection which varies depending on the type and numbers of bacteria located at each specific level (Table 2) (34).

The geographical arrangements of micro-organisms within the gastrointestinal tract account in part for the differences in septic complications that follow surgery on the upper and lower intestine. Sepsis that occurs after upper intestinal operation is generally less severe, with less morbidity and mortality than in sepsis that occurs following colonic surgery.

Gastroduodenal surgery

Prior to 1975, the most common indication for gastroduodenal surgery was for the treatment of chronic non-obstructing duodenal ulcer (14). Patients undergoing gastric resection for this indication rarely developed postoperative infection, which led to the generally accepted belief that the stomach contents were often sterile and that antibiotic prophylaxis was not indicated.

With the advent of modern medical treatment for chronic duodenal ulcer, the surgeon was called on less frequently to operate for this indication. Gastroduodenal operations are now frequently performed for the complications of duodenal ulcer, for gastric ulcer or malignancy. The common occurrence of postoperative infection in these cases has resulted in a reappraisal of the role of antibiotic prophylaxis in gastroduodenal surgery.

Risk of infection Published studies (14, 35) have defined two risk groups for the development of postoperative infections among patients undergoing gastric surgery. Low-risk patients (< 5% postoperative infection) are those who undergo operation for chronic non-obstructing duodenal ulcer in the face of normal gastric acid and motility. These patients have been found to have very low to absent micro-organisms in the gastric lumen at the time of resection (14). Another category of low risk includes patients operated on for perforative duodenal ulcer disease (36). The peritonitis encountered at operation in these cases is largely chemical, and a bacterial origin is noted only if a long delay occurs before surgical intervention.

High-risk patients (>10% postoperative infection) are those who undergo operation for indications of bleeding or obstructing duodenal ulcer or gastric ulcer or malignancy (14). Gastric colonizations with organisms that enter the stomach from saliva or reflux through the pylorus, are routinely isolated in these cases.

Prophylactic antibiotic recommendations Antibiotic prophylaxis is indicated in every high-risk patient (4, 5). Prospective randomized trials have shown the benefit of prophylaxis with a parenteral first- or second-generation cephalosporins in these patients (37, 38). The optimal regimen would utilize a 1 gram dose of either cefazolin or cefamandole given intravenously within 30 minutes of incision. No comparative studies of these two agents have been reported. The administration of 2–3 additional doses during the 24 hours after the start of operation would appear to be unnecessary unless the operative procedure is very complex and of long duration (>3 hours).

Although not generally recommended, one study has shown that the use of intermittent local intraoperative antibiotic irrigation of the operative site with antibiotics has also resulted in a postoperative low infection rate in patients not given parenteral antibiotic prophylaxis (39).

Elective colon resections

The human colon and distal small intestine contain an enormous reservoir of aerobic and anaerobic bacteria which are excluded from the body by the mucous membrane (40). When this membrane barrier is disturbed by disease or trauma, or if the colon is opened to the peritoneal cavity during surgery, bacteria may escape into adjacent tissues causing serious infection. For this reason, a reliable method of sterilizing colonic contents has been an objective of surgeons throughout this century. In the last 10 years results of clinical trials have shown clearly that in order to significantly reduce septic complications after elective colon surgery it is necessary to employ antibiotics which have activity against both colonic aerobes (*Escherichia coli*) as well as the anaerobes (*Bacteroides fragilis*) (41, 42). Controversy exists, however, concerning the optimal antibiotic regimen and route of administration (43). Future studies designed to test new techniques of preoperative antibiotic colon preparation should clearly not be compared with no-treatment controls (mechanical preparation alone), as every patient is at high risk for postoperative infection (44).

Prior to the 1970s the majority of surgeons utilized primarily mechanical cleansing before elective colon surgery (40). The oral antibiotics (neomycin, kanamycin, streptomycin and sulfonamides) that had been utilized up to that time most often only suppressed the aerobic colonic flora and were associated with high percentages of clinical failures (12). In addition, the use of these oral antibiotics for 3–5-day periods before elective colon resection was frequently associated with the overgrowth of staphylococci and yeasts within the patient's gastrointestinal tract. This finding rarely occurs when patients are given a short 1-day oral antibiotic preoperative preparation (45). Other investigators (46, 47) felt that the suppression of the normal colonic flora with intestinal antiseptics in patients undergoing colonic resection for carcinoma could favor the growth of tumor cells within the colonic lumen and in fact lead to a higher incidence of tumor implantation in the suture line. Most of these fears were subsequently dismissed when short-term efficacious oral antibiotic preoperative preparation schemes were introduced.

Mechanical preparation

Mechanical cleansing of the colonic lumen prior to elective colonic resection is a time-tested procedure which, when done appropriately, reduces the total fecal mass, thus allowing for easier operative manipulation of the colon as well as facilitating the action of oral antibiotics. The effect of vigorous mechanical cleansing alone utilizing either lavage techniques or the classic approach with dietary restrictions, enemas and cathartics have, however, not resulted in a significant reduction of micro-organisms recovered from residual colonic material (48–50). This microbiologic failure of mechanical cleansing alone also translates to clinical failure. More than 40% of patients undergoing elective colon resection developed septic complications following mechanical cleansing alone in two large prospective randomized, double-blind clinical trials investigating the efficacy of oral antibiotic prophylaxis (51, 52).

Today, approaches to mechanical cleansing vary considerably. The time-honored 5-day preoperative preparation utilizing dietary restriction, enemas and cath-

Table 3   *A suggested approach to preoperative preparation before elective colon resection*

Second day prior to surgery (AT HOME)
1. Dietary restriction — low residue or liquid diet
2. Magnesium sulfate 30 ml of a 50% solution (15 g) P.O. at 10:00 a.m., 2:00 p.m. and 6:00 p.m.
3. Fleet enemas until clear in the evening

Day of hospitalization (preoperative day) ADMIT IN THE MORNING
1. Clear liquid diet, i.v. fluids as needed
2. Magnesium sulfate in dosage as above at 10:00 a.m. and 2:00 p.m. *or*
2A. Whole gut lavage with Golytely 1 liter per hour for 2–4 hours until diarrhea effluent clear — before administration of oral antibiotic
3. No enemas
4. Neomycin and erythromycin base — 1 g each p.o. at 1:00 p.m., 2:00 p.m. and 11:00 p.m.

Day of surgery
1. Operation at 8:00 a.m.
2. *Optional* — one dose of antibiotic with aerobic-anaerobic activity given i.v. by anesthesia in the operating room just prior to incision

---

artics has long been abandoned for many good reasons. At the top of this list were the iatrogenically induced severe metabolic abnormalities which were reported on over 20 years ago (53). Modern approaches include standard mechanical cleansing which utilizes dietary restriction, cathartics and enemas for a 2-day period or whole-gut lavage with either an electrolyte solution, 10% mannitol or polyethylene glycol done on the day before operation (49, 54–56). A suggested schema for mechanical preparation is offered in Table 3.

Antibiotic preparation

The vast majority of surgeons today employ antibiotics as well as mechanical cleansing for preoperative preparation before elective colon resection. The antibiotics chosen should be effective in suppressing both the colonic aerobes and anaerobes (57). There continues to be interest concerning which agents are ideal and which route of administration is preferred (45). Those investigators who advocate oral antibiotic usage generally stress the importance of the reduction of microorganisms within the colonic lumen prior to opening the colon, while those who rely on parenteral agents stress the importance of adequate tissue levels of antibiotics.

Oral antibiotic agents   The 3 major requirements for an effective intestinal antiseptic were outlined by Cohn nearly 30 years ago (58). They include a rapid, highly bactericidal activity against gastrointestinal pathogenic organisms, low local and systemic toxicity, and limited absorption from the intestine. Many oral agents have been employed since Garlock and Seley reported on the use of sulfanilamide on surgery of the colon and rectum in 1939 (6). Most of these agents are no longer employed, due to either toxicity or inadequate suppression of the colonic microflora associated with clinical failure (40, 51, 52).

At present, 3 regimens of oral agents are utilized, including a combination of aminogycoside with either erythromycin base, metronidazole or tetracycline. The greatest experience in the United States has been with the neomycin-erythromycin base preparation which was introduced in 1972 (12) while the choice of kanamycin or neomycin and metronidazole is popular in Great Britain (59, 60). Authoritative reviews of antibiotic prophylaxis in colon surgery continue to support the value of the oral neomycin-erythromycin base in preventing infection following elective colon resection (4, 5). There appear to be no convincing data to recommend the use of metronidazole over erythromycin base in this clinical setting (5). The pharmacokinetics of the oral neomycin-erythromycin base bowel preparation have been studied in healthy volunteers (61) and in patients undergoing elective colon resection (62). The finding of these studies suggest that when adequate mechanical preparation is also used, significant intraluminal (local) and serum (systemic) levels of the oral agents are present and that both mechanisms may play a role in the prevention of infection after colon surgery. The timing of administration of these oral agents appears to be critical. It is recommended that 1 gram of each agent, neomycin and erythromycin base, be given at 1:00 p.m., 2:00 p.m. and 11:00 p.m. on the day prior to surgery (6 g total) (Table 3). Surgery should be scheduled to be at about 8:00 a.m. when utilizing this time sequence. If the time of operation is scheduled for later in the day, the time sequence of administration of the oral agents should be appropriately changed to preserve the 19 hours' preparation time. The use of more doses of oral antibiotic prophylaxis is unwarranted and can be associated with the emergence of resistant flora (5).

Parenteral antibiotic agents   The first prospective randomized, double-blind study published in 1969 on parenteral antibiotic prophylaxis in elective colon resection utilized perioperative intramuscularly administered cefaloridine (63). This study revealed a significant reduction in postoperative infections (30–7%) in the group of patients receiving antibiotics in addition to mechanical preparations when compared with mechanical preparation alone. Other clinical studies utilizing the same or similar first-generation cephalosporins for prophylaxis failed, however, to show the efficacy of this approach when compared with placebo (mechanical preparation alone) (64) or with oral neomycin and erythromycin base (65, 66). Clinical studies comparing parenteral cephalosporin alone in this setting showed lack of efficacy unless the antibiotic agent possessed aerobic and anaerobic activity (67, 68). Parenteral agents in this setting that have shown efficacy alone or in combination with an aminoglycoside include cefoxitin (67, 69–71), metronidazole (67, 71–73) or doxycycline (74, 75). One recent study reported by the Norwegian Study Group for Colorectal Surgery has advocated mechanical cleansing and a single preoperative parenteral dose of doxycycline (aerobic coverage) and tinidazole (anaerobic coverage) (76). Most investigators recommend the perioperative use of 1–5 doses of parenteral agents during the 24-hour period shortly before and after operation. Longer periods of usage of the parenteral agents have been associated with the development of antibiotic-resistant strains within the colonic lumen (77).

Combination of parenteral and oral antibiotic agents   Many surgeons presently utilize both oral and parenteral antibiotic agents in addition to mechanical cleansing as preoperative preparation before elective colon resection in the hope of further reducing the postoperative infection rate (78). In a survey of over 500 surgeons reported in 1979, only 8% utilized systemic antibiotics alone, 37% utilized oral antibiotics alone and 49% utilized oral plus systemic antibiotics prior to colon surgery (65). Despite the appeal of this dual approach providing both intraluminal bacterial suppression and high serum and tissue levels of antibiotics, the evidence remains debatable.

Condon et al (79) reported the results of a 5-year cooperative Veterans Administration Study of over 1 000 patients undergoing elective colon surgery, comparing oral neomycin-erythromycin base alone with parenteral perioperative cefalotin in addition to the oral agents. In this study the infection rate was not significantly different and was below 9% in both groups, which prompted the authors to conclude: 'There seems to be no discernible benefit from adding parenteral antibiotic prophylaxis when performing elective colon surgery if appropriate mechanical cleansing and oral neomycin and erythromycin therapy are employed.' Similar single hospital studies showed that the addition of systemic cefazolin to the oral neomycin-erythromycin base oral preparation did significantly reduce postoperative infections (80, 81), while others showed no additional significant benefit when adding older systemic antibiotics (82, 83).

Studies utilizing newer systemic agents with both aerobic and anaerobic coverage such as cefoxitin, cefonicid or ceftizoxime in addition to oral neomycin and erythromycin base have shown a low incidence of infections (84–86). It appears at this time, with somewhat conflicting evidence, that the addition of 1 dose of parenteral antibiotic with aerobic and anaerobic activity given intravenously within 30 minutes of incision added to mechanical and oral antibiotic bowel preparation may be beneficial.

Topical antibiotics   Although not recommended by this author, some surgeons have advocated the use of wound placement or irrigation with antibiotics in elec-

Table 4   *Parenteral antibiotic agents used for coverage of the aerobic and anaerobic components of the human colonic microflora*

Aerobic coverage — To be combined with a drug having anaerobic activity
Amikacin
Aztreonam
Ceftriaxone
Cefoperazone
Gentamicin
Netilmicin
Tobramycin

Anaerobic coverage — To be combined with a drug having aerobic activity
Carbenicillin
Chloramphenicol
Clindamycin
Metronidazole
Mezlocillin
Ticarcillin

Aerobic + anaerobic coverage — single agents
Ampicillin-sulbactam
Cefotaxime
Cefotetan
Cefoxitin
Ceftizoxime
Imipenem-cilastatin
Moxalactam
Piperacillin
Ticarcillin-clavulanic acid

---

tive colon surgery (87, 88). Anderson et al observed a significant reduction of wound sepsis in a group of patients in which 1 gram of ampicillin powder was applied to the subfascial and subcutaneous spaces before the fascial sutures were tied, compared to a similar group not receiving the local antibiotic placement. Others (89) have not identified the value of the local instillation of ampicillin to the wound in colon surgery.

Emergent colon surgery

Clinical conditions which most frequently dictate the necessity of emergent colonic surgery include acute bleeding, perforated diverticulum or carcinoma, ischemic intestinal disease, obstructed lesions, or penetrating or blunt abdominal trauma involving the colon. In this setting the operation is carried out on unprepared colon because the use of oral antibiotics and/or mechanical cleansing is not indicated and may in fact be harmful.

The mainstay for the prevention of infectious complications after emergent colon surgery are proper operative technique, sound judgment and the use of appropriately chosen and administered parenteral antibiotics (1). As in elective surgery, the antibiotics chosen should be active against both the aerobic and anaerobic populations of the colonic microflora (90–92). They should be started intravenously in appropriate doses shortly before operation and continued for 2–7 days postoperatively depending on the clinical findings and course. Many single agents and combinations appear to be equally efficacious and are presently advocated (3) (Table 4). The choice, therefore, depends on local hospital prices and the toxicity profile of the chosen agent or agents.

Small intestinal surgery

Because small intestinal contents are liquid and transit time is rapid, extensive preoperative mechanical preparation is unnecessary in elective surgery. There are no antibiotic prophylaxis studies available on surgery of the ileum, the site of most apparent risk for infection because of the complex intestinal flora present at this level (93). It seems prudent, however, to use the neomycin-erythromycin oral bowel preparation for such elective procedures. The use of parenteral agents effective against fecal aerobes and anaerobes would be advised in emergent procedures (Table 4).

Appendectomy

The pathologic state of the appendix is the most important determinant of postoperative infection. Appendectomy for perforative or gangrenous appendicitis has a 4–5 times higher rate of wound infection than it does for periappendicitis or a normal appendix. However, any incision of the appendix, even in the mildly inflamed state, exposes the patient to some risk due to contamination by the associated colonic microflora.

491

Since it is usually impossible to determine the pathologic state of the appendix prior to surgery, it is recommended that a dose of parenteral agents be given within 30 minutes of incision in every case (94, 95) (Table 4). If the appendix is only mildly inflamed, the single preoperative dose is sufficient. In the presence of perforative or gangrenous appendicitis, a 48–72-hour treatment regimen should be used.

Elective cholecystectomy

Cholecystectomy for chronic calculous cholecystitis is the only clinical setting where antibiotic prophylaxis is employed in biliary tract surgery. Operations for acute cholecystitis, empyema of the gallbladder, ascending cholangitis, or liver abscess require antibiotic treatment rather than prophylaxis.

The healthy human biliary tract rarely harbors significant concentrations of bacteria. In the presence of chronic calculous cholecystitis, bacteria have been isolated in bile in 15–30% of cases (96). The bacteria isolated are predominantly gram-negative bacilli. *Escherichia coli*, alone or mixed with another organism, is present in 50% of positive cultures. Other coliforms, e.g., *Klebsiella, Enterobacter* and *Proteus*, are less commonly isolated. Anaerobic micro-organisms are isolated in fewer than 20% of the cases, with *Clostridium perfringens* and *Bacteroides fragilis* the most common (97). A polymicrobial infection including both aerobes and anaerobes may be encountered in liver abscess or long-standing common duct obstruction due to choledocholithiasis.

Risk of infection Positive bile cultures collected at the time of cholecystectomy are associated with a higher risk of postoperative infection (33%) (98). Several studies have defined those clinical factors that favor bactibilia and therefore a corresponding increased risk of postoperative sepsis (99, 100). They are as follows: (a) age over 70; (b) past history or presence of jaundice; (c) previous biliary tract surgery; (d) chills or fever within 1 week of operation; (e) common duct pathology; (f) operations done within 1 month of an acute attack of cholecystitis; (g) diabetes mellitus.

Prophylactic recommendations Placebo-controlled studies have shown decreased postoperative infection rates when antibiotic prophylaxis is used for cholecystectomy in high-risk patients (one or more clinical risk factors) (101–104). Most studies have employed either a cephalosporin or gentamicin (101–104). No comparative studies of these regimens are available. Studies comparing first-generation with second-generation cephalosporins have shown no difference in effectiveness (4, 5). A recent report has recommended just one perioperative dose of parenteral cefazolin, administered during the 30 minutes prior to incision (104).

The primary controversy is whether only those patients with a clinical risk factor or positive intraoperative Gram stain should be given antibiotic prophylaxis perioperatively before elective cholecystectomy. One recent report recommends a single dose of cephalosporin in all patients undergoing cholecystectomy, regardless of clinical risk factors or Gram-stain results (105). This study revealed a high wound infection rate (18%) following assignment of antibiotics during surgery when positive Gram stains of bile were identified in patients without clinical risk factors.

Prostatectomy

When possible, proven urinary tract infections should be effectively treated before elective operations. This is frequently impossible in patients scheduled for prostatectomy due to the obstructive nature of benign prostatic hypertrophy. The authoritative committees (4, 5) therefore recommend the use of antimicrobial agents in all patients undergoing prostatectomy in the face of contaminated urine. The agent chosen should be based on the sensitivity of the offending micro-organism.

The use of prophylactic antimicrobial therapy in prostatectomy in patients with sterile preoperative urine cultures remains controversial at this time. It has been proposed that the prostatic tissue, when cut, is primarily responsible for postoperative bacteriuria in this clinical setting. Morris et al (106) identified positive prostatic chips in 64% of the patients who had sterile urine preoperatively. Despite these findings, other studies (107, 108) have not identified any benefit from antibiotic prophylaxis in this clinical setting. Most recently, Nielsen et al (109) have reported a significant reduction in bacteriuria at both 3 and 7 days postoperatively in patients treated with antibiotic prophylaxis. Further carefully designed studies utilizing appropriate antimicrobial agents and adequate bacteriology appear to be necessary to resolve this disagreement.

Hysterectomy

Studies concerning the use of prophylactic antibiotics in the obstetric patient have primarily concerned the patients with premature rupture of membrane and in cesarean section. This literature reveals a great disparity in reported findings, and further studies appear indicated before definite recommendations can be made (110).

A voluminous literature also has been reported concerning the efficacy of antibiotic prophylaxis in hysterectomy. Recently, Shapiro et al (20) have reported their finding of the risk factors for postoperative infection at the operative site after elective hysterectomy. In this study, short-term prophylaxis with a first-generation cephalosporin was found to be of significant benefit in both abdominal and vaginal hysterectomy. An increasing duration of operation was associated with a decreasing effect of antibiotic prophylaxis, the preventive fraction of which diminished from 80% at 1 hour to an unmeasurable effect at 3.3 hours. Based on these findings antibiotic prophylaxis appears to be indicated in both abdominal and vaginal hysterectomy. In operations requiring more than 2–3 hours of time, the antibiotic agent used should be repeated intraoperatively.

FUTURE DIRECTIONS

Much progress has been made in the last 10 years concerning the appropriate use of antibiotic prophylaxis in abdominal surgery. Today, the value of this technique when indicated and appropriately administered is without question and it appears, at least in the foreseeable future, to continue to be an integral part of the care of the surgical patient. Additions to our knowledge concerning antibiotic prophylaxis will come from carefully designed studies which primarily address the selection of resistant pathogens and the optimal choice of agents in each clinical setting.

REFERENCES

1. Nichols RL (1982) Postoperative wound infection. *N. Engl. J. Med., 307,* 1 701.
2. Nichols RL (1982) Techniques known to prevent postoperative wound infection. *Infect. Control, 3,* 34.
3. Nichols RL (1984) Prophylaxis for intraabdominal surgery. *Rev. Infect. Dis., 6,* S276.
4. Anonymous (1985) Antimicrobial prophylaxis for surgery. *Med. Lett. Drugs Ther., 27,* 105.
5. Kaiser AB (1986) Antimicrobial prophylaxis in surgery. *N. Engl. J. Med., 315,* 1 129.
6. Garlock JH, Seley GP (1939) The use of sulfanilamide in surgery of the colon and rectum: preliminary report. *Surgery, 5,* 787.
7. Bernard HR, Cole WR (1964) The prophylaxis of surgical infection: the effect of prophylactic antimicrobial drugs on the incidence of infection following potentially contaminated operations. *Surgery, 56,* 151.
8. Karl RC, Mertz JJ, Veith FJ, Dineen P (1966) Prophylactic antimicrobial drugs in surgery. *N. Engl. J. Med., 275,* 305.
9. Burke JF (1961) The effective period of preventive antibiotic action in experimental incision and dermal lesions. *Surgery, 50,* 161.
10. Alexander JW, Altemeier WA (1965) Penicillin prophylaxis of experimental staphylococcal wound infections. *Surg. Gynecol. Obstet., 120,* 243.
11. Dineen PA (1961) A period of unusual microbial susceptibility in an experimental staphylococcal infection. *J. Infect. Dis., 108,* 174.
12. Nichols RL, Condon RE, Gorbach SL, Nyhus LM (1972) Efficacy of preoperative antimicrobial preparation of the bowel. *Ann. Surg., 176,* 227.
13. Nichols RL (1981) Surgical bacteriology: an overview. In: Nyhus LM (Ed), *Surgery Annual, Vol 13,* p 205. Appleton-Century-Crofts, New York.
14. Nichols RL, Smith JW (1975) Intragastric microbial colonization in common disease states of the stomach and duodenum. *Ann. Surg., 182,* 557.
15. Gorbach SL, Nahas L, Plaut AG, Weinstein L, Patterson JF, Levitan R (1968) Studies of intestinal microflora. V. Fecal microbial ecology in ulcerative colitis and regional enteritis: relationship to severity of disease and chemotherapy. *Gastroenterology, 54,* 575.
16. Northey D, Adess ML, Hartsuck JM, Rhoades ER (1974) Microbial surveillance in a surgical intensive care unit. *Surg. Gynecol. Obstet., 139,* 321.
17. Cruse PJE, Foord R (1980) The epidemiology of wound infection: a 10-year prospecti-

ve study of 62,939 wounds. *Surg. Clin. North Am., 60*, 27.

18. Valentine RJ, Weigelt JA, Dryer D, Rodgers C (1986) Effect of remote infections on clean wound infection rates. *Am. J. Infect. Control, 14*, 64.

19. Balthazar ER, Colt JD, Nichols RL (1982) Preoperative hair removal: a random, prospective study of shaving versus clipping. *South. Med. J., 75*, 799.

20. Shapiro M, Munoz A, Tager IB, Schoenbaum SC, Polk BF (1982) Risk factors for infection at the operative site after abdominal or vaginal hysterectomy. *N. Engl. J. Med., 307*, 1 661.

21. Nora PF, Vanecko RM, Bransfield JJ (1972) Prophylactic abdominal drains. *Arch. Surg., 105*, 173.

22. Cerise EJ, Pierce WA, Diamond DL (1970) Abdominal drains: their role as a source of infection following splenectomy. *Ann. Surg., 171*, 764.

23. Magee C, Rodeheaver GT, Golden GT, Fox J, Edgerton MT, Edlich RF (1976) Potentiation of wound infection by surgical drains. *Am. J. Surg., 131*, 547.

24. Chodak GW, Plaut ME (1977) Use of systemic antibiotics for prophylaxis in surgery: a critical review. *Arch. Surg., 112*, 326.

25. Guglielmo BJ, Hohn DC, Koo PJ, Hunt TK, Sweet RL, Conte Jr JE (1983) Antibiotic prophylaxis in surgical procedures: a critical analysis of the literature. *Arch. Surg., 118*, 943.

26. Haley RW, Culver DH, Morgan WM, White JW, Emori TG, Hooton TM (1985) Identifying patients at high risk of surgical wound infection. *Am. J. Epidemiol., 121*, 206.

27. Westerman EL (1984) Antibiotic prophylaxis in surgery: historical background, rationale, and relationship to prospective payment. *Am. J. Infect. Control, 12*, 339.

28. Nichols RL (1984) Postoperative infections and antimicrobial prophylaxis. In: Mandell GL, Douglass Jr RG, Bennett JE (Eds), *Principles and Practice of Infectious Diseases, 2nd ed*, p 1 637. John Wiley and Sons, New York.

29. DiPiro JT, Bowden Jr TA, Hooks III VH (1984) Prophylactic parenteral cephalosporins in surgery: Are the newer agents better? *J. Am. Med. Assoc., 252*, 3 277.

30. Shapiro M, Townsend TR, Rosner B, Kass EH (1979) Use of antimicrobial drugs in general hospitals: patterns of prophylaxis. *N. Engl. J. Med., 301*, 351.

31. Crossley K B (1984) Antibiotic prophylaxis in surgery: improvement after a multihospital educational program. *South. Med. J., 77*, 864.

32. DiPiro JT, Cheung RPF, Bowden Jr TA, Mansberger JA (1986) Single dose systemic antibiotic prophylaxis of surgical wound infections. *Am. J. Surg., 152*, 552.

33. Alexander JW, Alexander NS (1976) The influence of route of administration on wound fluid concentration of prophylactic antibiotics. *J. Trauma, 16*, 488.

34. Nichols RL (1981) Use of prophylactic antibiotics in surgical practice. *Am. J. Med., 70*, 686.

35. Lewis RT (1977) Wound infection after gastroduodenal operations: a 10-year review. *Can. J. Surg., 20*, 435.

36. LoCicero J, Nichols RL (1980) Sepsis after gastroduodenal operations: relationship to gastric acid, motility, and endogenous microflora. *South. Med. J., 73*, 878.

37. Lewis RT, Allan CM, Goodall RG (1979) Discriminate use of antibiotic prophylaxis in gastroduodenal surgery. *Am. J. Surg., 183*, 640.

38. Nichols RL, Webb WR, Jones JW, Smith JW, LoCicero III J (1982) Efficacy of antibiotic prophylaxis in high risk gastroduodenal operations. *Am. J. Surg., 143*, 94.

39. Lord Jr JW, LaRaja RD, Daliana M, Gordon MT (1983) Prophylactic antibiotic

   wound irrigation in gastric, biliary, and colonic surgery. *Am. J. Surg., 145*, 209.
40. Nichols RL, Condon RE (1971) Preoperative preparation of the colon. *Surg. Gynecol. Obstet., 132*, 323.
41. Hirschmann JV, Inui TS (1980) Antimicrobial prophylaxis: a critique of recent trials. *Rev. Infect. Dis., 2*, 1.
42. Platt R (1984) Antibiotic prophylaxis in surgery. *Rev. Infect. Dis., 6*, s880.
43. Bartlett SP, Burton RC (1983) Effects of prophylactic antibiotics on wound infection after elective colon and rectal surgery: 1960 to 1980. *Am. J. Surg., 145*, 300.
44. Baum ML, Anish DS, Chalmers TC (1981) A survey of clinical trials of antibiotic prophylaxis in colon surgery: evidence against further use of no-treatment controls. *N. Engl. J. Med., 305*, 795.
45. Bartlett JG, Condon RE, Gorbach SL, Clarke JS, Nichols RL, Oche S (1978) Veterans Administration cooperative study on bowel preparation for elective colorectal operations: impact of oral antibiotic regimen on colonic flora, wound irrigation cultures and bacteriology of septic complications. *Ann. Surg., 188*, 249.
46. Vink M (1954) Local recurrence of cancer in the large bowel. *Br. J. Surg., 41*, 431.
47. Buinaukas P, McDonald GO, Cole WH (1958) Role of operating stress on the resistance of the experimental animal to inoculated cancer cells. *Ann. Surg., 148*, 642.
48. Beck DE, Harford FJ, DiPalma JA, Brady III CE (1985) Bowel cleansing with polyethylene glycol electrolyte lavage solution. *South. Med. J., 78*, 1414.
49. Nichols RL, Gorbach SL, Condon RE (1971) Alteration of intestinal microflora following preoperative mechanical preparation of the colon. *Dis. Colon Rectum, 14*, 123.
50. Crapp AR, Tillotson P, Powis SJA, Cooke WT, Alexander-Williams J (1975) Preparation of the bowel by whole-gut irrigation. *Lancet, 2*, 1 239.
51. Clarke JS, Condon RE, Bartlett JG, Gorbach SL, Nichols RL, Ochi S (1977) Preoperative oral antibiotics reduce septic complications of colon operations: results of prospective, randomized, double-blind clinical study. *Ann. Surg., 186*, 251.
52. Washington II JA, Dearing WH, Judd ES, Elveback LR (1974) Effect of preoperative antibiotic regimen on development of infection after intestinal surgery: prospective, randomized, double-blind study. *Ann. Surg., 180*, 567.
53. Trinkle JK, Fisher LJ, Ketcham AS, Berlin NI (1964) The metabolic effects of preoperative intestinal preparation. *Surg. Gynecol. Obstet., 118*, 739.
54. Beck DE, Harford FJ, DiPalma JA (1985) Comparison of cleansing methods in preparation for colonic surgery. *Dis. Colon Rectum, 28*, 491.
55. Jagelman DG, Fazio VW, Lavery IC, Weakley FL (1985) A prospective, randomized, double-blind study of 10% mannitol mechanical bowel preparation combined with oral neomycin and short-term, perioperative, intravenous Flagyl as prophylaxis in elective colorectal resections. *Surgery, 98*, 861.
56. Keighley MRB (1982) A clinical and physiological evaluation of bowel preparation for elective colorectal surgery. *World J. Surg., 6*, 464.
57. Nichols RL (1984) Update on preparation of the colon for resection. *Curr. Surg., 41*, 75.
58. Cohn Jr I (1958) Antibiotics for colon surgery. *Gastroenterology, 35*, 583.
59. Goldring J, McNaught W, Scott A, Gillespie G (1975) Prophylactic oral antimicrobial agents in elective colonic surgery. *Lancet, 2*, 997.
60. Matheson DM, Arabi Y, Baxter-Smith D, Alexander-Williams J, Keighley MRB (1978) Randomized multicentre trial of oral bowel preparation and antimicrobials for elective colorectal operations. *Br. J. Surg., 65*, 597.

61. Nichols RL, Condon RE, DiSanto AR (1977) Preoperative bowel preparation. *Arch. Surg., 112*, 1493.

62. DiPiro JT, Patrias JM, Townsend RJ, Bowden Jr TA, Hooks III VH, Smith RB, Spiro TE (1985) Oral neomycin sulfate and erythromycin base before colon surgery: a comparison of serum and tissue concentrations. *Pharmacotherapy, 5*, 91.

63. Polk Jr HC, Lopez-Mayor JF (1969) Postoperative wound infections. A prospective study of determinant factors and prevention. *Surgery, 66*, 97.

64. Evans C, Pollack AV (1973) The reduction of surgical wound infection by prophylactic parenteral cephaloridine. *Br. J. Surg., 60*, 434.

65. Condon RE, Bartlett JG, Nichols RL, Schulet WJ, Gorbach SL, Ochi S (1979) Preoperative prophylactic cephalothin fails to control septic complications of colorectal operations: results of controlled clinical trial — A Veterans Administration Cooperative Study. *Am. J. Surg., 137*, 68.

66. Edmondson HT, Rissing JP (1983) Prophylactic antibiotics in colon surgery. *Arch. Surg., 118*, 227.

67. Panichi G, Pantosti A, Giunchi G, Tonelli F, D'Amicis P, Fegiz G, Matrantonio PG, Luzzi I, Grandolfi ME (1982) Cephalothin, cefoxitin, or metronidazole in elective colonic surgery? A single-blind randomized trial. *Dis. Colon Rectum, 25*, 783.

68. Slama TG, Carey LC, Fass RJ (1979) Comparative efficacy of prophylactic cephalothin and cefamandole for elective colon surgery. *Am. J. Surg., 137*, 593.

69. Hoffman CEJ, McDonald PJ, Watts JM (1981) Use of perioperative cefoxitin to prevent infection after colonic and rectal surgery. *Ann. Surg., 193*, 353.

70. Kaiser AB, Herrington Jr JL, Jacobs JK, Mulherin Jr JL, Roach AC, Sawyers JL (1984) Cefoxitin versus erythromycin, neomycin, and cefazolin in colorectal operations: importance of the duration of the surgical procedure. *Ann. Surg., 200*, 525.

71. McDonald PJ, Karran SJ (1983) A comparison of intravenous cefoxitin and a combination of gentamicin and metronidazole as prophylaxis in colorectal surgery. *Dis. Colon Rectum, 26*, 661.

72. Eykyn S, Jackson BT, Lockhart-Mummery HE, Phillips I (1979) Prophylactic preoperative intravenous metronidazole in elective colorectal surgery. *Lancet, 2*, 761.

73. Feathers RS, Lewis AAM, Sagor GR, Amirak ID, Noone P (1977) Prophylactic systemic antibiotics in colorectal surgery. *Lancet, 2*, 4.

74. Nygaard K, Hognestad J (1980) Infection prophylaxis with doxycycline in colorectal surgery: a preliminary report. *Scand. J. Gastroenterol., Suppl, 59*, 37.

75. Ivarsson L, Darte N, Kewenter JG, Seeberg S, Norrby R (1982) Short-term systemic prophylaxis with cefoxitin and doxycycline in colorectal surgery. *Am. J. Surg., 144*, 257.

76. Norwegian Study Group for Colorectal Surgery (1985) Should antimicrobial prophylaxis in colorectal surgery include agents effective against both anaerobic and aerobic microorganisms? A double-blind, multicenter study. *Surgery, 97*, 402.

77. Kager L, Ljungdahl I, Malmborg AS, Nord CE, Pieper R, Dahlgren P (1981) Effect on the colon microflora and septic complications — a clinical model for prediction of the benefit and risks in using a new antibiotic in prophylaxis. *Ann. Surg., 193*, 277.

78. Peck JJ, Fuchs PC, Gustafson ME (1984) Antimicrobial prophylaxis in elective colon surgery: experience of 1,035 operations in a community hospital. *Am. J. Surg., 147*, 633.

79. Condon RE, Bartlett JG, Greenlee H, Schulte WJ, Ochi S, Abbe R, Caruana JA, Gordon HE, Horsley JS, Irvin III G, Johnson W, Jordan Jr P, Keitzer WF, Lempke R,

Read RC, Schumer W, Schwartz M, Storm FK, Vetto RM (1983) Efficacy of oral and systemic antibiotic prophylaxis in colorectal operations. *Arch. Surg., 118*, 496.

80. Stone HH, Hooper CA, Kolb LD, Geheber CE, Dawkins EJ (1976) Antibiotic prophylaxis in gastric, biliary and colonic surgery. *Ann. Surg., 184*, 443.

81. Portnoy J, Kagan E, Gordon PH, Mendelson J (1983) Prophylactic antibiotics in elective colorectal surgery. *Dis. Colon Rectum, 26*, 310.

82. Barber MS, Hirschberg BC, Rice CL, Atkins CC (1979) Parenteral antibiotics in elective colon surgery? A prospective controlled clinical study. *Surgery, 86*, 23.

83. Eisenberg HW (1981) The use of new antibiotics in colorectal surgery. *Am. J. Proctol., Gastroenterol. Colon Rectal Surg., 6*, 9.

84. Coppa GF, Eng K, Gouge TH, Ranson JHC, Localio SA (1983) Parenteral and oral antibiotics in elective colon and rectal surgery. *Am. J. Surg., 145*, 62.

85. Maki DG, Aughey DR (1982) Comparative study of cefazolin, cefoxitin and ceftizoxime for surgical prophylaxis in colo-rectal surgery. *J. Antimicrob. Chemother., 10*, 281.

86. Fabian TC, Mangiante EC, Boldreghini (1984) Prophylactic antibiotics for elective colorectal surgery or operation for obstruction of the small bowel: a comparison of cefonicid and cefoxitin. *Rev. Infect. Dis., 6*, S896.

87. Anderson B, Korner B, Ostergaard AH (1972) Topical ampicillin against wound infection after colorectal surgery. *Ann. Surg., 176*, 129.

88. Nash AG, Hugh TB (1970) Topical ampicillin and wound infection in colon surgery. *Br. Med. J., 1*, 471.

89. Juul P, Merrild U, Kronborg O (1985) Topical ampicillin in addition to a systemic antibiotic prophylaxis in elective colorectal surgery: a prospective randomized study. *Dis. Colon Rectum, 28*, 804.

90. Nichols RL, Smith JW, Klein DB, Trunkey DD, Cooper RH, Adinolfi MF, Mills J (1984) Risk of infection after penetrating abdominal trauma. *N. Engl. J. Med., 311*, 1 065.

91. Gentry LO, Feliciano DV, Lea AS, Short HD, Mattox KL, Jordan Jr GL (1984) Perioperative antibiotic therapy for penetrating injuries of the abdomen. *Ann. Surg., 200*, 561.

92. Jones RC, Thal ER, Johnson NA, Gollihar LN (1985) Evaluation of antibiotic therapy following penetrating abdominal trauma. *Ann. Surg., 201*, 576.

93. Nichols RL, Condon RE, Bentley DW, Gorbach SL (1971) Ileal microflora in surgical patients. *J. Urol., 105*, 351.

94. Busuttil RW, Davidson RK, Fine M, Thompkins K (1981) Effective prophylactic antibiotics in acute non-perforated appendicitis. *Ann. Surg., 194*, 502.

95. Campbell WB (1980) Prophylaxis of infection after appendectomy: a survey of current surgical practice. *Br. Med. J., 182*, 1 597.

96. Nichols RL (1977) Use of antibiotics in stomach, duodenal and biliary tract surgery. *J. Surg. Pract., 6*, 20.

97. England DM, Rosenblatt JE (1977) Anaerobes in human biliary tracts. *J. Clin. Microbiol., 6*, 494.

98. Delikaris PG, Michail PO, Klonis GD, Haritopoulos NC, Golematis BC, Dreiling DA (1977) Biliary bacteriology based on intraoperative bile cultures. *Am. J. Gastroenterol., 68*, 51.

99. Chetlin SH, Elliot D (1973) Preoperative antibiotics in biliary surgery. *Arch. Surg., 107*, 319.

100. Keighley MRB, Flinn R, Alexander-Williams J (1976) Multivariate analysis of clinical

and operative findings associated with biliary sepsis. *Br. J. Surg., 63*, 528.

101. Keighley MRB (1977) Prevention of wound sepsis in gastrointestinal surgery. *Br. J. Surg., 64*, 315.
102. Keighley MRB, Baddeley RM, Burdon DW, Edwards JAC, Quoraish AH, Oates GD, Watts GT, Alexander-Williams J (1975) A controlled trial of parenteral prophylactic gentamicin therapy in biliary surgery. *Br. J. Surg., 62*, 275.
103. Kaufman Z, Engelberg M, Eliashiv A, Reiss R (1984) Systemic prophylactic antibiotics in elective biliary surgery. *Arch. Surg., 119*, 1 002.
104. Lewis RT, Allan CM, Goodall RG, Marien B, Park M, Lloyd-Smith W, Wiegand FM (1984) A single preoperative dose of cefazolin prevents postoperative sepsis in high-risk biliary surgery. *Can. J. Surg., 27*, 44.
105. Murray WR, Bradley JA (1983) Antibiotic prophylaxis in elective biliary surgery. *Res. Clin. Forums, 5*, 97.
106. Morris MJ, Golovsky D, Guiness MDG, Maher PO (1976) The value of prophylactic antibiotics in transurethral prostatic resection: a controlled trial, with observations on the origin of postoperative infection. *Br. J. Urol., 48*, 479.
107. Plorde JJ, Kennedy RP, Bourne HH, Ansell JS, Petersdorf RG (1965) Course and prognosis of prostatectomy: with a note on the incidence of bacteremia and effectiveness of chemoprophylaxis. *N. Engl. J. Med., 272*, 269.
108. Gibbons RP, Stark RA, Correa Jr RJ, Cummings KB, Mason JT (1978) The prophylactic use — or misuse — of antibiotics in transurethral prostatectomy. *J. Urol., 119*, 381.
109. Nielsen OS, Maigaard S, Frimodt-Moller N, Madsen PO (1981) Prophylactic antibiotics in transurethral prostatectomy. *J. Urol., 119*, 381.
110. Sweet RL (1981) Perinatal infections: bacteriology, diagnosis and management. In: Iffy L, Kaminetzky HA (Eds), *Principles and Practice of Obstetrics and Perinatology*, p 1 035. John Wiley and Sons, New York.

CHAPTER 41

Therapy of *Pseudomonas aeruginosa* infections

E. RUBINSTEIN and B. LEV

Medical technology and modern therapy have created patient populations particularly susceptible to *Pseudomonas aeruginosa* infections.

In 1882 Gessard isolated *P. aeruginosa* from patients whose wounds showed 'blue pus' (1). The pathogenicity of this micro-organism was soon recognized by Hitschman and Fraenkel (2).

As a human pathogen, *P. aeruginosa* has been exceptional in its ability to infect various patient populations, in particular to cause nosocomial infections in debilitated patients, to infect patients with burns, cystic fibrosis, traumatic wounds and foreign bodies, and to cause blood-borne infections and endocarditis in intravenous drug abusers. Recently, various eye and skin infections caused by *P. aeruginosa* have been described in swimming pool and whirlpool users (3, 4).

The factors associated with its potential harm include the ability of *P. aeruginosa* to multiply in soil and water and, in the hospital setting, in reservoirs such as sinks, taps, flower vases, nebulizers, humidifiers, 'sterile' dialysis fluids and ophthalmic solutions, contact lens solutions, parenteral nutritional fluids and even certain disinfectants (5, 6). Its unique growth requirements (e.g. ability to grow over a wide temperature range and to use atmospheric CO_2 as its sole carbon source) allow it to grow under various conditions.

Approximately 3–6% of healthy individuals carry *P. aeruginosa* in the intestines (7). This rate increases in patients during stay in hospital (8). In neutropenic patients with bacteremia, due to *P. aeruginosa* the specific strain could be found concurrently in the gastrointestinal tract of 75% of patients (9).

Factors that correlate with *P. aeruginosa* colonization include antibiotic therapy, underlying diseases and length of hospitalization. The fact that only 8% of non-colonized patients (*vs* 21%) become septic (9) may be significant because prevention of colonization may decrease the incidence of *P. aeruginosa* infections. The unusual microbial virulence factors that *P. aeruginosa* possesses (Table 1), e.g. its ability to produce exotoxin A, elastase, alkaline protease and hemolysin as well

Antimicrobial Agents Annual 3
P.K. Peterson and J. Verhoef, editors
© Elsevier Science Publishers BV, 1988

as other proteases that enhance *P. aeruginosa* invasion and virulence, along with the presence of its pili-surface factors that mediate attachment, thereby facilitating subsequent invasion, and a polysaccharide capsule that protects *P. aeruginosa* from opsonization or phagocytosis or both, underlines its potential as an important pathogenic bacterium (reviewed in Ref. 7).

The role of *P. aeruginosa* infections is manifested by recent prevalence figures from various studies. In a report from the National Nosocomial Infections Study (NNIS) (10) *P. aeruginosa* accounted in 1980 for 8.6% of pathogens isolated from all infected sites and was third in rank to *Staphylococcus aureus* and *Escherichia coli*. In the lower respiratory tract and in surgical wounds it also ranked third (9.5% relative frequency).

The attack rate of *P. aeruginosa* in the year 1977–1978 per 10,000 discharges varied from 4–12 for blood-borne infections, 16–36 for urinary tract infections and 3–25 for lower respiratory tract infections (10). During 1980, data from a major burn institute showed that *P. aeruginosa* was recovered and ranked second among the pathogens (after *S. aureus*) and was 3 times more frequent than the next most frequent isolate (*Enterobacter cloacae*). During the same period *P. aeruginosa* was isolated most frequently (along with *S. aureus*) from biopsy specimens of burns. *P. aeruginosa* was the leading cause of death in patients with burns surviving the initial phase (11). In a cancer institute, *P. aeruginosa* bacteremia was responsible for 21% of the total number of cases with bacteremia and was the most frequent pathogen. It was associated with a case fatality rate of 65.0 and had an attack rate of 0.64 (10).

In 70–90% of patients with cystic fibrosis *P. aeruginosa* can be found in sputum samples and is the most common pathogen.

From the early report of Kerby (12) in 1972, it soon became evident that infections with *P. aeruginosa* were frequently seen in debilitated infants and in children with leukemia and that the infection carried a poor prognosis. Later surveys reported mortality rates ranging from 45 to 85% that were mainly dependent on the patient's underlying disease rather than on antimicrobial therapy (13, 14). The mortality rate is consistently high due to (a) severity of the underlying disease, the inability of antibiotics to cope with the infection, and (c) virulence characteristics of *P. aeruginosa* .

ANTIPSEUDOMONAL COMPOUNDS

β-Lactams

Two decades ago, the most common infections in immunocompromised hosts were caused by *P. aeruginosa*. At that time and under polymyxin therapy as single agent fewer than 20% of patients with *P. aeruginosa* septicemia responded, and the mortality rate approximated 90% (15). In the first study evaluating carbenicillin as single-drug therapy in neutropenic patients, the drug was efficacious in 54

Table 1   *Microbial virulence factors of P. aeruginosa*

Antigen	Characteristics and comments	Immunizing agent	Animal model	Results
Toxin A (84)	Protein, MW = 66,000; exotoxin heat-labile; interferes with protein synthesis by ribosylation of elongation factor 2 (resembling diphtheria toxin) (85–90); associated with virulence (91); produced by more than 85% of clinical isolates (92)	Antitoxin passive transfer	Burned mice	No enhancement of long-term survival when challenged with highly virulent strains (93), when challenged with intermediate virulent strain PA103; no protection under immunosuppressed conditions (94)
		Glutaraldehyde-treated toxoid + aluminium phosphate	Burned rats	No protection but elicited moderate levels of neutralizing antibodies (95)
			Burned mice	15% increase in survival (96)
		Formol-treated toxoid + MDP	Burned mice	Significant decrease in mortality rate following challenge with highly virulent strain; 50-fold increase in mean lethal dose (96)
Elastase	MW = 38,000–40,000; metalloprotease; elastolytic activity (97) causes tissue damage and hemorrhage in various models (98, 110); produced by more than 85% of clinical isolates (99a,b)	Detoxified elastase	Mink	High level protection against fatal hemorrhagic pneumonia (104)
		Elastoid	Murine burn	Enhanced survival in 1 study while no protection in 2 later studies (94, 105)

	Interferes with defense mechanisms by inactivation of complement components and thus decreases leukocyte activity (100) Acts also on α_1-protease inhibitor and IgG protease (101, 102); probably assists tissue invasion (103)	Anti-elastase (passive transfer)	Murine burn model	Ineffective (106)
Alkaline protease	MW-49,000, metalloprotease (107); dermonecrotic (108); addition of the enzyme to a strain with weak proteolytic activity reduces 10^3 mean lethal dose of *P. aeruginosa*			
Hemolysin	Phospholipase C (109), MW = 76,000–78,000; acts on tissues and provides nutrients for invading bacteria (110)			
Lipopolysaccharide (LPS)	LPS contains O-antigen polysaccharide and polysaccharide core linked to lipid A moiety by 2-keto-3-deoxyoctonic acid (KDO) (111); O-antigen responsible for serotype specificity; serotype specificity shared core region among *P. aeruginosa* strains (112)	Passive transfer of human gamma globulin raised against heptavalent LPS vaccine	Intraperitoneal challenge in mice	High-level protection against *P. aeruginosa* challenge administered in mucin (113); O-serotype-specific protection when given prior to or soon after challenge; protection decreases when administered late in infection (ineffective when given 3 hours after challenge) (114)

Table 1   *(continued)*

Antigen	Characteristics and comments	Immunizing agent	Animal model	Results
Lipopolysaccharide (LPS) *(continued)*		LPS 0.001–0.01 μg – > 1	Mice	Serotype-specific protection (115); cross-protection between Fisher immunotype 1 and 2 (suggesting 'shared' LPS determinants) (116)
		LPS 0.02 μg	Burn wound sepsis in rats	Protection against challenge of 10,000 LD_{50} of homologous strain (117)
		Passive transfer of anti-LPS	Burn wound model in mice	High-level protection (94)
			Burn wound model in rats and mice	High-level protection (94)
				Serospecific anti-LPS mean lethal dose 10^5-fold (even if administered after infection was established) (94)
		LPS	Immunosuppressed model in dogs	Protection: long-term survival, low bacteremia (118)
		LPS + granulocyte infusion	Immunosuppression model in dogs	Higher protection than granulocyte transfusion alone

		Passive transfer of anti-LPS	Immunosuppression model in dogs	No protection (119)
			Leukopenic mice	Prevents bacteremia and offers protection (106)
		LPS	Fetal acute pneumonia in guinea-pigs	Protection (120)
		Anti-LPS passive transfers		Enhanced bacterial clearing from lungs and reduced tissue damage (121)
High-molecular-weight polysaccharides (PS)	PS is non-toxic, less immunogenic than LPS (122)	PS	Mice	Creates protective immune response (116, 122); neutralizing antibodies
Flagella	Motility associated with virulence (123, 124)	Flagellar antigen (124)	Burn wound model in mice	40–100% protection; (protection associated with H(flagellar) antigen
		Antiflagellar antibodies; passive transfers		Immobilizes bacteria at infection site; reduces invasion (125)
Pilli	Mediate attachment to respiratory epithelium; homologous antipilus antibody prevents attachment in vitro	Purifies pilli	Burn wound model	Protection against homologous strain (117)

of 59 (91 %) cases of infection caused by *P. aeruginosa*. However, during the course of therapy 7% of *P. aeruginosa* strains developed resistance, 7% of patients only partly improved, and 10% relapsed as soon as therapy was discontinued (15). In addition, a very high rate of superinfections with *Klebsiella* and *Serratia* species occurred. A later study (16) found that carbenicillin alone in a dosage of 10 grams achieved a 50% cure of *P. aeruginosa* infections while the rate for gentamicin administered alone was only 55% (17). Ticarcillin administered alone in a daily dose of 20 grams failed to cure 2 of 5 *P. aeruginosa* infections. In one patient, relapse occurred soon after the drug had been discontinued. Overall, 16 of 20 infections caused by *P. aeruginosa* responded favorably to ticarcillin therapy. However, patients with pneumonia and bacteremia due to *P. aeruginosa* in immunocompromised patients responded poorly ($< 30\%$ response rate) (18).

In an early trial conducted in 1975 the efficacy of carbenicillin alone was compared with the combination of carbenicillin + gentamicin. The results showed among 22 patients with *P. aeruginosa* infections a slightly lower, but non-significantly different response rate for patients treated with carbenicillin alone (82%) than for those treated with the combination (91%) (19).

In non-neutropenic hosts with respiratory tract infection, including patients with cystic fibrosis, the efficacy of these two agents has been reported to be significantly better than that of polymyxins and aminoglycosides (20).

Therapy of *P. aeruginosa* endocarditis in heroin addicts using high doses of carbenicillin has been disappointing unless the infection was localized in the right side of the heart and antibiotic therapy was accompanied by surgical valve removal (21). Both carbenicillin and ticarcillin have proved to be effective when administered alone in the therapy of burn wound sepsis (22). However, combination therapy is currently recommended because of the rapid development of antibiotic resistance if a drug is used alone and because of the possible synergistic activity of the combination.

Necrotizing otitis externa was a lethal disease before the introduction of carbenicillin and ticarcillin when treated with aminoglycosides alone. Doubtless, the penicillins, probably because of their more favorable penetration into bone and cartilage, changed the prognosis of this disease (23).

Urinary tract infections caused by *P. aeruginosa* usually occur in patients with underlying abnormalities of the urinary tract. Ticarcillin and carbenicillin sterilize most infections while treatment is administered, if there is no indwelling urinary catheter present. However, relapses following the cessation of therapy have been common (20, 24).

Experience with infections of the central nervous system, particularly meningitis caused by *P. aeruginosa,* is incomplete. Kinetic data suggest that the spinal fluid levels of carbenicillin and ticarcillin are too low to provide adequate therapeutic levels (25). Similarly, eye fluid levels of antipseudomonal penicillins do not suggest that these agents will be effective in the therapy of *P. aeruginosa* endophthalmitis.

The introduction of the semisynthetic ureidopenicillins which have more marked activity than carbenicillin and ticarcillin against *P. aeruginosa* have renewed interest in therapy of *P. aeruginosa* infections with single agents. *Azlocillin* had a mean serum bactericidal activity of 1/32, 1 hour following a 5 gram intravenous infusion against 20 different strains of *P. aeruginosa* while that of mezlocillin and ticarcillin was 1/8 (25).

Azlocillin inhibits more than 80% of *P. aeruginosa* strains at a concentration of 64 mg/l or less. Its antipseudomonal activity is 4 times greater than that of mezlocillin and ticarcillin and 8 times greater than carbenicillin and is similar to that of piperacillin (26). All these penicillins are inactivated by plasmid-mediated β-lactamases present in *P. aeruginosa*. However, these compounds are most active against strains that lack these enzymes. All ureidopenicillins bind to numerous PBPs; however, PBP-3 is the major target, as suggested by the filamentation of *P. aeruginosa* when exposed to these agents. In a filamental form, rapidly developing cellular defects and blebs soon induce cell lysis (27). All ureidopenicillins have almost identical pharmacokinetics (28), which points to similar clinical results in comparative studies of these agents: e.g., in neutropenic patients with *P. aeruginosa* infections treated with low-dose mezlocillin (3 g q. 4 h) (29), high-dose mezlocillin (5.0 g q. 4 h) (30) and piperacillin (4 g q. 4 h) (31), response rates were 42, 50 and 60%, respectively, lower than that expected with the combination of an aminoglycoside and carbenicillin. Somewhat better, although not statistically significant, clinical results were observed when carbenicillin and azlocillin were compared in the therapy of cystic fibrosis patients (32). Ticarcillin was as effective as azlocillin in the treatment of patients with urinary tract infections (33, 34) and azlocillin was as effective as gentamicin in patients with serious infections of the skin, skin structures and lower respiratory tract caused by *P. aeruginosa* (35).

The failure to show differences in efficacy between therapeutic trials can be explained by the similar activity in vitro of many of the compounds used. Also, in many studies the number of patients was insufficient to give confident results (β-error). Often patients with a wide range of infections were included which precluded appropriate stratification.

In the last few years a number of new broad-spectrum cephalosporins with activity against *P. aeruginosa* have been introduced into clinical practice. *Moxalactam* has intermediate activity against *P. aeruginosa* with minimum inhibitory concentration for 70% of strains (MIC_{70}) of 25 μg/ml (36). Indeed, only 69% of 134 infections caused by *P. aeruginosa* were cured by moxalactam (37). Thus, this agent is sufficient in single-drug therapy of these infections. Interestingly, in combination moxalactam performed better than other combinations between β-lactams and aminoglycosides in the therapy of *P. aeruginosa* infections in leukopenic hosts.

Cefoperazone is another third-generation cephalosporin with outstanding gram-negative activity including *P. aeruginosa*. Despite the relatively low MICs of cefoperazone against *P. aeruginosa* ($MIC_{90} > 16$ μg/ml) (38) the clinical response during therapy of *P. aeruginosa* infections averaged only 55% in a large variety of infections in cancer patients (39). In patients without cancer, the overall satisfactory response rate was 71% (40).

Cefotaxime and *ceftizoxime* are third-generation cephalosporins, with MIC_{50} and MIC_{90} against *P. aeruginosa* of 19 and 61 µg/ml, respectively (41). However, the clinical results obtained with cefotaxime in combination with aminoglycosides were rather disappointing, as evidenced by the third study by the European Organization for the Research and Treatment of Cancer (EORTC) of infections caused by *P. aeruginosa* in granulocytopenic patients (82).

Cefsulodin was the first cephalosporin with antipseudomonal activity (MIC < 1.5 µg/ml for most strains) (42). In a multicenter study involving over 300 patients, cefsulodin eliminated only 64% of *P. aeruginosa* causing respiratory tract infections (excluding cystic fibrosis patients) and cured only 60% of patients with septicemia caused by *P. aeruginosa* (43). Thus, the efficacy of cefsulodin as sole antipseudomonal agent is limited and should be reserved for special situations such as urinary tract infections, bone infections etc. Cefsulodin may be particularly suitable for elderly patients with compromised renal function and congestive heart failure who cannot tolerate the sodium load administered with the penicillins and who are also likely to suffer from the toxic renal side effects of the aminoglycosides.

Ceftazidime is the most active cephalosporin against *P. aeruginosa*. The MIC_{90} is 4 µg/ml or less (44) and less than 5% of *P. aeruginosa* strains are resistant to this agent. The remarkable activity of ceftazidime against *P. aeruginosa* is probably due to the presence of both its carboxy-propyl-iminomethoxy side chain and the pyridine group present as the side chain of the dihydrothiazine ring (45). In clinical studies, ceftazidime cured some 60% of a variety of infections caused by *P. aeruginosa* (45–47). Remarkably, all 20 patients with *P. aeruginosa* bacteremia were cured, as were 87% of 79 patients with *P. aeruginosa* skin and soft tissue infections, and 86% of 35 patients with *P. aeruginosa* bone and joint infections. Only incomplete data exist with regard to therapy of *P. aeruginosa* infections in granulocytopenic patients treated with ceftazidime alone. In one study (48) ceftazidime alone cured all of granulocytopenic patients with *P. aeruginosa* infections. In an additional study all of 10 episodes of infections caused by *P. aeruginosa* in cancer patients (including 6 cases of bacteremia) were successfully cured with ceftazidime (49). When reviewing the literature, it is interesting to note that despite large studies of granulocytopenic patients the rate of *P. aeruginosa* infections in all studies was low, probably reflecting the very recent decrease of these infections in these patients.

Despite the unusual activity of the drug, the development of resistance has been reported in patients with cystic fibrosis during ceftazidime therapy (45).

Imipenem (*N*-formimidoyl thienamycin) is an extremely potent antipseudomonal agent with MIC_{50} of 1.67 and MIC_{90} of 3.8 µg/ml. MICs against carbenicillin-resistant and aminoglycoside-resistant *P. aeruginosa* strains are of the same order of magnitude (50). In patients treated with imipenem as well as with the above-mentioned agents the development of bacterial resistance has been observed (50); this phenomenon can easily be repeated in the test tube for imipenem as well as for other penicillins (50). Imipenem alone cured all of 25 patients with *P. aerugino-*

sa urinary tract infections (51) and all of 8 patients with *P. aeruginosa* bacteremia (52), as well as the majority of patients with *P. aeruginosa* osteomyelitis (53). Notably, in 2 of 34 (5.9%) patients with *P. aeruginosa* osteomyelitis imipenem-resistant strains could be cultured during therapy (53). This important observation may limit its use in the future as a single agent. Imipenem may become a valuable agent for therapy of mixed infections which include *P. aeruginosa*, because of its broader antibacterial spectrum and pronounced activity. Experience with the use of imipenem in leukopenic patients is still incomplete; however, theoretically one could expect this agent to be as successful as ceftazidime for this group of patients.

Monobactams

Aztreonam, a member of the monobactam group, has MIC_{50} and MIC_{90} values against *P. aeruginosa* of 16.0 and 32.0 $\mu g/ml$, respectively (54). It acts synergistically with the main aminoglycosides against the majority of *P. aeruginosa* strains (55). A particularly interesting feature of aztreonam is its lack of immunologic cross-reactivity with penicillins and cephalosporins, thus allowing its administration to patients with β-lactam allergy (56). Clinically, aztreonam cured all of 5 patients with *P. aeruginosa* osteomyelitis, 11 of 12 patients with other infections caused by *P. aeruginosa* (57), and 5 of 8 patients with *P. aeruginosa* nosocomial pneumonia (58). The microbiologic cure rate for *P. aeruginosa* in lower respiratory tract infections was 69% (compared with 50% with tobramycin) and 63% for urinary tract infections (59). There is little experience on the use of aztreonam in leukopenic patients with *P. aeruginosa* infections.

Quinolones

This group of novel antibiotics which can be administered orally as well as parenterally has recently emerged as a most important potential alternative to the 'classical' antipseudomonal antimicrobial agents. Whereas the older members of this group (nalidixic acid and oxolinic acid) had low or absent activity against *P. aeruginosa* and were indicated for the therapy of urinary tract infections only, newer agents such as enoxacin, pefloxacin, ofloxacin, ciprofloxacin, difloxacin and norfloxacin can be used for the therapy of *P. aeruginosa* infections that are not confined exclusively to the urinary tract. Representative MIC_{50} and MIC_{90} values for these agents against *P. aeruginosa* are: enoxacin 1.6 and 6.5 $\mu g/ml$, pefloxacin 1 and 4 $\mu g/ml$, ofloxacin 1 and 2.5 $\mu g/ml$, norfloxacin 0.5 and 2 $\mu g/ml$, difloxacin 2 and 4 $\mu g/ml$, and ciprofloxacin 0.5 and 1 $\mu g/ml$ (60). Among the quinolones, ciprofloxacin seems to exhibit the strongest in vitro anti-*P. aeruginosa* activity. Emergence of partial and complete cross-resistance of *P. aeruginosa* mutants against the various quinolones has been observed during therapy, particularly in patients with cystic fibrosis and chronic *P. aeruginosa* osteomyelitis (61). All quinolones are rapidly bactericidal against multiplying and stationary bacteria and are not adversely affected by inoculum size. Their outstanding pharmacokinetic properties, namely absorption following oral administration, adequate penetration into sputum, prostate and bone, and lack of serious side effects, make this group of antimicrobial agents prime candidates in the therapy of *P. aeruginosa* infections at these 'sanctuaries' (62). Favorable therapeutic results have been reported in the therapy of cystic fibrosis patients (28/35 patients), bone infections and urinary tract infections (62), the therapeutic success rate being equal to or better than conventional therapy. The development of quinolone-resistant *P. aeruginosa* mutants in patients with cystic fibrosis (62) and in patients with bone infections has been repeatedly observed (63) and may be a major concern in the future. Furthermore, rapidly developing cross-resistance by *P. aeruginosa* to quinolones may dictate the need for combined therapy with agents that cannot be administered orally. At any rate, the quinolones seem to offer a potentially important advantage in the therapy of such infections in the out-patient setting.

Aminoglycosides

Aminoglycosides have for many years been useful agents in the therapy of gram-negative bacillary infections and in particular of *P. aeruginosa* infections. The use of aminoglycosides as sole agents in therapy of severe *P. aeruginosa* infections, particularly in neutropenic patients, has been a source of major concern because of the need to administer high, potentially toxic doses to achieve therapeutic levels, and the lack of a postantibiotic effect when drug levels decline below the MIC (64). Aminoglycosides have proved successful in neutropenic patients when administered in a continuous intravenous infusion (65). Under such conditions, the continuous exposure of the eighth cranial nerve and the kidney to high aminoglycoside concentrations undoubtedly contributes to the high rate of untoward toxic side-effects. Indeed, recent data (66) suggest a direct relationship between the ratio of the height of the serum peak aminoglycoside concentration to the MIC of the infecting organism and the clinical response – favoring the administration of high doses of aminoglycosides. A major concern associated with aminoglycosides is the development of resistance by *P. aeruginosa* as well as other gram-negative bacilli. Whereas in some important centers the development of resistance by *P. aeruginosa* to gentamicin, tobramycin and amikacin was low and did not correlate with aminoglycoside usage (67, 68), in other centers it was found to be higher and to correlate directly with aminoglycoside usage and it was heralded by an increase in the frequency of aminoglycoside-inactivating enzymes (69, 70). Among the various aminoglycosides active against *P. aeruginosa* the rank of activity in vitro is: amikacin > tobramycin > gentamicin, amikacin being less susceptible to enzymatic inactivation by gentamicin-resistant *P. aeruginosa*. The use of an aminoglycoside as single agent for the therapy of *P. aeruginosa* infections is limited to non-life-threatening infections in systems in which high aminoglycoside levels are reached (e.g. urinary tract) and in infections that are unaccompanied by the presence of purulent material which inactivates aminoglycosides. Other than these few indications it seems that aminoglycosides should always be used in combinations, similar to the situation of ureidopenicillins. When piperacillin was used alone against infections caused by *P. aeruginosa,* 42% of the strains developed resistance. When piperacillin was administered with an aminoglycoside, the rate was only 17% (71). In *P. aeruginosa* bacteremia, combinations of antibiotics that offer synergistic interaction were associated with a significantly better survival (72, 73) both in immunosuppressed and normal hosts and in bacteremias secondary to endocarditis (74). Data from studies performed by the EORTC supports the superiority of aminoglycoside + carboxypenicillin synergistic combinations over non-synergistic combinations or single agents in the therapy of *P. aeruginosa* infections in leukopenic patients (75, 76).

The use of a combination of an aminoglycoside and β-lactam antibiotic became popular not only for the therapy of *P. aeruginosa* infections where synergy and decreased rate of development of resistance were demonstrable, but also for a variety of other clinical and microbiologic considerations (77). It soon became apparent, however, that intense aminoglycoside therapy in both immunocompetent and immunosuppressed hosts was associated with a high rate of nephrotoxic and ototoxic side effects (78, 79). Furthermore, the need to monitor aminoglycoside blood levels when intensive therapy is administered has not resulted in a significant decrease in the rate of adverse reactions but has complicated therapy and is a cause of increased costs as well. This has raised the question whether the use of two β-lactams with an additive antibacterial spectrum would have any advantages over the aminoglycoside + β-lactam combination, particularly in the reduction of the incidence of nephrotoxicity. The potential disadvantages of a double β-lactam combination include suppression of bone marrow, an enhanced adverse effect on the anaerobic intestinal flora, an increased susceptibility to fungal infections (80), and the induction of β-lactamases (81). Most clinical studies, however, have demonstrated little difference when double β-lactam combinations were compared with an aminoglycoside + β-lactam combination. Two studies have shown an excess mortality in patients treated with a combination of two β-lactam antibiotics (82, 83). In bacteremia in leukopenic patients both combinations had a similar success rate. In patients with *P. aeruginosa* infections the response rate was 65% for the double β-lactam combination and 60% for the β-lactam + aminoglycoside combination. Results of more recent trials show a decreasing response rate for the double β-lactam combinations, probably reflecting an increase in acquired resistance of *P. aeruginosa* to β-lactam antibiotics (80).

RECOMMENDATIONS

The preferred therapy of life-threatening *P. aeruginosa* infections (bacteremia, endocarditis, infection in leukopenic patients, burn wound sepsis, malignant external otitis, meningitis and nosocomial pneumonia) is: (a) a combination of an aminoglycoside + β-lactam that shows synergy in vitro; (b) alternatively, intravenous highly dosed ceftazidime or imipenem. For penicillin-allergic patients quinolones or the combination of aztreonam and an aminoglycoside can be used. In adult patients with *P. aeruginosa* meningitis, aminoglycoside should be administered intrathecally. These infections should be treated for a minimum of 14 days.

For chronic *P. aeruginosa* infections not immediately life-threatening (cystic fibrosis, chronic osteomyelitis, complicated urinary tract infections) we recommend the alternate use of effective single agents such as cefsulodin, ceftazidime, imipenem and quinolones after a fixed time-period. Care should be taken to alternate the drugs so as to diminish the emergence of resistance. Each course should not last for more than 21 days.

For minor infections (skin infections, conjunctivitis, external otitis, infections associated with whirlpools) a single agent for short periods of time, usually up to 10 days, will suffice.

Even under an optimal antibiotic regimen, failure of therapy is frequent. The following reasons may account for the high failure rate: (a) the severity of underlying disease; (b) the inability of antibiotics to cure the infections because of bacterial resistance, delayed onset of therapy, unfavorable pharmacokinetics; (c) bacterial virulence factors. The high failure rate of chemotherapy warrants the search for alternative solutions in selected patient populations. Bacterial factors associated with virulence of *P. aeruginosa* and which may thus become targets for future therapy are listed in Table 1.

VACCINES

Colonization of immunocompromised hosts by *P. aeruginosa* is a prerequisite for ensuing infection. Primary prevention of colonization in the immunocompromised host would therefore minimize the risk of overwhelming *P. aeruginosa* sepsis. Induction of protective immunity could be a preferred strategy to achieve this goal. This has led to the development of various vaccines and their evaluation in animal models and clinical trials (7).

Human serum is inefficient in clearing *P. aeruginosa* from the bloodstream since the majority of bacteremic isolates are resistant to the killing effect of serum. In addition to serum, the presence of phagocytic cells, opsonizing antibodies and complement are necessary for clearing of *P. aeruginosa* infection (126) (Table 1).

Survival after a bacteremic episode caused by *P. aeruginosa* was associated with a marked increase in opsonic antibody titers. Opsonic activity could be elicited by immunization with lipopolysaccharide (LPS). High titers of antibody against LPS and toxin A were associated with increased survival rates (127). Elevated titers to both were superior in terms of survival to elevation of antibody titers against either LPS or toxin A. Mortality was highest when there was no increase to either antigen. Survivors of *P. aeruginosa* bacteremia were found to have a 6-fold increase in antitoxin antibodies. Toxin-producing strains were more virulent than nontoxigenic strains. In patients infected with toxigenic *P. aeruginosa* strains, the absence of antibodies to toxin A and LPS was associated with higher mortality (128).

The following vaccines have been evaluated clinically for their preventive potential and antibody-eliciting capacity:

Whole-cell vaccines were first tried using a monovalent vaccine of a heat-killed *P. aeruginosa* strain isolated in a burn unit. Patients were treated with a combination of active immunization and hyperimmune human antisera. The mortality rate was lower in the immunized group (129). The fact that the study used historical controls makes the significance of these results questionable since the results could be attributed to improvement in burn wound management rather than to the effect of immunization. Another vaccine including 6 formalin-/heat-killed strains of *P. aeruginosa* and two strains of *S. aureus* resulted in prolonged survival and a lower rate of septicemia when compared with historical controls (130).

Heptavalent LPS vaccine composed of LPS of defined serotypes (131) (Fisher immunotyping system (132)) was used for vaccination of burn patients. A reduction from 14.1 to 3.1% in mortality due to *P. aeruginosa* bacteremia was observed. Three patients who died of *P. aeruginosa* sepsis had a low or absent antibody response to *P. aeruginosa* (133). Eight patients who developed *P. aeruginosa* sepsis after vaccination were treated with hyperimmune antiserum and survived (134). Hyperimmune gammaglobulin was found to offer protection against *P. aeruginosa* infection in an uncontrolled study in burn patients (135).

In cancer patients vaccination did not reduce the incidence of *P. aeruginosa* infection significantly nor did it prevent bacteremia. Mortality in bacteremic patients was usually related to neutropenia and to the lack of opsonic antibody in both vaccinated and non-vaccinated patients. Non-bacteremic fatalities were associated with a lack of antibodies rather than with neutropenia. Protection was associated with both circulating antibodies and granulocytes (136). Neither in acute leukemia (137, 138) nor in cystic fibrosis patients did the vaccine offer any protection or alteration of the clinical course (138). Vaccination in intensive-care-unit patients did not reduce the overall mortality and the rate of infection was not significantly altered (139). Adverse reactions to the vaccine occurred in up to 100% of immunized cancer patients and in 92% of cystic fibrosis patients (140). Burn patients tolerated the vaccine better than other vaccinated patient populations. Common reactions consisted of local pain, induration, fever, malaise and headache (138).

Polyvalent extract vaccine (PEV-01) contains formalin-inactivated antigens from 16 live serotypes of *P. aeruginosa*. The vaccine was found to be non-toxic in mice, although some components were toxic to embryonated chicken eggs. The PEV-01 vaccine has been evaluated in several animal models. In mice it offered protection against intraperitoneal challenge with a varying degree of cross-protection. In guinea-pigs immunization protected against fatal *P. aeruginosa* pneumonia and facilitated bacterial clearing from the lungs (141). In the chronic rat lung model, a reduction in tissue damage was observed even although the number of bacteria was not reduced, thus suggesting a protective effect offered by the vaccine against exotoxins of *P. aeruginosa* (142). The vaccine was found to be immunogenic in human subjects and clinical trials in burn patients revealed a marked reduction in mortality from *P. aeruginosa* sepsis, absence of positive *P. aeruginosa* blood cultures and decrease in *P. aeruginosa* wound colonization (143, 144). Immunized patients, however, had no advantage over non-immunized patients in overall mortality. *Original endotoxin protein (OEP)* is a substance consisting of protein, lipids, polysaccharides, 2-keto-3-deoxyoctonic acid (KDO) and hexosamines (145). Immunization of mice with OEP was protective against heterologous challenge. A vaccine composed of OEP detoxified elastase, alkaline protease and toxoid of toxin A is currently under clinical investigation (146).

The following vaccines are being currently evaluated and may prove to be efficacious:

Detoxified LPS and high-molecular-weight polysaccharide antigens elicit opsonizing antibodies in and cause no major side effects (detoxified *P. aeruginosa* LPS under alkaline conditions provokes an antibody reaction only when coupled covalently to a protein carrier such as *P. aeruginosa* pili or tetanus toxoid) (147, 148).

Toxin A toxoids (inactivated by formalin or glutaraldehyde) require adjuvants to evoke an immune response and thus are unsuitable for human use (97, 149). Alternatives include *P. aeruginosa* mutants containing immunologic cross-reacting non-toxic toxin A (150, 151, 159).

Detoxified elastase and alkaline protease are effective in veterinary use as part of a multicomponent *P. aeruginosa* vaccine (151). The heterogeneity of pili serotypes may diminish the value of these antigens as potential common immunogens (152, 159).

Live attenuated strains A temperature-sensitive strain (153) was tried as an aerosol immunogen in mice. It elicited an immune response and enhanced pulmonary clearing of bacteria (154). The vaccine may also have a role in eliciting a local immune response in the respiratory tract in man.

Ribosomal vaccines consist of RNA-protein complexes. Active or passive immunization induced serotype-specific protection in mice against peritoneal challenge (155, 156).

LPS-core vaccines are based on a mutant strain of *E. coli* that contains a LPS lacking in O-specific side chains. Immunization with this antigen elicits antibodies against the exposed core region of the LPS shared by various gram-negative bacteria. In animal models this immunogen has proved to be inferior to other multivalent *P. aeruginosa* vaccines. Clinical trials using antiserum raised against *E. coli* J5 reduced mortality when used for gram-negative bacteremia (157, 158).

THERAPEUTIC REGIMENS

Therapeutic regimens must be tailored to the specific host according to its immune capacity. Patients who are immunologically uncompromised, such as burn patients, may benefit from active immunization schedules in combination with passive immunotherapy. In the immunosuppressed host, passive transfer of hyperimmune sera with granulocyte transfusion may prove efficacious in reducing mortality from *P. aeruginosa* infections. Prevention of colonization of the respiratory tract by *P. aeruginosa* in cystic fibrosis patients may be the appropriate strategy, although the means to obtain this goal are not yet feasible. The combined use of intravenously administered immunoglobulins and antipseudomonal antibiotics may prove beneficial for *P. aeruginosa* infections in neutropenic hosts and in immunoglobulin-deficient patients.

At this point it seems that immunization in its present state of development has not reached the stage at which it could be recommended for clinical application. It is hoped that advances in biotechnology and molecular biology will contribute to better therapeutic results.

REFERENCES

1. Gessard C (1882) Sur les colorations bleue et verte des linges à pansements. *CR Séances Acad. Sci. (Sér. D)*, *94*, 536.
2. Fraenkel E (1897) Über Menschen-pathogenität des *Bacillus pyocyaneus* and zur Aetiologie des Ekthyma gangrenosum. *Wien. Klin. Wochenschr.*, *10*, 1893.
3. Gustafson TL, Band JD, Hutcheson RH, Schaffner W (1983) *Pseudomonas* folliculitis: an outbreak and literature review. *Rev. Infect. Dis.*, *5*, 1.
4. Insler MS, Gore M (1986) *Pseudomonas* keratitis and folliculitis after whirlpool exposure. *Am. J. Ophthalmol.*, *101*, 41.
5. Scheckelhoff DJ, Mirtallo JM, Ayers LW, Visconti JA (1986) Growth of bacteria and fungi in total nutrient mixture. *Am. J. Hosp. Pharm.*, *43*, 73.
6. Stephenson JR, Hecerrt SR, Richards MA, Tabaquachali S (1985) Gastrointestinal colonization and septicemia with *Pseudomonas aeruginosa* due to contaminated thymol mouth wash in immunocompromised patients. *J. Hosp. Infect.*, *6*, 369.
7. Cryz Jr SJ (1984) *Pseudomonas aeruginosa* infections. In: Germanier R (Ed), *Bacterial Vaccines*, p. 317. Academic Press, Orlando, FL.
8. Grogan JB (1966) *Pseudomonas aeruginosa* carriage in patients. *J. Trauma*, *6*, 639.
9. Schimpff SC, Moody M, Young VM (1970) Relationships of colonization with *Pseudomonas aeruginosa* to development of *Pseudomonas* bacteremia in cancer patients. *Antimicrob. Agents Chemother.*, *10*, 240.
10. Cross A, Allen JK, Burke J et al (1983) Nosocomial infections due to *Pseudomonas aeruginosa*. *Rev. Infect. Dis.*, *5*, Suppl 5 S837.
11. Pruitt Jr BA (1974) Infection caused by *Pseudomonas* species in patients with burns and in other surgical patients. *J. Infect. Dis.*, *130*, Suppl, 58.
12. Kerby GP (1947) *Pseudomonas aeruginosa* bacteremia: summary of the literature with report of a case. *Am. J. Dis. Child.*, *74*, 610.
13. Flick MR, Cluff LE (1979) *Pseudomonas* bacteremia: review of 108 cases. *Am. J. Med.*, *60*, 501.
14. Andriole V (1979) *Pseudomonas* bacteremia: can antibiotic therapy improve survival? *J. Lab. Clin. Med.*, *94*, 1960.
15. Fainstein V, Bodey GP (1985) Single agent therapy for infections in neutropenic cancer patients. *Am. J. Med.*, *79*, Suppl, 83.
16. Bodey GP, Roddriguez V, Luce JK (1969) Carbenicillin therapy of gram negative bacillary infections. *Am. J. Med. Sci.*, *257*, 408.

17. Klastersky J, Cappel R, Daneau D (1973) Therapy with carbenicillin and gentamicin for patients with cancer and severe infections caused by gram negative rods. *Cancer*, *31*, 331.
18. Rodriguez VK, Bodey GP, Horikoshi N, Inagaki J, McCredie K (1973) Ticarcillin therapy of infections. *Antimicrob. Agents Chemother.*, *4*, 427.
19. Bodey GP, Feld R, Burgess MA (1976) Beta lactam antibiotics alone and in combination with gentamicin for therapy of gram-negative bacillary infection in neutropenic patients. *Am. J. Med. Sci.*, *271*, 179.
20. Neu HC (1982) Carbenicillin and ticarcillin. *Med. Clin. North Am.*, *66*, 61.
21. Reyes MP, Brown WJ, Lerner AM (1978) Treatment of patients with *Pseudomonas* endocarditis with high dose aminoglycoside and carbenicillin therapy. *Medicine*, *57*, 57.
22. Yoshida T, Okimoto Y (1977) Fundamental and clinical studies on ticarcillin in plastic surgery. *Chemotherapy (Tokyo)*, *25*, 2681.
23. Zaky DA, Bentley DW, Lowy K (1976) Malignant external otitis: a severe form of otitis in diabetic patients. *Am. J. Med.*, *61*, 298.
24. Parry MF, Neu HC (1976) Ticarcillin for treatment of serious infections with gram-negative bacteria. *J. Infect. Dis.*, *134*, 476.
25. Coppens LK, Klastersky J (1974) Comparative study of anti-*pseudomonas* activity of azlocillin, mezlocillin and ticarcillin. *Antimicrob. Agents Chemother.*, *15*, 396.
26. Sanders C (1983) Azlocillin: a new broad spectrum penicillin. *J. Antimicrob. Chemother.*, *11*, *Suppl B*, 21.
27. Metzger K (1982) Killing of azlocillin and mezlozillin induced filamentous forms of *Pseudomonas aeruginosa* by decreasing concentrations of penicillin. *J. Antimicrob. Chemother.*, *9*, *Suppl A*, 11.
28. Meyers BR, Hirschman SZ, Strougo L, Srulevitch E (1980) Comparative study of piperacillin, ticarcillin and carbenicillin pharmacokinetics. *Antimicrob. Agents Chemother.*, *17*, 608.
29. Issell B, Bodey GP (1980) Mezlocillin for treatment of infections in cancer patients. *Antimicrob. Agents. Chemother.*, *17*, 1008.
30. Wade JC, Schimpff SC, Newman K, Fortner CL, Moody MR, Young VM, Wiernik PH (1980) Potential of mezlocillin as empiric single agent therapy in febrile granulocytopenic cancer patients. *Antimicrob. Agents Chemother.*, *18*, 299.
31. Jadeja L, Bolivar R, Fainstein V, Keating M, McCredie K, Hay M, Bodey GP (1984) Piperacillin plus vancomycin in the therapy of febrile episodes in cancer patients. *Antimicrob. Agents. Chemother.*, *26*, 295.
32. Huang NN, Palmer J, Keith H, Schidlow D, Braverman S, Goldberg M (1983) Comparative efficacy of and tolerance of study of azlocillin and carbenicillin in patients with cystic fibrosis. *J. Antimicrob. Chemother.*, *11*, *Suppl B*, 205.
33. Reed WP, Pulmer DL (1983) Comparison of azlocillin and ticarcillin in the treatment of urinary tract infections. *J. Antimicrob. Chemother.*, *11*, *Suppl B*, 189.
34. Cox C (1983) A comparison of azlocillin and ticarcillin in the treatment of complicated urinary tract infections. *J. Antimicrob. Chemother.*, *11*, *Suppl B*, 183.
35. Gonzalez M (1983) A comparison of azlocillin and gentamicin in the treatment of serious infections caused by *Pseudomonas aeruginosa*. *J. Antimicrob. Chemother.*, *11*, *Suppl B*, 169.
36. Goto S (1982) In-vitro and in-vivo antibacterial activity of moxalactam an oxabeta-location antibiotic. *Rev. Infect. Dis.*, *9*, *Suppl*, S501.

37. Kammer RB (1982) Moxalactam: clinical summary. *Rev. Infect. Dis.*, *4*, *Suppl*, S712
38. Bremner DA (1981) Susceptibility of clinical isolates to cefoperazone. *Drugs*, *22*, *Suppl 1*, 29.
39. Bolivar R, Feinstein V, Elting L, Bodey GP (1983) Cefoperazone for the treatment of infections in patients with cancer. *Rev. Infect. Dis.*, *22*, *Suppl 1*, S181.
40. Gerber AV, Craig WA (1981) Worldwide clinical experience with cefoperazone. *Drugs*, *22*, *Suppl 1*, 108.
41. Jones RN, Thornsberry C (1982) Cefotaxime: a review of in-vitro antimicrobial properties and spectrum of activity. *Rev. Infect. Dis.*, *4*, *Suppl*, S300.
42. Zak O, Konopka EA, Tosch W, Ahraens T, Zimmermann W, Kradolfer F (1979) Experimental evaluation of CGP 7174/E, a new injectable cephalosporin antibiotic active against *Pseudomonas aeruginosa*. *Drugs Intell. Clin. Res.*, *5*, 45.
43. Ahrens T (1981) Treatment of *Pseudomonas* infections with cefsulodin. In: *Abstracts, 12th International Congress of Chemotherapy, Florence, 1981*, p. 66.
44. Thornsberry C (1985) Review of in-vitro activity of third generation cephalosporins and other newer beta-lactam antibiotics against clinically important bacteria. *Am. J. Med.*, *79*, *Suppl 2A*, 20.
45. Neu HC (1985) Structure-activity relation of new beta lactam compounds and in-vitro activity against common bacteria. *Rev. Infect. Dis.*, *5*, *Suppl*, 9.
46. Clumeck N, Gordts B, Dab I, Jaspoor N, Van-Laethem Y, Butzler JP (1983) Ceftazidime as a single agent in the treatment of severe *Pseudomonas aeruginosa* infections. *J. Antimicrob. Chemother.*, *12*, *Suppl A*, 207.
47. *Ceftazidime Technical Monograph*. Glaxo, Greenford, U.K.
48. De Pauw BE, Kavw F, Mugtjens H, Williams KJ, Bothof T (1983) Randomized study of ceftazidime versus gentamicin plus cefotaxime for infections in severe granulocytopenic patients. *J. Antimicrob. Chemother.*, *15*, *Suppl A*, 93.
49. Fainstein V, Bodey GP, Elting L, Bolivar B, Keating MJ, McCredie KB, Valivieso M (1983) A randomized study of ceftazidime and tobramycin for the treatment of infection in cancer patients. *J. Antimicrob. Chemother.*, *12*, *Suppl A*, 101.
50. Kropp H, Gerckens L, Sundelof JG, Kahan FM (1985) Antibacterial activity of imipenem: the first thienamycin antibiotic. *Rev. Infect. Dis.*, *7*, *Suppl 3*, S389.
51. Cox C, Corrado ML (1985) Safety and efficacy of imipenem/cilastatin in treatment of complicated urinary tract infections. *Am. J. Med.*, *78*, *Suppl 6A*, 87.
52. Eron IJ (1985) Imipenem/cilastatin therapy of bacteremia. *Am. J. Med.*, *78*, *Suppl 6A*, 87.
53. Gentry LO (1985) Role of newer beta-lactam antibiotics in treatment of osteomyelitis. *Am. J. Med.*, *78*, *Suppl 6A*, 126.
54. Jacobus NV, Ferreira MC, Barza M (1982) In-vitro activity of aztreonam – a monobactam antibiotic. *Antimicrob. Agents Chemother.*, *22*, 832.
55. Sykes RB, Bonner DP (1985) Aztreonam: the first monobactam. *Am. J. Med.*, *78*, *Suppl 2A*, 2.
56. Adkinson NF, Swabb EA, Sugerman AA (1984) Immunology of monobactam aztreonam. *Antimicrob. Agents Chemother.*, *25*, 93.
57. Simons WJ, Lee TJ (1985) Treatment of gram-negative infections with aztreonam. *Am. J. Med.*, *78*, *Suppl 2A*, 27.
58. Schentag JJ, Vari AJ, Winslade NE, Swenson DJ, Smith IL, Simons GW, Vigano A (1985) Treatment with aztreonam or tobramycin in critical care patients with nosocomial gram-negative pneumonia. *Am. J. Med.*, *78*, *Suppl 1A*, 34.

59. Henry SA, Bendush CB (1985) Aztreonam: worldwide overview of the treatment of patients with gram-negative infections. *Am. J. Med., 78, Suppl 2A,* 57.

60. Rubinstein E, Segev S, Lev B (1986) The 4 quinolones: A promising new class of antibiotics. *Hosp. Ther., 2,* 39.

61. Barry AL, Jones RD (1984) Cross resistance among cinoxacin, ciprofloxocin, DJ 6783, enoxacin, nalidixic acid, norfloxacin and oxolonic acid after in-vitro selection of resistant population. *Antimicrob. Agents Chemother., 25,* 775.

62. Scully BE, Neu HC, Parry MF, Mandell W (1986) Oral ciprofloxacin therapy of infections due to *Pseudomonas aeruginosa. Lancet, 1,* 819.

63. Eron L, Harvey L, Hixon DL, Poretz DM (1985) Ciprofloxacin therapy of infections caused by *Pseudomonas aeruginosa* and other resistant bacteria. *Antimicrob. Agents Chemother., 27,* 3085.

64. Bundtzen RW, Gerber AV, Cohn DL, Craig WA (1981) Postantibiotic suppression of bacterial growth. *Rev. Infect. Dis., 3,* 28.

65. Valdivieso M, Feed R, Rodrigez V, Bodey GP (1975) Amikacin therapy of infections in neutropenic patients. *Am. J. Med. Sci., 270,* 453.

66. Moore RD, Lietman PS, Smith CR (1987) Clinical response to aminoglycoside therapy: importance of the ratio of peak concentration to minimal inhibitory concentration. *J. Infect. Dis., 155,* 93.

67. Young LS, Hindler J (1986) Aminoglycoside resistance: a worldwide perspective. *Am. J. Med., 80, Suppl 6B,* 15.

68. Gerding DN, Larson TA (1986) Resistance surveillance programs and the incidence of gram-negative bacillary resistance to amikacin from 1967 to 1985. *Am. J. Med., 80, Suppl 6B,* 22.

69. Gerding DN, Larson TA (1985) Aminoglycoside resistance in gram-negative bacilli during increased amikacin use. *Am. J. Med., 79, Suppl 1A,* 1.

70. Huovinen P, Gronroos P, Herva E, Karila ML, Renkonen OV, Toivanen P (1984) Aminoglycoside resistance among blood culture isolates. *J. Clin. Microbiol., 20,* 65.

71. Gribble MJ, Chow AW, Naiman SC, Smith JA et al (1983) Prospective trial of pipercillin monotherapy vs. carboxymethylpenicillin aminoglycoside combination regimens. *Antimicrob. Agents Chemother., 24,* 388.

72. Anderson ET, Young LS, Hewilt WL (1977) Antimicrobial synergism in the therapy of gram-negative rod bacteremia. *Chemotherapy, 24,* 45.

73. Klastersky J, Zinner SH (1982) Synergistic combinations of antibiotics in gram-negative bacillary infections. *Rev. Infect. Dis., 4,* 294.

74. Reyes MP, Lerner AM (1982) Current problems in the treatment of infective endocarditis due to *Pseudomonas aeruginosa. Rev. Infect. Dis., 4,* 45.

75. Klastersky YJ, Glauser M, Schimpff S, Zinner S, Gaya H (1986) Prospective randomized comparisons of three antibiotic regimens for empirical therapy of suspected bacteremic infections in febrile granulocytopenic patients. *Antimicrob. Agents Chemother., 29,* 263.

76. Klastersky J, Meunier-Carpentier F, Prevost JU (1977) Significance of antibiotic synergism for the outcome of gram-negative sepsis. *Am. J. Med. Sci., 273,* 157.

77. Siegenthaler WE, Bonetti A, Luthy R (1986) Aminoglycoside antibiotics in infectious diseases. *Am. J. Med., 80, Suppl 6B,* 2.

78. Smith CR, Baughman KL, Edwards CQ, Rogers JF, Lietman PS (1977) Controlled comparison of amikacin and gentamicin. *N. Engl. J. Med., 296,* 349.

79. Smith CR, Lipski JL, Laskin OL, Hellman DB, Mellits ED, Longstreth J, Lietman

PS (1980) Double-blind comparison of the nephrotoxicity and auditory toxicity of gentamicin and tobramicin. *N. Engl. J. Med., 302,* 1106.

80. DeJace P, Klastersky J (1986) Comparative review of combination therapy two beta-lactams verus beta-lactam plus aminoglycoside. *Am. J. Med., 80, Suppl 6B,* 29.
81. Sanders CC (1983) Novel resistance selected by the new expanded-spectrum cephalosporins. *J. Infect. Dis., 147,* 585.
82. The EORTC International Antimicrobial Therapy Project Group (1987) Three antibiotic regimens in the treatment of infections in granulocytopenic patients. *J. Infect. Dis., 137,* 14.
83. Gurwith M, Brunton JC, Lank B, Ronald AR, Harding GKM, McCullough DW (1978) Granulocytopenia in hospitalized patients: a prospective comparison of two antibiotic regimens in the empiric therapy of febrile patients. *Am. J. Med., 64,* 127.
84. Liu PV (1966) The role of various proteins of *Pseudomonas aeruginosa* in its pathogenesis III. Identity of the lethal toxins produced in vitro and in vivo. *J. Infect. Dis., 116,* 481.
85. Leppla SH (1976) Large scale purification and characterization of the exotoxin of *Pseudomonas aeruginosa. Infect. Immun., 14,* 1077.
86. Vasil ML, Kabat D, Iglewski BH (1977) Structure-activity relationships of an exotoxin of *Pseudomonas aeruginosa. Infect. Immun., 16,* 353.
87. Pavlovskis OR, Gordon FB (1972) *Pseudomonas aeruginosa* exotoxin: effect on cell culture. *J. Infect. Dis., 129,* 631.
88. Iglewski BH, Kabat D (1975) NAD-dependent inhibition of protein synthesis by *Pseudomonas aeruginosa* toxin. *Proc. Natl Acad. Sci. USA, 72,* 2284.
89. Chung DW, Collier RJ (1977) Enzymatically active peptide from the adenosine diphosphate-ribosylation toxin of *Pseudomonas aeruginosa. Infect. Immun., 16,* 832.
90. Pollack M, Taylor NS, Callahan LT (1977) Exotoxin production by clinical isolates of *Pseudomonas aeruginosa. Infect. Immun., 15,* 776.
91. Ohman DE, Burns RP, Iglewski BH (1980) Corneal injection in mice with toxin A and elastase mutant of *Pseudomonas aeruginosa. J. Infect. Dis., 142,* 547.
92. Sanai Y, Takeshi K, Homma JY, Kamata H (1978) Production of exotoxin, protease and elastase of *Pseudomonas aeruginosa* strains isolated from patients and environmental specimens. *Jpn. J. Exp. Med., 48,* 553.
93. Pavlovskis DR, Pollack M, Callahan LT, Iglewski BH (1977) Passive protection by antitoxin in experimental *Pseudomonas aeruginosa* burn infection. *Infect. Immun., 18,* 596.
94. Cryz Jr SJ, Furer E, Germanier R (1983) Protection against *Pseudomonas aeruginosa* infection in a murine burn wound sepsis model by passive transfer of antitoxin A, antielastase and antilipopolysaccharide. *Infect. Immun., 39,* 1072.
95. Walker HC, Mcleod Jr CG, Leppla SH, Mason Jr AD (1979) Evaluation of *Pseudomonas aeruginosa* toxin A in experimental rat burn wound sepsis. *Infect. Immun., 25,* 828.
96. Pavlovskis OR, Edman DC, Leppla SH, Wretlind B, Lewis L, Martin KE (1981) Protection against experimental *Pseudomonas aeruginosa* infection in mice by active immunization with exotoxin A. *Infect. Immun., 32,* 681.
97. Morihara K, Tsuzuki H, Oka T, Inone H, Ebats M (1965) *Pseudomonas aeruginosa* elastase. *J. Biol. Chem., 240,* 3295.
98. Kamaharajo K, Homma JY, Aoyama Y, Okada K, Morihara K (1975) Effects of protease and elastase from *Pseudomonas aeruginosa* on skin. *Jpn. J. Exp. Med., 45,* 79.

99a. Kamaharajo K, Abe C, Homma JY, Kamaro M, Gotoh E, Tanaka Y, Morihara K (1974) Corneal ulcers caused by protease and elastase from *Pseudomonas aeruginosa*. *Jpn. J. Exp. Med.*, *44*, 435.

99b. Wretlined B, Heden L, Sjoberg L, Wadstrom T (1973) Production of enzymes and toxins by hospital strains of *Pseudomonas aeruginosa* in relation to serotype and phage-typing pattern. *J. Med. Microbiol.*, *6*, 91.

100. Schultz DR, Miller KD (1974) Elastase of *Pseudomonas aeruginosa*: inactivation of complement and complement-derived chemotactic and phagocytic factors. *Infect. Immun.*, *10*, 128.

101. Morihara K, Tsuzuki H, Oda K (1979) Protease and elastase of *Pseudomonas aeruginosa*: inactivation of human plasma alpha-1 proteinase inhibitor. *Infect. Immun.*, *24*, 188.

102. Doring RJ, Obernesser HJ, Botzenhart HJ (1981) Extracellular toxins of *Pseudomonas aeruginosa*. II. Effect of two proteases on human immunoglobulins IgG, IgA and secretory IgA. *Zentralbl. Bakteriol. Microbiol. Hyg. (A)*, *249*, 89.

103. Snell K, Helder IA, Leppla SH, Sallinger CB (1978) Role of exotoxin and protease as possible virulence factors in experimental infections with *Pseudomonas aeruginosa*. *Infect. Immun.*, *19*, 839.

104. Homma JY, Abe C, Tanamoto K, Hirao Y, Morihara K, Tsuzuki H, Yanagaura R, Honda E, Aoi Y, Fugimoto Y, Goryo M, Imazeki N, Noda H, Ghoda A, Takeuchi S, Ishihara T (1978) Effectiveness of immunization with single and multicomponent vaccines prepared from a common antigen (OEP), protease and elastase toxoids of *Pseudomonas aeruginosa* on protection against hemorrhagic pneumonia in mink due to *Pseudomonas aeruginosa*. *Jpn. J. Exp. Med.*, *48*, 111.

105. Kawaharajo K, Homma JY (1977) Effects of elastase, protease and common antigen (OEP) from *Pseudomonas aeruginosa* on protection against burns in mice. *Jpn. J. Exp. Med.*, *47*, 495.

106. Pavlovskis OR, Wretlind BP (1979) Assessment of protease (elastase) as a *Pseudomonas aeruginosa* virulence factor in experimental mouse burn infection. *Infect. Immun.*, *24*, 181.

107. Morihara K (1963) Metalloprotease. I. purification and general properties. *Biochim. Biophys. Acta*, *73*, 113.

108. Esselman MT, Liu PV (1960) Lecithinase production by gram-negative bacteria. *J. Bacteriol.*, *81*, 939.

109. Berka RM, Vasil ML (1982) Phospholipase C (heat labile hemolysin) of *Pseudomonas aeruginosa*: purification and preliminary characterization. *J. Bacteriol.*, *182*, 239.

110. Kurioka S, Liu PV (1967) Effect of the hemolysin of *Pseudomonas aeruginosa* on phosphatides and on phospholipase activity. *J. Bacteriol.*, *93*, 670.

111. Wilkinson SG, Galbraith K (1975) Studies of lipopolysaccharide from *Pseudomonas aeruginosa*. *Eur. J. Biochem.*, *52*, 331.

112. Chester IR, Meadow PM, Pitt TL (1973) The relationship between the O-antigenic lipopolysaccharides and serological specificity in strains of *Pseudomonas aeruginosa* of different O-serotypes. *J. Gen. Microbiol.*, *78*, 305.

113. Fisher MW (1977) A polyvalent human gamma globulin immune to *Pseudomonas aeruginosa*: passive protection of mice against lethal infection. *J. Infect. Dis.*, *136*, *Suppl*, 181.

114. Pier GB, Sidberry HF, Sadoff JC (1981) High molecular-weight polysaccharice antigen from *Pseudomonas aeruginosa* immunotype 2. *Infect. Immun.*, *34*, 461.

115. Pier GB (1982) Cross protection by *Pseudomonas aeruginosa* polysaccharides. *Infect. Immun.*, *38*, 1117.

116. Young LS, Armstrong D (1972) Human immunity to *Pseudomonas aeruginosa*. I. In-vitro interaction of bacteria, polymorphonuclear leukocytes and serum factors. *J. Infect. Dis.*, *126*, 257.

117. Sadoff JC, Futrovski Sl, Sidberry HF, Iglewski BH, Seid RC (1982) Detoxified lipopo-lysaccharide-protein conjugates. In: Weinstein L, Fields BN (Eds), *Seminars in Infectious Disease*, p. 346. Thieme-Stratton, New York.

118. Harvath C, Andersen BR (1976) Evaluation of type-specific and non-type-specific *Pseudomonas* vaccine for treatment of *Pseudomonas* sepsis during granulocytopenia. *Infect. Immun.*, *13*, 1139.

119. Kazmierowski JA, Reynolds HY, Kaufman JC, Durbin WA, Graw Jr RG, Devlin HB (1977) Experimental pneumonia due to *Pseudomonas aeruginosa* in leukopenic dogs: prolongation of survival by combined treatment with passive antibody to *Pseudomonas* and granulocyte transfusions. *J. Infect. Dis.*, *135*, 438.

120. Penington JE (1979) Lipopolysaccharide *Pseudomonas* vaccine: efficacy against pul-monary infection with *Pseudomonas aeruginosa*. *J. Infect. Dis.*, *140*, 73.

121. Penington JE, Hickey WF, Blackwood LL (1981) Active immunization with lipopoly-saccharide *Pseudomonas* antigen for chronic *Pseudomonas* bronchopneumonia in gui-nea pigs. *J. Clin. Invest.*, *68*, 1140.

122. Pier GB, Sidberry HF, Zolyomi S, Sadoff JC (1978) Isolation and characterization of a high-molecular weight polysaccharide from slime of *Pseudomonas aeruginosa*. *Infect. Immun.*, *22*, 908.

123. McManus AT, Moody EE, Mason AD (1980) Bacterial motility: a component in ex-perimental *Pseudomonas aeruginosa* burn wound sepsis. *Burns*, *6*, 235.

124. Montie TC, Doyle-Hantzinger D, Craven RC, Holder IA (1982) Loss of virulence as-sociated with absence of flagellum in an isogenic mutant of *Pseudomonas aeruginosa* in burned mouse model. *Infect. Immun.*, *38*, 1296.

125. Holder IA, Wheeler R, Montie TC (1982) Flagellar preparation from *Pseudomonas aeruginosa*: animal protection studies. *Infect. Immun.*, *35*, 276.

126. Young LS, Armstrong D (1972) Human immunity to *Pseudomonas aeruginosa*. I. In vitro interaction of bacteria, polymorphonuclear leukocytes and serum factors. *J. Infect. Dis.*, *126*, 257.

127. Pollack M, Young LS (1979) Protective activity of antibodies to exotoxin-A lipopoly-saccharide at the onset of *Pseudomonas aeruginosa* septicemia in man. *J. Clin. Invest.*, *63*, 276.

128. Cross AS, Sadoff JC, Iglewski BH, Sokol PA (1980) Evidence for the role of toxin A in the pathogenesis of infection with *Pseudomonas aeruginosa* in humans. *J. Infect. Dis.*, *142*, 538.

129. Feller I, Pierson C (1968) *Pseudomonas* vaccine and hyperimmune plasma for burned patients. *Arch. Surg.*, *97*, 225.

130. Sachs A (1970) Active immunoprophylaxis in burns with new multivalent vaccine. *Lancet*, *2*, 959.

131. Hanessian S, Regan W, Watson D (1971) Isolation and characterization of antigenic components of a new heptavalent *Pseudomonas* vaccine. *Nature (London)*, *229*, 209.

132. Fisher MV, Devlin HB, Gnabasic F (1969) New immuno type schema for *Pseudomo-nas aeruginosa* based on protective antigens. *J. Bacteriol.*, *98*, 835.

133. Alexander JW, Fisher MW, MacMillan BG (1971) Immunologic control of *Pseudo-*

monas infection in burn patients: a clinical evaluation. *Arch. Surg.*, *102*, 31.

134. Alexander JW, Fisher M (1974) Immunization against *Pseudomonas* infection after thermal injury. *J. Infect. Dis.*, *130*, S152.

135. Jones CE, Alexander JW, Fisher M (1973) Clinical evaluation of *Pseudomonas* hyperimmune globulin. *J. Surg. Res.*, *14*, 87.

136. Young LS, Meyer RD, Armstrong D (1973) *Pseudomonas aeruginosa* vaccine in cancer patients. *Ann. Infect. Med.*, *79*, 518.

137. Haghbin MD, Armstrong D, Murphy ML (1973) Controlled prospective trial of *Pseudomonas aeruginosa* vaccine in children with acute leukemia. *Cancer*, *32*, 761.

138. Penington JE, Reynolds HY, Wood RE, Robinson RA, Levine AS (1975) Use of a *Pseudomonas aeruginosa* vaccine in patients with acute leukemia and cystic fibrosis. *J. Infect. Dis.*, *58*, 629.

139. Poll Jr HC, Border S, Aldrete JA (1973) Prevention of *Pseudomonas* respiratory infection in a surgical intensive care unit. *Ann. Surg.*, *177*, 607.

140. Alexander JW, Fischer MW (1976) Immunization against *Pseudomonas* in infection after thermal injury. *J. Infect. Dis.*, *130*, *Suppl*, 152.

141. Penington JE, Miler JJ (1979) Evaluation of a new polyvalent *Pseudomonas* vaccine in respiratory infections. *Infect. Immun.*, *31*, 73.

142. Klinger JD, Cash HA, Wood RE, Miler JJ (1983) Protective immunization against chronic *Pseudomonas aeruginosa* pulmonary infection in rats. *Infect. Immun.*, *39*, 1377.

143. Jones RJ, Roe EA, Gupta JL (1979) Controlled trials of polyvalent *Pseudomonas* vaccine in burns. *Lancet*, *1*, 977.

144. Jones RJ, Roe EA, Gupta JC (1980) Controlled trial of *Pseudomonas* immunoglobulin and vaccine in burn patients. *Lancet*, *2*, 1263.

145. Abe C, Tanamoto K, Homma JY (1977) Infection protective property of the common antigen (OEP) of *Pseudomonas aeruginosa* and its chemical composition. *Jpn. J. Exp. Med.*, *47*, 393.

146. Homma JY (1980) Role of exoenzymes and exotoxin in the pathogenicity of *Pseudomonas aeruginosa* and the development of a new vaccine. *Jpn. J. Exp. Med.*, *50*, 149.

147. Seid Jr RC, Sadoff JC (1981) Preparation and characterization of detoxified lipopolysaccharide-protein conjugate. *J. Biol. Chem.*, *256*, 7305.

148. Pier GP (1982) Safety and immunogenicity of high molecular weight polysaccharide vaccine from immunotype I *Pseudomonas aeruginosa*. *J. Clin. Invest.*, *69*, 303.

149. Cryz Jr SJ, Friedman RL, Pavlovskis OR, Iglewski BH (1981) Effect of formalin on *Pseudomonas aeruginosa* toxin A: biological, chemical and immunochemical studies. *Infect. Immun.*, *32*, 759.

150. Cryz Jr SJ, Friedman RL, Iglewski BH (1980) Isolation and characterization of a *Pseudomonas aeruginosa* mutant producing a nontoxic immunologically cross reactive (CRM) toxin A protein. *Proc. Natl Acad. Sci. USA*, *77*, 7199.

151. Cryz Jr SJ, Pavlovskis OR, Iglewski BH (1982) Chemical and genetic approaches to making *Pseudomonas aeruginosa* toxin A toxoid. In: Robbins JB, Hill JC, Sadoff JC (Eds), *Seminars in Infectious Disease, Vol 4. Bacterial Vaccines*, p. 70. Thieme-Stratton, New York.

152. Woods AE, Straus DC, Johnson Jr WG, Berry VK, Bass JA (1980) Role of pili in adherence of *Pseudomonas aeruginosa* to mammalian buccal epithelial cells. *Infect. Immun.*, *29*, 1146.

153. Hooke AM, Arroyo PJ, Oeschger MP, Bellanti JA (1982) Temperature sensitive mutants of *Pseudomonas aeruginosa*: isolation and preliminary immunological evaluation. *Infect. Immun.*, *38*, 136.

154. Sordelli DO, Cerquetti MC, Hooke AM, Bellanti JA (1983) Enhancement of *Pseudomonas aeruginosa* lung clearance after local immunization with a temperature-sensitive mutant. *Infect. Immun., 39,* 1275.

155. Lieberman MM (1978) *Pseudomonas* ribosomal vaccines: preparation, properties and immunogenicity. *Infect. Immun., 21,* 76.

156. Lieberman MM, Wright GL, Wolcott KM, McKissock-Desoto DC (1980) Polyvalent antisera to *Pseudomonas* ribosomal vaccines: protection of mice against clinically isolated strains. *Infect. Immun., 29,* 489.

157. Ziegler EJ, Douglas H, Sherman JE, Davis CE, Brande AI (1973) Treatment of *E. coli* and *Klebsiella* bacteremia in agranulocytic animals with antiserum to a UDP-gal epimerase-deficient mutant. *J. Immunol., 111,* 433.

158. Ziegler EJ, McCufchan JA, Douglas H, Brande AI (1975) Prevention of lethal *Pseudomonas* bacteremia with epimerase-deficient *E.coli* antiserum. *Trans. Assoc. Am. Physicians, 88,* 101.

159. Woods DE, Cryz Jr SJ, Friedman RL, Iglewski BH (1982) The contribution of toxin A and elastase to virulence of *Pseudomonas aeruginosa* in chronic lung infections of rats. *Infect. Immun., 36,* 1223.

CHAPTER 42

Monotherapy in neutropenic cancer patients

MARC RUBIN and PHILIP A. PIZZO

The concepts underlying the use of antibiotics in neutropenic cancer patients have not changed substantially since the early 1970s, when the importance of an empirical approach was first recognized. Indeed, some of the earliest empirical regimens consisting of aminoglycoside-containing antibiotic combinations remain viable therapeutic options today, and still represent the standard against which newer regimens must be measured. However, changes in the host at risk and the spectrum of infecting pathogens, along with the development of newer antimicrobial agents, have generated alternatives to aminoglycoside-containing combinations for empirical management of fever in granulocytopenic patients. These include combinations of β-lactam antibiotics, as well as selected single agents for use as 'monotherapy'. While the concept of empirical monotherapy in this population is not a new one, only in recent years have specific agents been developed with properties rendering them potential candidates for monotherapy. This Chapter will review the experience to date with the use of single-agent antibiotic therapy for the empirical treatment of febrile granulocytopenic cancer patients, and evaluate the current role for such an approach.

EMPIRICAL ANTIBIOTIC THERAPY – HISTORICAL PERSPECTIVE

During the 1960s, as cytotoxic chemotherapy became the primary therapeutic modality for the treatment of malignancy, a new population of patients was generated that was at increased risk for the development of serious infections. While many abnormalities in host defense contributed to the high risk of infection, granulocytopenia emerged as the most important predisposing factor (1). It quickly became apparent that delays in institution of antibiotic therapy until the infecting pathogen was identified often led to disastrous consequences, particularly if a gram-negative organism was responsible (2–6). Moreover, it became evident that when a granulocytopenic patient became febrile, routine clinical evaluation and diagnostic laboratory measurements could not reliably predict the presence or absence of infection (7).

Antimicrobial Agents Annual 3
P.K. Peterson and J. Verhoef, editors
© Elsevier Science Publishers BV, 1988

In that context, then, early institution of empirical antimicrobial agents became the standard of care when approaching a neutropenic patient with fever. While gram-positive bacteria (especially *Staphylococcus aureus*) were the organisms isolated most frequently from immunocompromised patients during the 1950s and the early 1960s (8–11), a shift occurred during the later 1960s and 1970s when gram-negative organisms emerged as the most commonly encountered pathogens. *Pseudomonas aeruginosa*, *Escherichia coli* and *Klebsiella pneumoniae* accounted for the majority of these isolates. Initial empirical antibiotic regimens were formulated, then, to provide maximal coverage against the gram-negative bacilli (12, 13) while maintaining a broad spectrum of activity against the diverse array of bacteria seen in this population. The goal, however, was not to provide effective therapy for all possible infecting micro-organisms, but to prevent the early morbidity associated with delayed or inadequate therapy of gram-negative pathogens.

In order to achieve the requisite bactericidal activity for effectiveness against these organisms (14) and to decrease the emergence of resistant isolates, most empirical regimens consisted of combinations of antibiotics. During the 1970s and early 1980s, this included an aminoglycoside (e.g. gentamicin, tobramycin or amikacin), in combination with an 'antipseudomonal' penicillin (e.g. carbenicillin or ticarcillin), and often with a β-lactamase stable or 'antistaphylococcal' β-lactam (e.g. nafcillin, oxacillin, or a first-generation cephalosporin) (15, 16). Central to the argument favoring the use of such combinations has been the large body of data demonstrating either improved efficacy in vitro or an improved clinical outcome when antibiotic combinations possessing synergistic activity against the gram-negative bacilli were employed (17–27). While a variety of highly effective combinations exist (15), no single regimen has been shown to be clearly superior. Moreover, it is unlikely that any new agent or combination of agents will be ideal in all settings.

ALTERNATIVES TO AMINOGLYCOSIDE-CONTAINING REGIMENS

Given these findings, are there still valid reasons to reconsider the role of aminoglycoside-containing regimens in the treatment of neutropenic patients and, if so, do viable alternatives exist? The answer to these questions is 'yes'. Firstly, the spectrum of infecting pathogens has again changed. During the 1980s, gram-positive organisms have re-emerged in many centers as the predominate organisms being encountered (28–39). Gram-negative isolates, while still important, have decreased in both a relative and absolute sense. At the same time, concomitant with their increased use, aminoglycoside-resistant isolates have increased in prevalence in some centers. In addition, the spectrum of neutropenic patients has become more varied, with more solid-tumor patients now receiving chemotherapeutic regimens causing granulocytopenia than was the case in previous years. As more potentially toxic drugs are employed in the management of the underlying malignancies, concerns about additive toxicities of aminoglycosides and these other agents (e.g. cyclosporin or cisplatin) arise. The need for monitoring aminoglycoside levels, as well as the expense and risk of error related to preparation and administration of combination regimens are also appropriate concerns. In this context, new antibiotic developments have provided us with possible alternatives to aminoglycoside-containing regimens. At present, these new regimens include 'double β-lactam' regimens (15, 40), as well as selected single agents for use as monotherapy (41–45). While certain β-lactam combinations are quite effective, potential disadvantages include antagonism (46) and increased cost. The advantages and possible drawbacks of monotherapy are discussed below.

MONOTHERAPY – THE EARLY EXPERIENCE AND CURRENT OPTIONS

The concept of using a single antibiotic for empirical therapy in granulocytopenic patients is not a new one. Early on, it was established that despite good sensitivity patterns *in vitro* against gram-negative organisms, aminoglycosides were not acceptable choices for single-agent therapy in neutropenic patients (47–51). Likewise, early studies demonstrated that carboxypenicillins (carbenicillin and ticarcillin) were insufficient as single agents (52–56). Failure was due primarily to their inadequate coverage of certain gram-negative aerobes (particularly *E. coli, Serratia* spp. and *Klebsiella*) (54–56), as well as to the development of resistant *Pseudomonas aeruginosa* isolates during therapy (52, 53).

It was hoped that the development of the ureidopenicillins (mezlocillin, piperacillin, azlocillin) would circumvent these deficiencies, since they have improved activity against these organisms (57–59). However, their advantages *in vitro* have not translated into clinical efficacy. The two published studies that utilized mezlocillin as monotherapy concluded that it was inadequate in this setting (60, 61). Unacceptably low response rates were seen not only with *Pseudomonas* infections, but also with other serious gram-negative as well as *Staphylococcus aureus* infections, often despite sensitivity in vitro. In addition, a high number of resistant organisms were isolated during therapy (61).

Although the other ureidopenicillins have not been studied as single agents in neutropenic patients, one study employed a combination of piperacillin and vancomycin (62), in which piperacillin provided the only coverage of gram-negative aerobes. Piperacillin alone offered inadequate gram-negative coverage, as the responses of *P. aeruginosa* infections were inadequate.

At present, certain third-generation cephalosporins are among the most promising for use as empirical monotherapy for febrile neutropenic patients. As a class, they have been the most extensively studied, primarily over the past 5 years. Other potential candidates whose efficacy has been less well characterized in this setting include the carbapenems (e.g. imipenem-cilastatin), the monobactams (e.g. aztreonam), and the quinolones (e.g. ciprofloxacin).

THE THIRD-GENERATION CEPHALOSPORINS

Many of the third-generation cephalosporins have, as a class, a broad spectrum of activity that includes predominantly the aerobic gram-positive and gram-negative bacteria (63, 64). There are, however, considerable differences among the specific agents. For example, certain agents possess some antianaerobic activity (e.g. moxalactam), while others have relatively little (e.g. ceftazidime). Some have potent antipseudomonal activity (e.g. ceftazidime, cefoperazone, cefsulodin), whereas others have virtually none (e.g. cefotaxime, ceftriaxone, ceftizoxime, moxalactam). Although the frequency of *Pseudomonas* infections appears to have decreased over recent years, good antipseudomonal activity is still an essential quality of an empirical regimen in a neutropenic patient, since untreated or inadequately treated infections due to *P. aeruginosa* can be rapidly fatal.

Despite their expanded activity against certain pathogens, there are some notable deficiencies in the antimicrobial spectrum of the third-generation cephalosporins that should be kept in the forefront when treating a neutropenic patient. Firstly, all are less active than the first-generation cephalosporins or 'antistaphylococcal' penicillins against gram-positive cocci. More specifically, none possesses any significant activity against methicillin-resistant staphylococci, the enterococci, or *Listeria monocytogenes*, all of which are potential pathogens in a granulocytopenic patient. It is likely, however, that these deficiencies will not vitiate their potential in this setting, as some of these gram-positive isolates are associated with relatively low morbidity, and can be treated after their isolation with expeditious addition of appropriate agents (as discussed below).

During the last 5 years, a number of studies have been published evaluating the use of third-generation cephalosporins as single agents in the treatment of oncologic patients. The specific agents that have been studied include ceftazidime (65–79), cefoperazone (80, 81), moxalactam (82, 83), cefotaxime (84), and ceftizoxime (85). Despite the number of published studies, many have been limited by one of several problems including: inadequate coverage provided by the study drug or control regimen, thus artificially 'favoring' one of the regimens; a non-random study design; and entry of only small numbers of patients, often with non-homogeneous characteristics (e.g. with regard to neutropenia or underlying disease). Furthermore, the methods of data assessment and evaluation that have been employed do not always cast the data in a context that is realistic for the neutropenic host. Reviews and critiques of many of the earlier studies mentioned above have been published (41, 43–47, 75).

THE RECENT EXPERIENCE

During the past year, two prospective randomized studies have been published evaluating the use of ceftazidime alone as empirical therapy for febrile granulocytopenic cancer patients (74, 78). We have recently reported our results from the

National Cancer Institute (NCI) comparing monotherapy using ceftazidime to combination therapy using cefalotin, gentamicin and carbenicillin (KGC) (74). While some investigators have argued that the definitive test of a new empirical antimicrobial regimen is the treatment of documented bacterial infections occurring in neutropenic patients (86), in our judgement the most salient objective with respect to the evaluation of efficacy is the impact on survival of the patient through the neutropenic episode. The rationale for empirical antibiotics is to prevent the early morbidity and mortality associated with untreated or inadequately treated infections, not to definitively treat all possible infections *per primum*. It is during the initial 72 hours of treatment, before the pre-treatment culture results are available, that the therapy is 'truly' empirical. After this time period, appropriate adjustment of the initial antibiotic regimen can be made, if necessary, based on sensitivity data, or changing clinical status. Accordingly, we evaluated patients with respect to success of therapy (alive *vs* dead) at 72 hours after entry, and also for the remainder of the neutropenic episode.

It is during this remaining period of neutropenia that patients are most likely to require some modifications of the initial regimen. Indeed, the need for modification, regardless of the initial regimen, is most likely to occur as the duration of the neutropenic episode increases (87). This is *not* necessarily a reflection of failure of the primary regimen *per se*, but instead representative of the limitations of any regimen in treating a patient at risk for development of multiple infectious complications. Examples of such modifications may include: the addition of an antianaerobic agent for patients who develop necrotizing gingivitis or perianal tenderness; addition of vancomycin for a resistant gram-positive infection; empirical addition of amphotericin B for persistent fever; addition of trimethoprim + sulfamethoxazole for suspected protozoal infection; or the addition of acyclovir for herpes simplex infections. In addition, patients were stratified for analysis according to whether their initial pre-treatment workup revealed a documented infection, or left the source of the fever undetermined (FUO).

In the NCI study, 550 episodes of fever in neutropenic patients were evaluated, with 268 randomized to receive combination therapy, and 282 to monotherapy. The mean age in both groups was approximately 28 years, with a range of 1–79 years, reflective of the fact that patients were enrolled from both the pediatric and adult cancer services. The two study groups were comparable with respect to the underlying neoplasm (40% *vs* 45% leukemia and lymphomas, 60% *vs* 55% solid tumors) as well as the mean initial granulocyte count (144 *vs* 157), with 60% of episodes in both arms having granulocyte counts of less than $100/mm^3$ at randomization. In terms of the initial diagnosis or cause of the presenting fever (documented infection *vs* FUO), 72% of the 550 episodes were classified as having an FUO, and 28% as documented infection. Among the microbiologically defined infections, 56% were gram-positive organisms, 40% were gram-negative, and 4% were anaerobes.

The comparative results of the two regimens at the 72-hour or 'early evaluation' are shown in Table 1. The overall success for both the combination and the mono-

Table 1   *Early evaluation of monotherapy versus combination therapy for episodes of fever in patients with neutropenia*

Status at early evaluation	Unexplained fever		Documented infections	
	Combination	Single agent	Combination	Single agent
		No. of episodes (%)		
Evaluable episodes	204	190	64	92
Afebrile at 72 hours	126 (62)	114 (60)	37 (58)	54 (59)
Success without modification	197 (97)	176 (93)	41 (64)	45 (49)
Success with modification	7 (3)	13 (7)	22 (34)	45 (49)
Addition of antibiotics	7 (3)	13 (7)	15 (23)	33 (36)
Addition of antifungal agent	0	1 (0.5)	0	1 (1)
Addition of antiviral agent	0	0	1 (2)	1 (1)
Crossover	2 (1)	1 (0.5)	3 (5)	4 (4)
Change to specific therapy	0	0	3 (5)	8 (9)
Failure	0	1 (1)	1 (2)	2 (2)
Total initial successes	204 (100)	189 (99)	63 (98)	90 (98)

The early evaluation was made after 72 hours of the randomly assigned therapy. 'Combination' denotes therapy with cefalotin, gentamicin, and carbenicillin; 'Single agent' denotes therapy with ceftazidime. Modified from Table 4, Ref. 74.

therapy groups was equally high (98–100%) regardless of whether patients presented with a documented infection or FUO. For episodes presenting with FUO, the vast majority had a successful outcome without the need for modification, in both the combination and single-agent groups (97% and 93%, respectively). Overall, episodes presenting with a documented infection required an early modification more often (67/167, 40%) than FUO episodes (20/394, 5%), and accounted for the majority (67/87, 77%) of all modifications made at the early evaluation point. The greater number of modifications made in the monotherapy group compared to the combination therapy group primarily reflected the need for additional gram-positive coverage with vancomycin (21/282, 7%, *vs* 10/268, 4%, respectively). In addition, more episodes in the monotherapy group were randomized on a separate study, to switch to pathogen-specific therapy for a microbiologically defined isolate, than were episodes in the combination-therapy group (9 *vs* 5, respectively); these episodes were also scored as 'modifications'.

The comparative results at the resolution of neutropenia are seen in Table 2. Again, the overall success for the monotherapy or combination therapy group was equivalent for those patients presenting with FUO (98% *vs* 91%, respectively), or

Table 2 *Overall evaluation of monotherapy versus combination therapy for episodes of fever in patients with neutropenia*

Status at overall evaluation	Unexplained fever		Documented infections	
	Combination	Single agent	Combination	Single agent
		No. of episodes (%)		
Evaluable episodes	204	190	64	92
Success without modification	159 (78)	147 (77)	20 (31)	28 (30
Success with modification	40 (20)	39 (21)	38 (60)	54 (59)
Addition of antibiotics	32 (16)	29 (15)	24 (38)	46 (50)
Addition of antifungal agent	23 (11)	21 (11)	12 (19)	11 (12)
Addition of antiviral agent	1 (0.5)	4 (2)	1 (2)	2 (3)
Crossover	8 (4)	14 (7)	7 (11)	15 (16)
Change to specific therapy	0	0	13 (20)	12 (13)
Failure	5 (2)	4 (2)	6 (9)	10 (11)
Total initial successes	199 (98)	186 (98)	58 (91)	82 (89)

The overall evaluation was made at the time of the resolution of neutropenia. Combination denotes therapy with cefalotin, gentamicin and carbenicillin; single agent denotes therapy and ceftazidime. Modified from Table 5, Ref. 74.

documented infection (89% *vs* 91%, respectively). Not unexpectedly, more modifications were made by the Overall Evaluation point than within the first 72 hours, regardless of the antibiotic regimen or the initial diagnosis. The majority of episodes in both treatment groups who presented with FUO were treated successfully without modifications (78% *vs* 77%). In contrast, the majority of the episodes presenting with documented infection required some modification during the course of neutropenia in order to achieve a successful outcome. It should be emphasized, however, that for this group, the need for modification was equivalent for the monotherapy and combination regimens (59% *vs* 60%, respectively), and did not reflect a specific deficiency in either regimen.

Thus, the data from this trial indicate that monotherapy with ceftazidime represent a viable option to more standard combination antibiotic regimens, such as cefalotin, gentamicin and carbenicillin. With appropriate modifications, equivalent numbers of patients in both groups can be treated successfully. Such modifications should be expected during the course of neutropenia, particularly for patients who present with a documented infection, irrespective of the initial empirical regimen.

The other recently published, randomized prospective study employing a monotherapeutic approach, treated 102 patients with fever and neutropenia with either ceftazidime alone or a combination of ceftazidime and cefalotin (78). The rationale for this particular combination was based upon the need for modifications of ceftazidime in some patients in earlier studies, due to resistant gram-positive isolates (66, 71). The results of the study found comparable clinical and bacteriologic cure rates for both regimens, with no specific advantages seen in either (clinical response 77% for monotherapy, 88% combination; bacteriologic clearance 70% for monotherapy, 79% for combination). Both regimens had an equivalently lower bacteriologic clearance rate for gram-positive organisms (60%; primarily *Streptococcus faecalis* and *Streptococcus sanguis*), but these were treated successfully with addition of vancomycin. The investigators concluded that ceftazidime as a single agent is effective for empirical therapy in this setting, and that one should be prepared to modify therapy, particularly for resistant gram-positive isolates.

CONCERNS

Despite these studies, two important issues that relate to potential deficiencies in ceftazidime for use as monotherapy have been raised by investigators. First, the increasing incidence of gram-positive organisms in this patient population, many of which are resistant to, or inadequately covered, by non-vancomycin-containing regimens (e.g. enterococci, coagulase-negative staphylococci, or CDC group JK corynebacteria), has led some investigators to recommend that additional gram-positive coverage be added routinely to such empirical regimens (65, 67, 69, 88, 89). Second, some authorities still feel that an aminoglycoside should be included in the initial regimen to maximize gram-negative coverage, add synergistic activity, and decrease emergence of resistance (86). In order to address these issues, we analyzed the use of vancomycin and aminoglycosides in the 550 episodes of fever and neutropenia described above.

A gram-positive pathogen was isolated in 75 of the 550 episodes (14%), and accounted for 63% of the microbiologically documented infections. Fifty-three of these 75 organisms were isolated from the pre-antibiotic evaluation (i.e. 'primary' infections); the remaining 22 were responsible for secondary infections (97).

Of the 53 primary gram-positive organisms, 36 were staphylococcal species (approximately equal numbers of coagulase-positive and -negative staphylococci), 13 were streptococcal species, and 4 were polymicrobial. Vancomycin was ultimately used in the treatment of 26 of 53 (49%) of these episodes, but was added only after the identification of the pathogen in 25 of 26 cases. All 26 patients were successfully treated, without morbidity due to the 'delay' in institution of vancomycin therapy. In the 27 episodes in which vancomycin was not used, the isolates were sensitive to antibiotics in the initial regimen.

The secondary gram-positive infections were most commonly due to streptococcal species (mostly Group D streptococci) and staphylococcal species (mostly coagulase-negative). Vancomycin was ultimately utilized in 17 of these 22 episodes (77%), but was added only after the microbiologic identification in 14 of these 17 episodes. There was no mortality and no significant morbidity associated with withholding the addition of vancomycin until the patient's clinical or microbiologic course indicated that it was necessary. Thus, it does not appear that the inclusion of vancomycin as part of the initial empirical therapy (i.e. with ceftazidime) would have improved the overall results. In our study, routine use would have overtreated the majority of patients, and promoted a significant increase in the cost of antibiotic therapy. At present, we feel that vancomycin need *not* be routinely included in the initial empirical antibiotic therapy of febrile neutropenic cancer patients, but that it should be used judiciously based on microbiologic data or clinical parameters. Routine empirical use may be warranted at centers with a high incidence of certain anaerobic infections (69, 89) or methicillin-resistant *Staphylococcus aureus*.

Of the 282 episodes of fever in patients initially randomized to receive ceftazidime, 36 (13%) required the addition of an aminoglycoside at some time during the neutropenia. Of these, 24 had the aminoglycoside added as part of a crossover to the combination regimen (as dictated by the protocol) in response to hypotension (11 episodes), a new pulmonary infiltrate (7 episodes), a breakthrough bacteremia (3 episodes), or progressive clinical symptoms (3 episodes). Another 9 had an aminoglycoside added as a component of a different regimen, and 3 had the aminoglycoside added with ceftazidime as part of their initial empirical coverage. Patients with a documented infection received an aminoglycoside in 16 of 92 episodes (17%), compared to 20 of 190 episodes (11%) for those with an FUO. Overall, 27 of 36 (75%) of patients receiving an aminoglycoside survived. Of the 9 deaths, 3 were due to respiratory failure and culture-negative hypotension, 3 to invasive or disseminated fungal disease, and one each to *Legionella* pneumonia, cytomegalovirus pneumonia, and pulmonary hypertension secondary to multiple pulmonary emboli (41).

Thus, the majority (87%) of episodes did not require the addition of an aminoglycoside, and routine use would have exposed them unnecessarily to the potential for added toxicity, as well as added inconvenience and cost.

OTHER MONOTHERAPEUTIC OPTIONS

The carbapenems

The carbapenems represent a new class of β-lactam antibiotic, of which imipenem (available in combination with cilistatin) is a prototype. The spectrum of activity of imipenem is broader than the third-generation cephalosporins (90). In addition to those organisms susceptible to ceftazidime, imipenem also has activity against some coagulase-negative staphylococci, *Listeria*, enterococci, and anaerobes (including *Bacteroides fragilis*). It is inactive against methicillin-resistant *Staphylo-*

coccus aureus, and most non-*aeruginosa* strains of *Pseudomonas*. Therefore, it has potential as an agent for monotherapy in the neutropenic population (91).

Thus far, only one study has been published using imipenem-cilastatin for empirical monotherapy in febrile cancer patients (92). It was non-random, and not all episodes involved neutropenic patients. In the 27 patients with initial neutrophil counts of < 100, the response rate was 74%. The overall response rate in the study was 67%, with 76% of the 45 documented infections responding. Failures were reported with *S. aureus* and polymicrobial septicemias. Gram-negative infections responded well, although one *P. aeruginosa* isolate developed resistance to imipenem during therapy. While these results are encouraging, it is difficult to draw meaningful conclusions because of the non-random design, small study size, and heterogeneous patient population.

Currently, at the National Cancer Institute, we are conducting a randomized prospective study comparing imipenem-cilastatin to ceftazidime as initial empirical therapy for febrile neutropenic cancer patients. The results are still preliminary, with 126 evaluable episodes randomized (ceftazidime 65, imipenem 61). Thus far, at the 72-hour evaluation point, 100% of the patients in both arms were alive. Of patients with FUO's, 88% in the ceftazidime arm and 75% in the imipenem arm have been treated successfully without modification at 72 hours. Of patients with documented infections approximately half of the episodes in each treatment group required early modifications. At the late evaluation point (resolution of neutropenia), of those patients randomized to ceftazidime, 96% with documented infection and 95% with FUO have been treated successfully, compared to 91% and 100% respectively for the imipenem group. Modifications were indicated in the majority of episodes presenting with documented infections in either arm (ceftazidime 75%, imipenem 62%), and in the minority of episodes presenting with FUO (ceftazidime 41%, imipenem 35%).

Thus, preliminary results suggest that imipenem may be comparable to ceftazidime as empirical monotherapy. Further study is needed, however, to firmly establish its ultimate role in this setting. Moreover, a cautionary approach must be maintained even in an investigational setting, particularly if *P. aeruginosa* infections are encountered, as development of resistance to imipenem has been reported with this organism (93). In addition, imipenem should be avoided in patients with a history of seizures or significant intracranial disease (e.g. brain tumors) placing them at increased risk for seizures (94).

Monobactams

The monobactams are a class of naturally occurring, structurally unique, monocyclic β-lactam antibiotics, of which aztreonam is the prototype. It has significant activity against most aerobic gram-negative bacilli, but is relatively inactive against the gram-positive and anaerobic bacteria (95). Resistant isolates of *Enterobacter* and *Acinetobacter* have been reported (96). At present, there are no published studies in which aztreonam is used as single-agent therapy in neutropenic patients. However, one study did utilize a regimen in which aztreonam was combined with vancomycin (thus providing the only aerobic gram-negative coverage) and compared it to the combination of aztreonam, amikacin and vancomycin, as well as moxalactam and ticarcillin. The investigators found the 3 regimens equally effective in treating documented gram-negative infections (87–94%). Clearly, aztreonam's nearly complete lack of gram-positive coverage will preclude its use as true monotherapy. Whether it will have a role as a single agent for gram-negative coverage, or for treatment of documented gram-negative infections in neutropenic patients, will require further study.

Quinolones

The quinolones represent a class of antibiotic distinct from other agents based on structure and mechanism of action. They exert their antibiotic effect through inhibition of DNA gyrase, a bacterial enzyme involved in the supercoiling of DNA. Nalidixic acid was one of the first quinolones used clinically. Subsequently, new fluorinated quinolone derivatives have been developed (e.g. ciprofloxacin, pefloxacin, enoxacin and others), possessing a broad spectrum of activity that encompasses most bacterial pathogens encountered in neutropenic patients. To date, there are only limited data regarding their use in this population, but studies are currently underway. Presently, at the National Cancer Institute, we are evaluating on oral quinolone, ciprofloxacin, in neutropenic patients who defervesce after 72 hours of parenteral antibiotics. Clearly, an effective oral antibiotic for this group of patients might have significant practical impact on overall management.

SUMMARY

In summary, certain newer antimicrobial agents have provided us with monotherapeutic alternatives to combination regimens in the empirical treatment of febrile neutropenic cancer patients. The third-generation cephalosporins (particularly ceftazidime) have been studied most extensively. Data have been generated that support their potential as a single agents in this setting, although some investigators have raised theoretical concerns in this regard. Other potential candidates for empirical monotherapy include imipenem-cilistatin, as well as the quinolones. Studies are currently underway to help define their future role in this population. As with many areas in medicine, there is no 'one best approach'. Rather, each clinician should know the appropriate options, and attempt to tailor his or her approach based on individual and institutional experience, as well as clinical parameters.

REFERENCES

1. Bodey GP, Buckley M, Sathe YS, Freireich ET (1966) Quantitative relationships between circulating leukocytes and infection in patients with acute leukemia. *Ann. Intern. Med., 64*, 328.
2. Bryant RE, Hood AF, Hood CE, Koenig MG (1971) Factors affecting mortality of gram-negative bacteremia. *Arch. Intern. Med., 127*, 120.
3. Freid MA, Vosti KL (1968) Importance of underlying disease in patients with gram-negative bacteremia. *Arch. Intern. Med., 121*, 418.
4. Schimpff SC, Greene WH, Young VM, Wiernik PH (1974) Significance of *Pseudomonas aeruginosa* in the patient with leukemia or lymphoma. *J. Infect. Dis., 130 Suppl*, 524.
5. Umsawasdi T, Middleman EA, Luna M, Bodey GP (1973) *Klebsiella* bacteremia in cancer patients. *Am. J. Med. Sci., 265*, 473.
6. Whitecar JP, Luna M, Bodey GP (1970) *Pseudomonas* bacteremia in patients with malignant disease. *Am. J. Med. Sci., 260*, 216.
7. Pizzo PA, Robichaud KJ, Wesley R, Commers JR (1982) Fever in the pediatric and young adult patient with cancer: a prospective study of 1001 episodes. *Medicine, 61*, 153.
8. Levine AS, Schimpff SC, Graw RG, Young RC (1974) Hematologic malignances and other marrow failure status: progress in the management of complicating infections. *Sem. Hematol., 11*, 141.
9. McGowan J (1985) Changing etiology of nosocomial bacteremia and fungemia and other hospital-acquired infections. *Rev. Infect. Dis., 7, Suppl 3*, S357.
10. McGowan JE, Barnes MW, Finland M (1975) Bacteremia at Boston City Hospital: occurrence and mortality during 12 selected years (1935–1972), with special reference to hospital-acquired cases. *J. Infect. Dis., 132*, 316.
11. Hersh EM, Bodey GP, Nies BA, Freireich EJ (1965) Causes of death in acute leukemia: a ten-year study of 414 patients, from 1954–1963. *J. Am. Med. Assoc., 193*, 105.
12. Schimpff SC, Saterlee W, Young VM (1971) Empiric therapy with carbenicillin and gentamicin for febrile patients with cancer and granulocytopenia. *N. Engl. J. Med., 284*, 1061.
13. Gaya H (1984) Rational basis for the choice of regimens for empirical therapy of sepsis in granulocytopenic patients. *Clin. Hematol., 13*, 573.
14. Sculier JP, Klastersky J (1984) Significance of serum bactericidal activity in gram negative bacillary bacteremia in patients with and without granulocytopenia. *Am. J. Med., 76*, 429.
15. Bodey GP (1986) Infection in cancer patients: a continuing association. *Am. J. Med., 81, Suppl 1A*, 11.
16. Schimpff SC (1985) Overview of empiric antibiotic therapy for the febrile neutropenic patient. *Rev. Infect. Dis., 7, Suppl 4*, S734.
17. DeJongh CA, Joshi JH, Newman KA, Moody MR, Wharton R, Standiford HC, Schimpff SC (1986) Antibiotic synergism and response in gram negative bacteremia in granulocytopenic cancer patients. *Am. J. Med., 80, Suppl 5C*, 96.
18. Anderson ET, Young LS, Hewitt WL (1978) Antimicrobial synergism in the therapy of gram negative rod bacteremia. *Chemotherapy, 24*, 45.
19. Moellering Jr RC, Eliopoulos GM, Allan JD (1986) Beta-lactam/aminoglycoside combinations: interactions and their mechanisms. *Am. J. Med., 80, Suppl 5C*, 30.

20. Lyon MD, Smith KR, Saag MS, Cloud GA, Cobbs CG (1986) In vitro activity of piperacillin, ticarcillin, and mezlocillin alone and in combination with aminoglycosides against *Pseudomonas aeruginosa. Antimicrob. Agents Chemother., 30,* 25.

21. Johnson DE, Thompson B (1986) Efficacy of single agent therapy with azlocillin, ticarcillin, and amikacin and beta-lactam/amikacin combinations for treatment of *Pseudomonas aeruginosa* bacteremia in granulocytopenic rats. *Am. J. Med., 80, Suppl 5C,* 53.

22. Jawetz E (1968) The use of combinations of antimicrobial drugs. *Annu. Rev. Pharmacol., 8,* 151.

23. Klastersky J, Cappel R, Daneau D (1972) Clinical significance of in vitro synergism between antibiotics in gram-negative infections. *Antimicrob. Agents Chemother., 2,* 470.

24. Klastersky J, Zinner SH (1982) Synergistic combination of antibiotics in gram-negative bacillary infections. *Rev. Infect. Dis., 4,* 294.

25. Kluge RM, Standiford HC, Tatem BA, Young VM, Greene WH, Schimpff SC, Calia FM, Hornick RB (1974) Comparative activity of tobramycin, amikacin, and gentamicin alone and with carbenicillin against *Pseudomonas aeruginosa. Antimicrob. Agents Chemother., 6,* 442.

26. Reyes MP, El-Khatib MR, Brown WJ, Smith F, Lerner AM (1979) Synergy between carbenicillin and an aminoglycoside (gentamicin or tobramycin) against *Pseudomonas aeruginosa* isolated from patients with endocarditis and sensitivity of isolates to normal human serum. *J. Infect. Dis., 140,* 192.

27. Rodriguez V, Whitecar JP, Bodey GP (1969) Therapy of infections with the combination of carbenicillin and gentamicin. *Antimicrob. Agents Chemother., 9,* 386.

28. Rubin M, Pizzo PA (1986) Should vancomycin be included in initial empiric management of febrile neutropenic cancer patients? In: *Program and Abstracts, 26th Interscience Conference on Antimicrobial Agents and Chemotherapy, New Orleans, 1986,* Abstract No. 222. American Society for Microbiology, Washington, DC.

29. Pizzo PA, Ladisch S, Simon RM, Gill F, Levine AS (1978) Increasing incidence of gram-positive sepsis in cancer patients. *Med. Pediatr. Oncol., 5,* 241.

30. Ladisch S, Pizzo PA (1978) *Staphylococcus aureus* sepsis in children with cancer. *Pediatrics, 61,* 231.

31. Kilton LJ, Fossieck Jr BE, Cohen MH, Parker RH (1979) Bacteremia due to gram-positive cocci in patients with neoplastic disease. *Am. J. Med., 66,* 596.

32. Sotman SB, Schimpff SC, Young VM (1980) *Staphylococcus aureus* bacteremia in patients with acute leukemia. *Am. J. Med., 69,* 814.

33. Wade JC, Schimpff SC, Newman KA, Wiernik PH (1982) *Staphylococcus epidermidis*: an increasing cause of infection in patients with granulocytopenia. *Ann. Intern. Med., 97,* 503.

34. Miser JS, Miser AW (1980) *Staphylococcus aureus* sepsis in childhood malignancy. *Am. J. Dis. Child., 134,* 831.

35. Carney DN, Fossieck Jr BE, Parker RH, Minna JD (1982) Bacteremia due to *Staphylococcus aureus* in patients with cancer: report on 45 cases in adults and review of the literature. *Rev. Infect. Dis., 4,* 1.

36. Grossi M, Green DM (1982) *Staphylococcus aureus* bacteremia in children and adolescents with acute lymphoblastic leukemia. *Oncology, 40,* 321.

37. Winston DJ, Dudnick DV, Chapin M, Ho WG, Gale RP, Martin WJ (1983) Coagulase-negative staphylococcal bacteremia in patients receiving immunosuppressive therapy. *Arch. Intern. Med., 143,* 32.

38. Friedman LE, Brown AE, Miller DR et al (1984) *Staphylococcus epidermidis* septicemia in children with leukemia and lymphoma. *Am. J. Dis. Child.*, *138*, 71.

39. Pizzo PA, Ladisch S, Witebsky FE (1978) Alpha-hemolytic streptococci: clinical significance in the cancer patient. *Med. Pediatr. Oncol.*, *4*, 257.

40. Dejace P, Klastersky J (1986) Comparative review of combination therapy: two beta-lactams versus beta-lactam plus aminoglycoside. *Am. J. Med.*, *80*, *Suppl 6B*, 29.

41. Hathorn JW, Rubin M, Pizzo PA (1987) Antibiotic therapy in the febrile neutropenic cancer patient: clinical efficacy and impact of monotherapy. *Antimicrob. Agents Chemother.*, *31*, 971.

42. Rubin M, Hathorn JW, Pizzo PA (1988) Controversies in the management of febrile neutropenic cancer patients. *Cancer Invest.*, *4*, in press.

43. Wade JC, Johnson DE, Bustamante CI (1986) Monotherapy for empiric treatment of fever in granulocytopenic cancer patients. *Am. J. Med.*, *80*, *Suppl 5C*, 85.

44. Fainstein V, Bodey GP (1985) Single-agent therapy for infections in neutropenic cancer patients. *Am. J. Med.*, *79*, *Suppl 2A*, 83.

45. Gaya H (1986) Combination therapy and monotherapy in the treatment of severe infection in the immunocompromised host. *Am. J. Med.*, *80*, *Suppl 6B*, 149.

46. Guttmann L, Williamson R, Kitzis M, Acar J (1986) Synergism and antagonism in double beta-lactam antibiotic combinations. *Am. J. Med.*, *80*, *Suppl 5C*, 21.

47. Bodey GP, Middleman E, Umsawaski T, Rodriguez V (1972) Infections in cancer patients: results with gentamicin sulfate therapy. *Cancer*, *29*, 1697.

48. Feld R, Valdivieso M, Bodey GP, Rodriguez V (1977) Comparison of amikacin and tobramycin in the treatment of infection in patients with cancer. *J. Infect. Dis.*, *135*, 61.

49. Valdivieso M, Feld R, Rodriguez V, Bodey GP (1975) Amikacin therapy of infection in neutropenic patients. *Am. J. Med. Sci.*, *270*, 453.

50. Valdivieso M, Horikoshi N, Rodriguez V, Bodey GP (1974) Therapeutic trials with tobramycin. *Am. J. Med. Sci.*, *168*, 149.

51. Young LS (1985) Use of aminoglycosides in immunocompromised patients. *Am. J. Med.*, *79*, *Suppl 1A*, 21.

52. Holmes KK, Clark H, Silverblatt F, Turck M (1969) Emergence of resistance in *Pseudomonas* during carbenicillin therapy. *Antimicrob. Agents* and *Chemother.*, 391.

53. Bodey GP, Whitecar JP, Middleman E, Rodriguez V (1971) Carbenicillin therapy for *Pseudomonas* infections. *J. Am. Med. Assoc.*, *290*, 62.

54. Klastersky J, Cappel R, Daneau D (1973) Therapy with carbenicillin and gentamicin for patients with cancer and severe infections caused by gram-negative rods. *Cancer*, *31*, 331.

55. Rodriguez V, Bodey GP, Horikoshi N, Inagaki J, McCredie, KB (1973) Ticarcillin therapy of infections. *Antimicrob. Agents Chemother.*, *4*, 427.

56. Bodey GP (1969) Carbenicillin therapy of gram negative bacilli infections. *Am. J. Med. Sci.*, *257*, 408.

57. Bodey GP, Pan T (1977) Mezlocillin: in vitro studies of a new broad-spectrum penicillin. *Antimicrob. Agents Chemother.*, *11*, 74.

58. Drusano GL, Schimpff SC, Hewitt WL (1984) The acylampicillins: mezlocillin, piperacillin, and azlocillin. *Rev. Infect. Dis.*, *6*, 13.

59. Fu KP, Neu HC (1978) Azlocillin and mezlocillin: new ureido-penicillins. *Antimicrob. Agents Chemother.*, *13*, 930.

60. Issell BF, Bodey GP (1980) Mezlocillin for treatment of infections in cancer patients. *Antimicrob. Agents Chemother.*, *17*, 1008.

61. Wade JC, Schimpff SC, Newman KA, Fortner CL, Moody MR, Young VM, Wiernik PH (1980) Potential of mezlocillin as empiric single agent therapy in febrile granulocytopenic cancer patients. *Antimicrob. Agents Chemother.*, *18*, 299.

62. Jadeja L, Bolivar R, Fainstein V, Keating M, McCredie K, Hay M, Bodey GP (1984) Piperacillin plus vancomycin in the therapy of febrile episodes in cancer patients. *Antimicrob. Agents Chemother.*, *26*, 295.

63. Barriere SL, Flaherty JD (1984) Third-generation cephalosporins: a critical evaluation. *Clin. Pharm.*, *3*, 351.

64. Neu HC (1982) The new beta-lactamase-stable cephalosporins. *Ann. Intern. Med.*, *97*, 408.

65. Darbyshire PJ, Williamson DJ, Pedler SJ, Speller DCE, Mott MG, Oakhill A (1983) Ceftazidime in the treatment of febrile immunosuppressed children. *J. Antimicrob. Chemother.*, *12*, *Suppl A*, 357.

66. De Pauw BE, Kauw F, Muytjens H, Williams KJ, Bothof TL (1983) Randomized study of ceftazidime versus gentamicin plus cefotaxime for infections in severely granulocytopenic patients. *J. Antimicrob. Chemother.*, *12*, *Suppl A*, 93.

67. Fainstein V, Bodey GP, Elting L, Bolivar R, Keating MJ, McCredie KB, Valdivieso M (1983) A randomized study of ceftazidime compared to ceftazidime and tobramycin for the treatment of infections in cancer patients. *J. Antimicrob. Chemother.*, *12*, *Suppl A*, S101.

68. Morgan G, Duerden BI, Lilleyman JS (1983) Ceftazidime as a single agent in the management of children with fever and neutropenia. *J. Antimicrob. Chemother.*, *12*, *Suppl A*, 347.

69. Ramphal R, Kramer BS, Rand KH, Weiner RS, Shands JW (1983) Early results of a comparative trial of ceftazidime versus cephalothin, carbenicillin, and gentamicin in the treatment of febrile granulocytopenic patients. *J. Antimicrob. Chemother.*, *12*, *Suppl A*, 81.

70. Reilly JT, Brada M, Bellingham AJ, Hart CA, Bennett C (1983) Ceftazidime compared to tobramycin and ticarcillin in immunocompromised haematological patients. *J. Antimicrob. Chemother.*, *12*, *Suppl A*, 89.

71. De Pauw B, Williams K, Neeff JD, Bothof T, De Witte T, Hodrinet R, Haanen C (1985) A randomized prospective study of ceftazidime versus ceftazidime plus flucloxacillin in the empiric treatment of febrile episodes in severely neutropenic patients. *Antimicrob. Agents Chemother.*, *28*, 824.

72. Viscoli C, Gargani G, Faaco F, Mantero E, Tuo P, Giachinno R, Campelli A, Nantron M, Perlino G (1985) Evaluation of ceftazidime in the treatment of 80 infectious episodes in compromised children. *Int. J. Clin. Pharmacol. Ther. Toxicol.*, *23*, 634.

73. Donnelly JP, Marcus RE, Goldman JM, Cohen J, Worsley AM, Catovsky D, Darrel JH, Want SV, Galton DAG (1985) Ceftazidime as first-line therapy for fever in acute leukemia. *J. Infect.*, *11*, 205.

74. Pizzo PA, Hathorn JW, Hiemenz JW, Brown M, Commers J, Cotton D, Gress J, Longo D, Marshall D, McKnight J, Rubin M, Skelton J, Thaler M, Wesley R (1986) A randomized trial comparing combination antibiotic therapy to monotherapy in cancer patients with fever and neutropenia. *N. Engl. J. Med.*, *315*, 552.

75. Hathorn, JW, Pizzo PA (1986) Is there a role for monotherapy with beta-lactam antibiotics in the initial empirical management of febrile neutropenic cancer patients? *J. Antimicrob. Chemother.*, *17*, *Suppl A*, 41.

76. D'Oliveira JJG, Pereira MEA, Mateus LM, Monteiro JMN, Parreira AS, Soares AD

(1986) Use of ceftazidime in febrile incidents in immunocompromised haematological patients. *J. Intern. Med. Res.*, *14*, 30.

77. Lagast H, Klastersky J, Kains JP, Van der Auwera PH, Meunier F, Woussen F, Thijs JP (1986) Empiric antimicrobial therapy with aztreonam or ceftazidime in gram negative septicemia. *Am. J. Med.*, *80, Suppl 5C*, 79.

78. Verhagen CS, De Pauw B, De Witte T, Janssen J, Williams K, De Mulder P, Bothof T (1987) Randomized prospective study of ceftazidime versus ceftazidime plus cephalothin in empiric treatment of febrile episodes in severely neutropenic patients. *Antimicrob. Agents Chemother.*, *31*, 191.

79. Verhagen C, De Pauw BE, Donnelly JP, Williams KJ, De Witte T, Janssen J (1986) Ceftazidime alone for treating *Pseudomonas aeruginosa* septicemia in neutropenic patients. *J. Infect.*, *13*, 125.

80. Bolivar R, Fainstein V, Elting L, Bodey GP (1983) Cefoperazone for the treatment of infection in patients with cancer. *Infect. Dis.*, *5, Suppl*, S181.

81. Piccart M, Klastersky J, Meunier F, Lagast H, Van Laetham Y, Weerts D (1984) Single-drug versus combination empirical therapy for gram-negative bacillary infections in febrile cancer patients with and without granulocytopenia. *Antimicrob. Agents Chemother.*, *26*, 870.

82. Alanis A, Rehm S, Weinstein AJ (1983) Comparative efficacy and toxicity of moxalactam and the combination of nafcillin and tobramycin in febrile granulocytopenic patients. *Cleveland Clin. Q.*, *50*, 385.

83. Bezwoda WR, Deman DP, Perkins S, Cassel R (1985) Treatment of neutropenic infection: a randomized trial comparing latamoxef (moxalactam) with cephradine plus tobramycin. *J. Antimicrob. Chemother.*, *15*, 239.

84. Friis H, Hoffman S, Hansen MM, Justesen T, Nissen NI (1983) Cefotaxime versus ampicillin, methicillin, and netilmicin in combination for treatment of febrile episodes in patients with haematologic malignancy. *Acta Med. Scand.*, *213*, 349.

85. Lawson RD, Baskin RC (1982) Ceftizoxime treatment of infection in neutropenic patients with malignancies. *J. Antimicrob. Chemother.*, *10, Suppl C*, 159.

86. Young LS (1986) Empirical antimicrobial therapy in the neutropenic host (Editorial). *N. Engl. J. Med.*, *315*, 580.

87. Pizzo PA (1987) After empiric therapy: what to do until the granulocyte comes back. *Rev. Infect. Dis.*, *9*, 214.

88. Karp JE, Dick JD, Angelopulos C, Charache P, Green L, Burke P, Saral R (1986) Empiric use of vancomycin during prolonged treatment-induced granulocytopenia: randomized, double-blind, placebo-controlled trial in patients with acute leukemia. *Am. J. Med.*, *81*, 237.

89. Kramer BJ, Ramphal R, Rand K (1986) Randomized comparison between two ceftazidime-containing regimens and cephalothin-gentamicin-carbenicillin in febrile granulocytopenic cancer patients. *Antimicrob. Agents Chemother.*, *30*, 64.

90. Kropp H, Gerckens L, Sundelof JG, Kahan FM (1985) Antibacterial activity of imipenem: the first thienamycin antibiotic. *Rev. Infect. Dis.*, *7, Suppl 3*, S389.

91. Wade JC, Standiford HC, Drusano GL, Johnson DE, Moody MR, Bustamante CI, Joshi J, De Jongh C, Schimpff SC (1985) Potential of imipenem as single-agent empiric antibiotic therapy of febrile neutropenic patients with cancer. *Am. J. Med.*, *78, Suppl 5A*, 62.

92. Bodey GP, Alvarez ME, Jones PG, Rolston KVI, Steelhammer L, Fainstein V (1986) Imipenem-cilastatin as initial therapy for febrile cancer patients. *Antimicrob. Agents Chemother.*, *30*, 211.

93. Quinn JP, Dudek EJ, DiVincenzo CA, Lucks DA, Lerner SA (1986) Emergence of resistance to imipenem during therapy for *Pseudomonas aeruginosa* infections. *J. Infect. Dis.*, *154*, 289.
94. Calandra GB, Wang C, Aziz M, Brown KR (1986) The safety profile of imipenem/cilastatin: worldwide clinical experience based on 3470 patients. *J. Antimicrob. Chemother.*, *18*, 3.
95. Sykes RB, Bonner DP (1985) Aztreonam: the first monobactam. *Am. J. Med.*, *78*, *Suppl 2A*, 2.
96. Hinkle AM, Bodey GP (1980) In vitro evaluation of RO 13–9904. *Antimicrob. Agents Chemother.*, *18*, S74.
97. Rubin M, Hathorn JW, Marshall D, Gress J, Steinberg SM, Pizzo PA (1988) Gram-positive infections and the use of vancomycin in 550 episodes of fever and neutropenia. *Ann. Intern. Med.*, *108*, 30.

CHAPTER 43

Antimicrobial agents in the management of travelers' diarrhea

CHARLES D. ERICSSON and HERBERT L. DUPONT

Recent literature on the use of antimicrobial agents in the management of travelers' diarrhea has emphasized the rational, practical and safe use of these agents. Antimicrobial agents have been used prophylactically for travelers at high risk for developing illness as well as for therapy. These approaches have been successful since much of the diarrhea among travelers to high-risk areas is caused by bacterial agents. A Consensus Development Conference Statement (1) concluded that prophylactic use of antimicrobial agents should be avoided in favor of aggressive, early treatment of the syndrome. In an editorial (2), we have presented a practical view of the role of patients and their physicians in assessing the risks and benefits of antimicrobial use in travelers' diarrhea. We have furthermore reopened the issue of the use of bismuth subsalicylate as a prophylactic agent (3), and these data are reviewed here because bismuth subsalicylate does appear to work, at least in part, as an antimicrobial agent (4). Work by Ericsson et al (5) has stressed the practical aspects of choosing patients for treatment with antimicrobial agents, and another study (6) suggests that an antimicrobial agent in combination with non-antibiotic therapy is especially efficacious. The carboxyquinolones, as exemplified by ciprofloxacin, are emerging as ideal agents for the therapy of travelers' diarrhea (7). Many authors continue to express concern about the development of antimicrobial resistance among enteropathogens, and recent evaluations of the problem by Murray and others (8–11) have helped to place the problem in perspective. Further, a study by Johnson et al (12) on the use of norfloxacin, a quinolone antibiotic, underscores the potential benefits of antimicrobial agents that do not have known plasmid-mediated antimicrobial resistance.

DEFINITIONS

Antimicrobial agents will include bismuth subsalicylate in this review. A study by Graham (4) has clearly shown that the agent has antimicrobial activity.

The definition of diarrhea continues to be a source of confusion. Some studies

Antimicrobial Agents Annual 3
P.K. Peterson and J. Verhoef, editors
© Elsevier Science Publishers BV, 1988

define diarrhea as the passage of unformed stools at twice the rate of normal stooling. We have often opted for a rigorous definition of diarrhea (4 or more unformed stools per 24 hours plus at least one additional symptom of enteric disease) which helps to eliminate much of the mild and non-infectious causes of symptomatology. Many studies use definitions of diarrhea that fall between these two. A problem is that study patients must wait to be declared a prophylaxis failure or wait to begin treatment until after they meet the study definition of diarrhea. Efficacy of early treatment might be higher than demonstrated to date and might compare more favorably with prophylaxis if patients were not required to meet study definitions of diarrhea before instituting therapy. Antimicrobial agents may or may not have a role in mild travelers' diarrhea depending in part on the definition of 'mild' (5, 7), especially because effective alternative therapy exists in the form of non-antibiotic medications (13).

HISTORICAL ASPECTS

Antimicrobial agents were suspected to be useful in the treatment of travelers' diarrhea when enterotoxigenic *Escherichia coli* were demonstrated to be the predominant cause of the syndrome. The heat-labile enterotoxin of *E. coli* is nearly identical to cholera toxin, and tetracycline had already been shown to be highly efficacious in treating cholera. Furthermore, the kinetics of action of *E. coli* toxins were not all-or-none like cholera toxin, implying that interruption of toxin production by killing the organisms might be expected to be followed by relatively prompt clinical relief. Kean et al (14) as early as 1962 demonstrated effectiveness of antimicrobial agents (phthalylsulfathiazole and neomycin sulfate) in preventing up to 62–71% of moderate to severe travelers' diarrhea. A later study by Turner (15) failed to demonstrate protection by neomycin-sulfonamides and showed only modest (28%) protection by Streptotriad. Turner raised the issue of the side effects of antimicrobial agents that needed to be weighed against the benefits.

Subsequent studies on prophylaxis were rationalized by the demonstration that most travelers' diarrhea is caused by bacterial agents. Concern has been raised in earlier studies that disturbance of fecal flora might encourage invasion by agents like *Salmonella* or *Campylobacter*, but in recent studies such has not been the case.

PROPHYLAXIS

Studies have been conducted with doxycycline in Kenya, Morocco, Honduras, Thailand and Mexico (16). As shown in Table 1, these placebo-controlled trials often involve small numbers of subjects with the exception of the study in Mexico where the duration of prophylaxis was only $^1/_2$–$2^1/_2$ days. Taken together however, the available studies report on 96 persons who received doxycycline at a dose of 100 mg/d for 21 days. The protection rate ranged from 59 to 86%. The drug was

Table 1   *Comparative efficacy of antimicrobial agents in the prevention of travelers' diarrhea*

Agent	Study location	Days of therapy	Daily dose of agent	No. of subjects with diarrhea/total no. (%)			Percent protection	P-Value
Doxycycline	Kenya	21	100 mg	A	1/18	(6)	86	0.01
				P	9/21	(43)		
	Morocco	21	100 mg	A	2/26	(8)	83	0.01
				P	11/24	(46)		
	Honduras	21	100 mg	A	7/22	(32)	68	0.001
				P	22/22	(100)		
	Thailand	21	100 mg	A	3/30	(10)	59	NS
				P	8/33	(24)		
	Honduras	21	100 mg*	A	8/24	(33)	27	NS
				P	10/22	(45)		
TMP+SMX	Mexico	$^1/_2$–$2^{1}/_2$	200 mg once then 100 mg	A	3/75	(4)	81	0.002
				P	15/70	(21)		
	Mexico	21	160/800 mg b.i.d.	A	11/67	(16)	71	<0.001
				P	44/80	(55)		
	Mexico	14	160/800 mg	A	1/57	(2)	95	<0.0001
				P	10/30	(33)		
TMP	Mexico	14	200 mg	A	8/58	(14)	59	<0.05
				P	10/30	(33)		
Bicozamycin	Mexico	21	500 mg q.i.d.	A	0/11		100	0.003
				P	10/19	(53)		
Amdinocillin (mecillinam)	Egypt and Far East	25	200 mg	A	5/38	(13)	75	<0.001
				P	19/36	(53)		
Erythromycin	Mexico	4–13	1.0 g	A	0/24		100	<0.005
				P	7/24	(29)		
Norfloxacin	Mexico	14	400 mg	A	4/54	(7)	88	<0.001
				P	34/57	(60)		

*twice weekly.

TMP+SMX = trimethoprim + sulfamethoxazole; A = active drug; P = placebo. Adapted from Refs 16 and 17.

well tolerated with expected gastrointestinal upset and sun-sensitivity rashes proving not to be reported problems. The lower ranges of protection (59 and 68%) were seen in Honduras and Thailand where resistance to doxycycline among enterotoxigenic *E. coli* approximated 50%. Also, only 27% protection was observed with twice-weekly doxycycline. This finding argues against a substantial role for subinhibitory levels of doxycycline interfering with adhesion and thereby preventing disease. Rather, the success of prophylactic doxycycline appears to be dependent on the susceptibility of the organism and stool levels of the antimicrobial agent.

Two studies (17) have been conducted in Mexico with trimethoprim + sulfamethoxazole (TMP + SMX) and one with trimethoprim alone (Table 1). The best protection (95%) was seen with one double-strength TMP + SMX tablet daily. A 1–3% incidence of cutaneous eruptions has been a consistent finding with use of TMP + SMX (or trimethoprim alone) in these studies.

Bicozamycin, a unique bicyclic non-absorbable antibiotic, with excellent activity against enteropathogens, was effective in a small number of subjects (18). Regrettably, bicozamycin is no longer being developed as an antibiotic for human use. Its focused activity and lack of systemic absorption or plasmid-mediated resistance made it an ideal candidate for an antidiarrheal agent.

As also shown in Table 1, amdinocillin (formally mecillinam) is effective as a prophylactic agent (16). The drug must be given as the pivaloyl ester as the drug is otherwise acid-labile. Theoretically, use of penicillins as prophylactic agents in the face of many alternatives probably should be discouraged to avoid the needless development of penicillin sensitivity.

Of theoretic interest, erythromycin was 100% effective in preventing diarrhea in a small group (n = 24) attending a conference in Mexico (16). Erythromycin has predictable activity against enteropathogens at the alkaline pH's of the gut and at the high concentrations found in stool. Gastrointestinal upset that is experienced by many persons taking the drug makes the widespread prophylactic use of erythromycin untenable.

Recently a trial of norfloxacin, 400 mg orally daily for 14 days, versus placebo was conducted in Guadalajara, Mexico, among recently-arrived U.S. adults (12). Norfloxacin is a member of a new group of antibiotics, the fluorinated carboxyquinolones. These DNA-gyrase inhibitors are quite broad spectrum in their activity and are especially active against enteropathogens including *Campylobacter jejuni*. Lack of demonstrated plasmid-mediated antimicrobial resistance and inconsistent activity against anaerobes make this group of agents theoretically appealing as antidiarrheal agents. Four of 54 patients (7%) developed diarrhea while taking norfloxacin compared to 34 of 57 (60%) taking placebo (P < 0.001). In contrast to the experience with TMP + SMX or trimethoprim alone, in which trimethoprim-resistant flora replaced stool flora during prophylaxis with the agents, use of norfloxacin was not associated with the emergence of resistant flora. In fact, 84% of 38 persons cultured on day 7 of the norfloxacin study showed no aerobic gram-negative bacilli in stool, and 92% of 37 subjects showed the same finding by day 14 of prophylaxis. Norfloxacin was well tolerated.

Bismuth subsalicylate (BSS) was shown to be effective in an earlier study that used the liquid formulation (19). In this study approximately 65% protection was realized. Inconvenience of the liquid and the dose required (one 8 oz. bottle per day) were limiting factors of this approach. The absorption of salicylate or bismuth were minor concerns of the Consensus Development Conference. Taking 8 oz. of BSS formulation is tantamount to taking 7–8 adult aspirins, so the potential for salicylate intoxication, especially if aspirin-containing compounds are taken concurrently, does exist. Bismuth is only absorbed to a limited degree, and documented serum levels have been well below those seen with bismuth intoxication.

Recently, two studies have examined the efficacy of tablet formulations of BSS in travelers. Under the circumstances of best compliance, the ingestion of a 2.1 g daily dose of BSS taken in two divided doses a day yielded 41% protection (20). In our most recent trial (3), BSS administration produced 65% protection with a 2.4 g daily dose of BSS taken as 2 tablets 4 times daily for three weeks. This efficacy rivaled that of the liquid formulation (8 oz. contains 4.2 g BSS). The data argue that both the total dose and spreading the dose throughout the day are important for optimizing efficacy. Also, an earlier study (21) showed that the best prevention of travelers' diarrhea by BSS was achieved when subjects also were careful where they ate.

What, if any, agent should be recommended for prophylaxis? The suggestion of the Consensus Development Conference that neither antimicrobial agents nor BSS formulations can be recommended seems unrealistic. DuPont et al (2) point to the risks versus benefits of prophylaxis, and the necessity of discussing the options with the patient. BSS is associated with minimal side effects when it is used in the recommended dosages and should be safe to administer to most travelers in whom salicylate is not contraindicated. Reves (personal communication) has demonstrated that antimicrobial prophylaxis (TMP+SMX or doxycycline) is more cost-effective than treatment options, but this argument may not be relevant for an affluent traveler. Excluding BSS, antimicrobial prophylaxis, if it is used at all, should probably be confined to use by persons on short and important trips and should probably be avoided in the very young and old due to lack of data and concerns about overdose.

TREATMENT

The Consensus Development Conference was disposed to favor avoidance of travelers' diarrhea in a developing nation by careful choice of food and drink and aggressive therapy if diarrhea developed despite taking precautions. One of the reasons for preferring this approach is the availability of effective antimicrobial agents to treat diarrhea of diverse causes, which is the case in travelers' diarrhea.

As can be seen in Table 2, several agents have previously been shown to be efficacious in travelers' diarrhea. TMP+SMX has emerged as the gold standard for therapy (22). Several potential problems exist with TMP+SMX. The drug is not

Table 2   *Comparative efficacy of antimicrobial agents in the treatment of travelers' diarrhea in Mexico*

Agent	Daily dose	Days of therapy	popula-tion size	Mean hours of diarrhea	Percent well at indicated time	
					48 h	72 h
Trial 1						
TMP+SMX	160/800 mg b.i.d.	5	37	29	78	89
TMP	200 mg b.i.d.	5	38	31	84	89
Placebo	b.i.d.	5	35	93	14	26
Trial 2						
Furazolidone	100 mg q.i.d.	5	47	57	55	74
Ampicillin	500 mg q.i.d.	5	47	72	32	49
Trial 3						
Ciprofloxacin	500 mg b.i.d.	5	60	29	72	ND
TMP+SMX	160/800 mg b.i.d.	5	59	20	93	ND
Placebo	b.i.d.	5	62	81	34	ND
Trial 4						
TMP+SMX	160/800 mg b.i.d.	3	31	24	85	90
Placebo	b.i.d.	3	33	59	50	65
Trial 5						
Bicozamycin	500 mg q.i.d.	3	72	28	85	94
Placebo	q.i.d.	3	68	64	47	62

ND = not done; TMP + SMX = trimethoprim + sulfamethoxazole. Adapted from Refs 6, 7, 22, 23, 24.

active against *Campylobacter jejuni* (which fortuitously has not caused much acute diarrhea in travelers in Guadalajara, Mexico). The use of the drug is consistently associated with a small percentage of patients who experience a self-limiting rash. Resistance to TMP+SMX among enteric isolates is beginning to emerge around the world (8–11).

Previously reported alternatives to TMP+SMX include bicozamycin and furazolidone (Table 2). Bicozamycin, a non-absorbable agent, was highly efficacious in a 3-day course of therapy, but the drug is no longer available (23). Furazolidone was marginally more effective than ampicillin (24). The latter cannot be considered a useful agent due to the high number of resistant enteric isolates. A limiting factor in the use of furazolidone among travelers was a disulfiram-type flushing reaction that occurred in 19% of subjects, who consumed alcohol while taking furazolidone despite having diarrhea and despite being forewarned of the reaction.

Ericsson et al (7) have reported favorable results of treatment of travelers' diarrhea for 5 days with ciprofloxacin, a potent fluorinated carboxyquinolone that achieves excellent stool concentrations (Table 2). TMP + SMX treatment was used as a positive control, and the mean duration of diarrhea of 20 hours in this study compares favorably with the 29 hours reported previously for 5 days of TMP + SMX therapy. Ciprofloxacin has the advantage of being active against *C. jejuni*; however, more research needs to be conducted before the efficacy of quinolones in *Campylobacter* disease can be determined.

Ciprofloxacin was efficacious compared with placebo in persons who reported to the clinic early (first 24 hours of illness) or late (48–72 hours) in the course of their disease (Table 3). Cramps were relieved compared to placebo by day 2 of therapy. Ciprofloxacin, compared to placebo, was effective in reducing the duration of diarrhea due to enterotoxigenic *E. coli* (33 *vs* 84 hours, P < 0.001), invasive enteropathogens, (27 *vs* 81 hours, P < 0.05) and no identified pathogens (27 *vs* 77 hours, P < 0.001). Only 3 of 59 ciprofloxacin-treated patients were declared treatment failures compared to 20 of 62 in the placebo group (P < 0.0001). Ciprofloxacin was reasonably well tolerated; one subject developed pruritus and swelling of hands, eyes and lips, and another subject developed a vaginal infection.

In this study, patients were stratified into mild-to-moderate and moderate-to-severe clinical presentations using an index of total diarrheal illness that included scores for diarrhea, nausea, vomiting, abdominal cramps and temperature elevation. Ciprofloxacin-treated patients benefited from antimicrobial use regardless of their initial presentation. Forty-one and 97% of mild to moderately ill subjects became well or improved at the end of 24 and 48 hours of treatment, respectively, compared with 46 and 82% of moderate to severely ill subjects. Coupled with the

Table 3   *Efficacy of ciprofloxacin compared to TMP + SMX in the treatment of travelers' diarrhea*

Agent	Mean hours of diarrhea after initiation of therapy when hour of diarrhea before therapy was (n):		
	0–24	24–48	48–72
Ciprofloxacin	30 (31)	34 (15)	23 (14)
TMP + SMX	23 (40)	13 (14)	7 (5)
Placebo	74 (35)	100 (18)	70 (9)

P < 0.01 for all values compared to respective placebo groups. TMP + SMX = trimethoprim–sulfamethoxazole. Adapted from Ref. 7.

finding that placebo-treated subjects became well at approximately the same pace regardless of their severity of clinical presentation, these data argue for the possibility of empiric antibiotic treatment for all presentations of travelers' diarrhea. These data, however, must be placed in context with recently reported data (5) that have shown that the duration of untreated mild diarrhea (as opposed to mild to moderate diarrhea as defined in the ciprofloxacin study) is, in fact, shorter than the duration of moderate to severe diarrhea. To complicate matters, clinical symptoms and fecal signs are not reliable predictors of the causal agent in travelers' diarrhea. The exception was *Shigella* dysentery which could be predicted accurately based on clinical findings. However, some mild presentations of travelers' diarrhea also proved to be shigellosis which ideally should be treated with an antimicrobial agent to prevent person-to-person spread. Also, very mild diarrhea (less than 4 unformed stools per 24 hours) has not been well studied. Mild to moderate diarrhea, as defined in the ciprofloxacin study, appears to benefit from antimicrobial therapy, but the disease is still relatively mild. Current recommendations are to begin therapy for mild disease with non-antibiotic treatment and to use antibiotic therapy only if indicated by an unfavorable clinical response or availability of stool culture results (5).

Combination therapy

Under the best of circumstances the mean duration of antimicrobial-treated diarrhea is approximately 1 day. One recently reported study (6) evaluated the use of symptomatic, non-antimicrobial therapy in combination with TMP+SMX (Table 4). The specific non-antibiotic agent was an experimental enkephalin-like pentapeptide (BW-942C) that has a rapid onset of antisecretory and anti-motility effects. The mean duration of diarrhea was virtually the same (24 hours) in the group treated with TMP+SMX (n=31) and combination therapy (n=31). However, combination therapy was associated with a lower frequency of stooling than

Table 4   *Treatment of travelers' diarrhea with an antimicrobial agent alone or an antimicrobial agent plus symptomatic therapy (BW-942C)*

Treatment group	Mean number of unformed stools passed during interval (h) after initiation of therapy	
	0–12	12–24
TMP+SMX	2.1	0.75
TMP+SMX plus BW-942C	1.5*	0.7
Placebo	3.0	1.4

*P=0.035 (compared to placebo).
TMP+SMX = trimethoprim + sulfamethoxazole; BW-942C, see text for explanation.
Adapted from Ref. 13.

therapy with TMP + SMX alone during the first 12 hours of therapy, when diarrhea was caused by enterotoxigenic *E. coli*. These data imply that non-antibiotic therapy may help to ensure relief from diarrhea in the first 12–24 hours following institution of therapy. After 24 hours no benefit from the addition of non-antibiotic therapy to TMP + SMX could be demonstrated.

The temptation might be to add available drugs such as bismuth subsalicylate or loperamide to antimicrobial therapy. Bismuth subsalicylate has been shown to decrease the intestinal absorption of doxycycline (25). Anti-motility agents, when used alone or with an antibiotic, have the potential, at least rarely, to prolong the course of bloody diarrhea (26). Further studies are necessary before combinations of available non-antibiotic therapy with antimicrobial agents can be endorsed routinely.

THOUGHTS FOR THE FUTURE

As spelled out in the Consensus Development Conference Statement, antimicrobial agents are as yet unstudied in prevention or treatment of travelers' diarrhea among children or elderly persons. Large-scale studies should be conducted to document uncommon but serious adverse effects of antimicrobial agents used in travelers' diarrhea, most importantly because travelers' diarrhea cannot be considered a life-threatening condition. The minimum effective doses remain to be determined for all antidiarrheal agents; conceivably single dose antimicrobial therapy might suffice.

Additional areas for research include clarifying the role of newer antimicrobials (e.g. quinolones) in the treatment of non-typhoidal salmonellosis and *Campylobacter jejuni* disease; antimicrobial agents may be effective when instituted very early in the course of disease. The use of antimicrobial agents with or without non-antibiotic therapy should be studied under the condition that patients institute therapy for themselves, rather than having them wait to come to the clinic or to meet study enrollment criteria. Finally, the selective pressure for the development of antimicrobial-resistant organisms among travelers using antimicrobial agents needs to be studied in more detail, and weighed against their use and abuse among indigenous persons in a developing world. It might be that resistant organisms present mostly a problem of transient colonization of the gut. Development of antimicrobial resistance should be studied where the traveling population is a substantial number compared with the indigenous population.

REFERENCES

1. Consensus Development Conference Statement (1986) *Rev. Infect. Dis., 8*, S227.
2. DuPont HL, Ericsson CD, Johnson PC (1985) Chemotherapy and chemoprophylaxis of travelers' diarrhea. *Ann. Intern. Med., 102*, 260.

3. DuPont HL, Ericsson CD, Johnson PC, Bitsura JAM, DuPont MW, Cabada FJ (1987) Prevention of travelers' diarrhea by the tablet formulation of bismuth subsalicylate. *J. Am. Med. Assoc.*, *257*, 1347.
4. Graham DY, Estes MK, Gentry LO (1983) Double-blind comparison of bismuth subsalicylate and placebo in the prevention and treatment of enterotoxigenic *Escherichia coli*-induced diarrhea in volunteers. *Gastroenterology*, *85*, 1017.
5. Ericsson CD, Patterson TF, DuPont HL (1987) Clinical presentation as a guide to therapy for travelers' diarrhea. *Am. J. Med. Sci.*, *294*, 91.
6. Ericsson CD, Johnson PC, DuPont HL, Morgan DR (1986) Role of a novel antidiarrheal agent, BW942C, alone or in combination with trimethoprim-sulfamethoxazole in the treatment of travelers' diarrhea. *Antimicrob. Agents Chemother.*, *29*, 1040.
7. Ericsson CD, Johnson PC, DuPont HL, Morgan DR, Bitsura JAM, Cabada FJ (1987) Ciprofloxacin or trimethoprim/sulfamethoxazole as initial therapy for travelers' diarrhea: a placebo-controlled, randomized trial. *Ann. Intern. Med.*, *106*, 216.
8. Murray BE (1986) Resistance of *Shigella, Salmonella*, and other selected enteric pathogens to antimicrobial agents. *Rev. Infect. Dis.*, *8*, S172.
9. Farrar WE (1985) Antibiotic resistance in developing countries. *J. Infect. Dis.*, *152*, 1103.
10. Murray BE, Alvarado M, Vorachit M, Kim KH, Levine MM, Jayanetra P, Prenzel I, Fling M, Elwell L, McCracken GH, Madrigal G, Odio C, Trabulsi LR (1985) Increasing resistance to trimethoprim/sulfamethoxazole among isolates of *Escherichia coli* in developing countries. *J. Infect. Dis.*, *152*, 1107.
11. Murray BE, Rensimer ER, DuPont HL (1982) Emergence of high-level trimethoprim resistance in fecal *Escherichia coli* during oral administration of trimethoprim or trimethoprim/sulfamethoxazole. *N. Engl. J. Med.*, *306*, 130.
12. Johnson PC, Ericsson CD, Morgan DR, DuPont HL, Cabada FJ (1986) Lack of emergence of resistant fecal flora during successful prophylaxis of travelers' diarrhea with norfloxacin. *Antimicrob. Agents Chemother.*, *30*, 671.
13. Ericsson CD, DuPont HL, Johnson PC (1986) Nonantibiotic therapy for travelers' diarrhea. *Rev. Infect. Dis.*, *8*, S202.
14. Kean DH, Schaffner W, Brennan RW, Waters SR (1962) The diarrhea of travelers. V. Prophylaxis with phthalylsulfathiazole and neomycin sulphate. *J. Am. Med. Assoc.*, *180*, 367.
15. Turner AC (1967) Travelers' diarrhoea: a survey of symptoms, occurrence, and possible prophylaxis. *Br. Med. J. 4*, 453.
16. Sack RB (1986) Antimicrobial prophylaxis of travelers' diarrhea: a selected summary. *Rev. Infect. Dis.*, *8*, S160.
17. DuPont HL, Ericsson CD, Johnson PC, Cabada FJ (1986) Antimicrobial agents in prevention of travelers' diarrhea. *Rev. Infect. Dis.*, *8*, S167.
18. Ericsson CD, DuPont HL, Galindo E, Mathewson JJ, Morgan DR, Wood LV, Mendiola J (1985) Efficacy of bicozamycin in preventing travelers' diarrhea. *Gastroenterology*, *88*, 473.
19. DuPont HL, Sullivan P, Evans DG, Pickering LK, Evans Jr DJ, Vollet JJ III, Ericsson CD, Ackerman PB, Tjoa WS (1980) Prevention of travelers' diarrhea (emporiatric enteritis): prophylactic administration of bismuth subsalicylate. *J. Am. Med. Assoc.*, *253*, 2700.
20. Steffen R, DuPont HL, Heusser R, Helminger A, Witassek F, Manhart MD, Schär M (1986) Prevention of travelers' diarrhea by the tablet form of bismuth subsalicylate. *Antimicrob. Agents Chemother.*, *29*, 625.

21. Ericsson CD, Pickering LK, Sullivan P, DuPont HL (1980) The role of location of food consumption in the prevention of travelers' diarrhea in Mexico. *Gastroenterology, 79*, 812.
22. DuPont HL, Ericsson CD, Reves RR, Galindo E (1986) Antimicrobial therapy for travelers' diarrhea. *Rev. Infect. Dis., 8*, S217.
23. Ericsson CD, DuPont HL, Sullivan P, Galindo E, Evans DG, Evans Jr DJ (1983) Bicozamycin, a poorly absorbable antibiotic, effectively treats travelers' diarrhea. *Ann. Intern. Med., 98*, 20.
24. DuPont HL, Ericsson CD, Galindo E, Wood LV, Morgan D, Bistura JAM, Mendiola JG (1984) Furazolidone versus ampicillin in the treatment of travelers' diarrhea. *Antimicrob. Agents Chemother., 26*, 160.
25. Ericsson CD, Feldman S, Pickering LK, Cleary TG (1982) Influence of bismuth subsalicylate on absorption of doxycycline. *J. Am. Med. Assoc., 247*, 2266.
26. DuPont HL, Hornick RB (1973) Adverse effect of Lomatil therapy in shigellosis. *J. Am. Med. Assoc., 225*, 1525.

CHAPTER 44

Treatment of diabetic lower limb infections: the fetid foot

ROBERT W. TOFTE

Soft tissue and osseous pedal infections, statistically more common in non-insulin-dependent diabetics over age 50, usually occur in previously neuropathic and ischemic lower limbs and are a major source of serious morbidity in these patients (1). Indeed, limb infections are second only to vascular complications as a reason for diabetic hospital admissions (2). Approximately US $ 200,000,000 annually in direct hospital costs are incurred in the treatment of these infections. Amputations in diabetics account for 50–70% of all non-traumatic below-knee amputations and many are probably performed needlessly because of common misconceptions about appropriate management of diabetic foot infections (3). The term 'fetid foot' encompasses a variety of suppurative processes including digital or pedal cellulitis, penetrating or mal perforans ulcers, plantar space abscesses, necrotizing fasciitis and osteomyelitis of the small bones. In nearly every instance, a potentially synergistic combination of aerobic and anaerobic bacteria can be isolated, necessitating treatment with broad-spectrum antibiotics in addition to surgical debridement, control of hyperglycemia and, in selected instances, vascular reconstruction.

Patients and physicians are mutually responsible for permitting apparently trivial cutaneous lesions to progress to frank mal perforans, ulceration or gangrene. Many diabetics are never taught proper methods for good foot care (daily inspection, use of skin emollients and wearing proper footwear) while others choose to ignore them. The sensory neuropathic changes unique to diabetics permit thick plantar calluses to develop over weight-bearing metatarsal-phalangeal joints as well as the heel and the toe interphalangeal joints, particularly in feet with an 'intrinsic minus' (claw toes/hammer toes) deformity. When an ulcer occurs in a previously fissured callus, relative or complete anesthesia permits repetitive vertical soft tissue trauma ultimately resulting in a deep undermining ulcer. Most patients have surprisingly few complaints of pain and a paucity of signs indicating the seriousness of the underlying infection. Physicians frequently underestimate the size, depth and extent of a mal perforans ulcer after casual inspection, potentially compounding the extent of injury if not treated initially by restricting weight-bearing.

Antimicrobial Agents Annual 3
P.K. Peterson and J. Verhoef, editors
© Elsevier Science Publishers BV, 1988

PATHOGENESIS

Factors which predispose diabetics to pedal infections include: (a) peripheral autonomic, sensory and motor neuropathies; (b) large and small vessel disease; (c) excessive and repetitive vertical trauma; and (d) leukocyte dysfunction (Table 1) (4–6). It is conjectural which of these factors is most important, although most authors feel that the neuropathy is of prime importance. The microangiopathic abnormalities deprive peripheral Schwann cells of important nutrients resulting in segmental demyelination. The attendant muscular atrophy creates subtle anatomic changes which, when coupled with sensory deficits and repetitive trauma, permit the development of thick calluses over the weight-bearing areas of the heel and metatarsal-phalangeal joints. Autosympathectomy leads to loss of cutaneous sweating, resulting in dry skin which is easily fissured. The colonizing cutaneous flora, which includes greater numbers of Group B streptococci and Enterobacteriaceae than are found on normal feet, gain easy access to the hypovascular deeper tissue compartments via these fissures, resulting in potentially serious suppurative lesions. Bacteria may also be introduced into the soft tissues when patients step on sharp objects, sustain cutaneous burns, or inadvertently cut themselves while trimming toenails.

BACTERIOLOGY

Despite the frequent occurrence and serious nature of diabetic foot infections, bacteriologic studies have received little scientific attention. In the era before anaerobic cultures were commonly available, *Staphylococcus aureus*, streptococci and

Table 1   *Diabetic fetid foot: predisposing factors*

a. Vascular insufficiency
    Large and small vessel occlusion

b. Neuropathy
    Motor: intrinsic minus deformity ('claw toes')
    Sensory: neurotropic ulcer, osteopathy
    Automatic: dry skin, fissured calluses

c. Excessive/Repetitive trauma
    Ulceration
    Charcot's joints

d. Leukocyte dysfunction
    Impaired chemotaxis, phagocytosis, killing (esp. *S. aureus, E. coli*)
    Impaired glycolysis

enteric gram-negative bacilli were reported to be the most common pathogens (7). More recent studies, however, have emphasized the importance of anaerobic, non-sporulating bacteria as a significant component of the complex microbial flora of pedal ulcers. Three prospective studies have clearly demonstrated that 5–6 bacterial species (40–50% anaerobes) can be consistently isolated from purulent or gangrenous lesions (Table 2) (8–10). In general, there is poor concordance between superficial swab and deep-tissue biopsy or aspirate cultures indicating that the superficial flora may not represent a true bacteriologic sampling of the deeper tissues. The aspirate and biopsy samples have reasonably good concordance. The needle-aspirate culture technique is easily performed with a minimum of trauma. One or 2 cc of non-bacteriostatic saline is injected through a 23-gauge needle introduced into normal tissue directing the bevel of the needle just below the base of the ulcer and aspirating. A few drops of fluid are sufficient to prepare a Gram's stain as well as aerobic and anaerobic cultures. Among the aerobic bacteria, Groups B and D (enterococci) streptococci, coagulase-positive and -negative staphylococci, Corynebacteria, *Escherichia coli, Proteus mirabilis* and *Enterobacter aerogenes* are the most commonly isolated species. *Pseudomonas aeruginosa* is an infrequent pathogen, isolated from only 1 of 20 patients in our study (10). Peptococci and *Bacteroides* species are the most frequently isolated anaerobic bacteria. We isolated *Clostridium perfringens* from a single biopsy specimen.

These diabetic foot infections are analogous to intra-abdominal abscesses or sacral decubitus ulcers with respect to their complex microflora. It is hypothesized

Table 2   *Diabetic foot ulcer bacteriology: comparative analysis*

	Author (Ref. No.)		
	Louie (8)	Sapico (9)	Tofte (10)
No. patients	20	13	20
Culture method	Curette	post-amputation tissue	aspirate/punch biopsy
Previous antibiotic treatment	none ≥ 30 d	12/13	none ≥ 30 d
Cellulitis-gangrene	8/20	9/17	18/20
Osteomyelitis	3/20	6/7	8/20
Predominant bacterial isolates			
Aerobic gram-positive	Enterococcus	Enterococcus	Enterococcus
gram-negative	*P. mirabilis*	*P. mirabilis*	*E. coli*
Anaerobic gram-positive	*Peptococcus* sp.	*Clostridium* sp.	*Peptococcus* sp.
gram-negative	*B. fragilis*	*B. fragilis*	*B. ureolyticus*
Mean isolates/specimen			
Aerobic	3.2	2.3	3.6
Anaerobic	2.6	2.4	2.4
Total	5.8	4.7	6.0

that the aerobic bacteria utilize available tissue oxygen permitting the anaerobic bacteria to survive and flourish. Mixed aerobic and anaerobic infections account for 90% of all pedal infections while exclusive isolation of aerobic bacteria occurs in only 10% of fetid foot ulcers. Important clues to the presence of anaerobes are a thin, feculent, seropurulent discharge and soft tissue gas with crepitation. Although *E. coli, Klebsiella* and *Enterobacter* species are capable of gas production under anaerobic conditions, anaerobic bacteria are much more commonly responsible for soft tissue gas production. Clostridial myonecrosis (gas gangrene) is extremely uncommon (11). Concurrent osteomyelitis may be demonstrated in up to 40% of mal perforans ulcers, but the osseous bacteriology has not yet been adequately defined.

CLINICAL PRESENTATION

In our series of 20 diabetic limb infections, there were 7 males and 13 females with a median age of 60 years (range 38–81 years) (10). Two-thirds had insulin-dependent diabetes with a median duration of 15 years (range 3–25 years). Ulcers were present a median of 3 months before clinical evaluation and 60% were 2 cm or smaller in diameter; 90% were located on the forefoot or toes. Pain (30%), fever (10%), leukocytosis (5%) and soft tissue crepitation (5%) were uncommon findings. Eighteen individuals had associated cellulitis and 65% of ulcers had a malodorous wound discharge. Two patients had gangrenous toes on presentation. Foot radiographs demonstrated soft tissue gas in 4 and osteomyelitis in 8 patients. None of our patients was critically ill or bacteremic.

CLINICAL EVALUATION

A thorough history and physical examination of the neurologic, vascular and integumentary systems is essential. Osteomyelitis should be suspected in association with chronically draining mal perforans ulcers, particularly if there is visible bone at the ulcer base. Significant neurologic deficits resulting in pedal hypesthesia or anesthesia as well as digital deformities invariably result in the development of subsequent neurotrophic ulceration unless corrective podiatric measures are applied.

The size and depth of the ulcer should be measured initially as well as serially to assess clinical improvement. A baseline roentgenogram of the foot will provide useful information regarding the presence of soft tissue gas, osteomyelitis, unsuspected fractures or Charcot joints. If osteomyelitis is clinically suspected but the X-ray is normal or non-diagnostic, a 3-phase bone scan or computed-tomographic (CT) scan may provide additional definitive diagnostic information. Bone scans are frequently abnormal in the presence of soft tissue inflammation and, as a result, rarely add useful clinical information. CT scans, although expensive, may confirm the presence of osteomyelitis if subtle osseous erosions are seen. Diabetic osteopathy due to excessive repetitive osseous trauma may be radiographically indistinguishable from osteomyelitis except for characteristic thinning of the metaphysis of the proximal phalanges in neuropathic feet (12). It is important to distinguish between these two entities in patients with mal perforans ulcers because their treatment and prognosis are quite different. It may be necessary to perform a Craig-needle bone biopsy to differentiate osteomyelitis from diabetic osteopathy. However, orthopedic surgeons have traditionally been reluctant to biopsy bones, contending that previously sterile bone could be contaminated during the biopsy procedure. Unfortunately, as with several other aspects in the diagnosis and management of diabetic limb infections, there are no well-controlled comparative clinical trials on which to base a number of important patient management decisions.

Assessment of adequate peripheral circulation is crucial to the management of the fetid foot since infected ischemic ulcers frequently do not heal with debridement and systemic antibiotics alone. Barnes et al (13) found that healing of below-the-knee amputations occurred in all patients with a below-the-knee systolic blood pressure of 70 mmHg, whereas Wagner reported that a calf-arm systolic pressure index of 0.45 or greater was a reliable predictor of wound healing. Cederberg and colleagues found no relationship between the calf systolic pressure or calf-arm systolic pressure index and the degree of wound healing in diabetics with severe peripheral vascular disease (14). Hauser and colleagues reported that Doppler-assisted blood pressure measurements in diabetic limbs was unreliable because of vascular calcification resulting in spuriously elevated pressure measurements (15). Using the heated Clark oxygen electrode to measure cutaneous oxygen tension and comparing this to a simultaneous chest wall measurement, they obtained a regional perfusion index (RPI). Normal pedal transcutaneous oxygen tension (65 ± 3 torr) is $91 \pm 2\%$ of a simultaneous chest measurement. RPI values less than $62 \pm 5\%$ indicate significant vascular disease and may predict poor wound-healing without vascular surgery or angioplasty.

MANAGEMENT OF THE FETID FOOT

Optimal management of the infected diabetic foot requires a team approach ideally including an endocrinologist, infectious diseases consultant, and an orthopedic surgeon or podiatrist. When financially feasible, the patient should be hospitalized initially for laboratory and radiologic analysis as well as for thorough debridement of all necrotic tissue serving as a potential nidus for persistent infection. Subsequently, moist, saline-soaked gauze pads can be applied to the ulcer base to prevent drying of the granulation tissues and to remove residual necrotic debris. Foot soaks serve little purpose except to insure adequate tissue hydration. The use of undiluted povidone iodine solutions ($>1\%$ concentration) is condemned since the iodine radicals are tissue-toxic. Topical application of enzymatic debriding agents or antibiotics is of no proven value. Ischemic ulcers, particularly in association with gangrene, are tetanus-prone and these individuals should be immunized with tetanus-diphtheria vaccine if appropriate (16). Pentoxyfylline (Trental) may improve peripheral circulation by decreasing blood viscosity and improving erythrocyte flexibility. However, no comparative studies in diabetics exist to support routine use of this agent. In severely ischemic limbs, angioplasty or vascular reconstruction may promote wound-healing by increasing tissue oxygenation. Hyperbaric oxygen is an expensive but intuitively appealing method to augment local tissue oxygenation. As with many other therapeutic modalities, there are no controlled studies in diabetics to document its effectiveness. Knighton and colleagues have described the use of individual patient platelet-derived wound healing factors (PDWHF) which promote wound fibroblastic proliferation and angiogenesis. They reported that PDWHF, incorporated into a paste and applied directly into the wound, resulted in complete healing of chronic ischemic ulcers in 7 diabetic renal transplant recipients in 13 weeks (17). Additional patient trials are required before this exciting and novel approach can be generally recommended.

Antiobiotic therapy

The selection of an initial antimicrobial regimen for diabetic lower limb infections is necessarily empiric but should include antibiotics with a broad spectrum of activity against both aerobic and anaerobic bacteria. A Gram's stain of the tissue aspirate can be used as a preliminary guide to the rational antibiotic selection based on the number and variety of bacteriologic morphologies identified microscopically. Potential initial antibiotic selections include agents with an acceptably broad spectrum of activity against the commonly isolated pathogens including cefoxitin, cefotetan, ceftizoxime, ticarcillin clavulanate, and imipenem/cilastatin. A combination of an aminoglycoside or β-lactam antibiotic plus an anti-anaerobic agent such as clindamycin, metronidazole or chloramphenicol is also popular. Combination chemotherapy is more expensive than monotherapy and regimens containing an aminoglycoside are potentially more ototoxic or nephrotoxic. The virtues of each of the potentially useful monotherapeutic agents including the second- and third-generation cephalosporins, ticarcillin clavulanate and imipenem/cilastatin have been extolled by representatives of the pharmaceutical industry. However, a dearth of clinical studies support such claims.

In one large open study, LeFrock and colleagues reported that cefoxitin, 8–12 grams daily, resulted in a clinical cure in 55 of 68 lower extremity infections, 49 of which required concomitant surgical debridement or abscess drainage (18). In the only published prospective, double-blinded, randomized clinical trial, Hughes et al (19) found no statistically significant difference in clinical response rates between ceftizoxime (23/28) and cefoxitin (17/25). Polymicrobial infections were present in over 80% of patients in both groups. Adverse effects were slightly more common among cefoxitin-treated patients (63% *vs* 49%). Six patients in each group who initially had a good response relapsed within 3 months.

In the absence of solid comparative clinical data to support the superior clinical effectiveness of any specific antimicrobial regimen, appropriate antibiotic selection must be determined by several factors including wound bacteriology, individual renal function and allergic status, antibiotic acquisition and delivery costs, ease and convenience of antibiotic administration, and previous physician experience. Although certainly not all-inclusive, Table 3 contains a tabulation of potentially useful antibiotic selections including relative merits and potential disadvantages of each. With the exceptions of ticarcillin clavulanate and imipenem/cilastatin, none of these single or combination therapies is active against enterococci. While com-

Table 3   *Treatment of diabetic fetid foot: possible antibiotic selections*

Antibiotic	Dose	Advantages	Disadvantages
Monotherapy			
Cefoxitin	1–2 g q. 6 h	good activity against *Bacteroides fragilis*	expensive, unpredictable activity against Enterobacteriaceae
Cefotetan	1–2 g q. 12 h	infrequent dosing, cost savings; good activity against *Bacteroides fragilis*	questionable activity *vs Bacteroides* spp. and Enterobacteriaceae; potential for hemorrhage with MTT side chain
Ceftizoxime	1–2 g q. 8 h	excellent activity against Enterobacteriaceae and most staphylococci; cheaper than cefoxitin	variable activity against *B. fragilis*
Ticarcillin clavulanate	3.1 g q. 6 h	broad-spectrum activity	expensive
Imipenem/cilastatin		extremely broad-spectrum activity including enterococci	expensive
Ciprofloxacin		oral or intravenous forms available	clinical inexperience; questionable activity *vs* streptococci
Combination therapy			
Gentamicin	80 mg q. 8 h	broad-spectrum activity	expensive; potential oto- and nephrotoxicity; risk of antibiotic-associated colitis
Clindamycin	800 mg q. 8 h		
Gentamicin	80 mg q. 8 h	more cost-effective than gentamicin and clindamycin	no activity against aerobic gram-positive cocci; potential aminoglycoside toxicity
Metronidazole	500 mg q. 8 h		
Ceftriaxone	2 g q. 24 h	cost-effective; easily administered on outpatient basis	questionable activity against staphylococci
Metronidazole	500 mg q. 8 h		

monly isolated, it is unlikely that this organism is a clinically significant pathogen in this particular setting, since many infections can be successfully treated with antibiotics possessing no intrinsic activity against enterococci.

Despite the common occurrence of diabetic lower limb infections, significant information gaps regarding optimal clinical management decisions remain and cannot be satisfactorily resolved until additional clinical and basic scientific research is performed.

REFERENCES

1. LeFrock JL, Joseph WS (1986) Lower extremity infections in diabetics. *Infect. Surg.,* *5*, 135.
2. Whitehouse F (1973) Infections that hospitalize diabetics. *Geriatrics, 28*, 97.
3. Lithner F, Tornblom N (1980) Gangrene localized to the lower limbs in diabetics. *Acta Med. Scand., 208*, 315.
4. Lippmann HI (1982) The foot of the diabetic. In: Brodoff BN, Bleicher SJ (Eds), *Diabetes Mellitus and Obesity*, p 712. Williams and Wilkins, Baltimore.
5. Brand PW (1979) Pathomechanics of diabetic (neurotrophic) ulcer and its conservative management. In: Bergin JJ, Yao JST (Eds), *Gangrene and Severe Ischemia of the Lower Extremities*, p 829. Grune and Stratton, New York.
6. Greenbaum D, Richardson PC, Salmon MJ, Urich H (1964) Pathological observations on six cases of diabetic neuropathy. *Brain, 87*, 201.
7. Pratt TC (1965) Gangrene and infection in the diabetic. *Med. Clin. N. Am., 49*, 987.
8. Louie TJ, Bartlett JG, Tally FP, Gorbach SL (1976) Aerobic and anaerobic bacteria in diabetic foot ulcers. *Ann. Intern. Med., 85*, 461.
9. Sapico FL, Canawati HN, Witte JL, Montgomerie JZ, Wagner FW, Bessman AN (1980) Quantitative aerobic and anaerobic bacteriology of infected diabetic feet. *J. Clin. Microbiol., 12*, 413.
10. Tofte RW, Sidwell E (1983) A prospective bacteriologic evaluation of diabetic foot ulcers comparing three culture methods. In: *Abstracts, 23rd Interscience Conference on Antimicrobial Agents in Chemotherapy, Las Vegas, 1983*. American Society for Microbiology, Washington, DC.
11. Bessman AN, Wagener W (1975) Non-clostridial gas gangrene: report of 48 cases and review of the literature. *J. Am. Med. Assoc., 233*, 958.
12. Friedman SA, Rakow RB (1971) Osseous lesions of the foot in diabetic neuropathy. *Diabetes, 20*, 302.
13. Barnes RW, Shanik GD, Slaymaker EE (1976) An index of healing in below-knee amputation: leg blood pressure by Doppler ultrasound. *Surgery, 79*, 13.
14. Cederberg PA, Pritchard DJ, Joyce JW (1983) Doppler-determined segmental pressures and wound-healing in amputations for vascular disease. *J. Bone Jt Surg., 65*, 363.
15. Hauer CJ, Klein SR, Mehringer CM, Appel P, Schoemaker WC (1984) Assessment of perfusion in the diabetic foot by regional transcutaneous oximetry. *Diabetes, 33*, 527.
16. Stroud II WH, Yarbrough III DR (1980) Ischemic gangrene: an indication for tetanus prophylaxis. *Arch. Surg., 115*, 1401.

17. Knighton DR, Fiegel VD, Austin LL, Ciresi KF, Butler EL (1986) Classification and treatment of chronic nonhealing wounds. *Ann. Surg., 204*, 322.

18. LeFrock JL, Blais F, Schell RF, Carr BB, Jacobs RL, Wirth CR, Kowalsky SF, Tillotson JR (1983) Cefoxitin in the treatment of diabetic patients with lower extremity infections. *Infect. Surg., 2*, 361.

19. Hughes C, Johnson C, Bamberger D, Reinhardt J, Peterson L, Mulligan M, Gerding D, George L, Finegold S (1985) A randomized double-blind trial of ceftizoxime vs. cefoxitin for therapy of lower extremity infections in patients with diabetes mellitus and/or peripheral vascular disease. In: *Abstracts, 14th International Congress of Chemotherapy, Kyoto, 1985*. American Society for Microbiology, Washington, DC.

CHAPTER 45

Home parenteral antibiotic therapy

TEMPLE W. WILLIAMS Jr and JOAN M. LOOS

The cost of health care in the United States has increased at 3 times the inflation rate. The political promise of quality medical care for all has turned out to be a promise that is larger than the public purse can meet. To reduce the rate of growth in health care costs, a prospective payment system was devised to replace the cost-reimbursement system. The system, known as 'Diagnosis-Related Groups' (DRG), is the clinical basis for determining payment (1–5). DRG is an acronym which is becoming as familiar as the FBI or the IRS.

These prospective pricing systems are now the law of the land and will, in one form or another, shape an entirely new economics of hospital care. Concerns have been voiced that certain DRGs within the area of infectious diseases do not provide the reimbursement necessary to ensure quality care. An example is DRG No. 126, acute and subacute endocarditis, which reimburses for a mean stay of 18.4 days. This, in most cases, is hardly enough to ensure an adequate course of parenteral antibiotic therapy, much less diagnosis as well as treatment.

The pressures exerted on physicians and hospitals by DRGs for expedient discharge of patients in addition to the escalating costs of medical care have served as impetus to move long-term parenteral antibiotic treatment into the outpatient arena. The mushrooming of hospital-based and commercial home-health-care programs in the United States over the last 5 years has facilitated this transition from inpatient to outpatient therapy.

There is historical evidence that outpatient therapy is not only therapeutically successful and cost-effective but an extremely popular option to hospitalization.

HISTORICAL SURVEY

The first reported experience with outpatient intravenous antibiotics was the experience of Ruker and Harrison (6) at the Texas Institute for Rehabilitation and Research in Houston in 1974. In 62 patients with cystic fibrosis, intravenous antibiotics (gentamicin and colistin) were given via a heparin lock for a total of 127 treatment courses. No major complications were noted and no difficulties were

Antimicrobial Agents Annual 3
P.K. Peterson and J. Verhoef, editors
© Elsevier Science Publishers BV, 1988

encountered in administration of the antibiotic by patient or parent. In 68% of these episodes, hospitalization was avoided with considerable savings in medical costs and lack of disruption of family routine as well as, in some cases, continuation of education or employment. In the failures, adjunctive measures of therapy were required once the patient was hospitalized, suggesting that parenteral antibiotics alone were not adequate treatment even in the hospital setting. They concluded that the convenience, patient acceptability, lack of complications, prevention of hospitalizations, and effectiveness entitled this mode of therapy to a place of importance in the management of cystic fibrosis.

Gilbert and associates (7) in Portland expanded this concept to include outpatient therapy of 13 patients with osteomyelitis, bacteremia or infective endocarditis once the patient's infection had responded clinically to treatment and the patient had been afebrile for 5 days. They then discharged selected patients to continue their parenteral antibiotic therapy at home with proper education and close supervision and found that this plan of management was effective. Antibiotic-related complications in the outpatient group were similar to those in a control group of 7 hospitalized patients. The most dramatic result was the reduction in costs when the treatment was given at home. The reduction in average daily cost was from US $234.22 to US $69.35 with an average overall saving of some US $3700.00 per patient. They concluded that outpatient parenteral antibiotic self-administration was no more dangerous and no less efficacious than inpatient parenteral antibiotic treatment provided patient selection and education were appropriate.

Stiver et al (8) from Winnipeg reported their results in the treatment of 23 patients not only with bone and joint infections, bacteremia and endocarditis, but also several patients with systemic fungal infections requiring amphotericin B therapy. Their method was much more like the system we use today. The majority of the care and follow-up was accomplished by trained home-care nurses who delivered the medications to the home and were responsible for maintaining the intravenous access and for monitoring the patient for adverse effects. In this way the patients were required to see the physician only weekly as opposed to the Portland system which required the patient to return every third day to see the physician and pick up supplies. Their study likewise documented that once a patient's infection had begun to resolve and the patient no longer required hospitalization, continued intravenous antibiotic therapy could be given at home with safety, therapeutic efficacy and considerable cost savings (US $2231.00 savings per patient per treatment course).

In 1979, Kind et al (9) from Minneapolis reported a substantial monetary saving (at least US $1600.00 per patient) in the treatment of 15 patients at home. They felt that this method of treatment was safe and effective and, in addition, the patients were much more comfortable and productive outside of the hospital environment. They, like Gilbert and Stiver, were impressed with the potential savings, but were unable to convince all insurance carriers, particularly Medicare, of the advantages of this system.

In 1981, Swenson (10) reported a successful home intravenous infusion program in a medium-sized primary-care hospital in Renton, Washington. His estimated cost savings was US $2371.00 per patient and the treatment at home was considered successful in all 8 patients.

In 1982, Portez et al (11) reported the largest series of outpatients treated with intravenous antibiotics at home. Their method was much like that of Gilbert (7) with patients returning for follow-up every Monday and Friday, at which time they picked up their supplies and were seen by a physician at least weekly. Their series included 150 patients with a variety of infections, the majority being bone and joint infections. Cost reductions were calculated to be US $142.00 per day. They concluded that this treatment plan was safe, practical and cost-effective if patients were screened for reliability before entering the program and if careful appropriate monitoring was conducted during the treatment period. Moreover, the patients were more comfortable and productive (many were able to return to school or work) and the hospitals were able to utilize their acute-care beds more prudently.

Rehm and Weinstein (12) organized a multidisciplinary team to facilitate home therapy at the Cleveland Clinic Hospital. In 1983, they reported the treatment of 48 patients for an average of 19 days with an average savings of US $5728.00. They concluded that the team approach was an efficient use of the resources of specialized health professionals (infectious disease physicians, social workers, pharmacists, and specialty nurses) for the selection, training and follow-up of patients to receive home intravenous antibiotic therapy.

Poretz, Eron and associates have continued to expand their experience in the treatment of outpatients in a variety of settings (13, 14). They have successfully applied their system to the treatment of pediatric patients with similar success (15). They have more recently become involved in clinical trials of new long-acting cephalosporins, particularly ceftriaxone, in the outpatient treatment of bone and joint and other infections (16–18).

Subsequent release of other second- and third-generation cephalosporins which can be administered once or twice daily has made outpatient treatment even more convenient. Eisenberg and Kitz (19) utilized cefonicid in the treatment of osteo-

Table 1   *Outpatient parenteral antibiotics (HMSS data, 1982–1986)*

	The Methodist Hospital Houston, Texas	Houston, total	National
Patients	280	889	3489
Treatment courses	317	1048	3773
Female/Male	80/200	292/597	1283/2206
Age range (avg.)	12–90 (46)	1–93 (41)	1–93 (41)
Average treatment course (days)	25	21	19

myelitis. Their analysis suggested that substantial savings were available from a program of early discharge and continued outpatient parenteral antibiotic therapy for patients with osteomyelitis, but the implications depend upon whose perspective is used to measure the savings. Their calculated savings per patient ranged from US $510.000 to US $22,232.00 and depended upon different sources of data to estimate total hospital costs including both direct and indirect costs of the illness.

OUTPATIENT PARENTERAL TREATMENT – THE HOUSTON AND NATIONAL HMSS EXPERIENCE

Poretz and associates' success and enthusiasm led us in 1982 to try outpatient parenteral antibiotic treatment in selected patients who were ready for discharge except for the need to complete a prolonged course of parenteral antibiotics. We elected to utilize the services of Home Medical Support Services, Inc. (HMSS) as our home-care provider. Our system is patterned after the 'Stiver approach' with the HMSS nurses visiting the patients at home on a regular basis to deliver the supplies, to monitor for toxicity and clinical response, and to maintain the intravenous access. The data to follow include not only our Methodist Hospital experience over the past 5 years, but also the total HMSS experience from a number of centers (Beaumont, Texas; Chicago, Illinois; Cincinnati, Ohio; Columbia, Maryland; Dallas, Texas; Denver, Colorado; Houston, Texas; Kansas City, Kansas; Minneapolis, Minnesota; Philadelphia, Pennsylvania; Tampa, Florida) in an effort to illustrate the efficacy and applicability of this approach in a variety of geographic settings.

Since 1982, we have treated a total of 280 patients with parenteral antibiotics at home. As seen in Table 1, our experience is quite similar to the total Houston and national experience of HMSS with the exception that we do not treat children and our average age is some 5 years older.

As can be seen from the total number of patients treated by this one provider, this form of therapy is becoming a popular and effective means of treatment of a number of infections (Table 2) as well as an innovative answer to the DRGs. The key to success, however, as pointed out very early by Gilbert (7), is prudent patient selection and education. A physician familiar with the clinical circumstances and a trained person from the health-care provider will need to carefully select and train patients for this form of treatment.

The first criteria is that patients be medically stable. We do not send patients home until they have responded clinically to the treatment of their infection and until we have arrived at the appropriate antibiotic or combination of antibiotics to be used at home based on culture data and antibiotic levels. We switch to the antibiotic regimen to be used at home at least 1 day prior to discharge from the hospital. In this way we avoid the hazard of an anaphylactic reaction from the first dose of a new antibiotic outside the hospital setting. An alternative is to start treatment in the office or an emergency room if the patient does not require hos-

Table 2   *Outpatient parenteral antibiotics: diagnostic categories treated (HMSS data, 1982–1986)*

Abdominal abscess/Infection	132
Bacteremia/Endocarditis	271
Brain abscess/Meningitis	74
Intravenous catheter-related infections	12
Systemic fungal infections	99
Herpes/Cytomegalovirus	60
Infected prostheses	76
Osteomyelitis/Septic arthritis/Bursitis	1539
Pelvic inflammatory disease	39
Pneumonia/Lung abscess/Empyema	349
Pre- and post-instrumentation prophylaxis	17
Pyelonephritis/Prostatitis/Epididymitis	212
Sinusitis/Otitis	100
Soft tissue/Wound infections	505
Venereal diseases	26

pitalization initially, or if antibiotics need to be changed during a course of treatment at home because of development of toxicity.

The second criterion, and unfortunately sometimes the most influential, is whether the patient has insurance coverage or the personal finances to pay for outpatient services. Medicare patients are currently not covered. This poses a serious dilemma with DRGs since retirees frequently cannot incur the personal debt. Medicaid patients, likewise, are exempt from outpatient coverage. Some insurance companies still fail to acknowledge the cost-effectiveness of outpatient services, but hopefully this is on the decline. Patients will not be interested in home care if they themselves have to incur the full cost.

The third criterion is patient motivation and ability. Physical impediments such as immobility, decreased motor skills or visual acuity can often be overcome by teaching a significant other person or having a nurse infuse the antibiotic. Likewise, the patient's intellectual capacity to learn aseptic technique must be evaluated. Patients who speak a foreign language offer a real challenge. We frequently have Spanish-speaking patients but are fortunate to also have a large population of Spanish-speaking nurses. In addition, we utilize educational brochures written in Spanish. We also have interpreters available for many other languages, however, which generally extends the educational process. Patients with history of alcohol or intravenous drug abuse are not automatically excluded as home candidates but are evaluated on an individual basis.

Virtually any antibiotic can be utilized in outpatient therapy, as is evident in Table 3. Single antibiotics are used most frequently, but up to 25% of patients received more than one antibiotic during a course of treatment and 1 patient received 4 antibiotics simultaneously. Obviously, antibiotics with a long half-life are

Table 3   *Antibiotics administered at home (HMSS data, 1982–1986)*

Acyclovir	Cloxacillin
Amikacin	Doxycycline
Amphotericin B	Erythromycin
Ampicillin	Ganciclovir (DHPG)
Azlocillin	Gentamicin
Carbenicillin	Imipenem-cilastatin
Cefalotin	Methicillin
Cefamandole	Metronidazole
Cefapirin	Moxalactam
Cefazolin	Nafcillin
Cefonicid	Netilmicin
Cefoperazone	Oxacillin
Ceforanide	Penicillin G
Cefotaxime	Pentamidine
Cefotetan	Piperacillin
Cefoxitin	Streptomycin
Ceftazidime	Ticarcillin
Ceftizoxime	Ticarcillin-clavulanate
Ceftriaxone	Tobramycin
Cefuroxime	Trimethoprim-sulfamethoxazole
Chloramphenicol	Vancomycin
Clindamycin	

ideal since they can be given once or twice a day and patients can easily maintain their work or school schedule. Antibiotics requiring dosing every 4–6 hours interfere with sleep and have a tendency to decrease compliance. In general, fewer daily doses reduce the cost of drug preparation and administration.

An area which is often overlooked in the selection and cost of antibiotics is the monitoring of patients for drug side effects. The most obvious example is the aminoglycosides. Frequent renal function tests and antibiotic blood level estimations may be more costly than the antibiotic. Cephalosporins containing the methylthiotetrazol ring (cefamandole, cefoperazone, cefmetazole, cefotetan, moxalactam, cefmenoxime) may cause prolongation of the prothrombin time. Monitoring for and treating hypoprothrombinemia becomes a hidden cost of using these antibiotics. Although not related to cost, the antabuse-like effect of these same cephalosporins with alcohol ingestion becomes a real hazard in the outpatient setting. HMSS data show antibiotic toxicity to be acceptable (Table 4) with only 465 antibiotics having to be discontinued or an alternate antibiotic substituted in 3773 treatment courses (12%).

The total cost savings vary as reported by the various investigators. To illustrate the cost savings in our hospital, we picked 4 representative treatment regimens that we have utilized and compared the total cost for the treatment in the hospital

Table 4 *Outpatient parenteral antibiotics: antibiotic toxicity – 3773 treatment courses (HMSS data, 1982–1986)*

Side effects	No.	(%)
Allergic reactions	267	(7)
Gastrointestinal intolerance	137	(4)
Nephrotoxicity	30	(1)
Ototoxicity	20	(1)
Hematologic toxicity	11	(0.3)

and at home as provided by HMSS (with identical monitoring for toxicity). These are summarized in Table 5. The more complex the treatment regimen and its studies to monitor for toxicity, the less the savings in overall cost. Nevertheless, the patient is at home and most prefer to be there even if they are unable to return to school or work.

Goldenberg (20) cited medicolegal issues associated with outpatient therapy, a fertile ground for malpractice litigation. Herein lies the importance of quality care by the home health agency. Employing personnel knowledgeable and experienced in this relatively new field is critical in avoiding problems subject to litigation. Likewise, continued follow-up by the physician after discharge is mandatory. We maintain contact with all our patients weekly to assess progress, evaluate side effects, and determine satisfaction with home services. We maintain contact with HMSS daily. Although informed consent for outpatient services is obtained, drug side effects are explained, and a list of patient rights is issued. We believe the rapport established by frequent direct contact between the patient, physician, and home health-care worker is still the best deterrent to litigation.

Table 5 *Parenteral antibiotics: hospital versus home administration – cost comparison (The Methodist Hospital, Houston, Texas)*

1. Vancomycin 500 mg q. 6 h × 20 days
   Hospital US $7300.00   Home US $4472.00
2. Cefazolin 1 g q. 8 h × 20 days
   Hospital US $5500.00   Home US $3075.00
3. Piperacillin 3 g q. 4 h × 20 days
   +
   Tobramycin 80 mg q. 8 h × 20 days
   Hospital US $9965.00   Home US $8134.00
4. Amphotericin B 50 mg/d × 20 days
   Hospital US $4950.00   Home US $2295.00

CONCLUSIONS

Like our predecessors, we have found outpatient parenteral antibiotic therapy to be a safe, efficient and cost-effective alternative to continued hospitalization which is welcomed by patients and their families.

REFERENCES

1. Iglehart JK (1982) The new era of prospective payment for hospitals. *N. Engl. J. Med., 307,* 1288.
2. Iglehart JK (1982) New Jersey's experiment with DRG-based hospital reimbursement. *N. Engl. J. Med., 307,* 1655.
3. Ginzberg E (1983) Cost containment – imaginary and real. *N. Engl. J. Med., 308,* 1220.
4. Platt R (1983) Cost containment – another view. *N. Engl. J. Med., 309,* 726.
5. Shakno R (Ed) (1984) *Physicians Guide to DRGs,* p 232. Pluribus Press, Chicago.
6. Rucker RW, Harrison GM (1974) Outpatient intravenous medications in the management of cystic fibrosis. *Pediatrics, 54,* 358.
7. Antoniskis A, Anderson BC, Van Volkinburg EJ, Jackson JM, Gilbert DM (1978) Feasibility of outpatient self-administration of parenteral antibiotics. *West. J. Med., 128,* 203.
8. Stiver HG, Telford GO, Mossey JM, Cote DD, Van Middlesworth EJ, Trotsky SK, McKay NL, Mossey WL (1978) Intravenous antibiotic therapy at home. *Ann. Intern. Med., 89,* 690.
9. Kind AC, Williams DN, Persons G, Gibson JA (1979) Intravenous antibiotic therapy at home. *Arch. Intern. Med., 139,* 413.
10. Swenson JP (1981) Training patients to administer intravenous antibiotics at home. *Am. J. Hosp. Pharm., 38,* 1480.
11. Poretz DM, Eron LJ, Goldenberg RI, Gilbert AF, Rising J, Sparks S, Horn CE (1982) Intravenous antibiotic therapy in an outpatient setting. *J. Am. Med. Assoc., 248,* 336.
12. Rehm SJ, Weinstein AJ (1983) Home intravenous antibiotic therapy: a team approach. *Ann. Intern. Med., 99,* 388.
13. Poretz DM (1983) The private practice of infectious diseases. *J. Infect. Dis., 147,* 417.
14. Eron LJ (1984) Intravenous antibiotic administration in outpatient settings. *Infect. Dis., 14,* 4.
15. Goldenberg RI, Poretz DM, Eron LJ, Rising JB, Sparks SB (1984) Intravenous antibiotic therapy in ambulatory pediatric patients. *Pediatr. Infect. Dis., 3,* 514.
16. Eron LJ, Parks CH, Hixon DL, Goldenberg RI, Poretz DM (1983) Ceftriaxone therapy of bone and soft tissue infections in hospital and outpatient settings. *Antimicrob. Agents Chemother., 23,* 731.
17. Eron LJ, Goldenberg RI, Poretz DM (1984) Combined ceftriaxone and surgical therapy for osteomyelitis in hospital and outpatient settings. *Am. J. Surg., 148,* 1.
18. Poretz DM, Woolard J, Eron LJ, Goldenberg RI, Rising JB, Spark S (1984) Outpatient use of ceftriaxone: a cost-benefit analysis. *Am. J. Med., 77,* 77.
19. Eisenberg JM, Kitz DS (1986) Savings from outpatient antibiotic therapy for osteomyelitis: economic analysis of a therapeutic strategy. *J. Am. Med. Assoc., 255,* 1584.
20. Goldenberg RI (1985) Pitfalls in the delivery of outpatient intravenous therapy. *Drug Intell. Clin. Pharm., 19,* 293.

Subject index